Handbook of Sensory Physiology

Volume VI/2

Vestibular System Part 2: Psychophysics, Applied Aspects and General Interpretations

By

A.J. Benson · N. Bischof · W.E. Collins · A.R. Fregly · A. Graybiel F.E. Guedry · W.H. Johnson · L.B.W. Jongkees · H.H. Kornhuber · R. Mayne D.L. Meyer · E. Peitersen · W. Precht · K.P. Schaefer

Edited by

H.H. Kornhuber

With 198 Figures

Springer-Verlag Berlin · Heidelberg · New York 1974

ISBN 3-540-06864-3 Springer-Verlag Berlin · Heidelberg · New York
ISBN 0-387-06864-3 Springer-Verlag New York · Heidelberg · Berlin

Library of Congress Cataloging in Publication Data. Kornhuber, Hans. Vestibular System. (Handbook of Sensory Physiology, v. 6/1-2). Contents: pt. 1. Basic Mechanisms — pt. 2. Psychophysics, Applied Aspects and General Interpretations. 1. Vestibular Apparatus. I. Bagger-Sjöbäck. II. Title. III. Series. [DNLM: 1. Vestibular Apparatus. 2. Vestibular Nuclei. WL700 H236 v. 6] QP351.H34 vol. 6/1-2 [QP471] 591.1'82'08s [591.1'82]. 74-14870.

Typesetting and printing: Roth sel. Ww., München; Binding: Brühlsche Universitätsdruckerei, Gießen

Preface

The function of the vestibular system is not as obvious as those of vision, hearing, touch or smell. Vestibular dysfunction, however, is clearly apparent where lesions are present. It is probably for this reason that the vestibular sense was not discovered until the nineteenth century and that clinicians have continued to play a major role in basic vestibular research right up to the present. The relationship between basic and clinical research is certainly stronger in the vestibular field than in that of tactile sensation, for instance, as testified by the work of clinicians as MENIÈRE, BREUER, BÁRÁNY, DEKLEIJN and FRENZEL. In this respect the situation is similar in vestibular physiology and in endocrinology, and for the same reason.

This second part of the vestibular volume of the Handbook of Sensory Physiology will be of interest to neurologists, otologists, neurosurgeons, ophthalmologists and physiotherapists on the one hand, and psychologists, physiologists, engineers and aviation specialists on the other. For a full understanding of Part 2, it is necessary to have assimilated the basic anatomy, physiology, and biochemistry of Part 1.

Each sensory system has some motor aspects. Nociceptors, for instance, have a special relation to the spinal flexion reflex and to flexion spasticity after spinal cord lesions. Tactile afferents are strongly engaged in the regulation of voluntary finger, hand, lip, and tongue movements. However, there is no other sensory system where the motor aspects are as important as in the vestibular. The cerebellum has evolved out of the vestibular system; the cerebellar nuclei are analogous (in function and in their connections to the cerebellar cortex) to the vestibular nuclei. The study of the role of vestibular mechanisms in body posture and eye movements has made a substantial contribution to the theory of the motor system. The simpler organization of active eye movements as compared to limb movements has facilitated understanding. This book takes these facts into account.

It is hoped that this volume may represent a small step toward an understanding of this part of Nature's secrets and at the same time facilitate clinical knowledge about the vestibular system.

Ulm, June 1974 HANS HELMUT KORNHUBER

List of Contributors

BENSON, A.J., Neurobiology Section, R.A.F. Institute of Aviation Medicine, Farnborough, Hampshire, England

BISCHOF, N., California Institute of Technology, Division of Biology, Pasadena, Calif. 91109, USA

COLLINS, W.E., Psychology Laboratory, Civil Aeromedical Institute, P.O. Box 25082, Oklahoma City, Oklahoma 73125, USA

FREGLY, A.R., Naval Education and Training Support, Code N 213, Building 45, Naval Air Station, Pensacola, Florida 32508, USA

GRAYBIEL, A., Naval Aerospace Medical Center, Pensacola, Florida 32512, USA

GUEDRY, F.E., Naval Aerospace Medical Center, Pensacola, Florida 32512, USA

JOHNSON, W.H., Dept. of Otolaryngology and Physiology, University of Toronto, Toronto, Canada

JONGKEES, L.B.W., Academisch Ziekenhuis bij de Universiteit van Amsterdam, Keel-, neus-en oorheelkundige kliniek, Amsterdam-Oud west, Eerste Helmerstraat 104, Holland

KORNHUBER, H.H., Abt. f. Neurologie der Universität, D-7900 Ulm, Steinhövelstraße 9, Germany

MAYNE, R., Arizona State University, Faculty of Electrical Engineering, Tempe, Arizona 85281, USA

MEYER, D.L., Universitäts-Nervenklinik D-3400 Göttingen, v. Siebold-Str. 5, Germany

PEITERSEN, E., University E.N.T. Clinic, Rigshospitalet, Blegdamsvej, DK-2100 Copenhagen Ø, Denmark

PRECHT, W., Max-Planck-Institut für Hirnforschung, Neurobiologische Abt. D-6000 Frankfurt-Niederrad, Deutschordenstraße 40, Germany

SCHAEFER, K.P., Universitäts-Nervenklinik, D-3400 Göttingen, v. Siebold-Str. 5, Germany

Vestibular System

Part 2: Psychophysics, Applied Aspects and General Interpretations

Contents

E. Psychophysics

F. Applied Aspects

G. General Interpretations

Part 1: Basic Mechanisms

Contents

E. Psychophysics

frequency of about 3 Hz while fixing the eyes on the palm of the hand held still at a distance of about 25 cm (MELVILL JONES, 1966a). The lines in the palm remain clearly visible. If the head is held fixed while the palm is oscillated in a like manner, visibility of the lines in the palm is very poor. BENSON (1972) has recently demonstrated that there are comparable effects with whole-body passive oscillation which depend upon vestibular function. This is an illustration of how the vestibular system participates in the control of coordinated movement, i.e., without conscious awareness of the vestibular input. During head oscillation, the vestibular system reflexly stabilizes the eyes. In this task there is no awareness of vestibular sensations, but there is an obvious awareness of visual data.

The vestibular system has been likened to a component in an inertial guidance system (MAYNE, 1950a, b, 1951, 1969; BARLOW, 1964, 1970). It is fairly well developed at birth in man (GALEBSKY, 1927; TIBBLING, 1969; GROEN, 1963, 1965). The extent of our awareness of vestibular sensations as we are carried about for the first year or so of our lives, and later as we begin to develop skill in control of voluntary movement is an interesting area for speculation (ORNITZ, 1970; PETO, 1970) and scientific inquiry. As part of the postural control system, it participates in an influence on vital functions such as respiration and heart rate, signs which are used as measures of emotions. The fact that we have built-in emergency reactions (startle reactions) to falling and that startle reactions are easily conditioned suggests that genetic factors as well as early imprinting or learning may shape the magnitude of our reactions to unnatural vestibular inputs and may even influence emotional and cognitive aspects of development (GUEDRY, 1972). Further, it has been proposed that deprivation of early motion experience may also alter normal emotional and cognitive development (PETO, 1970; ORNITZ, 1970; PRESCOTT, 1971). There are pronounced differences among infants of 2 to 4 years in emotional reactions to unexpected passive motion (SMITH and SMITH, 1962). Moreover, it has been indicated that passive gentle oscillation of premature infants contributes to general health as well as cognitive development (NEAL, 1968). As part of an inertial guidance system, the nonauditory labyrinth provides information which must aid in early discrimination among whole-body movement, movement of surroundings, and movement of the eyes alone. Thus its contribution may be important in the development of concepts of "self" (SCHILDER, 1933; ORNITZ, 1970).

Whereas the visual and auditory systems respond to energies from the external environment and serve to describe "things" in the environment, the vestibular system in natural movement responds to self-generated movements of the body and serves to convey information about the state of orientation and motion of the head relative to the environment. Although stimulated by voluntary movement, it cannot be turned off and on in the obvious way that visual, auditory, tactile, and olfactory messages can be voluntarily controlled, respectively, by closing the eyelids, plugging the ears, moving a finger, or holding the nose. It also is never directed toward a particular environmental object, as other systems are, in turning to see, hear, touch, or smell something; yet in each of these actions it is stimulated in the course of a volitional act. During these actions, attention is directed toward the various sensory channels which have been voluntarily directed toward something in the environment, many of which also provide correlated orientation and

I. Introduction

During natural movement on the earth's surface, we are seldom aware of vestibular sensations, and when we do become aware of them, they usually signify an unnatural stimulus or an abnormality of vestibular function. With specially contrived conditions of observation, relationships between acceleratory stimuli and vestibular sensations and perceptions can be described quantitatively and qualitatively. These relationships constitute the primary subject matter of this chapter, but to appreciate this material in relation to daily experiences, we must first consider why vestibular sensations do not typically achieve conscious awareness during natural voluntary head and body movement.

The control of body transport movements and of concomitant head and eye orientation is vital to survival on or near the surface of the earth. The vestibular, tactile, and kinesthetic systems provide synergistic feedback data on the state of motion and orientation of the body in relation to the earth while the visual system provides not only immediate feedback but also immediate assessment of *future* requirements; e.g., visually detected slopes, obstacles, et cetera, project upcoming needs for changes in this state of motion. The auditory and even olfactory systems also project immediate as well as future requirements by their ability to localize and identify things in the environment.

To be effective in vital life functions, control of movement must become skilled, and it is well established (Kimble and Perlmuter, 1970) that as skill develops, those sequential components of movement sequences that can become automatic tend to recede from conscious awareness. Some integral components of whole sequences of skilled movement are neither purposely initiated nor monitored, yet they occur with precision (Mayne, 1951). The vestibular system is ontogenetically and phylogenetically an old system that participates in sensory feedback during skilled movement. Its dimensions vary among species in a way which adjusts its frequency response of velocity transduction to the range of natural movement of the animal (Melvill Jones and Spells, 1963; Mayne, 1965), a finding that suggests its importance to survival of species. Without a major muscle group of its own, it reflexly influences a number of motor systems throughout the body, and in man the oculomotor influence is especially apparent. An illustration of typical vestibular participation in voluntary movement is available to anyone who will oscillate his head back and forth smoothly through an arc of about 20 degrees (as in signifying "yes" or "no" by persistent head oscillation) at a

Chapter I.

Psychophysics of Vestibular Sensation*

By

FRED E. GUEDRY, JR., Pensacola, Florida (USA)

With 39 Figures

Contents

* Opinions or conclusions contained in this report are those of the author. They are not to be construed as necessarily reflecting the view or the endorsement of the Department of the Navy.

motion information. So without a monopoly on orientation or motion information, the vestibular system fairly early in the life cycle makes its unique contribution to the voluntary control of motion and orientation as a silent partner. Awareness of its sensory messages becomes apparent during unusual voluntary movement, as in the spinning games children play, or during vestibular pathology or during unnatural passive motion on ships, aircraft, et cetera. In the latter case, energies from the environment supply the vestibular stimulus, and the motion perceived is that of the body and vehicle moving as a unit relative to an external fixed reference which perceptually is the earth and the direction of its gravity.

A. Vestibular Sensations

In view of the preceding considerations, it is not surprising that questions have been raised as to whether we have true vestibular sensations. Two alternatives have been considered: 1) that perceptual experiences associated with vestibular stimulation arise indirectly from the various reflexes set off by this system (GELDARD, 1972); or 2) that the sensations of motion and orientation can be produced directly by the system itself (WENDT, 1951). The position that seems to be evolving today is one that was anticipated by MACH, BREUER, POLLAK, DE LAGE, NAGEL and JAMES (MACH, 1902). They regarded the labyrinth as a specific sense department which produces sensations, but they stressed that it cooperates in the maintenance of the equilibrium with the senses of pressure, the muscle sense as well as sight. In addition, most of these authors, whose conclusions were reached toward the end of the nineteenth century, included the influence of the "will" or, as it is referred to today, reafference (neural traces from voluntary commands to action) on the processing of incoming information from the eyes, the muscles and the vestibular sense in a way which would permit discriminations among movement of the eyes, movement of the body, and movement of the environment. The results of these early workers with deaf mutes and with operated animals indicated that the maintenance of equilibrium is possible without labyrinthine sensations, although the sense of rotation during and immediately after spinning about the vertical axis was absent, and they indicated that delicate problems of balance were not skillfully performed (cf. MACH, 1902).

More recently, there have been several lines of investigation which strengthen the argument for the presence of direct vestibular sensations. First, monophasic potential changes have been recorded in specific cerebral cortical areas following vestibular stimulation with a latency sufficiently short to suggest a primary cortical projection of the vestibular system (WALZL and MONTCASTLE, 1949; MICKLE and ADES, 1952; ANDERSON and GERNANDT, 1954). Second, direct application of gentle electrical currents to the cerebral cortex in man has elicited sensations of spinning, sinking and swinging (PENFIELD, 1957; CROSBY et al., 1962). Third, certain cortical lesions have produced larger than normal errors in perceptual judgments related to spatial orientation (BARLOW, 1970; TEUBER, 1960; cf. MCNALLY and STUART, 1967; HOWARD and TEMPLETON, 1966, pp. 267–271).

Cerebral cortical vestibular representation has been fairly clearly established. Cortical-evoked potentials have been recorded between the first and second somatic areas in the cat along a narrow strip of cortex comprising the anterior bank of the anterior ectosylvian gyrus and the posterior bank of the anterior suprasylvian gyrus. These findings by MICKLE and ADES (1952) confirmed earlier evidence of vestibular cortical activity and have since been confirmed by other workers (KEMPINSKI, 1951; WALZL and MONTCASTLE, 1949; ARSLAN and MOLINARI, 1965; SPIEGEL et al., 1968a, b). Comparable findings have been reported by FREDRICKSON et al. (1966) for the rhesus monkey, and the short response latencies suggest a fairly direct vestibular projection. Vestibular afferent projection to the motor cortex has also been indicated by evoked potentials of longer latency than those found in the primary projection area.

As FREDRICKSON et al. (1966) pointed out, the location of this projection area is in the postcentral gyrus of the monkey, not in the temporal lobe. PENFIELD (1957) reported eliciting sensations of spinning, sinking, swinging, et cetera, in a series of 108 temporal lobe explorations in man. He also reported eliciting reports of specific rotation (clockwise) and appropriate nystagmus in a patient by stimulation of an area between the occipital and parietal cortex. Because of the variety of explored areas that produced motion sensations, PENFIELD only tentatively located an area in the temporal lobe as being a vestibular projection area. CROSBY et al. (1962) elicited turning sensations in patients by stimulation of the superior temporal gyrus in man and also reported that stimulation of an area in the parietal lobe produces a sensation of dizziness in which the world revolves around the patient. Because closing the eyes altered the sensation, it was concluded that ocular as well as vestibular factors were involved.

Lesions in the parietal lobe of man have been found to produce deficits in various tests of spatial orientation (CRITCHLEY, 1953; TEUBER and MISHKIN, 1954; TEUBER, 1963; SEMMES et al., 1955). Without vestibular function, blindfolded individuals led over various paths are unable to reproduce the paths later with vision permitted (BERITOV, 1959). According to BARLOW (1970), however, individuals with lesions of the nondominant parietal lobe but with intact vestibular organs are unable to retraverse paths normally, even with the aid of vision during the initial path exploration (cf. TEUBER, 1960). Since individuals with normal vestibular and central function can perform such tasks quite well, it appears that there is a cortical area which requires vestibular inputs for forming images of spatial maps which can be stored and reconstructed later in the reproduction task.

Arguments for the presence of vestibular sensations per se are multiple. Individuals without vestibular function do not have turning sensations when visual and other motion cues are masked or eliminated. Individuals with vestibular function treated in like manner do have turning sensations. With functioning vestibular systems there are of course all of the reflex actions that this system sets off. However, patients with different neurological deficits have been used in attempts to clarify this point. For example, patients with normal vestibular function but with bilateral abducens paralysis do not have horizontal vestibular nystagmus, but they still experience the vestibular turning sensations (VAN DISHOECK et al., 1954). Individuals with spinal injuries involving complete spinal transections in the cervical region have normal sensations of linear velocity (presumably otolithic in origin) on the parallel swing (WALSH, 1961a). This kind of information coupled with the strong evidence for primary cortical projection based on recordings of cortical-evoked potential and on sensation reports induced by stimulation of cortical areas, plus the dysfunctions that are produced by cortical lesions, support the contention that the vestibular system has at least some sensations of its own.

It is of course difficult, if not impossible, to specify all of the necessary and sufficient neurophysiological conditions for the occurrence of any sensory experience. However, this inquiry into vestibular sensations is instructive in that it shows that this phylogenetically and ontogenetically old system has a small direct representation in the highest level of the nervous system and that it has indirect representation in a number of other cortical areas representing systems such as the visual system with which it is functionally interrelated. The integration of afferent data from vestibular and somatosensory systems in an overlapping cortical projection area is consistent with the functional interplay necessary among these systems. The vestibular structures are located in the head, which can move relative to the body, which can move relative to the earth. Therefore, it is clear that sensory data from the vestibular system become useful for equilibration only when integrated with afferent data from the muscles and joints.

The relevance of the foregoing considerations to a description of dynamic relationships between acceleratory stimuli and vestibular sensations and perceptions should be noted. It lies in the interpretation of this kind of information. Because of the number of different systems which contribute to the perception of orientation and motion, it is apparent that a number of auxiliary cues must either be masked or controlled in order to estimate the vestibular component. This is very difficult (especially in the case of the otolith system) because whole-body manipulation is involved. Moreover, the elimination or distortion of a number of normally correlated inputs may influence the dynamics of the response; i.e., the perceptual response may not follow the dynamics of the sensory inflow from the end-organ because of unnatural patterns of accompanying stimuli, or because of their unnatural absence. Due to the role of the vestibular system in development and its potential relation to emotional reactivity (GUEDRY, 1972), a strong immediate reaction to a specially contrived stimulus does not necessarily reflect a sensory input of abnormal intensity. Nevertheless there are functional reasons to believe that vestibular sensations and reactions should be reasonably accurate in direction and magnitude relative to an external reference during natural movement. Their use by the body demands a degree of accuracy relative to the external inertial reference system, but a high degree of accuracy may not be necessary because one system which, for example, can bring the head approximately into level is backed up by several other systems which may make finer adjustments. Finally, the pervasive physiological effects of unnatural vestibular stimuli complicate the study of adaptation and habituation to these stimuli because there are so many changes that occur, not all at the same rate, and the rate of change of reaction components may well be influenced by how the vestibular signals are paired with signals to other naturally interacting systems.

1. Plan and Scope of Chapter

The general plan of this chapter is to provide 1) a description of vestibular stimuli; 2) a description of subjective responses and related effects produced by simple stimuli to the semicircular canals; 3) a description of subjective measures and stimulus situations used in attempts to assess otolith function; 4) a description of responses dependent upon sensory interactions between the semicircular canals, otoliths, and visual systems; and 5) summarizing comments on several forms of adjustment to unusual vestibular stimulation.

B. Describing Acceleratory Stimuli to the Vestibular Structures

Analysis of the inertial forces and torques which displace the utricular and ampullar sensory detectors involves a branch of mechanics referred to as kinetics, but these forces and torques are proportional to linear and angular accelerations of the head. Therefore, the simple and more commonly used kinematic descriptions of linear and angular accelerations of the head are sufficient for specifying vestibular stimuli. Linear and angular accelerations are vectors that must be specified in relation to anatomical coordinates of the head in order to be properly described as vestibular stimuli. A nomenclature for this specific purpose has been developed in some detail by Hixson et al. (1966), and some of its salient features are presented here.

C. Nomenclature

The planes and cardinal axes of the head as defined by this nomenclature are shown in Fig. 1. These head axes do not correspond to the primary sensing axes of the semicircular canals or of the otolith systems. However, they provide a clear anatomical reference to which stimulus parameters can be related.

It is necessary to designate the sign (or sense) of an acceleration, its line of action, and its magnitude. For example, consider a person who is seated facing forward in a train that starts from a station and increases speed at constant rate

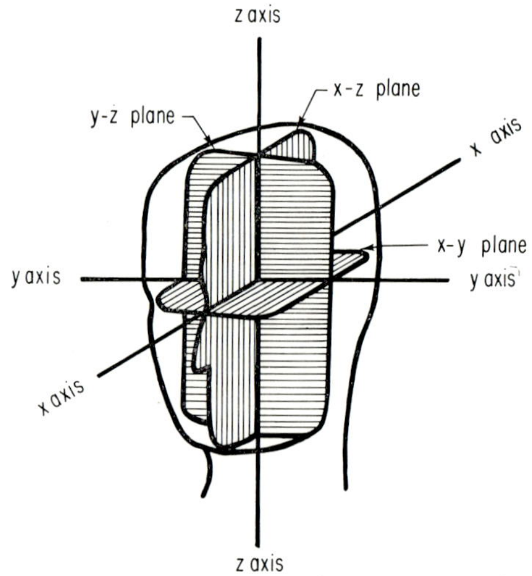

Fig. 1. Nomenclature for head axes and planes. Adapted from Hixson et al. (1966)

for 10 sec along a straight track until a velocity of 60 mph is attained. The train imparts a linear acceleration to the man along his x-axis, and it has a magnitude of $\frac{88 \text{ ft/sec}}{10 \text{ sec}} = 8.8 \text{ ft/sec}^2$. The sign (or sense) of this acceleration relative to the man is defined as positive, and the magnitude is indicated by the length of the vector. If the acceleration of gravity is used as unit magnitude, then the length of the arrow would be $\frac{8.8}{32.2}$ or 0.275 of the length of the arrow designating the magnitude of gravity. Thus the linear accelerations along the head axes are $A_x = +.275$ g-unit, $A_y = 0$ and $A_z = +1$ g-unit. Once specified in this way, the stimulus can be projected, if desired, to the planes of the utricle and saccule, at least to the limits of accuracy that the otolith planes have been related to visible anatomical landmarks of the skull.

Gravity is often considered to be the stimulus to the otoliths. Therefore, it is important to recognize the equivalence of the effects of linear acceleration and gravity. Einstein states this in his equivalence principle: "A gravitational field of force at any point in space is in every way equivalent to an artificial field of force resulting from acceleration, and no experiment can possibly distinguish between them." (White, 1940, p. 678). In the above example, A_z is the acceleration of gravity, and the total resultant linear acceleration is obtained by the vectorial resolution of A_x (the "artificial field of force resulting from acceleration") with A_z (the "gravitational field of force"). Just before the train started, the only force was gravity, and due to it, the seat was applying an upward force (as though the man were being accelerated upward); but as the train accelerated, the total resultant acceleration changed direction relative to the man. It changed from alignment with his z-axis toward his x-axis. In other words, it *rotated* in his x-z plane (sagittal plane) about his y-axis, through the angle designated as $\varnothing_y$, as

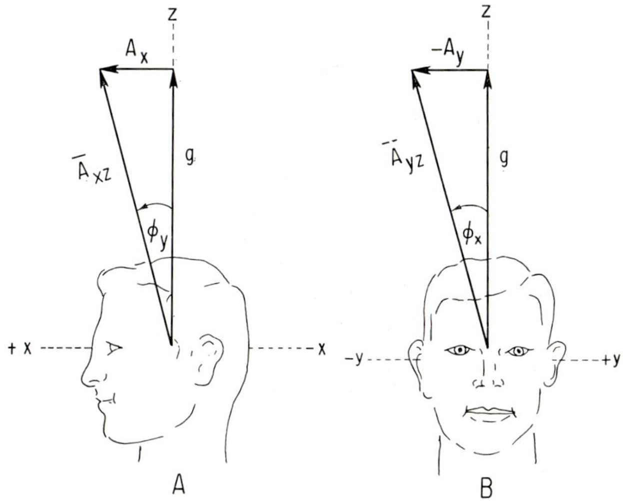

Fig. 2. Illustrating changes in resultant vector relative to two men, A and B, fixed in different orientations in a vehicle accelerating on an earth-horizontal track

illustrated in Fig. 2. It is important to note here that the man in this example has remained upright relative to the direction of gravity, but the resultant acceleration has rotated relative to the man. Because only linear accelerations have been used, the semicircular canals would not have been stimulated during this "rotation" but the otolith system would detect the new direction of the resultant vector (and perhaps the increased magnitude).

Now consider another man, B, seated on a sideseat of a club car and traveling with his right ear leading. While the train is accelerating, his linear acceleration can be described by $A_x = 0$, $A_y = -.275$ g-units, and $A_z = +1.0$ g-units. In B, the resultant has moved from his z-axis toward his y-axis; it has rotated in the y-z plane about the x-axis as shown in Fig. 2. This resultant vector $\bar{A}_{yz}$ makes an angle $+\varnothing_x = 15.376$ degrees with the man's z-axis. The positive sign of $\varnothing_x$ can be established by the right-hand rule of rotation as depicted in Fig. 3. When the thumb of the right hand is pointed along the +x head axis, the curl of the fingers and the direction or sense in which they are pointing determine the positive sign of rotation of $|\bar{A}_{yz}|$, the resultant acceleration, away from the +z head axis, through the angle $+\varnothing_x$.

In the two cases just considered, there was no angular acceleration; only linear accelerations were involved. However, B could be rotated about his x-axis in a tilt chair (in a stationary laboratory) about an earth-horizontal axis. In this case, if he is rotated 15.4 degrees so his left side is downward, then there is an angle of $+\varnothing_x = 15.4$ degrees between the direction of gravity and his z-axis. There are, however, important differences in the way the "tilt" conditions were produced

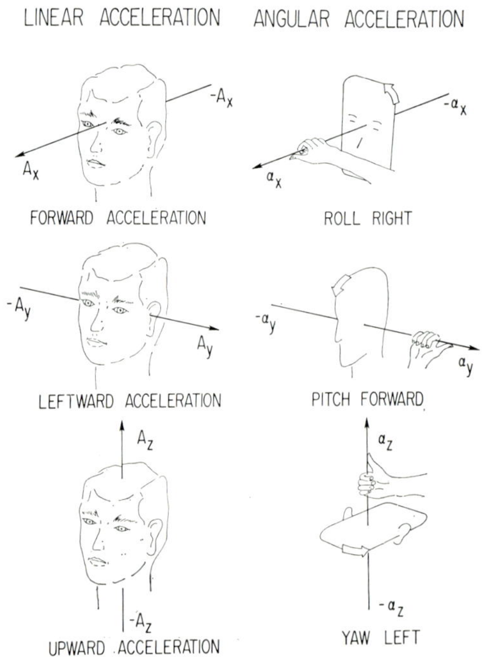

Fig. 3. Polarity conventions for head-referenced linear and angular acceleration vectors after Hixson et al. (1966)

by the train in one case and by the chair in the other. If the train rapidly attained a linear acceleration of 8.8 ft/sec² as it started, then the shift in the resultant vector through the angle $\varnothing_x$ would be rapid, but angular acceleration to stimulate the canals would be absent. On the other hand, if the angle $\varnothing_x$ were achieved quickly with the tilt chair, angular accelerations about the x-axis, a_x, would stimulate the semicircular canals and provide additional information about the 'tilting movement,' i.e., canals and otoliths would both signal the change in $\varnothing_x$.

Angular acceleration (a) is the rate of change of angular velocity (ω), and it also can be represented as a vector. If the angular velocity (the rotation rate) changes rapidly, then the magnitude of the angular acceleration is greater than when the angular velocity changes more slowly. The magnitude of the angular acceleration is represented by the length of the vector, and it is expressed in units such as degrees/second² or radians/second². The orientation of the vector relative to the head is either parallel to or colinear with the axis of rotation, and the sign or sense of the vector is again found by the right-hand rule. For example, if the head is rotated counterclockwise (CCW) as viewed from above about the z-axis (or about an axis parallel to the z-axis[1]), as the rate of rotation increases, there is an angular acceleration, $+a_z$, which is represented by a vector pointing upward along the +z-axis. If the thumb of the right hand points toward +z, the curl of the fingers corresponds to the direction of *increase* of angular velocity. Now, if this CCW angular velocity is decreased, the sign of the angular acceleration is reversed; it would be $-a_z$ and the vector would point downward along the —z axis. When angular velocity is increased in the clockwise (CW) direction, if we curl the fingers of the right hand in the direction of the increased speed, the thumb will point toward the —z axis and the angular acceleration is again $-a_z$. Conversely, when the CW angular velocity is decreased, the angular acceleration is $+a_z$. The same rules apply to the other axes illustrated in Fig. 3. These rules for designating the sign of the angular acceleration follow standard rules of mechanics, and the signs correspond to the effects of angular acceleration; for example, $+a_z$ produces the same cupula deflection, irrespective of whether the $+a_z$ is produced by deceleration from a CW angular velocity or by acceleration to a CCW angular velocity.

To specify the angular acceleration stimulation in a practical situation, the anatomical landmarks in this nomenclature system must be located relative to the axis of rotation of the stimulating device, and the angular acceleration of the device can then be projected to the x, y, and z coordinates of the head. If the angular acceleration lies in one of the three cardinal planes, 1) frontal or yz; 2) sagittal or xz; or 3) horizontal or xy, then the angular acceleration vector can be located relative to the head by the same system as was used for linear accelerations. Vectors intermediate between the main planes can also be located precisely (HIXSON et al., 1966).

D. Resolution of Acceleratory Stimuli by the Vestibular Sensors

The linear and angular acceleration stimulus vectors are sensed and located relative to the skull and relative to gravity by the vestibular sensors. In this

1 Parallel axis theorem (cf. SHAMES, 1960).

section the classical division of function within the vestibular system is assumed to be essentially correct, i.e., the semicircular canals are assumed to be especially sensitive to angular acceleration and relatively insensitive to linear acceleration while the otolith system, especially of the utricle, is assumed to act like a density-difference linear accelerometer, signaling angular position relative to gravity and also responding differentially to various resultant vectors of which linear accelerations and gravity are components.[2]

1. The Semicircular Canals

The three semicircular canals of each ear lie in a very hard portion of the temporal bone. The membranous canals are small tubes, filled with endolymph, which form closed loops by virtue of connecting at each end with a larger tube, the utricle. At one end, each canal expands into a spheroid chamber, the ampulla, just before it enters the utricle. The ampulla contains the cupula and crista, which constitute the sensory element of the canal. The cupula is a gelatinous fan-shaped structure whose edges fit closely to the inner surface of the ampulla, and it sits astride the crista which is a ridge of sensory hair cells. These sensory cells project cilia into the gelatinous cupula. The crista serves as a hinge upon which the cupula swings like a close-fitting valve in the ampulla as endolymph is displaced in the membranous tube.

Although each of the loops (formed by the canal, the ampulla and the utricle) is not perfectly in a single plane, each loop represents a mean plane, and these mean planes of the three canals in a single ear are nearly orthogonal to one another, like the planes of the walls in the corner of a room. The planes of the two vertical canals in a single ear are approximately 45 degrees from the sagittal plane of the skull; the lateral canal is in a plane defined by lines drawn from the outer canthi to the tragi.

The cupula substance is presumed to be exactly the same or very nearly the same specific gravity as the endolymph. This means that the cupula-endolymph system should not be influenced by linear acceleration or by its orientation relative to gravity, but it should be influenced by angular acceleration, i.e., by angular acceleration about an axis perpendicular to the mean plane of the canal.

During angular acceleration of the head, the ring of fluid in the canal accelerates at a lesser rate than the membranous tubes due to inertia of the fluid. Thus the relative movement between endolymph and the canal walls results in deflection of the cupula, whose elasticity resists displacement and provides a restorative force. It is usually assumed that displacement of the cupula controls the rate of neural inflow of the ampullary nerve which, in turn, affects the magnitude of the vestibular response under investigation, for example, subjective angular velocity.

The canals of the two ears are arranged approximately in three coplanar pairs. The lateral canals of the left and right ears form one pair, the superior right and inferior left form another pair, while the third pair comprises the superior left and inferior right canals. Each pair lies in one of three orthogonal planes, and the canals in a pair are complementary in that both respond to angular acceleration in the common average plane that they share.

---

2 Evidence relating to deviations from this classical subdivision of function is the subject of Section F.IV. by Benson in this volume.

In the horizontal (or lateral) pair of canals, deflection of the cupula toward the utricle (utriculopetal deflection) causes depolarization in the crista and increased rate of neural discharge in the ampullary nerve (TRINCKER, 1962). Deflection of the cupula away from the utricle (utriculofugal deflection) causes hyperpolarization in the crista and a decreased rate of neural discharge. The neural firing rate can either increase or decrease because there is a spontaneous discharge in the ampullary nerves even in the absence of stimulation. This important property of increasing or decreasing firing rate relative to a spontaneous level of activity (cf. LOWENSTEIN, Section A.II. this volume) permits a single canal to signal either direction of angular acceleration within its plane. By virtue of this property and the orthogonal arrangement of the three canals, one functional ear is capable of signaling the orientation of the axis of the angular acceleration relative to the skull (head) and also the direction (the sign) of rotation relative to that axis. Individuals who have lost the function of one ear can correctly discriminate the axis and direction of angular acceleration, although during recovery from sudden unilateral loss, they are severely disoriented.

The stimulus delivered to any one canal depends upon the orientation of the canal to the angular acceleration, and can be described in terms of the relative orientations of the canal and the rotation planes. However, because the angular acceleration vectors are perpendicular to the rotation plane (i.e., aligned with or

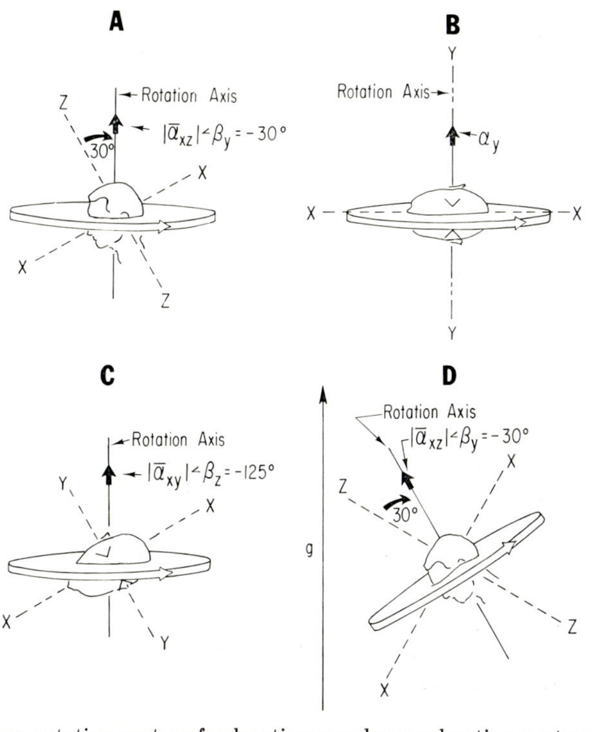

Fig. 4. Illustrating notation system for locating angular acceleration vectors relative to the head after HIXSON et al. (1966)

parallel to the axis of rotation), it is convenient to envision a canal axis perpendicular to its plane and to describe the relationship between the angular acceleration vector and the canal axis. When there is some angle, β, between the canal axis and the angular acceleration vector, a, then the effective stimulus, a_e, is given by $a_e = a \cos \beta$. In A and D of Fig. 4, a is aligned with the axis of the horizontal canals; thus the pattern of neural input from the canals in A and D would be a change in spontaneous rate proportional to $a \cos 0° = a$ in the two lateral canals and to $a \cos 90° = 0$ in the two vertical canals. This pattern is sufficient to determine the alignment of the stimulus vector relative to the head, while the fact that input from the left lateral increased while that from the right lateral decreased determines the sense (or sign) of the rotation. In B and C of Fig. 4, there would be no change in the spontaneous input from the lateral canals because they are 90 degrees displaced from the stimulus, but there would be changes from the vertical canals. In B, the angle β is 45 degrees for all four vertical canals and the change from all four would be proportional to $a \cos 45° = .707\ a$. This pattern locates the stimulus vector on the y-axis, and the fact that there would be a decreased rate from the two anterior canals and an increased rate from the two posterior canals determines the sign of rotation as "backward tumble" relative to the man's y-axis. In C, the proportionate changes would be: $-a \cos 15° = -.966\ a$ from the right anterior vertical; $-a \cos 75° = -.259\ a$ from the left anterior vertical; $+a \cos 75° = .259\ a$ from the right posterior vertical; and $+a \cos 15° = .966\ a$ from the left posterior vertical. In all of these cases, if the magnitude of the angular acceleration stimulus were greater, the relative patterns would remain the same, but the changes produced would be greater. Thus, according to the classical descriptions of semicircular canal function, the canals signal 1) the orientation of the axis of angular acceleration relative to the head; 2) the magnitude of the angular acceleration[3]; and 3) the sense (or sign) of rotation about the axis of angular acceleration. Also by classical concepts the canals *do not* indicate the axis of rotation relative to the earth; e.g., the canal signals in A and D would be identical.

2. The Otolith System

Whereas the semicircular canal system can locate the angular acceleration vector relative to the head, the otolith system can relate the orientation of the head to gravity.

In man, there are two otolithic receptor systems in each ear, one in the utricle and the other in the saccule. The sensory maculae in the utricle and saccule consist of hair cells covered by a gelatinous layer with a surface of calcite crystals. These crystals have a specific gravity of 2.71 (CARLSTROM, 1963), much greater than the specific gravity of endolymph, 1.003, which fills the utricle and saccule. Between the otolith 'membrane' and the surface of the hair cells are gelatinous strata into which sensory hairs project.

During linear acceleration or when the otolith surface is repositioned relative to gravity, the difference in density between the otoliths and the surrounding

3 The stimulus is, of course, a function of magnitude and time, which is discussed in a later section.

media results in a displacement of the otolith membrane relative to the hair cells. The amount of displacement depends upon 1) the stimulus, i.e., the magnitude and direction of the total resultant linear acceleration relative to the otolith surfaces, and 2) properties of the receptor organs, i.e., the density difference between the otoliths and the surrounding media and the elastic and viscous properties of the substances resisting the displacement. This displacement bends the sensory hairs which signal the orientation of the total resultant linear acceleration relative to the head.

The spatial relations of the utricular and saccular maculae relative to the skull defy simple verbal description. In man, the average plane of the utricular macula, is approximately parallel to that of the horizontal canals. However, the surface is concave and the anterior third curves upward fairly abruptly and is wider than the posterior position; its area is between 3.5 and 4.5 mm^2 (Quix, 1925; Corvera et al., 1958). The saccular macula is an elongated oval with its anterior end curling and perhaps twisting slightly. The saccular plane corresponds very roughly to the plane of the ipsilateral anterior semicircular canal. It has a surface area of about 2.2 mm^2 in man (Igarashi, 1966; Corvera et al., 1958). The angle between the saccular and utricular maculae has been variously estimated between 70° and 110°.

Because of the extremely small surface area being measured, and because the sensory epithelium of the utricle is not directly attached to the bone, the curvature and spatial relations indicated in a variety of publications are not in perfect agreement. There is, however, potential functional significance in these spatial relations. The maculae in the utricle and saccule have been examined in detail with the electron microscope, and the hair cells appear to have a systematic topographical orientation as indicated by the relative positions of kinocilia and sterocilia on each hair cell. In the saccule, the kinocilia are consistently directed away from a single curved dividing line. In the utricle the kinocilia are consistently directed toward a single curved dividing line. There is evidence indicating that deflection of hairs in the kinocilial direction produces an increased rate of neural activity, whereas bending the hairs away from the kinocilia produces a decreased rate of neural activity relative to a spontaneous level (Spoendlin, 1966). Considering these characteristics in relation to the curvature of the various otolithic maculae, it would appear that a single macula could produce distinctive patterns of neural input, each of which would be unique for each of a variety of directions and magnitudes of inclination relative to gravity.

There is not, however, general agreement on how the otolith system signals the direction of gravity. The possibility that the saccular and utricular organs form two primary sensing planes which provide coordinates for determining direction and magnitude of various tilts was suggested by Breuer (Mach, 1902, p. 156) and cannot be ruled out, but there are questions about the function of the saccule. Some have suggested that it is a vestigial organ in man (cf. Howard and Templeton, 1966), but this is not generally accepted (Jongkees, 1950, 1968, 1969; McNally and Stewart, 1967; Fluur, 1970). Some of the confusion may be attributable to different functional roles in different species and may also arise from the possibility that the saccule may have functional roles slightly different from those tested in some experiments involving surgical insult to the system; e.g., it may respond dynamically to changes in linear acceleration of fairly high frequency, and serve to stabilize and orient the head and eyes during trotting or jogging, rather than to act primarily as a static position sensor.

Despite this lack of general agreement on exactly how the otoliths signal orientation relative to gravity, it is generally accepted that they perform this sensory function. In addition to position indication (angular position relative to gravity), other functions of the otolith organs have been suggested by recorded electrical activity of the utricular and saccular nerves. Some units respond maximally to a particular position, but others respond to vibration, and still others respond specifically to a change in position (LOWENSTEIN and ROBERTS, 1949). Units responding to movement of the otoliths, rather than to a position, suggest that the otoliths may contribute to the perception of linear velocity by contributing velocity information during a changing linear acceleration which would not stimulate the semicircular canals. From assessment of electrophysiological recordings (LOWENSTEIN and ROBERTS, 1949), ROBERTS (1967) concluded that the otoliths provide sufficient information to enable the central nervous system to deduce not only angle of tilt, but also axis of rotation about which the tilt has taken place. Thus, in natural movement the otoliths and canals work synergistically.

The following points are presented in partial summary of preceding sections:

1. The primary natural function of the vestibular system is to assist in efficient movement and positioning of the head and body in relation to the earth, and except under special conditions, vestibular sensations do not reach "conscious awareness."

2. During head movement, the semicircular canals localize the angular acceleration vector relative to the head and contribute the sensory input for a) appropriate reflex action relative to an anatomical axis, and b) for perception of angular velocity about that axis.

3. Perception of how this axis is oriented relative to the earth depends upon sensory inputs from the otolith and somatosensory systems, and thus appropriate reflex actions relative to the earth depend upon these other systems working synergistically with the canals.

4. The otoliths provide both static and dynamic orientation information (relative to gravity) and probably contribute to the perception of tilt and also to perception of linear velocity.

5. The perception of linear velocity derives from a *combination* of a) change-in-position information from the otoliths and b) the absence of angular velocity information from the canals. The otoliths provide change-in-position information when the cilia are in motion, and the stimulus required is a change in linear acceleration without concomitant angular acceleration, for example, the *onset* of horizontal linear acceleration or horizontal linear oscillation.

II. Subjective Reactions to Semicircular Canal Stimulation by Simple Angular Acceleration

When the head is fixed very near the center of a turntable which has a vertical axis of rotation, angular acceleration of the turntable delivers a relatively simple stimulus to the semicircular canals. This is the stimulus under consideration in this section; it avoids the otolithic and somatosensory stimulation that occurs when the rotation axis is tilted or when the head is appreciably displaced from the rotation center. It is not an unnatural stimulus because the head is frequently turned in natural movement about an axis, especially the z-axis, which is very nearly aligned with gravity.

The direction, magnitude, and duration of vestibular stimuli must be specified, and in the case of the semicircular canals, the temporal aspects of the stimulus, especially the changes in acceleration with respect to time, are of major importance. By structural considerations alone, it is clear that the cupula-endolymph loop is some kind of a damped spring system, and a considerable body of investigation, including measures of structural characteristics (MELVILL JONES and MILSUM, 1965, 1967; MAYNE, 1950a, 1965), neural activity (GROEN et al., 1952; FERNÁNDEZ and GOLDBERG, 1971), vestibular nystagmus, and vestibular sensations (VAN EGMOND et al., 1949), indicates that the system reacts to angular acceleration like a highly damped torsion pendulum. A review of pertinent literature, including consideration of several alternative hypotheses, has been made recently by OUTERBRIDGE (1969). In general, the alternatives do not question whether the cupula-endolymph loop has some characteristics of a damped spring system, but rather they question what kind of a spring system is involved and how complex it is. Many characteristics of these stimulus-response relationships are predicted by a cupula-endolymph system that reacts to stimuli like a simple, overcritically damped torsion pendulum, but there are some clearly discrepant findings, and these have prompted alternative considerations primarily in three directions: 1) the basic torsion pendulum model has been assumed to be inadequate, 2) the basic model has been assumed to be adequate but various forms of hysteresis change its mechanical response to abnormal stimuli, 3) the basic model has been assumed to be adequate but the central nervous system, through feedback loops, and at various way stations, reshapes the stimulus-response relationship. To be viable, alternative hypotheses must account not only for the "discrepant findings" but also for the very many relationships which are consistent with the older hypothesis when a large number of stimulus waveforms are used. From this point of view, the third alternative seems the more viable, and it probably represents a consensus of current opinion.

In dealing with the psychophysics of semicircular canal sensations, some set of original assumptions regarding the dynamic response of the endorgan is involved merely in selecting stimuli. The vestibular response to a constant angular acceleration has a gradual rise time. When such a stimulus terminates without being followed by acceleration of the opposite sign, the vestibular response decays gradually and thus outlasts the stimulus by a considerable period. These response characteristics complicate many of the kinds of psychophysical comparisons of stimuli which are used in investigations of other sensory systems. Thus for planning purposes alone, it is necessary to estimate the sensory input which a given stimulus is likely to introduce. In this chapter, it is assumed that the basic torsion pendulum analogy to an overcritically damped torsion spring system is an adequate first approximation model for stimulus definition. It is a particularly useful starting point for considering semicircular canal stimuli because once values have been estimated for three parameters of the appropriate differential equation, then the expected sensory input and its phase relation to any angular acceleration waveform can be described precisely.

A. Four Typical Stimulus Patterns

The four stimulus patterns shown in Fig. 5 have been used frequently in the study of semicircular canal function. Each is illustrated by the simultaneous time-course changes of angular acceleration and angular velocity. Also shown are the corresponding time-course changes of cupula displacement calculated from the torsion pendulum (TP) model. The "angular impulse" or velocity-step stimulus is essentially a high-magnitude angular acceleration applied for a short time, and its magnitude is proportional to the total angular velocity change. For example, the angular impulse delivered by a very sudden arrest (sudden stop) from a 60 deg/sec angular velocity is twice that delivered by a sudden (rapid) stop from 30 deg/sec. Van Egmond et al. (1949) introduced the practice of referring to such stimuli as angular velocity impulses, e.g., a "60 deg/sec angular impulse." This form of stimulus control was widely used before the ready availability of devices that control angular acceleration.

In Fig. 5, the time scale used for the "angular impulse" stimuli and for the angular velocity ramp ("acceleration-step") stimuli shows 180-sec time segments whereas the scale used for the triangular and sinusoidal stimulus waveforms show only 2-sec time segments. With both the impulse and ramp sequences, the initial and final angular accelerations are separated by long periods of constant angular velocity, a sequence which almost never occurs in natural movement. Under these circumstances the response is clearly elicited by the angular accelerations, and it decays during the periods of constant velocity. In these cases the response is more or less "on acceleration" and false information occurs during constant velocity. On the other hand, the short triangular and sinusoidal stimulus waveforms are much closer approximations to natural turning movements, in which the angular acceleration that starts the turn is immediately followed by an opposite angular acceleration that stops the turn. Under these circumstances the negative angular acceleration serves to return the deflected cupula to zero position, and very little cupula overshoot is predicted at the end of turns that are completed in less than 2 or 3 sec.

It is important to note in Fig. 5 that the cupula waveforms calculated for the short stimulus waveforms look like the stimulus waveforms of angular velocity and not like those of angular acceleration. Plots of neural activity and of nystagmus slow-phase velocity during such stimuli give waveforms which also look like the stimulus angular velocity waveform. For this reason the semicircular canals are frequently referred to as angular velocity transducers (Mayne, 1950a, b; Melvill Jones, 1966a, b). This is not a denial that the adequate stimulus to the semicircular canals is angular acceleration, but it simply means that during stimulus waveforms with periods (and frequencies) like those of natural movement, the dynamic response of the end-organ is such that its output (presumed to be proportional to cupula displacement) copies the stimulus velocity waveform. If one imagines the acceleration-step (velocity-ramp) stimulus waveform of Fig. 5 to be a repeating cyclic event, one can visualize that the cupula response will copy

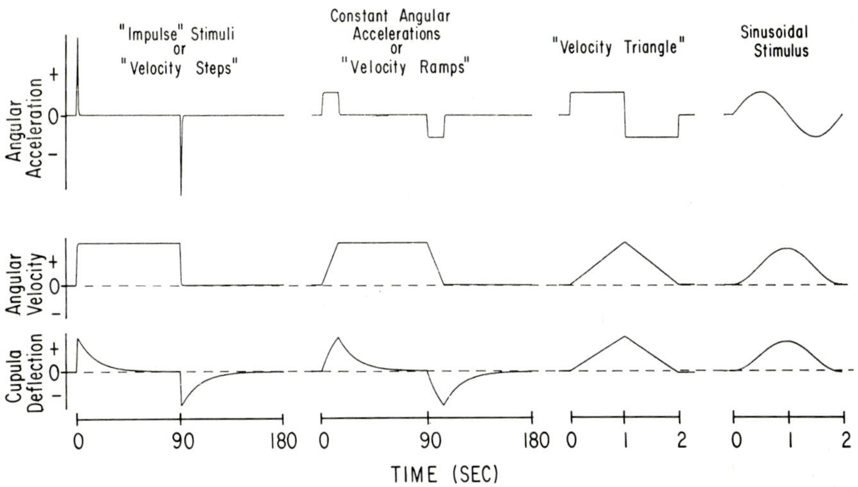

Fig. 5. Angular acceleration, angular velocity and expected cupula deflection during four stimulus patterns

the angular acceleration waveform during very low frequency (long wavelength) sinusoidal stimulus waveforms. The semicircular canals are said to be angular acceleration transducers during very low frequency periodic stimulation. Note, however, that the immediate (instantaneous) response at any particular time during the stimulus waveform is still regarded as angular velocity information (i.e., the velocity of nystagmus is measured or the person at any instant feels he is turning at some 'rate'), so with very low frequency stimulation, this velocity information coincides with the acceleration waveform. With such stimuli, reflexes would be inappropriate and velocity perceptions would be inaccurate, as they are in the constant velocity segments of the "long wavelength" stimuli shown in Fig. 5. Thus, with a change in frequency of a sinusoidal stimulus from waveforms which approximate natural stimuli to very low frequency (long wavelength) stimuli, there is a shift of the response waveform from one that corresponds to the stimulus velocity waveform in the first case to one that corresponds to the stimulus acceleration waveform in the second case.

B. Measurable Aspects of Subjective Reactions to Simple Angular Acceleration

It is with unnatural stimuli like the 180-sec stimulus sequences of Fig. 5 that man discovers he has vestibular sensations, and this kind of stimulus is convenient for illustrating some of the available options in measuring vestibular sensations. Shortly after the beginning of a controlled constant angular acceleration (velocity ramp), rotation is experienced even in the absence of auditory and visual cues to motion. As the angular acceleration continues, the sensed "speed of turning" increases. It continues to increase as the angular acceleration is maintained, although with velocity ramps longer than 5 to 10 sec, the turning sensation increases at a lesser rate of increase than the stimulus velocity.[4] When the angular acceleration terminates and constant angular velocity is maintained, the experienced speed of turning gradually diminishes and finally terminates. This portion of the reaction to angular acceleration has been referred to as the primary reaction, and it is followed by a secondary reaction of reversed sign which will be discussed later under probable adaptation effects. At this point in time the calculated cupula deflection is nearly zero. (The assumption of 'overcritical damping' predicts no cupula overshoot in this situation.) When deceleration begins, the cupula-endolymph ring tends to continue its rotation by virtue of its angular momentum while the head speed is reduced, and thus cupula deflection in opposite direction begins and increases until the viscous damping and spring action balance the offsetting inertial torque, or until deceleration stops. During deceleration a sensation of turning in opposite direction commences and increases until deceleration is completed, and then it declines gradually to zero. The response to deceleration is similar to the acceleration response except that it is reversed in direction. Because these sensations of turning have both magnitude and direction, subjective angular velocity seems appropriate to designate the instantaneous perception of motion.

C. The Oculogyral Effect and the Somatogyral Effect

The subjective turning sensations just described have been observed in two basic situations, one in total darkness and the other with a visual target fixed in front of the rotating observer. In both situations, the observer is usually encapsulated so that external visual reference is prevented, and efforts are made to reduce or mask auditory, vibratory, and other cues to movement. With such precautions, the sensations experienced in total darkness have usually been accepted as vestibular (van Dishoeck et al., 1954), but the origin of sensations experienced with the fixed visual reference have been subject to more controversy. They have been attributed (Graybiel et al., 1946) to the visual information generated by movement of images over the retina of the eye during the slow phase of nystagmus, the fly-back fast phase being regarded as too fast for visual information. The term, "oculogyral illusion," was coined to name the effect (Graybiel and Hupp, 1946). Although the terms *oculogyral* or *optogyral* remain in common use, the explanation has not been completely accepted and will be considered in a later section. A number of authors (Mann et al., 1951; van Dishoeck et al., 1954; Byford, 1963) pointed out that the perception of body rotation relative to an unseen fixed external reference occurs with or without a target light, and any directional sensory datum, a light, a touched object, or a sound (Mayne, 1952; Arnoult, 1950; Clark and Graybiel, 1949), that is perceived in fixed relation to the vertiginous observer will be perceived as moving with the observer relative to an unseen external reference. *Oculogyral effects* (OGy) are present even when movement of the retinal image is stopped or distorted by a variety of methods (van Dishoeck et al., 1954; Mann et al., 1951; Byford, 1963), and in general the sensation of rotation in the dark, which herein will be called the *somatogyral effect* (SGy), has a similar, though not identical, time-dependent magnitude change in response to

4 When velocity ramps are maintained for more than 25 sec, the sensation begins to diminish, presumably due to adaptation effects.

angular acceleration. During moderate semicircular canal stimulation with a target light present, visual suppression usually overrides vestibular nystagmus so that it may not be detectable (BYFORD, 1963), and smooth turning sensation of body and target light together are usually reported. Under such conditions, the oculogyral effects are generally not regarded as simply an epiphenomenon of moving retinal images, but rather as perceptual sequences dependent upon vestibular messages, but also dependent upon visual-vestibular interactions which in the "ideal" observation conditions detailed by CLARK and STEWART (1969) seem to sensitize the observer to the perceptual task. With stronger vestibular stimulation that overrides visual control, image movement contributes a readily perceived target drift and jerk-recovery which are superimposed on a sensation of over-all turning and, with further increases in stimulation, a blurring of vision (GUEDRY, 1968). Also, apparent displacement of the target (lead or lag) relative to perceptual "dead-ahead" (GRAYBIEL and HUPP, 1946; BROWN et al., 1949) and apparent tilting of a target line (WAPNER et al., 1951) have been reported. However, unless especially noted, the effects referred to in this section are the subjective angular velocity of light and body considered together as a unit (in the OGy case) or of the body alone (in the SGy case).

D. Thresholds of Perception of Angular Acceleration

An excellent review of experimental determinations of thresholds for perception of angular acceleration by CLARK (1967) shows various estimates of mean threshold values between 0.035 deg/sec^2 and 4.0 deg/sec^2 for rotation about an earth-vertical axis. This considerable range of mean values is attributable to a combination of factors such as individual differences among subjects, small samples of subjects, variations in psychophysical procedures, and differences in equipment used for producing and measuring the stimuli and also the responses (cf. EK et al., 1959).

When very sensitive angular accelerometers are attached to devices which "control" angular acceleration, it is typical to find some rather long rise times (e.g., 0.5 to 1 sec) and fairly large oscillatory transients before the device settles down to the programmed constant angular acceleration, and even then there is continuous noise (high frequency transients) about a mean acceleration. The transients are somewhat obscure in typical recordings of velocity-indicating tachometers and position-indicating potentiometers, and they can also be hidden in recordings of some angular accelerometers that do not follow the transients in the stimulus. Thus, differences among various experiments in the dynamic response characteristics of rotating devices and recording systems probably account for some of the differences in thresholds reported. Such problems and their effects on threshold determination are difficult to assess in the available literature, but with a few exceptions, they may not be the major cause of the reported variations. The frequency response of the semicircular canal system itself is probably such that it does not respond to all of the stimulus transients. In many experiments employing long velocity ramps, the mean constant angular acceleration has probably been a sufficient indication of the stimulus for practical purposes, especially when the desired angular velocity was attained in the programmed time. However, this statement is based upon assumptions about cupula dynamics, and so even here with long duration of the adequate stimulus, essentially the same assumptions are involved in assessing probable effects of stimulus duration and the ever-present "errors" in stimulus control and measurement. Moreover, since extravestibular systems can respond to fast transients and vibration, the assumption that a given response is dependent upon canal input is sometimes based on the dynamic characteristics of the response itself (cf. VON BÉKÉSY, 1940). This kind of reasoning is circular, but it is defensible within limits. For example, individuals apparently without vestibular function can correctly indicate direction of rotation during angular accelerations of sufficient magnitude and duration (MANN, 1951), but when constant velocity is attained the normal rotation experience and exponential response decay are not reported (cf. MACH, 1902, p. 159f). They typically report either continuous rotation if they make intellectual use of vibration cues, or they report cessation of rotation very soon after constant velocity is attained. During deceleration they may simply report stopping or they may report rotation in the other direction, depending on their use of the extravestibular cues during constant velocity, but in either case when deceleration terminates, there is no postrotational effect. Thus the dynamics of the response serve to establish that the reported sensations were probably extravestibular.

1. Threshold Estimates from Constant Angular Acceleration

Several strategies for estimating thresholds from velocity ramps (sometimes called "acceleration steps" or simply constant angular accelerations) have been

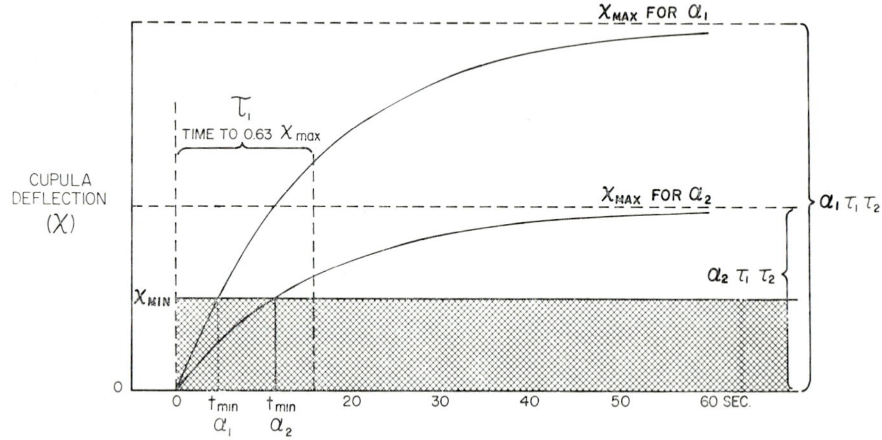

Fig. 6. Cupula deflection during constant angular accelerations according to the TP model

employed, and within each of these strategies, many variations of specific rules for subjective reporting are possible. Several representative methods are indicated herein, but other variations have been used in the threshold studies listed in Table 1 which is an adaptation from CLARK (1967).

Table 1. *Thresholds for detection of angular acceleration in man* (adapted from CLARK, 1967)

Author	Principal Rotation Axis	Perceptual Mode	Threshold Values deg/sec²
MACH (1875)	z-axis	SGy	0.5 (calculated by GROEN and JONGKEES)
DODGE (1923)	z-axis	SGy	1–2
TUMARKIN (1937)	z-axis	SGy	0.2
CHRISTIAN (1939)	z-axis	SGy and OGy	0.13–2.0
CLARK et al. (1948)	—	OGy	0.2
GRAYBIEL et al. (1948)	z-axis	OGy	0.12
GROEN and JONGKEES (1948a)	z-axis	SGy	0.18–2.0
MACCORQUODALE (1948)	—	SGy	0.1–0.15
DEVRIES (1949)	z-axis	SGy	0.9–4.0
HALLPIKE et al. (1952)	z-axis	SGy and OGy	0.2–2.0
HILDING (1953)	z-axis	SGy	0.25–3.0
DEVRIES and SCHIERBEEK (1953)	z-axis	SGy	0.9–1.7
v. BÉKÉSY (1955)	z-axis	SGy	0.4–1.5 (calculated in text)
SADOFF et al. (1955)	y-axis	SGy	5.3–8.2
MANN and RAY (1956c)	z-axis	SGy	.035–0.13
MONTANDON and RUSSBACH (1956)	z-axis	SGy	0.5–1.0
ROGGEVEEN and NIJHOFF (1956)	z-axis	SGy and OGy	1.3–1.8
CLARK and STEWART (1962)	z-axis	SGy	0.12–0.17
v. DIRINGSHOFEN et al. (1964)	z-axis	SGy	.26–1.0
MEIRY (1965)	z-axis	SGy	0.1–0.2
MEIRY (1965)	x-axis	SGy	0.5

Each of the main strategies is easily understood from the point of view of the theoretical cupula dynamics expressed in Eq. (1) and illustrated in Fig. 6. According to the torsion pendulum theory, during constant angular acceleration, a, cupula deflection, x, approaches an asymptotic deflection, $a\,\tau_1\,\tau_2$, at a rate determined by:

$$x \cong a\tau_1\tau_2\,(1 - e^{-\frac{t}{\tau_1}}) \tag{1}$$

$$\dot{\psi} \cong Kx \tag{1a}$$

where τ_1, the "long time constant," is the ratio of the viscous term to the spring term, τ_2, the "short time constant," is the ratio of the inertial term to the viscous damping term in a second-order linear differential equation, and K is a constant of proportionality relating cupula deflection to a response, $\dot{\psi}$, such as subjective angular velocity.[5]

5 The symbols used by VAN EGMOND et al. (1949) are Π/Δ for τ_1 and θ/Π for τ_2.

Thus, if the value of the long time constant is 16 sec, the cupula will reach 63% of asymptotic deflection for any given acceleration in 16 sec, about 85% in 30 sec, and about 98% in 60 sec. If cupula deflection controls input and if it is presumed that some minimum input is required to elicit a response, then low magnitude accelerations must be applied for a fairly long time to be sure that the minimal cupula deflection, x_{min}, has been exceeded. Then because, unaided, the cupula returns to "zero position" from any deflection, however small, along the same time course (see Eqs. 4 and 5 below), long rest intervals must be interpolated or else the second of two stimuli will be influenced by the first.

Mann and Ray (1956c) followed a procedure in which they selected a given low magnitude acceleration and varied stimulus duration and direction, the latter randomly. The observer was required to make a direction guess at the time the stimulus ended. If two successive guesses were correct, the stimulus duration was decreased by one-sixth and the sequence repeated, errors being followed by increases and correct responses by decreases in stimulus duration. The criterion for "latency" threshold was the duration that yielded 75% correct responses in 60 trials. Then a new magnitude acceleration was selected and the whole sequence repeated. When the response latency for four or five near-threshold accelerations had been so determined, an empirical curve was fitted to the observer's data. On the assumption that subjective responses peak at about 30 sec of constant acceleration, the absolute threshold estimates obtained from the curves ranged between .03 and .06 deg/sec^2. The possibility that these extremely low threshold values for somatogyral effects resulted from extra-vestibular cues was considered (Mann and Ray, 1956c).

Clark and Stewart (1962, 1968a, b), in an extensive series of threshold studies, chose to hold duration of angular acceleration constant at 10 sec while varying magnitude and direction, the latter randomly, between trials. They compared several methods including the generally accepted but very time-consuming method of constant stimuli, and found (1968a) that it gave essentially the same results as a quicker forced choice "double staircase" method. A threshold magnitude was estimated from initial practice trials and then two starting steps were selected six steps (of 0.1 log unit each) above and below the threshold estimate. For example, with a 0.5 deg/sec^2 threshold estimate, the initial upper and lower starting steps would be 1.6 and 0.1 deg/sec^2, respectively. If two successive presentations of the upper step, 1.6 deg/sec^2, were correctly judged, then the next stimuli to be presented in the "descending staircase" were two steps down, i.e., 1 deg/sec^2. An error on either stimulus in a step causes a one-step increase for the next presentation in the descending series. On the other hand, starting from the lowest step, 0.1 deg/sec^2, of the "ascending staircase," if a judgment error was made in either of two presentations, then the next step was two steps higher (toward the estimated threshold value), whereas two correct judgments caused a stimulus decrease of one step. This is simply a systematic but apparently random (from observer viewpoint) method to approach the threshold from supra- and subthreshold stimuli. After the staircases intersected, the same rules were followed except that all subsequent changes were in two-step units and threshold was taken as the mean of some requisite number of observations (60 or 120) after the intersection. By this procedure, somatogyral thresholds ranging between 0.05 deg/sec^2 and 2.2 deg/sec^2 were found in 33 men with a mean of 0.42 deg/sec^2, a median of 0.29 deg/sec^2, and 10 observers below 0.20 deg/sec^2. Considering the fact that CLARK and STEWART used only 10-sec durations throughout, these thresholds are not far out of line with those reported by MANN and RAY for longer stimulus application. Because by other methods it has been shown that sensation increases for about 30 sec of suprathreshold constant angular acceleration, there is reason to suspect that lower thresholds would be obtained with longer stimulus application, although results obtained by DOTY (1969) might be interpreted otherwise.

2. Thresholds by Extrapolation of Supraliminal Response Curves

It is clear from empirical evidence that the time required for detection of a given acceleration is inversely related to its magnitude (GUEDRY and RICHMOND, 1957; MOWRER, 1935). By setting x in Eq. (1) equal to some minimum cupula deflection, x_{min}, and solving for t, response latency, (t_{min}) for any given acceleration is given by:

$$t_{min} = \tau_1 \ln \left(\frac{\tau_1 \tau_2 a}{\tau_1 \tau_2 a - x_{min}}\right) \tag{2}$$

Data obtained by MEIRY (1965) are shown in relation to a curve generated by Eq. (2), using values for τ_1 and τ_2 determined by other kinds of experiments[6] and

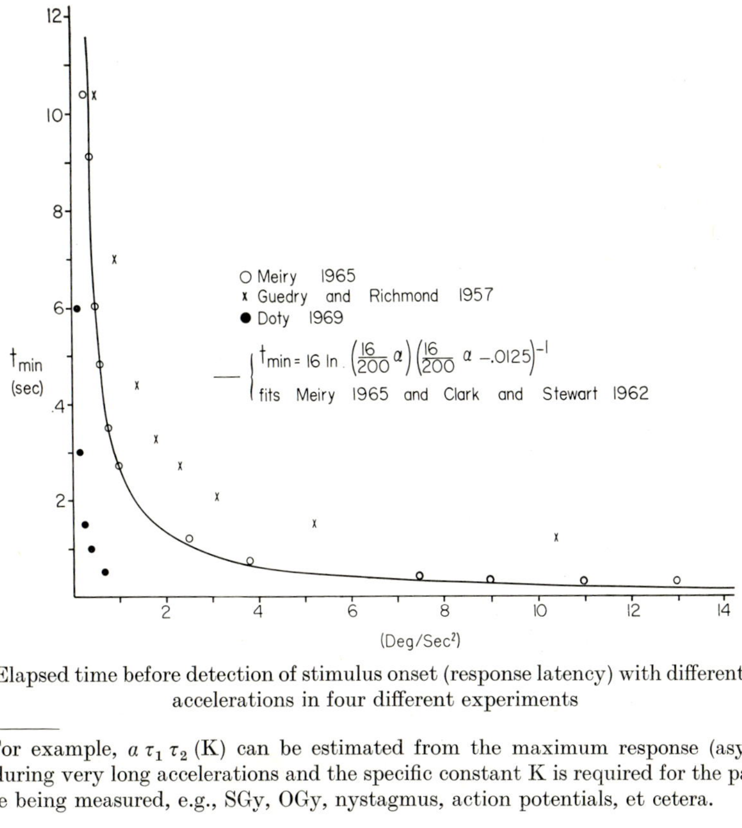

Fig. 7. Elapsed time before detection of stimulus onset (response latency) with different angular accelerations in four different experiments

6 For example, $a\, \tau_1 \tau_2$ (K) can be estimated from the maximum response (asymptotic value) during very long accelerations and the specific constant K is required for the particular response being measured, e.g., SGy, OGy, nystagmus, action potentials, et cetera.

a value of x_{min} selected to give a best "least squares" fit (Fig. 7). The fit is good except for the low magnitude accelerations where the measured latencies (ignored in the statistical fit) are less than the calculated values. Essentially the same results were reported by CLARK and STEWART (1962) and the one curve approximates their data as well. By extrapolating this curve to very long response latencies, one obtains a threshold estimate of about 0.3 deg/sec². This is greater than the 0.14 deg/sec² threshold determined directly by MEIRY (i.e., the point falling below the curve) and also by CLARK and STEWART; but it is a little less than the SGy threshold determined by CLARK and STEWART (1969) in another experiment. Also plotted in Fig. 7 are points from DOTY (1969) and from GUEDRY and RICHMOND (1957). Although both of the latter experiments used the OGy situation, which in all direct comparisons with SGy is the more sensitive indicant, it is apparent that the GUEDRY and RICHMOND latencies are consistently longer (while those of DOTY are consistently shorter) than corresponding points on the SGy curve based on MEIRY's data. The striking difference in results of these two OGy experiments is largely attributable to differences in methods. GUEDRY and RICHMOND initiated the acceleration stimuli from a 15 deg/sec base angular velocity which was maintained for a random duration anywhere from about 33 to 133 sec before the acceleration stimulus commenced. Continuous vibratory cues during constant base velocity served to disguise stimulus onset transients, and this with the random onset time probably contributed to the longer latencies in this study. Moreover, only one direction of rotation was used in the experiment, and since autogyral effects are experienced with prolonged exposure to any rotary device, observers soon recognized that they had to discriminate "real" acceleration effects from autogyral effects, thus introducing some decision time. In the experiment of DOTY, a ready signal was given just before each stimulus presentation, and thresholds, determined by the "force-choice random double staircase" procedure described above, were found for each of the six stimulation durations plotted in Fig. 7. Each of these "latencies" is a threshold for responding with slightly better than chance accuracy very soon after a ready signal which, from the point of view of alertness, should optimize signal detection and incidentally optimize the information value of transients. Here, then, is a study carried out with modern stimulating and recording equipment with as careful attention to psychophysical method and detail as is feasible, but nevertheless some of the questions that troubled earlier investigators remain. By selecting particular stimulus times and using the same criterion of threshold accuracy for each, DOTY has apparently avoided the reaction time problem, but the potential problem of biased transients serving as stimuli to the vestibular or somatosensory systems remains a matter for conjecture. In the history of threshold estimation from response latencies during ramp velocities, these problems of reaction time, stimulus transients, and extravestibular cues have been frequently mentioned, which is one reason why other approaches were considered.

GROEN and JONGKEES (1948a) were disturbed about reaction time with latency measures of thresholds and about extravestibular sensations with "impulse stops" from "minimal detectable" angular velocities (ω_{min}) and therefore suggested determination of thresholds by extrapolation from what have come to be known as sensation cupulograms. According to the torsion pendulum theory (VAN EG-

MOND et al., 1949), a rapid stop from some constant angular velocity produces cupula deflection, x_i, equal to the angular velocity just before the stop times the short time constant, τ_2; thus

$$x_i = \omega \tau_2 \tag{3}$$

To obtain some intuitive appreciation for this approximation formula, $x_i = \omega \tau_2$, derived by GROEN and JONGKEES (1948a), it should be recalled that $\tau_2 \simeq \theta / \Pi$ where θ is a constant representing the moment of inertia of the endolymph ring and Π is the moment of viscous retardation per unit angular velocity of the fluid relative to the canal walls. During constant angular velocity (ω), the endolymph ring acquires an angular momentum approximated by $\omega\theta$. With sudden stopping, the cupula deflection is directly proportional to the angular momentum $\omega\theta$ and inversely proportional to the viscous retardation, Π. The retarding effect of cupula spring action was considered to be negligible for small rapid displacements produced under this condition.

The cupula return from x_i deflection would be given by:

$$x = x_i e^{-t/\tau_1} \tag{4}$$

The duration of the sensation expected following the x_i deflection is dependent upon the cupula's elastic restoring force during constant (or zero) velocity and can be calculated by setting $x = x_{min}$ in Eq. (4), $x_i = \omega \tau_2$ and solving for t, which in this special case is called t_u:

$$t_u = \tau_1 \ln \frac{\omega \tau_2}{x_{min}} = \tau_1 \ln \omega + \tau_1 \ln \frac{\tau_2}{x_{min}} \tag{5}$$

Thus a plot of the durations of the primary after-sensation, t_u, against the logarithm of the angular velocity just before stopping should produce a linear relationship with a slope of τ_1. Such relationships were called cupulograms by VAN EGMOND et al. (1949). Mean cupulograms from large numbers of observers have been obtained (HULK and JONGKEES, 1948; ASCHAN et al., 1952), and by extrapolation from such curves, it appears that no response is produced in the average person by impulse stops from angular velocities on the order of 2.5 to 4.5 deg/sec. Substituting in Eq. (3) for ω_{min}, we obtain $x_{min} = \omega_{min}\tau_2 \approx 2.5$ deg/sec τ_2. Now, as indicated earlier, x_{min} can also be produced by a very low magnitude angular acceleration, a_{min}, applied for a long time, and can be calculated from Eq. (1), $x_{min} = a\tau_1\tau_2 (1 - e^{-t/\tau_1})$, which approaches its asymptotic value, $a\tau_1\tau_2$, when t is very long. Therefore, $x_{min} = \omega_{min}\tau_2 = a_{min}\tau_1\tau_2$ and the threshold acceleration is:

$$a_{min} = \frac{\omega_{min}}{\tau_1} = \frac{2.5 \text{ deg/sec}}{\tau_1} \tag{6}$$ [7]

From the slope of sensation cupulograms, a value of $\tau_1 \approx 10$ sec was estimated and the calculated threshold would be 0.25 deg/sec^2. However, these cupulogram estimates of τ_1 may have been low due to adaptation effects which seem to in-

7 Note that an estimate of τ_2 was not necessary in calculating the threshold because it cancels out of Eq. (6), but is it required for calculation of cupula deflection. VAN EGMOND et al. (1949) estimated $\tau_2 \approx 0.1$ sec, which would mean a threshold cupula deflection of about 0.25 degrees. However, other estimate of τ_2 are much shorter (BELANGER and MAYNE, 1965; OUTERBRIDGE, 1969).

fluence the sensation time-course. Recently Dockstader (1971) reported high values for thresholds extrapolated from sensation cupulograms, but his estimates would be considerably lower if calculated according to Eq. (6). It should be noted that the low threshold estimates of Meiry (1965) and Clark and Stewart (1962, 1968a, b) obtained by more conventional psychophysics with ramp accelerations are inconsistent with the latencies in response reported by Meiry to higher magnitude accelerations, in that if the lower threshold estimates are fitted by Eq. (2) then the predicted latencies to the higher magnitude accelerations are too short. This probably indicates the intrusion of methodological factors beyond the scope of the torsion pendulum model, because Doty's results (1969) actually reverse this discrepancy; i.e., if Doty's "threshold" latency with lower magnitude acceleration is fitted by Eq. (2), then the predicted latencies for the higher magnitude accelerations are too long (cf. Ek et al., 1959).

2.1. "Mulder's Constant or Mulder's Law"

Mulder (1908) used brief ($\approx$ .8 sec) angular accelerations and found that velocity changes of about 2 deg/sec or less were not detectable. This is sometimes taken to mean that the threshold cupula deflection, $x_{\min}$, is constant and proportional to the angular velocity change, $\omega_{\min}$, irrespective of the angular accelerations involved. The theoretical constancy of a given value of $at = \omega_{\min}$ in producing a given cupula deflection with different values of a is dependent upon estimates of τ_1 and τ_2 and also upon the range of a values selected. For values of a less than 0.5 deg/sec^2, cupula deflection calculated from Eq. (1) or from the more complex version of Eq. (1) (presented below in a summary of working equations) is not constant.

"Mulder's Law" as described by van Egmond et al. (1949, p. 9) refers to the fact that during short angular displacements with velocity profiles like those of natural movement, observers are able to estimate angular displacement fairly accurately. During such movements, the theoretical cupula displacement curve looks like the stimulus velocity curve. Thus it appears that observers must have accurate velocity information which they can integrate to obtain displacement estimates, and that, within limits, subjective angular velocity, $\dot{\psi}$, must be approximately equal to at. Note, however, that the accelerations involved in natural head movement far exceed threshold magnitudes. This topic will be discussed in a later section.

3. Thresholds Estimated from Sinusoidal Oscillation

The peak angular acceleration, $a_{\max}$, during any sinusoidal oscillation is given by the product of the square of the cyclic frequency, ω_f, times the amplitude of oscillation, Θ, so that $a_{\max} = (\omega_f)^2\ \Theta$, where the cyclic frequency is expressed in radians/sec rather than in cycles/sec, and Θ is expressed in any convenient angular unit such as degrees. Mach (1875) found that he could just barely detect rotation during oscillation with a period of 14 sec and an amplitude of 10 degrees. With this period and amplitude of sinusoidal oscillation, the peak angular acceleration is 2 deg/sec^2, and Mach referred to this as a threshold value. However, because this peak acceleration occurred for only an instant in each cycle of the stimulus, it is apparent that some estimate of the cupula response to this stimulus waveform would be necessary in order to compare this threshold estimate with values obtained by other stimuli methods. GROEN and JONGKEES (1948a) calculated the threshold deflection for frequencies between 0.6 and 1.3 rad/sec, a frequency range which they believed to be near the natural frequency of the cupula-endolymph system. Within this frequency range, responses such as nystagmus slow-phase velocity compensate for stimulus velocity, i.e., they are "on velocity," and the ratio of response velocity output to stimulus velocity input is theoretically maximum and fairly constant. According to the torsion pendulum model (GROEN and JONGKEES, 1948a), the peak cupula deflection under such circumstances is given by:

$$\mathrm{x} \approx [\omega_f\,(\Theta)]\,\tau_2 \tag{7}$$

from which $\mathrm{x}_{\min}$ can be calculated when the stimulus is on the threshold of detection. By substituting this value into the asymptotic expression for Eq. (1), which is $\mathrm{x}_{\min} = a\tau_1\tau_2$, Eq. (8) is obtained.

$$\mathrm{x}_{\min} = [\omega_f\,\Theta]_{\min}\,\tau_2 = a_{\min}\,\tau_1\,\tau_2, \text{ and}$$
$$a_{\min} = \frac{[\omega_f\,\Theta]_{\min}}{\tau_1} \tag{8}$$

Again τ_2 drops out of the threshold calculation but τ_1 remains. With the values of τ_1 used by GROEN and JONGKEES (1948a), these authors estimated that an angular acceleration of 0.5 deg/sec^2 was a representative threshold value for their own data as well as for the data of MACH. With $\tau_1 = 16$ sec, the threshold estimate would change to 0.3 deg/sec^2. In the GROEN and JONGKEES report, the representative threshold estimate for thirty observers is probably based on several methods, including latency measures with ramp velocities, minimum detectable impulse stops, extrapolation of sensation cupulograms, and minimum detectable oscillation as amplitude declined at each of several frequencies. However, the data for two of the observers for three procedures are shown and are the basis of calculated thresholds in Table 2.

Table 2. *Threshold estimates in deg/sec^2 for two observers using different methods*

	Latency	Impulse Stop $\omega_{\min}$	Cupulogram	Oscillation
G	0.19	0.16	—	0.18
J	0.56	0.51	0.41	0.24

The values in Table 2 were calculated from $\tau_1 = 8.3$ sec, used by GROEN and JONGKEES, but if $\tau_1 = 16$ sec were used, each value would be fractionated by the ratio 8.3/16, i.e., about 1/2 the indicated values.

3.1. Some Necessary Theoretical Considerations for Threshold Measurements from Sinusoidal Oscillation

During suprathreshold "steady state" sinusoidal oscillation, the observer senses rotation in one direction in one half of the cycle and rotation in opposite direction in the other half of the cycle. If directional reports were obtained from observers, it would be possible to determine the magnitude of stimulation which yields 75% correct identification of stimulus direction and to use such values for threshold estimates. It appears that GROEN and JONGKEES simply used a yes-no

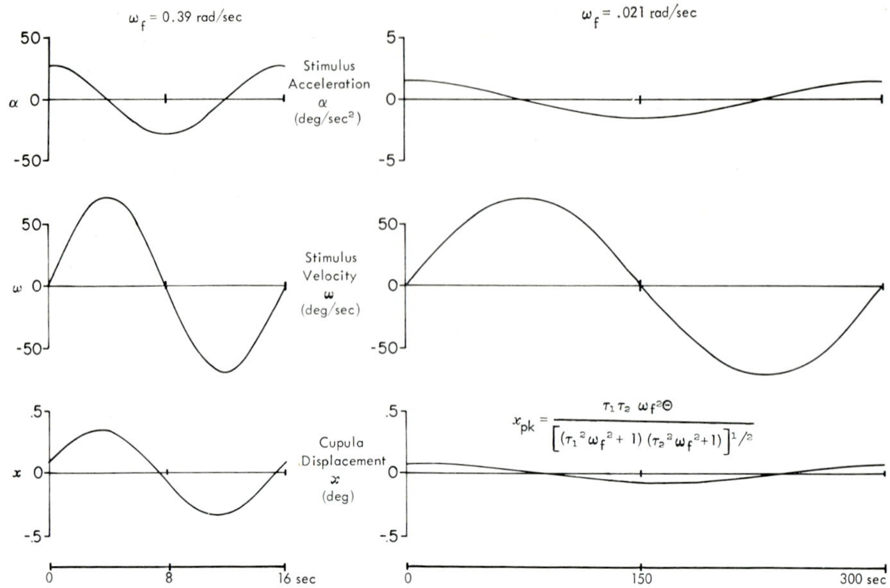

Fig. 8. Cupula displacement (x) during "steady state" sinusoidal variation in angular acceleration. Assumed values of τ_1 and τ_2 were 10 sec and .005 sec respectively. With the low frequency stimulus, the cupula response is almost 'on acceleration' but with the higher frequency stimulus, the response is almost 'on velocity'

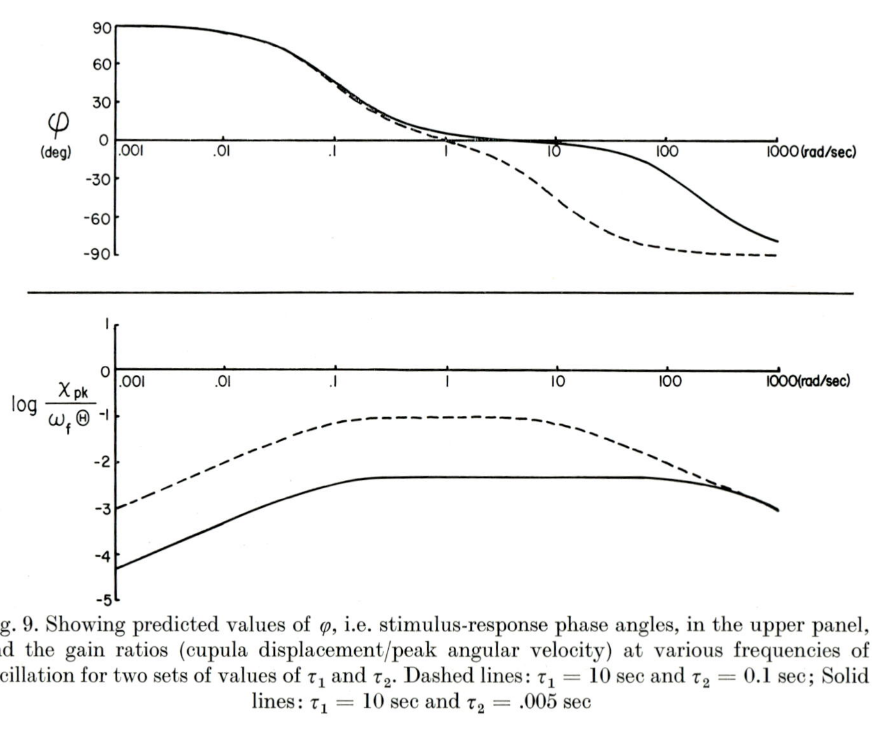

Fig. 9. Showing predicted values of φ, i.e. stimulus-response phase angles, in the upper panel, and the gain ratios (cupula displacement/peak angular velocity) at various frequencies of oscillation for two sets of values of τ_1 and τ_2. Dashed lines: $\tau_1 = 10$ sec and $\tau_2 = 0.1$ sec; Solid lines: $\tau_1 = 10$ sec and $\tau_2 = .005$ sec

criterion and thus their values might be still lower if a 75% accuracy criterion had been used. Only a little of this kind of threshold estimation has been done (DE VRIES, 1949), but nevertheless it is important to consider some of the stimulus-response phase and gain relations with different frequencies of oscillation and their potential role in threshold determination.

Figure 8 illustrates theoretical stimulus-response relations during continuous oscillation at two frequencies, .39 rad/sec and .021 rad/sec. With the higher stimulus frequency, the response curve crosses the zero baseline a little before the stimulus velocity, and it is phase advanced by about 1/24 of a cycle (or 15 degrees) relative to stimulus velocity, but relative to the stimulus acceleration, it has a phase lag of 75 degrees. For this frequency, it is clear that if any interval of forced choice responses were required in threshold determination, the interval should commence several seconds before peak stimulus velocity and end shortly after it. In other words, at this frequency, directional responding during the interval $a_{max} \pm 2$ sec would clearly miss the predicted peak response and would include the response zero crossing and thus both directions of response. Clearly such considerations are of paramount importance to the reasonable application of psychophysical methods. With the lower stimulus frequency, there is a response lead relative to stimulus velocity of 78.2 degrees and *ipso facto* a phase lag relative to stimulus acceleration of only 11.8 degrees. The theoretical response at this frequency is much more nearly "on acceleration."

The phase angle (φ) between the response magnitude and stimulus velocity predicted by the torsion pendulum model is given by:

$$\varphi = \frac{\Pi}{2} - \tan^{-1} \omega_f \tau_1 - \tan^{-1} \omega_f \tau_2 \tag{9}$$

and its theoretical relationship to stimulus frequency is shown in Fig. 9 for several estimates of the τ_1 and τ_2 parameters. The "steady state" frequency which produces zero phase angle is considered to be an estimate of the undamped natural frequency of the system.

With a damped spring system, maximum response is obtained at a stimulus frequency that is equal to the undamped natural frequency of the spring. In Fig. 8, when $\omega_f = .39$ rad/sec, the ratio of the maximum response to the peak velocity is .05, whereas when $\omega_f = .021$ rad/sec, the ratio is .002. A plot of these output-input ratios relative to frequency is called a Bode plot and as can be seen in Fig. 9, the ratio is constant for a range of frequencies that include the natural frequency, but it diminishes at either end. From this it is apparent that according to the torsion pendulum model, stimulus frequency as well as amplitude is an important determiner of response magnitude and must be considered in the threshold determination or in any measure of response magnitude.

VAN EGMOND et al. (1949) and VON BÉKÉSY (1955) estimated the natural frequency of the canal system by recording the zero sensation points, i.e., points of reversal, between the two directions of rotation sensed in each oscillation cycle (also see CRAMER, 1964). By holding peak velocity, $\omega_f \Theta$, constant and gradually increasing frequency within the approximate range of 0.1 to 1.0 rad/sec, VON BÉKÉSY found that phase angle (between zero subjective velocity and zero stimulus velocity) changed between 45 degrees and 0 degrees.

There were large individual differences in the phase-angle curves of different observers, but the results essentially substantiated the observations of VAN EGMOND et al. (1949) and showed a frequency-dependent change in phase angle as expected from Eq. (9) and Fig. 9. It was from such determinations of the approximate natural circular frequency of the canals that appropriate stimulus frequencies could be selected for the investigation of thresholds. In other words, knowing that near the natural frequency, the response gain should be at its asymptotic maximum value, as shown in Fig. 9, GROEN and JONGKEES (1948a) and VON BÉKÉSY (1955) selected stimulus frequencies in an appropriate range for threshold determination.

VON BÉKÉSY determined thresholds by selecting a 10-sec period of oscillation, $\omega_f = .628$ rad/sec, giving the observer control of the direction of change in amplitude of oscillation and automatically recording the instantaneous amplitude setting. Observers increased amplitude at a fixed rate (.15 deg/sec) by pressing a switch until the rotation was just sensed, and then by releasing the switch, decreased amplitude at the same fixed rate until the sensation disappeared, and over a period of 10 to 30 min of these up-down series, they produced continuous records that wobbled about threshold, comparable to records obtained from the VON BÉKÉSY recording audiometer. VON BÉKÉSY found some large individual differences in threshold, large threshold shifts over time in some individuals (especially after rest), improved stability of thresholds after brief vigorous exercise, and some major shifts in threshold depending on the particular sensation reported. In the latter connection, about half of VON BÉKÉSY's observers indicated that they could detect rotation before they could identify its direction and before they could appreciate angular displacement. In a sample record, one "insensitive" observer is shown shifting from average amplitude settings of about 11 degrees to average amplitude settings of about 37 degrees in changing from "rotation detection" to "displacement detection." These amplitudes with the 10-sec period of oscillation correspond to calculated threshold changes from 0.69 deg/sec^2 to 2.4 deg/sec^2 if $\tau_1 = 10$ sec is used in Eq. (8), or from .43 deg/sec^2 to 1.5 deg/sec^2 if $\tau_1 = 16$ sec is used.

Each of these observations on threshold shifts may be interpreted in relation to the well-established intimate neurophysiological interplay between the vestibular system and the reticular activating system. Conscious awareness of the presence of passive motion can set off quick assessment of other sensory inputs which together can produce a directionally appropriate reaction; brief vigorous exercise may regularize the functional interplay between these systems to facilitate consistent reflex action, needed for movement control and not needed in rest, whereas prolonged exposure to oscillation at a natural frequency, which may eventually be sleep-inducing, may first lower the sensitivity for detection of the motion. In any event, thresholds obtained by VON BÉKÉSY seemed to increase during 30-min testing periods from .08 to 0.16 deg/sec^2 (calculated from Eq. (8) with $\tau_1 = 16$ sec) in one "sensitive stable" subject, while in the case of a less sensitive subject, they ranged from about 0.2 deg/sec^2 to 1.2 deg/sec^2.[8]

8 VON BÉKÉSY also estimated difference limens, comparable to the traditional psychophysical approach, by using increasing amplitude sinusoidal oscillation.

4. Thresholds Estimated from the Oculogyral and Somatogyral Reactions

Thresholds determined with OGy have been consistently lower than SGy thresholds in experiments where both effects have been measured under the same conditions with the same observers. It is particularly significant that this finding has been confirmed by extrapolated thresholds from cupulograms (MANN and CANELLA, 1956; VAN DISHOECK et al., 1954) as well as by several procedures involving minimal detectable stimuli (CLARK and STEWART, 1969, 1972b; HALLPIKE and HOOD, 1953a; ROGGEVEEN and NIJHOFF, 1956). The cupulogram findings seem to eliminate the possibility that the greater sensitivity with a target light (OGy) could be solely attributable to stimulus transients which might impart small relative movements between the head and target because the cupulogram is based on the endpoints of sensations following the stimulus by an appreciable time. In other words, the observer has been stopped for some little time when he signals the endpoint. Thus, the presence of the target light in an otherwise dark room sensitizes the observer (CLARK and STEWART, 1969) so that, as compared with the SGy situation, he experiences the angular velocity a little longer following a stimulus and also a little sooner when the cupula is offset from null state by a low-magnitude angular acceleration.

There are many possible explanations for these differences in OGy and SGy thresholds. It has been suggested (HALLPIKE and HOOD, 1953a) that unrecordable minute eye movements may contribute retinal movement information, and even if the visual fixation should ever totally suppress vestibular nystagmus (which would be present without vision), it is possible that this suppression generates information (WHITESIDE et al., 1963, 1965) which contributes to the movement sensation. With onset of above-threshold acceleration, normal observers experience an angular displacement from dead-ahead of the light as well as over-all rotation of light and body together. BYFORD (1963) reported the absence of the target displacement in observers whose retinal movement information was absent due either to an optically stabilized image or to absence of the external rectus muscle, even though the over-all subjective angular velocity of light and body was apparently not changed. This indicates an information contribution from the visual suppression of vestibular nystagmus that could influence threshold judgments with the target light and that would not be available in the SGy situation. Finally, the direction of attention to a visual target rotating together with the body involves different systems from the SGy situation, and it is possible that we are aware of lesser vestibular signals in this operating mode, even when all systematic retinal movement information is absent.

5. The Concept of Threshold

Signaling when a sensation begins or when it ends as the sensory input gradually increases or decays involves a difficult decision. It is comparable to the difficulty involved in deciding when nystagmus begins or ends from continuous eye movement records made over a fairly long interval which includes a brief period of mild angular acceleration. To discriminate the precise beginning or end of the nystagmus response from random eye movements is difficult, although the regular pattern in the middle of the response is readily discernible. The problem with signaling sensations of turning is similar. An observer encapsulated in a rotation device will frequently perceive rotation when none has occurred. This autogyral effect of body and visual reference seems more dependent upon the observer's belief that "real movement can occur" than is the visual autokinesis of a target in a dark room,[9] but in rotation threshold experiments this effect contributes to the difficulty of judgments involving either the onset or end of gradually changing signals.

Thus the individual criterion for signaling is an important determiner of results, and this can be influenced by a number of variables. Certainly the criterion can be influenced by instructions "to wait and be sure" or to "signal as quickly as possible," and if instructions are not explicit, the observer will instruct himself one way or another. There appear to be idiosyncratic differences in judgments of gradually decaying signals as indicated by significant positive correlations of the reported persistence of the motion after effects of moving visual fields (such as a spiral), the perceived persistence of gradually decaying auditory signals, and vestibular aftereffects (REASON and BENSON, 1968; NILSSON and HENRIKSSON, 1967; HENRIKSSON et al., 1968). Moreover, there is evidence that suggests that instructions and demeanor of the experimenter may influence the magnitude of the sensation itself and not just the criterion for reporting it. BENSON et al. (1966) found that "strong" (loud, definite) instructions influence sensation and nystagmus decay curves. Although nystagmus cannot be regarded as a faithful indicator of sensation, the fact that nystagmus as well as sensation cupulograms were influenced by instructions certainly makes it conceivable that sensation, *per se*, and not just signaling criteria, could be influenced by instructions and other subtle factors. There are many observations that clearly show a relationship between arousal and vestibular nystagmus (BENSON and BRAND, 1966; COLLINS, 1964), and between personality and vestibular function (REASON, 1969; ANDERSSON et al., 1972).

For reasons such as these, the usefulness of the traditional threshold concept has been challenged in recent years, and alternative approaches have been extensively explored (CORSO, 1963; LICKLIDER, 1959; SWETS, 1961; PRICE, 1966). One of these, *signal detection theory*, emphasizes 1) the fact that sensory signals occur in a background noise level, internal as well as external, and 2) the fact that the subject's response depends upon his willingness to make a mistake in saying whether or not the signal was present. These points, of course, have been long recognized in "threshold studies" but the signal detection theorists manipulate: 1) the probability that a signal will be presented and inform the subject of this probability, 2) the "risk function" or "payoff matrix" by instructions concerning the relative costs of mistakes and correct responses, and 3) the signal-to-noise ratio. The exact procedures of the signal detection theorist are difficult to use in vestibular studies because of practical difficulties in presenting frequent brief stimuli and of obtaining frequent brief responses, although short wavelength triangular or sinusoidal stimulus waveforms could be used for such purposes because their aftereffects are relatively short.

Vestibular threshold experiments are not available in which 1) the noise level has been manipulated by introducing either extraneous cues to motion or random

9 Healthy observers simply do not experience whole-body rotation when they are in an obviously stationary room except in some sensory deprivation experiments (HEBB, 1949).

vestibular cues, 2) the probability of body motion has been manipulated and known to the subject, and 3) the subject's "risk criterion" has been manipulated. From a practical point of view, the detection of vestibular signals while the observer is performing some other task would also be important (SADOFF et al., 1955), especially since vestibular signals seldom reach conscious awareness in natural body movement. Such studies would certainly supplement the application of available threshold information to vestibular sensations experienced by man during the onset and recovery from pathological conditions as well as to the understanding of performance in various motion conditions such as the aerospace environment.

6. Summary of Threshold Methods and Working Equations

In adapting any set procedure, i.e., traditional psychophysics or methods of signal detection theory, to the study of the semicircular canals, it is necessary to take into account the dynamics of stimulus response relationships. There are some fairly well-established discrepancies from the predictions of the torsion pendulum theory, a number of which appear to be attributable to adaptation effects, although some remain a puzzle. Nevertheless, the torsion pendulum theory remains the best available first approximation of sensory inflow to the central nervous system. Its principal predictions of response waveforms and stimulus-response phase relations with many different stimuli have in general been sufficiently accurate for rational planning of experimental procedures, and at least when discrepant findings occur, they can be recognized as discrepant and not as just another interesting curve in an infinite catalog of empirical findings. Moreover, a viable alternative, which makes specific predictions about phase relations and about per- and poststimulus time-dependent response changes with any of the many possible stimulus waveforms, has never been proposed. For these reasons this section on threshold has included a number of working equations that provide specific estimates of expected sensory inputs with different stimulus waveforms. A summary of the equations introduced in this section follows.

1. Cupula deflection (x) and dependent responses ($\dot{\psi}$) during constant angular acceleration (a):

   a) $x \approx a \tau_1 \tau_2 (1 - e^{-t/\tau_1})$ when $t > 1$ sec and

   b) $\dot{\psi} \approx K a \tau_1 \tau_2 (1 - e^{-t/\tau_1})$ where $\dot{\psi} = Kx$.

   c) $\dot{\psi} \approx K a \tau_1 \tau_2$ when $t \gg \tau_1$, but for any value of t,

   d) $$x = \frac{a \tau_1 \tau_2}{\tau_1 - \tau_2} \left[\tau_1 (1 - e^{-t/\tau_1}) - \tau_2 (1 - e^{-t/\tau_2}) \right]$$

2. Response latency (t_{min}) with given a:

   $$t_{min} = \tau_1 \ln \left(\frac{\tau_1 \tau_2 a}{\tau_1 \tau_2 a - x_{min}} \right)$$

   where x_{min} is "threshold" cupula deflection.

3. Cupula deflection produced by fast stop from constant velocity (ω):

   a) $x \approx \omega \tau_2$

   b) $x_{min} \approx \omega_{min} \tau_2$

   where ω_{min} is the greatest velocity that yields no response to a fast stop.

4. Cupula recovery during period (t_ω) of constant velocity from some initial deflection x_i:

$$\text{a) } x = x_i\,(e^{-t/\tau_1} - e^{-t/\tau_2})$$

$$\text{b) } x \approx x_i\, e^{-t/\tau_1}$$

5. Response duration (t_u) following an initial, x_i, deflection:
This is the equation for sensation cupulograms:

$$t_u = \tau_1 \ln x_i - \tau_1 \ln x_{min}$$

When x_i is produced by stops from ω:

$$t_u = \tau_1 \ln \omega + \tau_1 \ln (\tau_2/x_{min})$$

Where τ_1 is the slope of a $t_u/\ln \omega$ plot and the intersection with the axis of the abscissa provides an estimate of ω_{min}.

6. To estimate threshold acceleration, a_{min}, solve 1c and 3b simultaneously:

$$\omega_{min}\,\tau_2 \approx x_{min} \approx a\tau_1\,\tau_2$$

$$a_{min} = \frac{\omega_{min}}{\tau_1}$$

7. During steady state sinusoidal oscillation of a simple damped spring system, the phase angle φ is zero at the "undamped natural frequency" of the driven system and near this frequency, the output/input ratio is at its asymptotic maximum for a given amplitude (Θ) as shown in Fig. 10. The undamped natural frequency, ω_o, is:

$$\omega_o \approx \left(\frac{1}{\tau_1\,\tau_2}\right)^{1/2}$$

Peak cupula deflection, x_{pk}, at frequencies near ω_o is:

$$x_{pk} \approx \Theta\,\omega_f\,\tau_2$$

where $\omega_f\Theta$ is the peak stimulus velocity and $\omega_f^2\Theta$ is the peak stimulus acceleration.

8. To estimate threshold acceleration, a_{min}, from the minimum detectable oscillation:
   a) Select a frequency, $\omega_f \approx \omega_o$, i.e., where the phase angle is small.
   b) Determine the least detectable amplitude (Θ_{min}) of oscillation.
   c) Solve Eqs. (1c) and (7) simultaneously:

$$\Theta_{min}\,\omega_f\,\tau_2 = x_{min} \approx a_{min}\,\tau_1\,\tau_2$$
$$a_{min} = \Theta_{min}\,\omega_f/\tau_1$$

9. The stimulus response phase angle φ during steady state oscillation is given by:

$$\text{a) } \varphi = \frac{\Pi}{2} - \tan^{-1} \omega_f\,\tau_1 - \tan^{-1} \omega_f\,\tau_2$$

$$\text{b) } \varphi \approx \frac{\Pi}{2} - \tan^{-1} \omega_f\,\tau_1$$

In these equations the constants τ_1 and τ_2 appear repeatedly. They can be estimated from calculations based on physical characteristics of the cupula-endolymph system (MAYNE, 1965; MELVILL JONES and MILSUM, 1965, 1967; MELVILL JONES and SPELLS, 1963) and also from stimulus-response relationships. Estimates of τ_1 have been obtained from slopes of cupulograms (Eq. 5) and from measures of stimulus-response phase angles (Eq. 9). In the experiments reviewed, response measures have involved primarily the temporal characteristics of responses in relation to the stimulus, i.e., the beginning or end or point of reversal of responses in relation to the time-course stimuli. Where response magnitude has been considered, it has been in relation to occurrence-nonoccurrence or percent correct identification with different magnitude stimuli, and when stimulus duration or frequency was such that maximum cupula deflection was theoretically attenuated in relation to the angular acceleration of the stimulus waveform, then τ_1 was used to estimate from the "attenuated" response, thresholds that would have occurred if stimuli had been used that would have maximized the ratio of response magnitude to angular acceleration. τ_1 can also be estimated from characteristics of the time-dependent magnitude change in response during and after various stimulus waveforms, which is taken up in the following section. In most of the equations for estimating threshold, τ_2 became negligible or factored out of the final working equation. However, many of these working equations are theoretically appropriate only within certain time limits, and very short durations of acceleration and very short intervals after accelerations are not within these limits.

Estimates of τ_2 from stimulus-response relationships are not obtained as readily as are estimates of τ_1. τ_2 can be estimated from the upper break frequency in Fig. 9, i.e., the high frequency at which the ratio of response magnitude to the peak stimulus velocity begins decreasing. In practice, responses at these higher frequencies have not behaved as expected (FERNÁNDEZ and GOLDBERG, 1971; BENSON, 1970; HIXSON, 1969).

E. Measurement of the Magnitude of Subjective Angular Velocity

A number of techniques have been devised to measure the magnitude of subjective angular velocity throughout the course of reactions to semicircular canal stimulation and to the extent that the measures are reliable, they offer an opportunity to compare the time-dependent magnitude changes of sensation with other continuous responses, such as nystagmus or neural activity, and also with predicted cupula responses.

1. Magnitude Estimation

The magnitude of subjective angular velocity, i.e., how fast a person feels he is spinning, appears to be a suitable application of a psychophysical procedure which STEVENS (1960) has called "magnitude estimation". This procedure has been used to measure a wide variety of subjective reactions with the typical result (STEVENS, 1966) that the relationship between the subjective measures, $\dot{\psi}$,[10] and the stimulus, S, can be fairly well described by a power function, $\dot{\psi} = kS^N$, which is sometimes referred to as "Stevens' Power Law." The observer's task is to estimate the apparent intensity or magnitude of his subjective impressions relative to a standard set either by himself or by the experimenter. More specifically, he attempts to assign numbers appropriate to the magnitude of the attribute or sensation that is being investigated. Applied to the sensation of rotation,

10 The magnitude of subjective angular velocity and of subjective angular displacement will be designated by $\dot{\psi}$ and ψ, respectively.

if a person felt that he was spinning very fast, he might assign the number 50 to this sensation and later when his sensation of rotation has declined, he might assign the number 25 to the sensation. The magnitude estimates can be called for at specific intervals or at the subject's discretion. Whether or not a standard stimulus is assigned a number by the experimenter "to set the scale" seems to influence the power function obtained (ENGEN and ROSS, 1966; POULTON, 1968).

This procedure has been used recently by several investigators, and data collected by PARSONS (1970), reproduced in Fig. 10, illustrate that the method yields curves during and after angular acceleration that are similar in form to

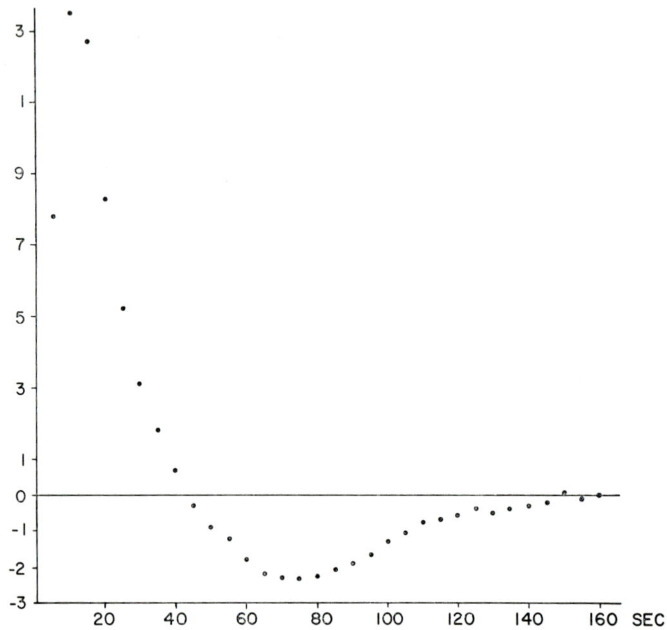

Fig. 10. "Magnitude estimates" of subjective angular velocity during and after a 9 deg/sec² angular acceleration applied for 9 sec (adapted from PARSONS, 1970)

those obtained by other methods and to plots of other canal-dependent reactions such as nystagmus slow-phase velocity. In their general aspects the data conform to the torsion pendulum theory although the secondary reaction, which is well substantiated by all methods, and the continued response increase immediately after angular acceleration, which has been noted with other methods, do not follow the simple torsion pendulum model without some assumptions about other intervening variables.

One problem in the application of power functions to vestibular turning sensation is the definition of the stimulus. It is clear from a number of considerations already presented that the semicircular canal stimulus involves magnitude,

a, and duration, t, of angular acceleration and that some assumptions about the dynamics of the cupula response to angular acceleration must be made if "the stimulus" is to be raised to some power. Both BROWN (1966) and PARSONS (1970) found equivalent magnitude estimates when different values of angular acceleration, a, were used to attain the same final velocity, ω. Approximately equal response magnitudes for equal at products are predicted by the torsion pendulum theory for the conditions used in these experiments. If, within certain limits of t, cupula deflection is approximately proportional to the product at (angular acceleration x time), then because this product is equal to the instantaneous angular velocity (ω), Stevens' power law would give $\psi = k\omega^n$ where ω is the instantaneous angular velocity during some angular acceleration, a, which is sustained within some time limits.

Figure 11a illustrates that the magnitude data tabulated by PARSONS (1970) can be fit very well by a power function, $\psi = 1.13\ \omega^{.58}$. PARSONS used accelerations of 9, 6, 3, and 2 deg/sec² each applied for 1, 3, 6, and 9 sec and each followed by a long period of constant velocity. The "least squares" fit of PARSONS' tabulated data is closer (Fig. 11a) than that provided by the torsion pendulum model (Fig. 11b), but the latter is reasonably close, even without adjustments for threshold at products.

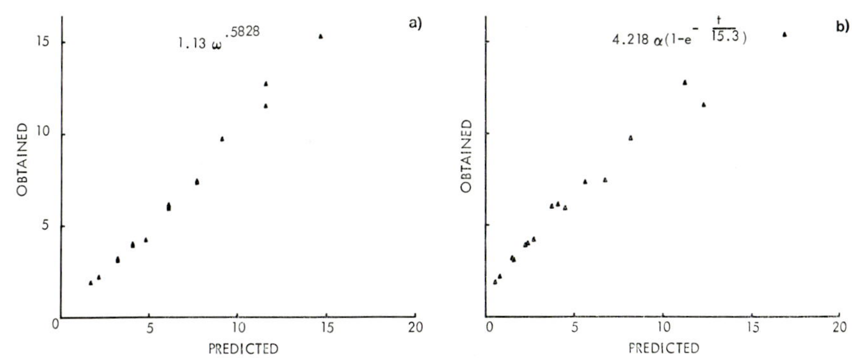

Fig. 11. Showing "least squares" fits to data collected by PARSONS (1970) using a power function (left panel) and the TP model (right panel)

The method of magnitude estimation, because it provides data throughout the course of a reaction, can be used to estimate the long time constant, τ_1, of the torsion pendulum model from 1) the rate of increase of the rise curve, 2) from the rate of decay of the declining curve, and 3) from the duration of aftereffects. From the rate of increase in sensation during the acceleration, a value of $\tau_1 = 15.3$ sec was estimated from PARSONS' data by differentiating Eq. (1) and using slopes calculated between contiguous reports of ψ to substitute into:

$$\ln \frac{\ddot{\psi}}{a} = \ln \frac{K}{\tau_1} - \frac{1}{\tau_1}(t) \tag{10}$$

where $\ddot{\psi}$ is the rate of change of $\dot{\psi}$ and t is the midpoint of the interval during which the slope was calculated.

From PARSONS' average decay curves following 9 deg/sec^2 angular accelerations of 9 sec, 6 sec, 3 sec, and 1 sec duration, τ_1 values calculated from Eq. (4) were, respectively, 9.2 sec, 9.5 sec, 11.3 sec, and 17.8 sec. These values are fairly consistent with τ_1 estimates from other procedures, if adaptation effects are considered. Adaptation effects (YOUNG and OMAN, 1969; MALCOLM and MELVILL JONES, 1970) are presumed to progressively diminish the sensation as a function of the total immediately preceding response of like direction and therefore, the rate of response decay following the longer applied accelerations should be increased, yielding a lesser τ_1 estimate for the longer stimuli. If, however, Eq. (5) is used to calculate τ_1 from the durations of first effects reported by PARSONS for various magnitude stimuli, then the calculated values do not match average values reported by any investigator whose observers were asked only to signal the end of the aftereffects. Thus, it appears that observers who are attempting to indicate the magnitude of vestibular turning sensations will typically indicate different duration after-reactions than will observers who are set to signal the end of a turning sensation. This kind of a difference in reporting criterion may well account for some of the individual variation reported by DOBIE (1969) in a recent study of sensation cupulograms obtained from 1,000 observers whose only task was to signal sensation endpoints.

Contrary to PARSONS' findings, BROWN (1966), CLARK and STEWART (1972a) and ELSNER (1971) all reported magnitude estimation data fit by a power function with an exponent greater than 1. BROWN's z-axis data (when t was less than 20 sec) can be fit by $\dot{\psi} = .06\ (at)^{1.3}$; CLARK and STEWART found $\dot{\psi} = .07\ (at)^{1.44}$ for the x-axis, $\dot{\psi} = 0.08\ (at)^{1.39}$ for the y-axis, and $\dot{\psi} = .06\ (at)^{1.44}$ for the z-axis; ELSNER found for the z-axis $\dot{\psi} = 0.1\ (at)^{1.41}$ for SGy and $\dot{\psi} = .20\ (at)^{1.25}$ for OGy. Significant differences would not be expected on the basis of the torsion pendulum analogy among the x-, y-, and z-rise curves for the 5-sec stimuli used by CLARK and STEWART (1972a), and none was found. Differences in the rates of decay of responses following these stimuli would be expected, but were omitted from this study of the "power law", which cannot predict poststimulus events unless some model, like the torsion pendulum model, is used to estimate, as BENSON (1968a) did, the decay in the "stimulating position" of the cupula. Differences between OGy and SGy have also routinely been reported and ELSNER did find some small but statistically significant differences between these two effects with his magnitude estimation procedure.

It should be clear that power functions where at carries an exponent greater than 1 can only be descriptive of vestibular turning sensations within certain limits of t because it is well known that the *rate of increase* of all semicircular canal reactions, sensation, nystagmus, et cetera, begins diminishing when an angular acceleration is maintained for more than about 15 sec. Actually, BROWN's data are fit by an exponent of 1.3 between $t = 0$ and $t = 15$ sec, but for $t > 15$ sec, the exponent would be less than 1.

The implications of the discrepancy between the "power law" fit to PARSONS' data and to the magnitude estimate data of the others are apparent if we select any value of at and use a constant such that the $\dot{\psi}$ sensation is in deg/sec units. For example, at $at = 2$ deg/sec, $\dot{\psi}$ is 1.8 in the power fit to PARSONS' data; thus the constant is 1.11 deg/sec. Using this constant at $at = 80$ deg/sec, $\dot{\psi}$ is only 16.6 deg/sec, i.e., only about 21% of the actual velocity. The same procedure applied to BROWN's data (1966), wherein $\dot{\psi} = .06\ (at)^{1.3}$, gives a constant of 10 deg/sec when $at = 2$ deg/sec. However, using this constant at $\omega = 80$ deg/sec yields a $\dot{\psi}$ estimate of 205 deg/sec, i.e., about 256% of the actual velocity. This in effect means that the use of STEVENS' magnitude estimation method, and "power law" fits to data so obtained do not constitute a panacea which eliminates apparent inconsistencies among different sets of subjective data.

2. Other Methods of Measuring Subjective Angular Velocity

A number of other methods have been used in attempts to measure subjective angular velocity. These may be roughly dichotomized into a) methods in which subjective velocity was reported directly, or b) methods in which angular displacement, ψ, was signaled and subjective angular velocity, $\dot{\psi}$, derived by calculation from the time required for the estimated displacement.

2.1. "Direct Measures" of Subjective Angular Velocity[11]

Magnitude estimation, as just described, is one of the "direct measures" of $\dot{\psi}$. Various forms of velocity estimation had been used earlier, one of which required the observer to move a pointer on a dial according to the immediately sensed speed so that the pointer was to be advanced as speed increased, held constant when speed remained constant, and returned toward "zero position" as sensed speed declined (GUEDRY and CERAN, 1958). This method, like recent forms of magnitude estimation, yields curves of the same form as those obtained by displacement methods. It permits comparison of relative magnitudes during the time course of a single response and during iterative stimulation, but the method does not permit comparison between observers of response magnitude. "Magnitude estimation" data are analogous to readings obtained from an uncalibrated tachometer or speedometer; the speed can be observed to be increasing or decreasing or constant, but its magnitude is unknown. Thus, between-subject comparisons can be made on rate of change of "subjective magnitude" or in regard to relative peak magnitudes with different stimuli, but there is no basis on which to decide whether or not one subject has a response of greater magnitude than another at a comparable point during the course of a stimulus. This is true aside from any consideration of the difficulty of the subject's task; the "magnitude-estimation" methods simply do not provide this information.

However, there have been attempts to measure the subjective angular velocity by "velocity-matching" procedures. HOOD (in CAWTHORNE et al., 1956; HALLPIKE and HOOD, 1953a) used two techniques in which the observer adjusted the velocity of a light oscillating in direction relative to him until the compensatory velocity direction seemed to cancel the ongoing OGy. The recording of velocity of the light then produced time-dependent response changes of a form similar to curves

11 Not to be confused with STEVENS' distinction between direct-scaling procedures and indirect-scaling procedures typified by the "just-noticeable differences" approach. All of the methods used to estimate subjective velocity are direct-scaling procedures according to STEVENS' definitions.

obtained by other methods, and from these results, estimates of the long time constant, τ_1, were derived that were similar but slightly longer than those found by conventional (time measures) sensation cupulometry. The magnitude of the maximum compensating light velocity was between 20% and 25% of the peak stimulus velocity, and slight individual differences in "gain" as well as the τ_1 constant were noted.

A similar method was employed by GUEDRY et al. (1969, 1971a) in which the observer controlled the angular displacement of the target light so as to keep it fixed at a constant compass heading while he experienced a turning sensation. In this case, the observer controls angular displacement of the light relative to himself (instead of having a "velocity control") in order to match his immediately perceived angular velocity relative to the earth. The form of the curves was also similar to that obtained by other methods, but again the magnitudes recorded were considerably lower than the true angular velocities (or the αt products).

Still another similar method requires the observer to move his hand to compensate for experienced rotation (TRAVIS and DODGE, 1928; VON BÉKÉSY, 1955), and VON BÉKÉSY made the important point that the observer's task differs depending on whether he is attempting to a) keep his hand fixed relative to the unseen but imagined room, or b) move his hand with the speed of the perceived rotation but in the opposite direction. Such subtle differences in the observer's mode of operation appear to be very important (GUEDRY et al., 1971a). These various "velocity-matching" methods have not been used extensively or compared with one another among fairly large groups of observers. Potentially they provide measures of individual differences in response magnitude as well as of time-dependent magnitude changes, but of course, whether or not the output response is reliably representative of the experience is a matter of conjecture because the observer's task is difficult.

2.2. Derivation of Subjective Angular Velocity from Angular Displacement Estimation

The repeated judgment of angular displacement during the course of a stimulus and its aftereffects is a method that has been used rather extensively for studying subjective angular velocity (VON BÉKÉSY, 1955; VAN EGMOND et al., 1949; GROEN and JONGKEES, 1948b; GUEDRY and LAUVER, 1961; BENSON, 1968a, COLLINS, 1964). Typically the observer has been asked to signal each time he has rotated through some prescribed angle, e.g., 45, 90, 180, or 360 degrees. Time between successive signals has been used to calculate mean subjective velocity within intervals. The observer is either encapsulated or in the dark, and therefore he must imagine an external reference point from which to commence his displacement estimate. He may do so by attempting to signal each time he faces a wall in an imagined rectangular room or by attempting to signal each time he has traversed some angle, e.g., the arc from straight ahead to one shoulder; but in either case, the task requires the observer to integrate angular velocity data over time, to maintain a fixed concept of whatever angle is prescribed for estimation, to signal when this angle has been traversed, and then to imagine anew another reference point from which to recommence his angle estimation task. The prolonged maintenance of a fixed external reference and shifting to new points of reference seem to be sources of difficulty. The instruction to "signal every time you rotate through

90 degrees," although apparently simple, demands a fairly difficult set of judgments from the observer. Lengthy instruction and practice are required before many observers gain confidence in the judgments and before the responses produced conform approximately to the theoretical expectations. Such procedures are acceptable for experimental purposes, but they are not practical if subjective data are to be useful in evaluating large numbers of people.

However, the judgment of angular displacement has the advantage that the natural experience of the individual provides a concept of magnitudes of angular displacement. Most observers have well-developed concepts of the navigational consequences of a quarter-turn, a half-turn, or a full-turn. This perceptual information undoubtedly has had survival value in man as well as in lower animals. Thus, if two people signal that they have turned in 1 second through different angles, e.g., a quarter-turn versus a full-turn, then there is reason to believe that the magnitude of the average subjective angular velocity was greater in one person than in the other.

GROEN and JONGKEES (1948b) employed this procedure to plot the sensation decline following "impulse stimuli" and found time constants of decay, τ_1, to be similar (8.3 sec) to those found from temporal measures of sensation endpoints. The ratio of $\dot{\psi}_{max}/\omega_{max}$ was approximately 1.0, although apparently there were instances of ratios as high as 1.5 (GROEN and JONGKEES, 1948b; BENSON, 1968a). The method was considered unsuitable for routine clinical use because of the difficulty of the task for a number of observers.

Using highly practiced observers, GUEDRY and CERAN (1958) obtained similar results with this method in a study of adaptation effects during prolonged accelerations. Because of the long duration stimuli, the decay rate of after-sensations in this experiment is not a reasonable basis for estimating τ_1, but from the sensation rise curves during the first 20 sec of the stimuli, $\tau_1 = 7.4$ sec and $K = 16.0$ sec have been calculated from a least squares fit of the data to Eq. (10) which provides a good fit to the data. Like the findings of GROEN and JONGKEES, the mean subjective velocity, $\dot{\psi}$, was about 1.5 times the true velocity during the first 15 sec of the stimulus. However, this experiment was conducted over the course of four daily sessions. Considering only the fourth session, then the parameter estimates derived from the data are $\tau_1 = 13.4$ sec and $K = 19.8$ sec, and in this case the mean subjective velocity and the actual velocity were in fairly close correspondence (Fig. 12). The τ_1 estimate from the fourth session is comparable to values found by several other authors (GUEDRY et al., 1971b; BENSON and GUEDRY, 1971; MELVILL JONES et al., 1964). A power function $\dot{\psi} = 2.4\ (\alpha t)^{.69}$ also provides a good description of the over-all data when $t < 20$ sec, and for the data from the fourth session ($t < 20$ sec), $\dot{\psi} = 1.18\ (\alpha t)^{.88}$ provides a good fit.

BENSON (1968a) also used displacement estimates to measure the decline in subjective velocity following impulse stimuli in a group of eight observers. Estimates of τ_1 and K based on these data are on the order of 35 sec and 44.4 sec, i.e., considerably different from those estimated in several other experiments with the same method (GROEN and JONGKEES, 1948b). In this experiment the ratio of $\dot{\psi}_{max}/\omega_{max}$ was on the order of 3/1 for the lower magnitude angular impulse stimuli. The power function which described the peak $\dot{\psi}$ after impulse stops of various magnitudes was $\dot{\psi} = K(\omega)^{0.49}$.

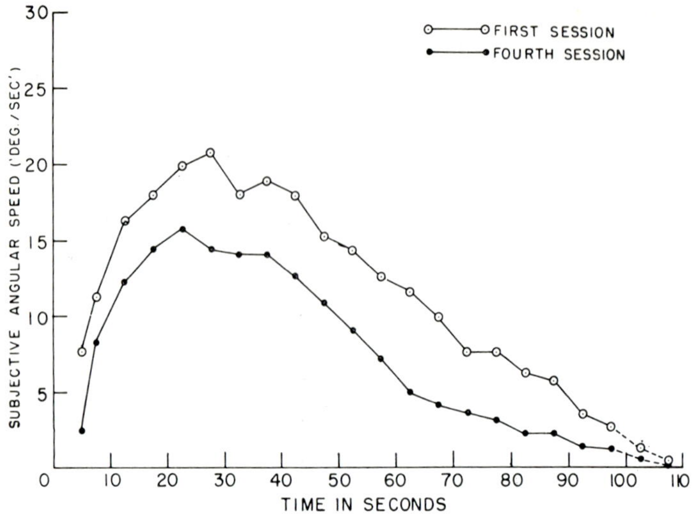

Fig. 12. Subjective angular velocity ($\dot{\psi}$) derived from signals of 90-deg arcs of turn (GUEDRY and CERAN, 1958)

It is likely that the differences between these various experiments are attributable to the differences in the amount of practice and instruction given to the observers (COLLINS, 1964, p. 21; BROWN, 1966, p. 171) as well as to the fact that GROEN and JONGKEES dealt with selected observers and considered the task unsatisfactory for others. The typical problem is that most observers at first find the task very difficult, and, for example, when key-press responses are used to signal when prescribed angles have been traversed, some observers respond with an apparently autogenous rate which they maintain until shortly before they signal stop. If one then obtains verbal descriptions of the experience or a description by one of the several methods of magnitude estimation from these latter observers, the descriptions so obtained usually do not correspond at all with the picture obtained from the calculations based on the repetitive signaling. The problem with this method then lies in the fact that it is difficult to specify the kind and amount of instruction necessary to obtain what appear to be reasonable results, and it is therefore impractical for any routine clinical application.

3. Measurement of Subjective Data during Stimuli Approximating Natural Movements

Some of the inconsistencies in subjective results when different methods and/or different training procedures have been used can probably be considerably reduced by standardizing procedures, but the differences obtained thus far are instructive. It is desirable to compare whether or not similar response durations are obtained when observers are signaling stops and when they are signaling magnitude. These kinds of checks will in time show what man does in different modes of operation.

Part of the inconsistencies in results between methods as well as the discrepancies from theoretical expectations may well be attributable to the unnatural subjective tasks. At least part of this difficulty can be overcome by using stimuli which approximate natural movement, thus permitting observers to operate in an accustomed range of stimulation. Several recent experiments indicate that reliable measures of vestibular sensations can be obtained during such stimuli when a particular method of subjective reporting is used.

Triangular waveforms of brief duration approximate the type of stimulus received by the canals during natural movement. Under these circumstances the form of the theoretical cupula displacement curve is believed to be similar to the form of the stimulus angular velocity curve as shown in Fig. 13a. If the semicircular canals provide angular velocity information like that shown in Fig. 13a,

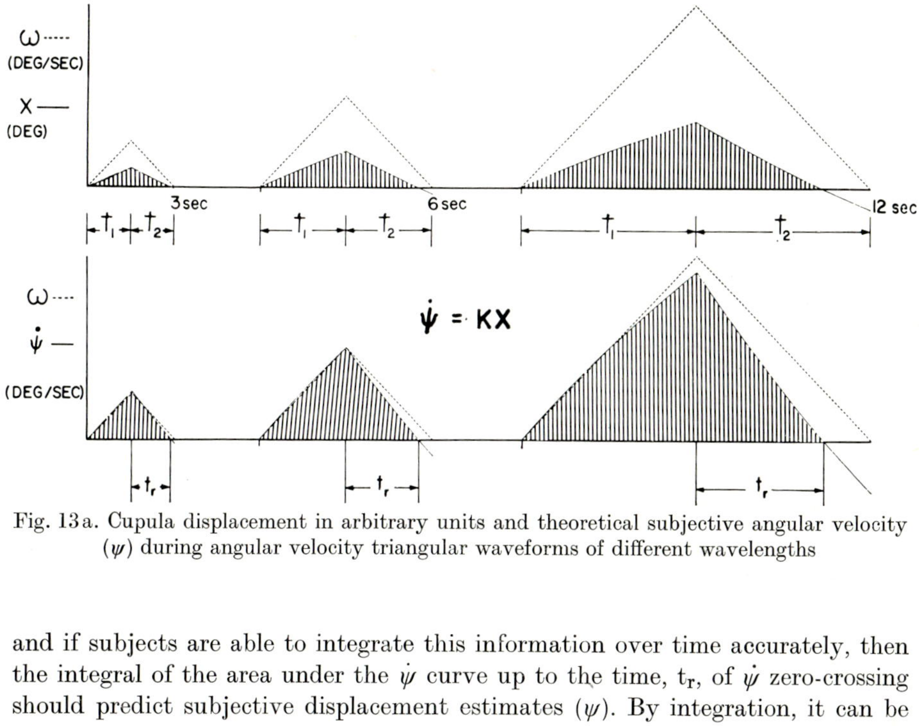

Fig. 13a. Cupula displacement in arbitrary units and theoretical subjective angular velocity ($\dot{\psi}$) during angular velocity triangular waveforms of different wavelengths

and if subjects are able to integrate this information over time accurately, then the integral of the area under the $\dot{\psi}$ curve up to the time, t_r, of $\dot{\psi}$ zero-crossing should predict subjective displacement estimates (ψ). By integration, it can be shown (GUEDRY et al., 1971a) that, according to the torsion pendulum theory,

$$\psi = a \mathrm{K} (t - t_r) \tag{11}$$

when the positive and negative accelerations in triangular velocity waveforms are of equal magnitudes and durations.

The time (t_r) from the beginning of deceleration until the response "zero crossing" is given by:

$$t_r = \tau_1 \ln (2 - e^{-t/\tau_1}). \tag{12}$$

Although we are primarily concerned with the measurement of sensation, the nystagmus response provides a convenient illustration (Fig. 13b) of the particular response characteristics for which the above equations were developed. $\dot{\psi}$, ψ, and t_r each has nystagmus and sensation analogs. The slow phase velocity ($\dot{\psi}_n$) curve

(Fig. 13 b) is probably similar in form to its subjective angular velocity ($\dot{\psi}$) analog, although the latter is difficult to measure as we have just seen. The other two response characteristics, t_r and ψ, seem to offer opportunities for reliable measurement in both the nystagmus and sensation. The reversal of nystagmus during deceleration apparent in Fig. 13b provides a fairly definite measure of t_r. Its

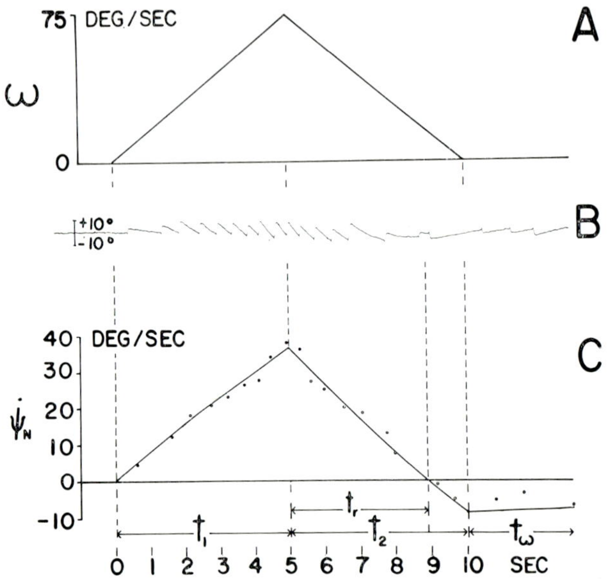

Fig. 13b. Illustrating nystagmus slow-phase velocity ($\dot{\psi}_N$) and t_r in Panel C, the nystagmus tracing in Panel B during a 10-sec triangular wave form of angular velocity (Panel A) (GUEDRY et al., 1971a)

subjective counterpart can be obtained from signaled points of reversal of apparent rotation, and such measures correspond fairly closely to nystagmus measures when stimulus wavelength is short (GUEDRY, 1965a). The subjective t_r is more consistently reported in the OGy than in the SGy situation.

Two methods were used in obtaining subjective displacement measures from a stimulus series of 20 triangular waveform stimuli separated one from another by 30-sec rests (GUEDRY et al., 1971a). Each stimulus waveform comprised angular accelerations and decelerations of equal magnitude and duration. Two accelerations were used, 5 and 15 deg/sec², and each was combined with five stimulus durations to give ten displacements that ranged from 5 to 375 degrees. Each of the ten displacements was given in both the clockwise and counterclockwise direction. Order of presentation of stimuli within series was scrambled, but was the same for each subject.

Method A. A spot of light was projected approximately at eye level onto a white strip that conformed to the inner wall of the cylindrical enclosure. Observers were instructed to turn the light source in a compensatory direction so that the spot would remain at a fixed position in space. In the event that the perceived turn exceeded the excursion limit of the light source (120 degrees), observers were to reposition the light and recommence tracking.

Method B. The observer viewed a circular dial (10 inches in diameter) marked off in 10-degree intervals. The enclosure was dimly illuminated by a small overhead light. The face of the dial was in the earth-horizontal plane and was viewed with a downward-directed gaze and at a reading distance of about 14 inches. Observers were instructed to move a pointer on the dial in a compensatory direction so that the pointer would maintain a fixed compass heading.

Eleven men participated in the experiment. Six were administered the stimulus first using Method A and again using Method B. The order of the methods was reversed for the other five men.

Two results were apparent in the data (Fig. 14). Method A yielded much smaller estimates than Method B, and angular displacements generated by ± 5 deg/sec² stimuli were more underestimated than were displacements generated by the

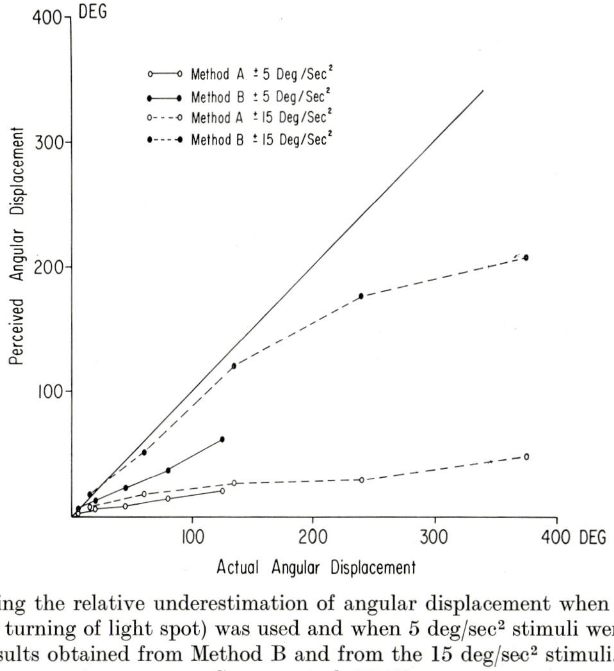

Fig. 14. Showing the relative underestimation of angular displacement when Method A (the compensatory turning of light spot) was used and when 5 deg/sec² stimuli were used as compared with results obtained from Method B and from the 15 deg/sec² stimuli. Adapted from GUEDRY et al. (1969)

± 15 deg/sec² stimuli. According to Eq. (11), more underestimation with the 5 deg/sec² stimuli was expected, but the obtained values were lower than the predicted values if the same constants, τ_1 and K, are used in the equation for both 5 deg/sec² and 15 deg/sec² stimuli.

An important feature of the results is that both methods yielded a progressive underestimation of angular displacement as actual displacement increased. This result might be considered a sign of adaptation, but the way different observers performed their tasks suggested a different interpretation. It was apparent that many observers moved the pointer simultaneously with the changing subjective velocity, but some delayed until the stimulus was completed or was almost completed before making an estimate. The latter case constituted retrospective displacement judgments, whereas the former amounted to velocity-matching judgments at least part of the time. Concurrent velocity matching involves a different process than does retrospective displacement matching, and furthermore, the concurrent psychomotor performance required in velocity matching could interfere with the processing of incoming sensory data.

In a second experiment, this ambiguity in the observers' mode of operation was avoided by instructing them to wait until the initial effect was completed before giving their displacement estimates. In addition, because there is some sensation of reversed motion following the stimulus, they were specifically instructed to make judgments quickly just after the point of reversal and to ignore the sensation of reversed motion. Method A (movement of the light spot) was discarded and Method B (movement of the pointer on the circular dial) was used exclusively in the second experiment.

As before, the stimuli were triangular waveforms of angular velocity with the increase and decrease in speed in any one waveform accomplished by angular acceleration of the same magnitude and duration. Angular accelerations of two magnitudes, 10 and 15 deg/sec^2, were used to produce the velocity changes. Twenty-six men participated in the second experiment.

The results, shown in Fig. 15, illustrate that the mean estimates of angular displacement were nearly accurate. Separate theoretical curves were plotted for the 10 and 15 deg/sec^2 stimuli to illustrate the fact that only slight differences in ψ_s were expected for these two stimulus magnitudes within the range of stimulus wavelengths used. These curves were calculated from Eq. (11) assuming $K = 19.9$ sec and $\tau_1 = 16$ sec. These values of K and τ_1 are comparable to those derived from the practiced observers in the study by GUEDRY and CERAN (1958) and to the τ_1 value derived from PARSONS (1970).

Results from three men are shown in Fig. 16. It is apparent that each of these individuals gave consistent responses, but differed markedly from one another in the relationship of their responses to actual angular displacement. These three individuals are fairly representative of the range of responses of the entire sample. Individual consistency within series is indicated by high correlations between actual and perceived displacement. Mean correlation was 0.95, indicating an orderly increase in displacement estimates as actual displacement was increased for most individuals tested.

To estimate test-retest reliability, slopes of the lines of best fit through the raw data points of each observer were determined for the first series of stimuli and the second. The correlation between slopes from the first and second series was 0.93 for clockwise trials and 0.87 for counterclockwise trials. When the estimates from clockwise and counterclockwise trials were combined, the correlation between slopes obtained from the 26 observers for the two series was 0.94. Thus it is clear that, within one experimental session at least, when an observer yields a given slope in one series, he is apt to yield a similar slope in a second series.

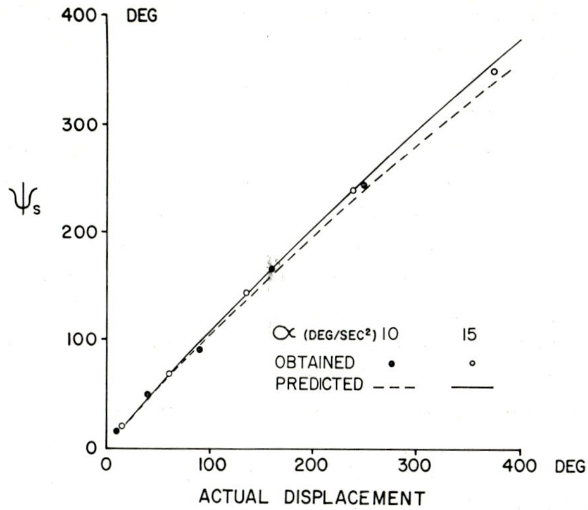

Fig. 15. Mean results obtained when *retrospective displacement estimation* was used with triangular velocity waveforms. The solid and dashed curves were generated by equation 11 with K = 19.9 sec (GUEDRY et al., 1971a)

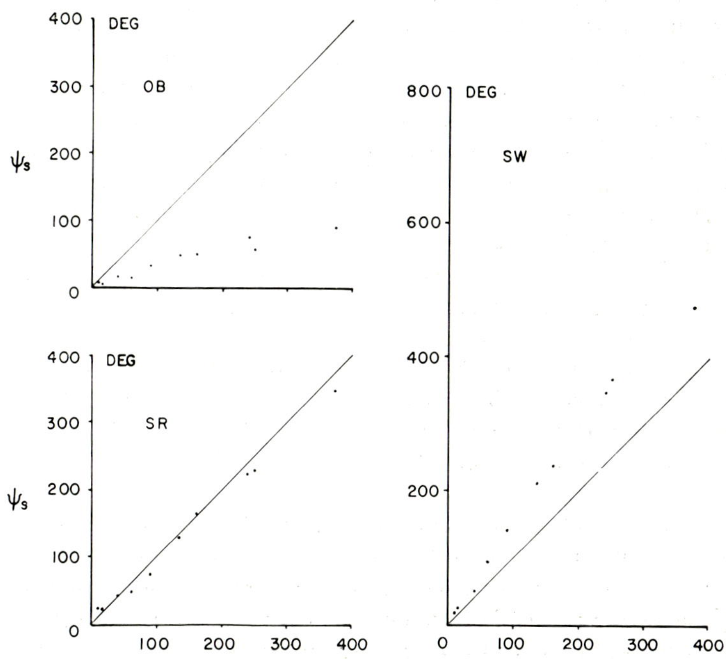

Fig. 16. Differences in results yielded by three individuals using the retrospective displacement estimation task (GUEDRY et al., 1971a)

The close correspondence between actual and mean estimated displacement found in the second experiment (Fig. 15) is to be compared with the results from the first experiment when Method B (movement of the pointer on a dial) was also used (Fig. 14). The two sets of data for the ± 15 deg/sec^2 stimuli diverge as the angular displacement increases. The mean estimates of the 375-degree displacement were 206 degrees and 351 degrees in the first and second experiments, respectively, and this difference is statistically significant ($t = 3.45$; $df = 35$; $p < .01$). It appears likely that the improved accuracy in the second experiment is attributable to the requirement to make retrospective judgments, i.e., to delay judgment until the apparent initial displacement was complete.

Triangular waveforms were selected as test stimuli because they approximate stimuli that are frequently experienced in natural movement, permitting observers to operate within a range of stimulation and judgment for which they are naturally practiced. The accuracy of the ψ measures by the method of retrospective displacements suggests that the mean subjective angular velocity profiles may be fairly accurate matches to the stimulus triangular waveforms of angular velocity.

Moreover, the sequence of experiments illustrates clearly that seemingly slight differences in the method of obtaining subjective data can generate major differences in results. The very low displacement estimates obtained with Method A are comparable to the values obtained by HOOD (CAWTHORNE et al., 1956; HALLPIKE and HOOD, 1953a) when a similar method with moving light was used to measure subjective velocity, and they are comparable to the Aubert-Fleischl paradox (cf. TEUBER, 1960). It is possible that counterrotation of the light spot diminished subjective angular velocity because as it moved in the same direction as nystagmus slow phase velocity, it failed either to suppress vestibular nystagmus (as an observer-fixed target would) or to produce appropriate slippage of the retinal image (GUEDRY et al., 1971a, p. 443). The low estimates of displacement obtained with 5 deg/sec^2 stimuli should be further verified because they were obtained before the retrospective displacement estimation method was adopted. It may not be the low magnitude of the 5 deg/sec^2 accelerations, but rather the longer integration time required for a given displacement which governs the perceived displacement.

4. Comparison of Responses to Stimulation of the Vertical and Horizontal Semicircular Canals

There are differences in the dimensions of the vertical and horizontal semicircular canals that should introduce characteristic differences in cupula response characteristics during and after angular acceleration (MELVILL JONES et al., 1964). Such differences have been noted in nystagmus as well as in subjective responses. During constant angular acceleration about the y-axis, nystagmus slow phase velocity ($\dot{\psi}_n$) asymptotes at a lower slow phase velocity than does $\dot{\psi}_n$ during z-axis stimulation. In the torsion pendulum analogy, this means that both τ_1 and K in Eq. (1) are less for vertical canal stimuli than for horizontal canal stimuli. The lesser τ_1 value for vertical canal responses means that response decay rates following angular acceleration should be greater and that the stimulus-response phase advance during low-frequency "steady state" sinusoidal stimuli should also be greater for responses set off by vertical canal stimulation than for responses set off by horizontal canal stimulation; these expectations have been confirmed

(MELVILL JONES et al., 1964; BENSON and GUEDRY, 1971; COLLINS and GUEDRY, 1967).

The differences in expected response characteristics for the vertical and horizontal semicircular canals afford an opportunity to test the method of retrospective displacement estimation, and this was done with a group of forty observers (GUEDRY et al., 1971b).

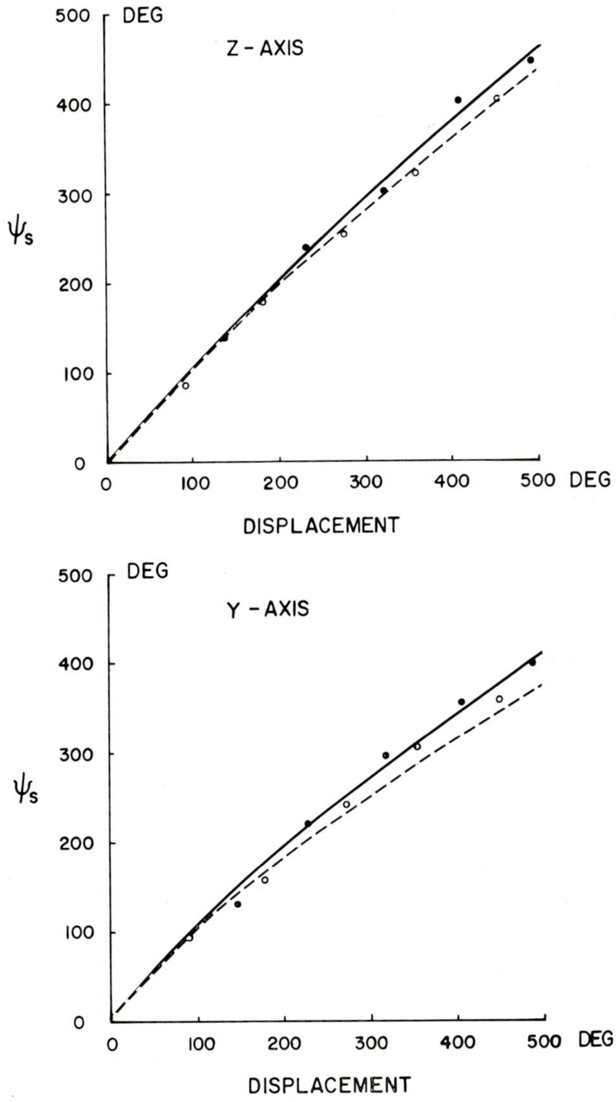

Fig. 17. Mean angular displacement estimates from triangular velocity waveforms about the z-axis compared with y-axis responses. Solid lines and solid circles are, respectively, predicted and obtained results for the ± 15 deg/sec^2 stimuli and dashed lines and open circles are respectively, predicted and obtained results for the ± 10 deg/sec^2 stimuli (GUEDRY et al., 1971b)

Observers were seated upright in one series with the z-axis and the axis of rotation in alignment to stimulate the horizontal canals; in another series they were positioned right-side-down with the y-axis and the rotation axis in alignment to stimulate the vertical canals. Half were tested in the right-side-down position first, and the other half upright first. As before, series of 20 triangular waveform stimuli were presented and two accelerations were used, 10 and 15 deg/sec^2, each combined with five stimulus durations to give ten displacements that ranged from 90 to 495 degrees in both the clockwise and counterclockwise directions. Unlike the previous experiment, judgments of angular displacement (ψ) were reported verbally in degrees, but observers were instructed to make retrospective judgments; i.e., to delay judgment until apparent displacement was completed, and to avoid concurrent velocity estimates.

Mean subjective displacement judgments (ψ) were approximately correct throughout the range of stimuli under all conditions of the experiment, as shown in Fig. 17. As stimulus wavelength was increased, displacement estimates in the y-axis series (vertical canals) became progressively smaller than displacement estimates in the z-axis series (horizontal canals). This difference was statistically significant, indicating that the method was sufficiently sensitive to detect expected differences between the vertical and horizontal canal response systems.

Equation (11) was used to generate the smooth curves in Fig. 17. Values of $K = 19.9$ sec and $\tau_1 = 16$ sec fit the z-axis data, the same values that provided a close fit in the previous study (Fig. 15 above). Values of $K = 10.5$ sec and $\tau_1 = 7.2$ sec were used to fit the y-axis data. The τ_1 values found for the z- and y-axes are consistent with values determined by other methods (BENSON and GUEDRY, 1971; MELVILL JONES et al., 1964), and although previous estimates of K are not available for the y-axis, the ratio of the K values for the y- and z-axes is consistent with an analogous ratio derived from the nystagmus asymptotes in the data of COLLINS and GUEDRY (1967). Thus it appears from several sources that there is a clear difference in the τ_1 parameter for the z- and y-axis responses, but that there is also a compensatory difference in the respective K constants, which works to approximately equate subjective velocity information for z- and y-axes when the stimulus waveforms are short.

Although there were large individual differences, each individual gave internally consistent responses. The internal consistency of individual responses was not quite so good as that obtained with the dial used previously (Fig. 15), but it was certainly superior with relatively little instruction to subjective data obtained by other methods.

Individuals tended to give similar judgments for rotation about both the y- and z-axes; i.e., a subject who gave large estimates for z-axis stimuli also tended to give large estimates for y-axis stimuli. The slopes of responses for the two axes were significantly correlated ($r_{yz} = 0.62$, $n = 40$), a result which may indicate that individuals tend to have "matched sets" of canals, but which may also be indicative of a common gain factor. Nevertheless there were consistent and significant differences between the z- and y-axis data as expected.

Figure 18 illustrates two triangular waveform stimuli and the theoretical subjective velocity during these stimuli. It is apparent that the areas under the subjective velocity curve [given by Eq. (11)] are about equal for the z- and y-axes

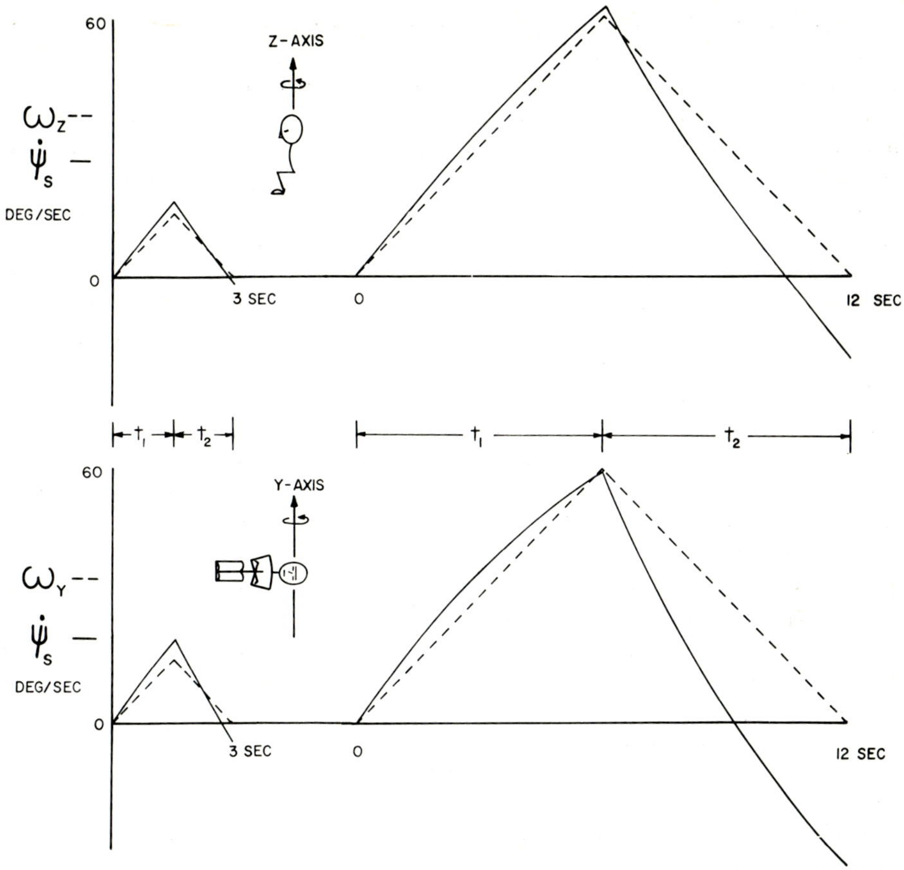

Fig. 18. Illustrating theoretical differences between z-axis and y-axis responses to triangular waveforms of different wavelengths

with the shorter wavelength stimulus, and thus the expected displacement estimates should be about equal, as they were. For the longer wavelength stimulus, the areas are not equal for the z- and y-axis responses and hence different displacement judgments were expected and were also obtained. For the greater wavelength stimulus, the peak stimulus velocity for 10 deg/sec^2 acceleration was 60 deg/sec, and for 15 deg/sec^2 (not shown in Fig. 18) it was 90 deg/sec. As shown in the figure, the magnitude of $\dot{\psi}$ predicted for the y- and z-axes at the end of the initial acceleration is almost identical. This is relevant to the data of Clark and Stewart (1972a) who obtained $\dot{\psi}$ magnitude estimates during x-, y-, and z-axis ramp stimuli generated by various magnitude angular accelerations applied for 5 sec. There were no significant differences in the maximum $\dot{\psi}$ measures for the different axes, but with these stimuli, significant differences would not necessarily be expected according to the torsion pendulum theory. Thus the findings of Clark and Stewart are not in conflict with other experiments where differences were found in the response decay or in the response rise during prolonged stimuli.

With the longer stimulus waveforms in Fig. 18, two other aspects of the responses for the z- and y-axes differ appreciably, one is time of zero-crossing and the other is the amount of overshoot. Signals of zero-crossing, t_r measures, differ significantly from one another for the z- and y-axes, like the difference illustrated in Fig. 18, especially with the OGy situation, and observers spontaneously report that the overshoot (the sensation of reversed rotation) is greater for the y-axis than for the z-axis stimuli (GUEDRY et al., 1971b). These differences in response with triangular waveform stimuli have also been shown with nystagmus measures (GILSON et al., 1973b), and measures of t_r from either sensation reports or nystagmus recordings can be used as means of estimating τ_1[12], although the wavelength of the stimulus is critical because if it is too short, then small errors in measurement imply large changes in τ_1, whereas if the wavelength is too long, then adaptation effects are encountered (GUEDRY et al., 1971a; YOUNG and OMAN, 1969; MALCOLM and MELVILL JONES, 1970).

In summary, except for the data of PARSONS, the rise curves from magnitude estimation are fit fairly well by a power function with an exponent greater than 1, assuming αt to be "the stimulus." The torsion pendulum model cannot give a close fit to the positively accelerated curves, those with exponents appreciably greater than 1, although it can provide a reasonably good fit simply by using a value of τ_1 from other experiments and finding the best fitting K value. A better fit could be obtained by using very long τ_1 values, but this would simply be an exercise in curve fitting, and to do so destroys the generality of the model for different semicircular canal stimuli and different time segments of responses to particular stimuli. When displacement estimation has been used to derive subjective velocity during the course of an angular acceleration, the rise curves can be fit by either a power function or the torsion pendulum model (Fig. 11). The exponent of the power function with these judgments is less than 1, and the values of τ_1 and K found in the rise curves give a reasonable fit by the torsion pendulum model to the decay curves as well. The so-called power law has no generality to other parts of response curves or to other stimulus waveforms unless the torsion pendulum or some other model is accepted and a power function is applied to 'the cupula input' stimulus as defined by the model. Thus without some additional assumptions, the power law cannot predict decay curves or second effects or displacement estimates with various triangular waveforms or peak responses to different frequencies of angular oscillation or temporal characteristics of responses to single or interacting ramp stimuli (CLARK and GRAYBIEL, 1952; GUEDRY, 1957); it simply has nothing to say about such things without some model of "the stimulus."

5. Information Theory and Subjective Angular Velocity

There have been recent attempts (BECHINGER et al., 1969; KONGEHL and KORNHUBER, 1969, 1970) to determine the "channel capacity" for perception of angular acceleration by methods of statistical information theory (GARNER and

---

12 With nystagmus and symmetrical triangular waveform stimuli, the ratio of the peak overshoot velocity to the peak velocity during acceleration also affords a measure of τ_1, but analogous instantaneous measures of sensation magnitude are probably not sufficiently reliable for this purpose.

HAKE, 1951; GARNER, 1962). In general, the procedure involves giving observers several different magnitude stimuli, requiring magnitude estimates of some kind and then determining the frequency of coincidence of particular estimates with particular stimulus magnitudes. From the probability of occurrence of the stimulus, of the response, of joint occurrences, et cetera, the amount of information transmitted can be calculated from stimulus-response matrices (GARNER and HAKE, 1951) and this is expressed in *bits*. One bit of information is the amount of information necessary to distinguish correctly between two equally likely alternatives, whereas two bits of information would indicate correct decisions among four equally likely alternatives. The number of bits of information is the power to which 2 must be raised to give the number of equally likely alternatives that can be correctly categorized. In studies of judgment of pitch and many other subjective continua, it has been found that the "channel capacity" is about 2.5 bits. In other words, within a range of 100 to 8000 cps, no more than about 6 tones can be categorized without error by the "average" listener. This approximate channel capacity was observed in so many scales of subjective ratings that MILLER (1956) refers to the "magical number seven, plus or minus two" in a review of the topic. The method provides a means of comparing information content of various sensory channels.

Fifty observers were investigated with 600 series of stimuli, each consisting of 40–100 randomized stimuli in 4–10 categories of angular acceleration between 0 and 8 deg/sec^2 with stimulus duration always 5 sec (KONGEHL and KORNHUBER, 1970). Apparently, attempts were made to optimize distributions of stimuli by selecting equal intervals along different stimulus response scales as described by best-fitting power, exponential, and linear functions, and also by analyzing information transmission in different parts of the stimulus-response range investigated. The maximum information transmission was found to be 1.7 bits for magnitude estimates of angular acceleration, and 1.5 bits for displacement estimates.[13] This would mean that the typical observer can categorize accurately less than four different magnitudes of angular acceleration and only two or three different angular displacements ($2^{1.5} = 2.83$ categories) on the basis of z-axis semicircular canal information.

This low channel capacity relative to that found with many other sensory modalities is interesting, and it may reflect a feedback system that participates in the control of movement with only meager cerebral cortical representation, or in other words, a system which, by itself, yields little accurate conscious awareness of natural movement. Before conclusions of this kind are considered, however, it would seem highly desirable to estimate channel capacity with several methods of subjective reporting, including retrospective displacement estimation when higher magnitude angular accelerations are used to generate stimulus waveforms that approximate natural movement. Discrete triangular or sinusoidal velocity waveforms (like those in natural movement) comprising higher magnitude angular accelerations theoretically generate more angular displacement information for a given stimulus angular displacement (cf. Eq. 11 and Figs. 14 and 15); the time over which input must be integrated is reduced, and in addition, there is experi-

13 The available descriptions of this work are brief, and the exact task of observers is not clear to the writer.

mental evidence indicating that angular displacements produced by triangular velocity waveforms comprising ± 5 deg/sec^2 angular accelerations were more underestimated than were a comparable range of displacements produced by ± 15 deg/sec^2 accelerations (GUEDRY et al., 1969). Thus, there are several reasons to increase the magnitude of angular accelerations beyond the BECHINGER, KONGEHL, and KORNHUBER experiments, which were limited by available equipment, and to change from ramp stimuli to discrete natural waveforms. The latter change may provide information gain analogous to that attained by "chunking" (cf. MILLER, 1956) in other sensory channels. Further exploration along these lines should permit specification of stimulus magnitudes, waveforms and wavelengths that optimize the information content of semicircular canal inputs. Such information may well have important implications for the natural function of the system and perhaps for its interrelations with other sensory systems involved in the control of movement.

6. Evidence of Adaptation in Prolonged Responses to Angular Acceleration

Prolonged responses to semicircular canal stimulation by angular acceleration deviate from responses expected from the torsion pendulum model in a number of ways. That many of these deviations can be considered manifestations of adaptation is based on the assumption that the sensory input is in fact controlled by a cupula-endolymph system that responds like an overcritically damped torsion spring. However, some of the response deviations are independent of this assumption. For example, when an angular acceleration of constant magnitude is applied for a long time (e.g., 60 sec), the magnitude of subjective velocity, after attaining some maximum, begins to decline (DODGE, 1923; GRAYBIEL et al., 1948; GUEDRY and CERAN, 1958; EK et al., 1960; GUEDRY and LAUVER, 1961; CLARK and STEWART, 1968c). In this case, the decline in response cannot be attributed to a return of the end-organ toward its initial condition because a constant inertial torque is being applied when the decline occurs. According to the torsion pendulum model of the cupula response, the decline could be attributable to a lowered cupula velocity as asymptotic deflection is approached, but an uncomplicated relationship between cupula velocity (relative to the skull) and response magnitude is unlikely in view of the substantial evidence that during steady state sinusoidal oscillation, cupula velocity, according to the same model, approaches maximum as the response magnitude approaches zero. This response decline and other discrepancies from the torsion pendulum model, such as a slight continued increase of the primary reaction[14] after the acceleration ends and the secondary post-acceleratory response, could be indicative of undercritical damping (ROHRER, 1922; CAPPEL, 1966) instead of neurophysiological hysteresis, but this explanation seems question-

14 "Overshoot" phenomena, a continued response increase beyond the end of constant acceleration, have been reported for a number of response measures. These phenomena have not been considered in adaptation models and they may be in part artifacts of measurement. Many subjective measures involve an unavoidable reporting lag since the experience must occur *before* it can be reported. Measures of nystagmus slow phase velocity can also involve artifactually displaced peak velocities, e.g., when averages over intervals of 1–5 sec are obtained, or when changes in slow phase slopes within single beats are ignored. When stimulus records come from the drive motor shaft and not the rotary structure itself, there can be substantial lags between the real stimulus and the recorded "stimulus."

able in view of the frequency response of the system (GROEN et al., 1952; OUTERBRIDGE, 1969, pp. 46–55). The cupula response may be more complex than is usually assumed (TEN KATE, 1969), but the simplest explanation for the response decline during prolonged angular acceleration appears to be some kind of adaptation effect in the central nervous system and perhaps the crista. Since the secondary effects occur more prominently with the longer stimuli that also produce the response decline during acceleration and also shorter primary after-reactions, it would appear that all of these effects may be different manifestations of adaptive mechanisms that alter the relationship between stimulus and response. It is, therefore, reasonable to accept the simple model as a means of estimating the sensory input for short duration response waveforms and to assume that observed deviations from predictions with longer response waveforms are attributable to adaptation.

6.1. Indications of Adaptation during Prolonged Stimulation

As just indicated, results from a number of experiments have indicated that responses at first increase and then decrease during a period of prolonged constant angular acceleration, but a particularly important finding is that sensation peaks earlier and declines more rapidly than does the nystagmus reaction, as is shown in Fig. 19. This time-dependent magnitude change in sensation has been repeatedly

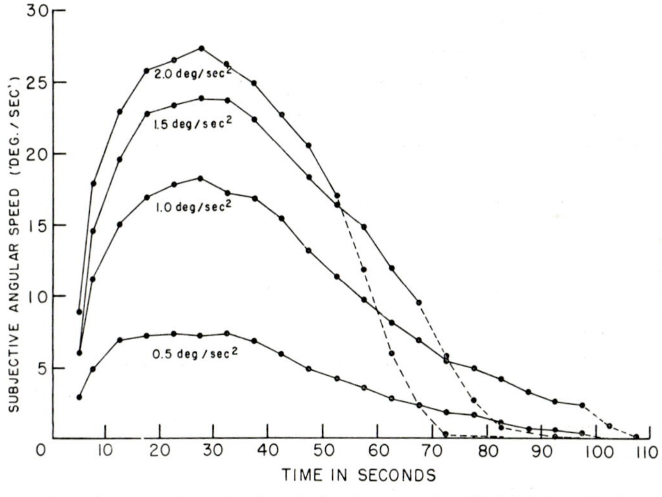

Fig. 19. Mean subjective angular velocity derived from signalled 90-deg displacements during constant angular accelerations sustained until the point where the dashed lines commence (From GUEDRY and LAUVER, 1961)

verified with a variety of procedures (GUEDRY and CERAN, 1958; BROWN, 1966, 1968; CLARK and STEWART, 1968c), and the peak occurs at about 25 sec. The nystagmus decline commences sufficiently late so that in some earlier experiments (GUEDRY and LAUVER, 1961; COLLINS and GUEDRY, 1962), where acceleration was maintained for 40 to 60 sec, it was concluded that the slight declines in nystagmus occasionally noted might be attributable to "loss of arousal." However, nystagmus declines have been noted during long stimuli with sustained high arousal levels (Malcolm and Melvill Jones, 1970; Brown and Wolf, 1969).

The decline in nystagmus also occurs even in the absence of a continuous response. This can be observed in restrained squirrel monkeys that exhibit nystagmus during long sustained angular acceleration only when a variety of extraneous (auditory and cutaneous) alerting stimuli are used. Interpolated alerting signals at selected intervals reveal a few beats of nystagmus, and from these it can be seen that a rise and decline of response is occurring, even though very little preceding nystagmus has occurred (Guedry, 1965a, p. 83). In this way, a secondary nystagmus can also be observed in the absence of any clear primary nystagmus. It appears that the oculomotor response per se is not a necessary condition for these signs of adaptation and also that they occur during sustained arousal. Thus, this form of response modification is probably not dependent upon state of arousal even though its measurable manifestation is dependent upon arousal state.

"Single cell recordings" at various levels show overshoot responses, but others show early declines (Goldberg and Fernández, 1971; Crampton and Gall, 1971; Melvill Jones and Milsum, 1967; Shimazu and Precht, 1965; Lowenstein, 1955, 1956). Ledoux (1958, 1961) reported changes in the mass discharge of ampullary nerve of frog, suggesting adaptation effects. Because the nystagmus and sensation curves in man clearly differ (Guedry and Lauver, 1961), it would not seem likely that both these manifestations of adaptation are attributable to peripheral changes, although it is possible that the "adapting" peripheral elements ascend predominantly to centers that influence sensation as opposed to oculomotor activity (Guedry, 1965a; Goldberg and Fernández, 1971). It also should be noted that signs of adaptation are more pronounced and occur earlier in nystagmus of the alert cat than in the nystagmus of the alert man (Collins and Guedry, 1967; Guedry and Collins, 1968) and therefore these sensation measures, considered indicative of adaptation, may be shaped in higher centers in man than in lower forms.

6.2. Indications of Adaptation during Post-Acceleration Primary Reaction

Nystagmus recorded in darkness persists beyond the end of the sensation, especially with stimuli that produce long reactions (van Egmond et al., 1949; Aschan et al., 1952; Guedry and Lauver, 1961). Following ramp stimuli involving very large angular velocity changes, stops are sometimes signaled when the slow phase velocity of the primary reaction is of the order of 20–40 deg/sec (Guedry et al., 1968). Differences in the slopes of nystagmus and sensation cupulograms are a manifestation of this fact, and such phenomena led Groen to theorize that a central inhibitory mechanism suppresses "in a specific manner all labyrinthine information of too long a duration converging on the central vestibular nuclei. Sensation is more strongly influenced by this inhibitory tendency than nystagmus is, but both show the marks of this curtailing process" (Groen, 1961b, p. 60). There have been suggestions that cupula stiffness (Groen, 1961b) or hair cell generator potential may be under corticofugal influence, but if so, then the clear difference between nystagmus and sensation indicates that there is additional central suppression specific to sensation.

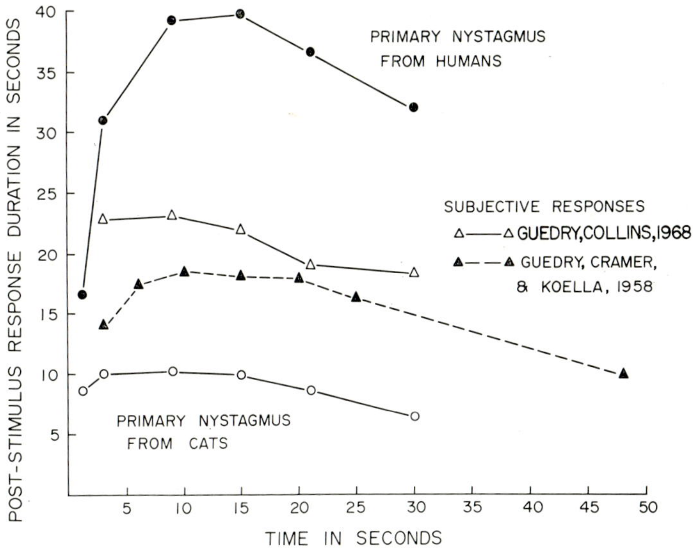

Fig. 20. Duration of after-responses plotted as a function of the duration of the angular acceleration stimulus. Accelerations maintained longer than 15 sec yielded shorter after-responses than 15-sec stimuli. Nystagmus data (open and closed circles) from GUEDRY and COLLINS (1968)

The effect of duration of the over-all reaction on the primary after-reaction is illustrated by experiments in which the same magnitude acceleration was applied for a number of different durations (cf. GUEDRY, 1965b, pp. 72–83). Accelerations maintained for more than 15 sec produced shortened primary after-sensations and as a matter of fact, some observers occasionally signaled cessation of rotation during the longer applied accelerations (GUEDRY et al., 1958; GUEDRY and COLLINS, 1968). Since the longer applied accelerations could not produce lesser cupula deflection than the shorter stimuli (of equal magnitude) unless some corticofugal process changed cupula stiffness, these shortened primary after-sensations must surely signify adaptation. As shown in Fig. 20, the beginning of the decline in sensation duration occurs with shorter stimuli than does the decline in primary nystagmus duration in man, and the sensation duration curve more closely resembles the nystagmus duration curve of cat than of man.

The form of the slow phase velocity decay curves following a stimulus can also be considered indicative of adaptation. An example is provided by data from BROWN and CRAMPTON (1964) who used 9-sec angular accelerations of various magnitudes. Equation (1) derived from the torsion pendulum model provides an excellent fit to the rise curves of BROWN and CRAMPTON during the 9-sec accelerations when $\tau_1 = 15.5$ sec and $K = 8$ sec[15] are used. These K and τ_1 values were obtained from another experiment with stimulus waveforms designed to

15 The best fitting simple power function for these data is $\dot{\psi}_n = at^{1.17}$, but the fit is not as good as that provided by $\dot{\psi}_n = (8\text{ sec})\,(a)\,(1 - e^{-t/15.5})$. BROWN and CRAMPTON (1964) found a more complex equation which yielded an excellent fit to the data.

minimize adaptation effects (GILSON et al., 1973b). In the primary post-acceleration reactions, the torsion pendulum model predicts that a plot of the natural logarithms of the nystagmus slow phase velocity against time after the acceleration will be a straight line. As shown in Fig. 21, the values of $\tau_1 = 15.5$ sec and K = 8 sec also provide excellent fits to primary after-reactions for about 20 sec, and thereafter the responses appear suppressed relative to the theoretical curves. Such departures of responses from the expected decay rates have sometimes been taken as signs of adaptation (GROEN, 1956–1957, 1957; MALCOLM and MELVILL JONES, 1970).

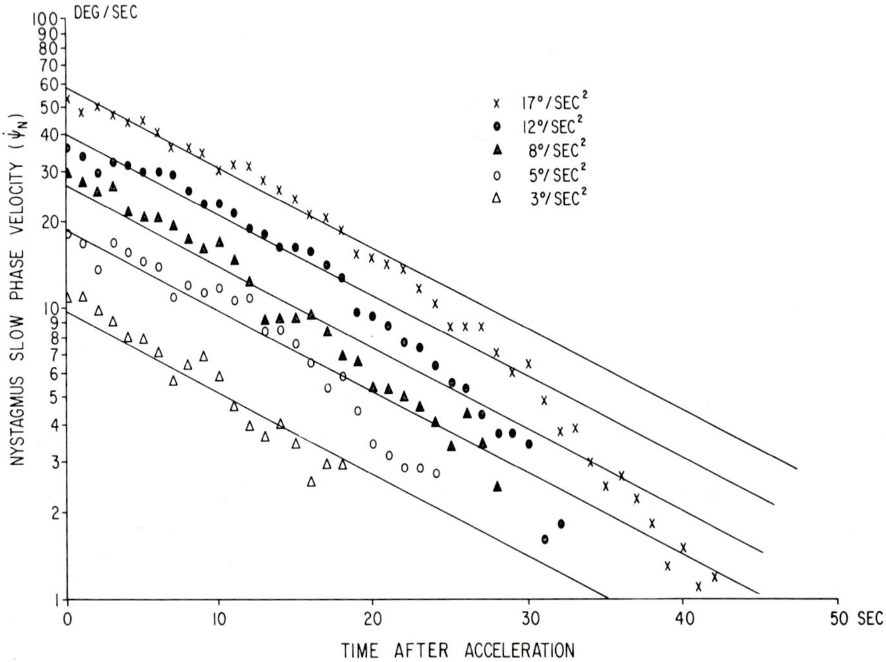

Fig. 21. Decay in nystagmus slow-phase velocity in man following 9-sec angular accelerations of various magnitudes. The decay rate is constant for about 20 sec and thereafter the decay rate increases. Adapted from BROWN and CRAMPTON (1964)

6.3. Secondary Reactions as a Sign of Adaptation

During constant angular velocity and after the primary reaction subsides, a secondary reaction of reversed sign occurs in sensation, nystagmus (BÁRÁNY, 1907; BUYS, 1924; ASCHAN and BERGSTEDT, 1965), and neural activity (GROEN et al., 1952; LEDOUX, 1961; GOLDBERG and FERNÁNDEZ, 1971). The ratio of the peak secondary to peak primary nystagmus reaction is higher in the cat than in man (COLLINS and GUEDRY, 1967; GUEDRY and COLLINS, 1968), but in either case, its magnitude appears directly related to the total amount of immediately preceding unidirectional stimulation.

A direct relationship between magnitude and duration of the primary stimulus and magnitude of secondary sensations has also been found with the use of magnitude estimation methods (CLARK and STEWART, 1968c; PARSONS, 1970) and by studies of the effects of an initial stimulus on immediately following stimuli. HALLPIKE and HOOD (1953b) studied subjective effects during the secondary reaction by applying a "standard" test stimulus 40 sec after a prolonged angular acceleration. They reported a diminution in the after-sensation of turning produced by the standard test stimulus when the latter and the preceding stimulus were of the same direction. If the directions of the two stimuli were opposite, the reaction to the test stimulus was reported to be unchanged. A similar procedure was employed by GUEDRY et al. (1958) who varied both the duration of the "conditioning" stimuli and the interval of delay before the standard stimuli were presented. The results of HALLPIKE and HOOD (1953b) were confirmed, but in addition, it was found that when the "conditioning" stimuli were of 40 or 50 seconds' duration, then primary reactions to contradirectional test stimuli were slightly increased in duration, but the increase was not nearly so great nor so persistent as the decrease which occurred with ipsidirectional stimuli.

In an effort to clarify the relation between secondary nystagmus and the subjective reaction, an experiment was carried out in which triangular velocity waveforms (8-sec period) were presented at one-minute intervals starting one minute after a constant angular acceleration of 15 deg/sec^2 maintained for 16 seconds (GUEDRY et al., 1968). When the first triangular waveform was presented (60 sec after the end of the conditioning stimulus), most observers were experiencing a secondary sensation and also had secondary nystagmus. For the series (Series A) in which the primary reaction to the triangular waveform was in the same direction as the ongoing secondary reaction, observers experienced an increase in the "secondary sensation," then a decrease to a stop (which they signaled) and then brief rotation in opposite direction; this was followed by resumption of the secondary sensation. The stop was signaled near or very shortly after nystagmus velocity passed through the bias level of the secondary nystagmus, and the brief apparent rotation in opposite direction occurred while nystagmus was of the same direction but of less magnitude than the level of the normal secondary reaction. A comparable result was obtained in Series B when the triangular waveforms reversed the direction of the ongoing secondary reaction (Fig. 22). In this case, shortly after the beginning of the first triangular waveforms, observers experienced a cessation of the secondary reaction[16], then a rise and decline of apparent rotation in opposite direction, then a stop (which they signaled), and then a resumption of the secondary reaction. Again the average time of subjective zero corresponded very closely with the time at which mean nystagmus slow phase velocity passed through the "bias level" of the secondary reaction. It appears from the nystagmus curves that at least 240 sec were required before the secondary response approached zero bias. There was a slight increase in average response time from the peak of triangular stimulus waveform when stimuli were contradirectional (i.e., when the ongoing secondary reaction and the primary reaction to the triangular stimulus were ipsidirectional) and there was a slight

16 This first subjective stop was not recorded because some observers found it difficult to signal twice in a relatively short interval.

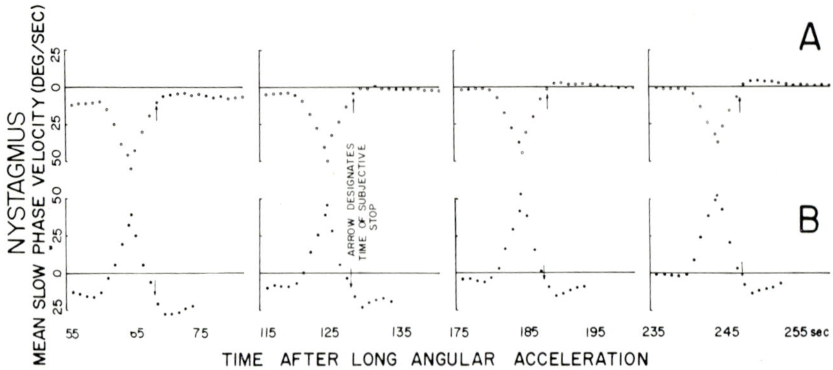

Fig. 22. Showing average subjective stops (arrows) signalled by subjects when triangular velocity stimulus waveforms were administered at various intervals after a prolonged constant angular acceleration. The subjective stop occurs very near the point where the nystagmus slow-phase velocity (closed and open dots) reaches the apparent level of the secondary nystagmus reaction (Previously unpublished data from GUEDRY et al., 1968)

decrease in the average t_r response when they were contradirectional. The changes in response durations were small as compared with those found previously (HALLPIKE and HOOD, 1953b; GUEDRY et al., 1958) because the cupula would pass through the shifted zero reference at a fairly high rate as compared with the slow return expected with ramp stimuli. It was expected that the smaller difference would be compensated by easier judgments, but unfortunately the judgments during secondary reactions proved to be difficult for the relatively unpracticed observers, and some failed to render judgments. Nevertheless, the median subjective zero points of 11 observers in Series B (and the mean of 14 observers tested only under Series A conditions) indicate that the subjective zero reference level operates around the nystagmus secondary level. This is comparable to individuals with spontaneous nystagmus whose sensation seems normal during rotation testing, and it may well be that the functional adjustment toward subjective normalcy during a secondary reaction is a sign of the readiness of the central nervous system to accommodate for a new level of sensory inflow.

6.4. A Proposed Adaptation Model

Several authors have independently proposed equivalent models to account for the various "adaptation effects" during and after prolonged semicircular canal responses (YOUNG and OMAN, 1969; MALCOLM and MELVILL JONES, 1970). They have accepted the basic model of the canals as an overcritically damped spring system and have assumed that response output at any moment depends upon the difference between cupula-controlled neural inflow and a shifting reference level. The rate of change of the reference level is assumed to have a direction so as to minimize the difference between sensory input and the reference level and a magnitude proportional to the magnitude of the difference. This idea can be expressed mathematically when the simple torsion pendulum model is used to predict neural input from cupula displacement. Similar ideas have been presented in the past by a number of authors (GROEN, 1961a; GUEDRY and COLLINS, 1968), but the mathematical expression offers the advantage of explicitly indicating that measurement of only one new parameter, an adaptation time constant, τ_a, can be used along with the basic torsion pendulum model to predict the general form of the various nystagmus adaptation effects described above, as well as other as yet unobserved response changes during various sequences of stimuli. By assuming that there is a shorter adaptation time constant for sensation than for nystagmus, the general form of most of the subjective signs of adaptation, as well as the differences between subjective and nystagmus manifestations, can also be predicted. Thus, once a few basic parameters have been determined, this relatively simple mathematical statement is descriptive of a wide range of observations, and of course its prediction of responses to all angular acceleration stimuli, irrespective of waveform or frequency, can be tested.

To test this model, an experiment was conducted by using triangular velocity waveforms of various wavelength as stimuli and measuring the time, t_r, during deceleration when the subjective and nystagmus responses reached zero and then reversed (STOCKWELL et al., 1973). The basic predictive equation for t_r, wherein $t_r = \tau_1 \ln (2 - e^{-t/\tau_1})$ becomes more complex, when the adaptation model is included:

$$t_r = (\tau_a^{-1} - \tau_1^{-1})^{-1} [\ln (2 - e^{-t/\tau_a}) - \ln (2 - e^{-t/\tau_1})] \tag{13}$$

As shown in Fig. 23, both nystagmus and subjective t_r are predicted fairly well by the complex model when $\tau_1 = 16$ sec and $\tau_a = 50$ sec for sensation and $\tau_a = 150$ sec for nystagmus.

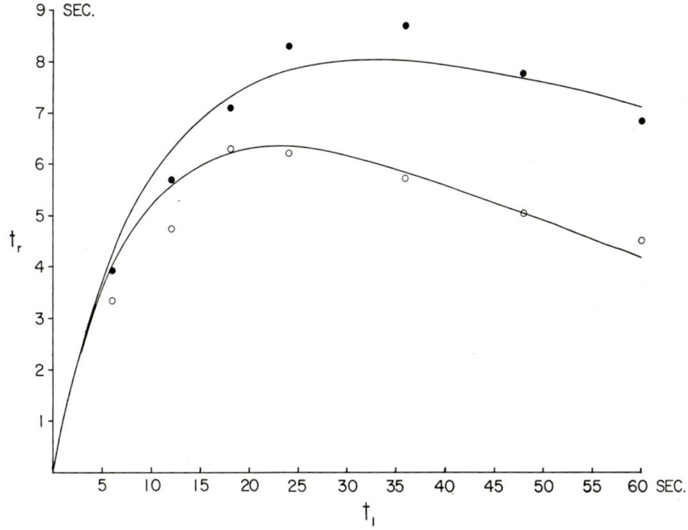

Fig. 23. The time (t_r) from peak velocity until the response reaches zero during triangular velocity waveforms of different wavelengths. Subjective and nystagmus responses are represented respectively by open and closed circles. The decline in t_r when t_1 was longer than 20 sec is an apparent sign of adaptation

It was expected that t_r for sensation and nystagmus would be fairly easily measured for the longer waveforms because during the deceleration of the long wavelength stimuli, the cupula is being driven through the "theoretically shifted" reference level at a fairly high rate. This could be expected to produce more rapid reversals of nystagmus and "sharper" endpoints than when the transition through the reference level is more gradual. However, such was not the case for either the nystagmus or the subjective transitions. The longer waveforms seemed to produce longer transition zones and more difficult judgments of both nystagmus and subjective endpoints.

The proposed model describes fairly well the decline in sensation and the lesser decline in nystagmus during prolonged constant angular acceleration; the more rapid decay of sensation than nystagmus after acceleration (which includes the differences in sensation and nystagmus cupulograms), as well as the sensation endpoints following various duration accelerations; the second effects of both sensation and nystagmus, and the change in estimates of the long time constant, τ_1, by "sinusoidal cupulometry" with various frequencies of oscillation and various peak accelerations at a given frequency (NIVEN and HIXSON, 1961; HIXSON and NIVEN, 1962). However, the model does not appear to predict subjective endpoints following standard test stimuli (velocity ramps) which in turn follow unidirectional stimuli unless some permanent dead zone is assumed; it does not predict the findings with contradirectional test stimuli (ramps), nor does it completely account for the data with discrete velocity triangles of varying wavelengths. It remains, however, the best available unifying concept for describing this range of observations.

7. Arousal Effects and Changes in Relationships between Nystagmus and Subjective Angular Velocity

The previous section described changes in both nystagmus and sensation in a direction to reduce any prolonged primary reaction. The adaptive suppression and recovery rate is different for nystagmus and sensation reactions, and these differences produce changes in relationships between nystagmus and subjective reactions. The effects seem to build up in spite of differences in arousal states during the primary reactions so that the process is at least partially independent of arousal state and also partially independent of the occurrence of the oculomotor reaction itself.

However, changes in arousal can alter the nystagmus reaction almost as though a switch had been thrown in the nervous system to activate or deactivate a circuit. Therefore, arousal effects can substantially alter the relationship between vestibular nystagmus recorded in darkness and concurrent subjective angular velocity. After a few repetitions of ramp stimuli (COLLINS, 1964; GUEDRY, 1965a) or a mild caloric stimulus (COLLINS, 1965) or during sinusoidal stimuli (WENDT, 1951), nystagmus typically diminishes as the observer becomes more relaxed and less aroused by the situation. Both the slow and fast phases of nystagmus are changed. Slow phase velocity may diminish and become less regular while the transition from slow and fast phases is more gradual. Both may diminish and even disappear during formerly adequate stimuli. During prolonged sinusoidal oscillation, the fast phase may disappear while the slow phase remains, yielding a sinusoidal eye movement without nystagmoid appearance (Kennedy, 1972; cf. Groen, 1970).

When observers are instructed to attend to and report sensations of rotation, the act of reporting the vestibular sensations may be sufficiently arousing at first to sustain nystagmus, but after a few trials the nystagmus may diminish and almost disappear even though the observers continue to make systematic and apparently meaningful subjective reports. If the subjective task, such as continuous angular displacement estimation, is fairly difficult, then the nystagmus may be sustained for more trials, but even with this task and while subjective reporting remains systematic, the nystagmus diminishes. When it has thus diminished, a change of mental tasks will reinstate the nystagmus to its initial form and intensity (Collins, 1964) but with familiarization, the effectiveness of new tasks diminishes.

One of the more effective mental tasks in sustaining vestibular nystagmus is arithmetic computation. This seems paradoxical in that mental arithmetic which distracts the attention from the vestibular sensation actually increases vestibular nystagmus. By contrast, with other sensory systems, distraction by extra-system arousal sources tends to suppress the response of the particular system. For example, Hernández-Péon and Donoso (1957, 1959) have reported that photic-evoked potentials recorded from electrodes from visual radiations were markedly smaller during arithmetic calculations and recovered when solutions were reached. It is curious, then, that vestibular nystagmus which is diminished after a few stimulus repetitions (when the observer is no longer aroused by the stimulus) can be reinstated by mental arithmetic. This apparent paradox may well be due to the fact that in natural movement, the vestibular system typically functions as a silent partner in contributing adequate reflex actions when the person's attention is focused on something else. For example, in the act of pursuing game, vestibular reflex contributions to coordinated skilled movement must be at their peak while attention to vestibular sensations is minimal. Whereas other systems inform of things in the environment, the vestibular system automatically provides dynamic orientation feedback information which sets off postural and oculomotor reflexes while the attention is focused on something else such as visual and auditory information. In this context, it is not surprising that mental arithmetic enhances vestibular nystagmus, though it distracts attention from vestibular sensations.

III. Response to Linear Acceleration Considered in Relation to Otolith Function

Perceptual events which have been studied in relation to otolith function may be divided into two general classes. The first involves static as opposed to dynamic stimuli; the linear acceleration stimulus is fixed in magnitude and direction relative to the head of the observer. The simplest example of this form of stimulus is a stationary, tilted observer; the gravity vector is constant in magnitude and in its direction relative to the observer's head. The response is measured after the position has been attained, and it is usually assumed that there are no residual influences on the response from the acceleratory stimuli which were used to achieve the orientation of the stimulus vector relative to the head. The second involves dynamic stimuli which change in magnitude and/or direction relative to the head.

The responses typically studied with static stimuli are perception of verticality (or perception of tilt) and ocular counterrolling (cf. Section 9.2). The responses typically studied in connection with dynamic otolith stimuli are subjective linear velocity, signals of reversal in apparent motion, signals of selected positions relative to gravity, perception of tilt, and "otolith nystagmus", which has been called "dynamic counterrolling" when induced by rotation about the x-axis.

A. Mechanics of the Otolith System

Toward the end of the nineteenth century, Breuer (in Mach, 1902, p. 156) formulated ideas of otolith mechanics which are conceptually similar to current ideas: "For every position of the head there is only one definite combination of four magnitudes of gravitation of the otoliths in the four maculae. When, as we suppose, the gravitation of the otoliths is felt, then every position of the head is characterized by a definite combination of these sensations." Breuer was referring to that component of gravity which would produce a "sliding movement" in each of the utricular and saccular maculae. Today, the component of gravity which would produce a sliding movement of the otolith membrane is called the "shear component" in contrast to compression or traction components.

1. Shear-Directed Force as a Stimulus to the Otoliths

Since Breuer's time, some writers have favored *compression* and others have favored *traction* (Magnus, 1924; Quix, 1923, 1925; Mygind, 1948) as the "stimulating" component of the force field, but most authors seem to agree today that the *shear* component is the most effective component of the stimulus (von Holst, 1950a, b; Meiry, 1965; Schöne, 1964; von Békésy, 1966).

Ulrich (1934–1935) and others (Trincker, 1959; see reviews by Trincker, 1962; McNally, 1955; McNally and Stuart, 1942) found that reflex eye movement could be reliably produced when the utricular membrane was probed with calibrated filaments directed to produce shearing movements, but compression, local force applied perpendicularly to the otolith surface, had no effect. Ulrich reported lateral shear produced reliable eye displacement responses, whereas medial shear did not. Trincker obtained similar results using pressure, traction, and shearing forces and recording bioelectric changes in the macula as a sign of end-organ stimulation. Trincker found changes in potential for either medial or lateral shear. These findings are sometimes cited as evidence that shear is the important component of the stimulus, but they also raise several issues that require clarification. Trincker applied perpendicular pressures sufficient to destroy sensory cells and yet did not obtain responses. This amount of pressure certainly must have deflected underlying cilia, and deflection of cilia is believed to be the necessary and sufficient condition for triggering underlying hair cells. Moreover, local pressure of this magnitude would produce shearing forces in the surrounding area (cf. von Békésy, 1966). Why were responses not recorded when cilia must have been deflected? Apparently *topically* applied pressure did not fire cells in a sufficient number or in an adequate pattern to produce responses detectable by the recording methods and conditions used by either TRINCKER or ULRICH, but in the case of TRINCKER, some cell activity must have been triggered. Nevertheless, the results indicate that the otolith membrane slides easily and that shear is an efficient stimulus. It seems possible that mechanical probing directed to produce shear may produce a sliding movement of the otolith membrane, thereby producing a good approximation of a physiological stimulus, whereas a local compression or traction force normal to the surface would not accomplish this.

The otolith surfaces are curved. The curvature is sufficiently great that a force field which is directed to produce "compression" in one part of the macula will produce a significant shear component in another part of the same macula. This is especially true considering the utricular maculae of the two ears, since the "average" planes of these two maculae are not in the same plane, and both are curved surfaces. It may be sufficient to assume that a simple average plane represents a single curved surface, but how adequate this is for dynamic stimuli remains to be seen. For example, following horizontal linear acceleration with head upright, the restoration of a planar otolith membrane would depend solely upon elastic properties of the end-organ, whereas restoration of a concave surface would depend not only upon elasticity, but upon components of the gravity vector as well.

Based upon the information available on the topographical arrangement of the hair cells in the utricle (ENGSTRÖM and WERSÄLL, 1958; SPOENDLIN, 1966; LINDEMAN, 1969; FLUUR and MELLSTRÖM, 1970a, b) it appears that a single macula is capable of yielding distinctive patterns which would signal orientation of the head relative to gravity, at least within limited angular displacements. However, it is also possible that the perceived orientation is based upon central nervous system integration of a pattern of sensory signals from both utricles and as BREUER assumed, it may depend upon the two utricular and the two saccular organs. For these various reasons, it is possible that attempts to understand perceptual events on the basis of the estimated mechanical response of a single idealized utricular plane may be an unwarranted oversimplification.

2. Dynamics of the Otoliths

The otolith end-organs have the apparent structural characteristics of density-difference accelerometers. Attempts to examine more or less directly the mechanical response of the otoliths have included direct manipulation of the otoliths (STEINHAUSEN, 1934–1935; ULRICH, 1934–1935; SZENTÁGOTHAI, 1952), x-ray photographs of otoliths displacement in fish (DE VRIES, 1950; VILSTRUP and VILSTRUP, 1952), recordings of bioelectric potentials in the sensory macula during direct manipulation (TRINCKER, 1962), and recordings of neural activity (MELVILL JONES, 1967; SCHOEN, 1957; LOWENSTEIN and ROBERTS, 1949; DUENSING and SCHAEFER, 1959; ADRIAN, 1943; LEDOUX, 1949).

Based upon x-ray photographs of sharks, VILSTRUP and VILSTRUP (1952) estimated maximal tangential displacements of the utricular otolith membrane of approximately 15 μ to either side of "normal position" during static tilts up to 90 degrees relative to gravity. Assuming a depth from otolith surface to hair cell surface of approximately 70 μ to 120 μ[17], the angular displacement imparted to

17 Estimated by VILSTRUP and VILSTRUP.

cilia, if they were initially perpendicular to the hair cell surface, would be between 7 degrees and 12 degrees. Using forces up to 11 g-units and x-ray techniques, De Vries measured tangential displacements in the saccular otoliths of fish as great as 0.25 mm. A displacement of this magnitude far exceeds the estimated distance between hair cells and otoliths, and De Vries assumed that such forces produced some displacement of the membranous saccules. Although De Vries indicated that measurements of the utricular otolith were difficult, he estimated that all otoliths are displaced by about .006 mm by a force of 1 dyne. This would produce an estimated displacement of .005 mm (i.e., 5 μ) in the small utricular otoliths in fish during static tilt relative to gravity. This value is of the same order of magnitude as that measured by Vilstrup and Vilstrup in the shark.

From measures of x-rays made during oscillatory stimulation, De Vries estimated that the motion of the otolith is critically damped and thus there would not be a long time of "creeping" following application of constant force. The "time of indication" was estimated to be .02 sec for the sacculus and about .005 sec for the smaller utricular otolith. In other words, upon applying a constant force to the utricular otolith, final displacement is reached within .005 sec. He estimated the coefficient of internal friction of the gelatinous substance to be about 500 times that of water and the natural frequency of the sacculus to be about 40 cycles/sec.

The measurements based on x-ray photography were difficult and undoubtedly contained some error of estimation. Aside from resolution of detail in x-ray photography, some error may have resulted from the fact that edges of the otolith membrane were measured. As De Vries pointed out, the individual crystals are large enough to introduce error if they should change orientation. Engström et al. (1966) indicated that statoconia (otoliths) vary in size between 1 μ and 30 μ in several species, with the largest being near the margins of the macula. If the crystals in fish have a similar range, the potential errors of measurement of edges would be important.

Unknown in these measurements is the degree to which the otolith membrane moves as a whole and also the effect of orientation relative to gravity on the dynamic response. The orientation of the otolith macula relative to gravity will change the resultant direction of any vibratory stimulus relative to the receptors and may also change the shape of the entire supporting structure. With changes in shape, the same maculae may have different response characteristics. Whether or not these speculations are reasonable depends upon intimate structural details that are not known.

Ulrich (1934–1935) reported that lateral displacement of the otolith membrane was produced by a fine hair calibrated to yield forces between 3 and 7 mg and that eye deviation was sustained while the lapillus was laterally displaced, but the eyes returned *promptly* to normal position as soon as the pressure was released. Since Ulrich's observations of the utricular lapillus were aided by Steinhausen's staining technique, which permitted descriptions of structural features of the gelatinous portions of the utricle, it is possible that a slow repositioning of the lapillus following removal of the stimulus would have been visible. A slow return was not mentioned. Instead, it was reported that eye deviation increased slowly when gentle shearing forces were applied gradually, quickly when forces were increased quickly, and that repositioning of the eyes was *instantaneous* when the stimulus was released. It does not appear that there was any observable slow recovery either in the end-organ response or in the eye movement response similar to that which STEINHAUSEN (1933) had observed in the cupula of the pike. In relation to these observations, the estimates made by DE VRIES seem reasonable to retain.

Recordings from neural projections of the otolith organs have indicated position sensing units whose activity declines with sustained tilt (ADRIAN, 1943; MELVILL JONES, 1967) and in the ray, LOWENSTEIN and ROBERTS (1949) reported some slowly adapting units and other fast adapting units. It is possible that different elements in the sensing system are attuned to different frequencies or rates of change of position. It has been suggested that the saccule, in some species at least, is responsive to higher frequency stimulation than the utricular system (LOWENSTEIN and ROBERTS, 1951).

2.1. Some Subjective Responses Considered in Relation to Otolith Dynamics

From fairly direct methods of estimating otolith response characteristics in fish, it would appear that the otolith structure is critically damped and has a "long time constant" which is short. This means that after a sudden angular displacement relative to gravity, otolith displacement would be achieved quickly with little or no creeping into final position, and there would be no overshoot and oscillation about the newly achieved position. Hence, we should not feel a gradual creeping into final position when we are suddenly tilted, nor should we feel an oscillation once we have attained the tilt, nor should we feel sustained linear velocity (or tilt) in opposite direction following a sudden arrest from constant linear velocity.

MEIRY (1965) attempted to evaluate "the frequency response of the utricle" by having subjects indicate, with a light spring-located stick, direction of motion during horizontal linear oscillation within the frequency range 0.02 cps to 0.9 cps. Actually, the turning point of the stick was measured relative to the turning points of the stimulus (peak horizontal linear accelerations), thus permitting an estimate of stimulus-response phase relations. Assuming the saccule to be irrelevant, MEIRY devised a 'utricle' model to fit his measured phase relations during oscillatory stimuli. The model also fit a set of measures of response latencies based upon time elapsed from onset of horizontal linear acceleration until the observer signaled detection of the motion. MEIRY attributed differences in results with upright and supine positions to differences in the utricular shear component of the imposed acceleration in the two positions. However, this interpretation must be reconciled eventually with the findings of WALSH (1960), who reported equivalent thresholds for a variety of positions in which the utricular shear component was varied considerably. On the basis of his findings, WALSH concluded that the saccule had a significant influence on his results. Moreover, the time constant of the otoliths based on MEIRY's model was very long as compared with those estimated by DE VRIES (1950) and others (JONGKEES and GROEN, 1946, p. 533–534).

A revised model by YOUNG and MEIRY (1968) included a static component and provided a better fit to a greater range of observations. However, the revised time constant of 5.3 sec (the time to achieve 63% of maximum otolith displacement for a particular constant stimulus) is still long as compared with estimates by De Vries of a .005-sec "indication time." The static sensitivity of 0.4 which was introduced into the revised model implies that after about 20 sec of sustained tilt, a person will experience only 40% of the true tilt. This appears inconsistent with findings of Clark and Graybiel (1962, 1966b) on prolonged exposure to a tilted resultant force (the "Oculogravic Illusion"), but it finds support in some neurophysiological indications of rapidly adapting units, 'change in position' units, and slowly adapting units. There is also some perceptual evidence of adaptation to tilt (Mann, 1950; Mann and Passey, 1951; Mann and Ray, 1956a, b). Passey and Guedry (1949), using a tilt device, found that observers after being maintained in a position of tilt showed signs of adaptation when they returned to perceptual vertical. Comments by observers in this experiment indicated that judgments following 60 sec of exposure to tilt were more difficult to make than those involving immediate resetting. Some observers occasionally felt they were gradually being returned to upright during sustained tilt. Following delay and upon being instructed to right themselves, some failed to move the device at all, and in a few instances increased the degree of tilt. The manifestation of such effects is probably dependent upon the observers remaining as motionless as possible throughout the adaptation period, being aware that the experimental device is capable of very smooth orientation change, considering such change a fairly likely event, and perhaps thinking about something else during the period of delay. There has been disagreement as to the occurrence of such effects. In some experiments, 'delays' in tilted positions have not yielded signs of adaptation, as is made manifest by increasing errors in returning the body to the upright (Clegg and Dunfield, 1954a, b; Pearson and Hauty, 1960). Different rates of turn to and from upright influence judgments (Fleishman, 1953a) and probably account for some of the differences, since very low rates of turn might yield as much adaptation to tilt as a fixed tilt position. It is also possible that other variables (see reviews by Howard and Templeton, 1966; Clark, 1970; Schöne and Udo de Haes, 1971) account for different findings.

There have also been findings of adaptation to a preceding body tilt as indicated by continuous adjustment of a line of light (the 'visual vertical') to vertical immediately following returning the body to upright. The aftereffect is an error in the direction opposite to the preceding body tilt, and it decays with a time constant of about 120 sec (Benson, 1968b; Day and Wade, 1966; Wade and Day, 1968). Wade (1969), using various alignments and tilts of the head and trunk, attributed the adaptation to cervical rather than otolithic change, although vestibular-cervical interplay is a complex two-way interaction (Gernandt, 1967; Frederickson and Swartz, 1970). Thus, the perceptual signs of adaptation to tilt are not necessarily otolithic in origin, but by the same token, those experiments finding no evidence of perceptual adaptation do not prove the absence of adaptation in the peripheral and central otolithic neural processes. During natural tilting there is a considerable inflow of rate (or change in position) and position information from the otoliths and semicircular canals, and after completion of the tilting, otolith-related neural activity declines according to almost all available studies of neuronal activity of this system. The initially perceived tilt may be sustained by the memory of the dynamic tilt information plus some sustained

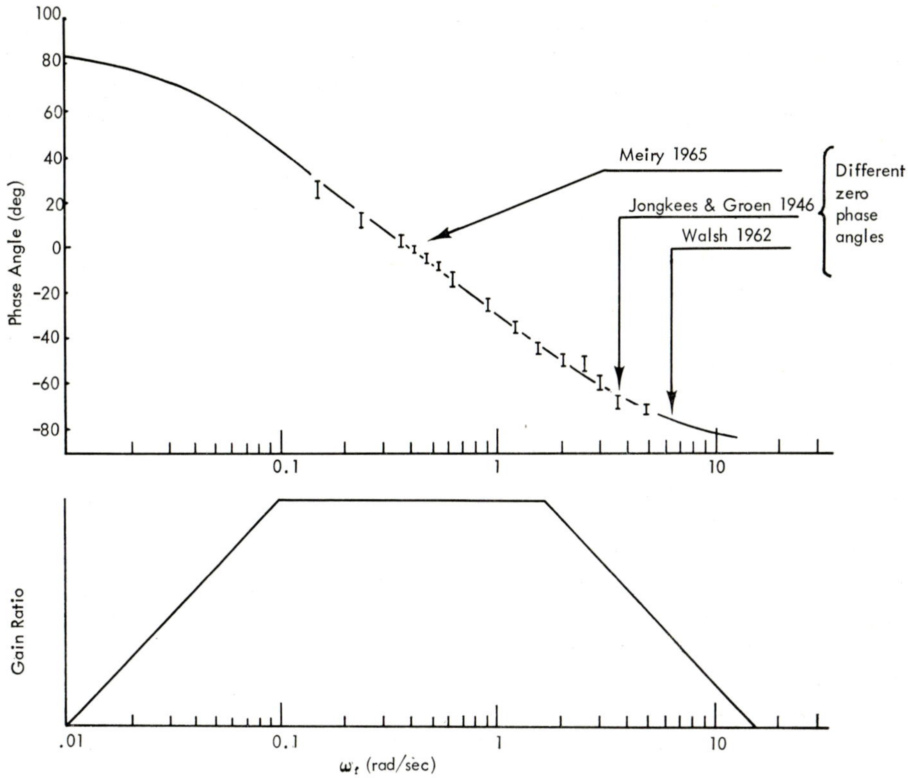

Fig. 24. Upper Panel: Phase angles reported by Meiry (1965) between actual and subjectively indicated motion reversal during linear oscillation at different frequencies. Results of Walsh (1962) and Jongkees and Groen (1946) are discrepant if corresponding stimulus derivatives were used in each study. Lower Panel: A theoretical bode plot for the otolith model proposed by Meiry (1965)

information from a number of sensory systems, perhaps enhanced by minor unrecorded movements of the observer. With a large number of interacting factors only partially experimentally manipulated, it appears that the perceptual studies of static tilt are not by themselves sufficient to infer otolith response dynamics.

There are also some inconsistencies among some of the dynamic studies, as illustrated in Fig. 24. Stimulus response phase angles at different stimulus frequencies were not consistent among the studies of Meiry (1965), Walsh (1962), and Jongkees and Groen (1946).[18] Meiry's experiments represent a well-organized sequence of tests based upon established principles of engineering analysis, but Walsh also made an interesting series of observations, and although the series did not include an extensive examination of frequency effects, Walsh did include some important psychophysical checks. For example, having ascertained when linear velocity in a given direction was sensed, Walsh instructed observers to open their eyes immediately thereafter. With the stimulus frequency of .111 cps (which is 0.69 rad/sec), observers found themselves going in one direc-

18 Assuming that the same stimulus derivatives were used in these studies.

tion (as shown by visual relative motion cues) while their immediately preceding linear velocity sensation with the eyes closed was of opposite sign. The immediacy of the comparison afforded the observer, and his surprise at the comparative perceptions, provide increased confidence in the recorded data which indicated subjective linear velocity in one direction while the linear velocity of the device (and body) was in the opposite direction. The extent to which Meiry (1965) and Walsh (1959, 1960, 1961a, b, 1962) applied checks of this nature is not clear from their reports. Obviously there are substantiating data for the Meiry-Young models, but there are remaining inconsistencies that require further evaluation.

Introspective observation of turning points during horizontal linear oscillation indicates that there is a curious temporal discrepancy between sensations of linear velocity and linear displacement that may affect decision time in signaling turning points. This paradox may be attributable to phase angles between sensory inputs from different systems, e.g., otolithic and somatosensory inputs, a possibility that Mach (1875) entertained as a potential contributor to motion sickness. Although the measurement of phase angle between driving and driven systems is a valuable tool in studying a response system, if the turning point of the response system is not accurately measured, the analysis is misleading. There may be an alternative to total reliance on temporal measures in estimating otolith dynamics from subjective data. During horizontal linear oscillation, observers have an immediate sensation of linear velocity which increases and decreases in a sinusoidal fashion. Subjects can integrate this velocity signal and make estimates of linear displacement which appear to be systematic. During steady state oscillation, the observer can estimate the displacement during each of several cycles, and there is no urgent requirement for the observer to convey the information at a particular instant in time. The maximal displacement of the otolith during any one cycle in steady state oscillation should be dependent upon the frequency of the driving function and also upon the characteristics of the otolith structures. If the rate of otolith displacement controls subjective linear velocity which can be integrated by the observer into displacement estimates, these displacement estimates should be frequency-dependent, and should provide the basis of a Bode plot like that shown in Fig. 24. At low stimulus frequencies, the subjective linear displacement estimates are systematic with a gain of about 1, and they appear to be dependent upon vestibular function (Guedry and Harris, 1963; Guedry, 1965a). At higher stimulus frequencies, von Békésy (1940) showed an almost linear relationship between stimulus amplitude and displacement estimates, with observers standing on a vertically vibrating platform, for frequencies below 4 cps. At about 0.5 cps there was fairly good agreement between actual and estimated displacement. This finding is inconsistent with the Bode plot from Meiry's model shown in Fig. 24, which indicates that there should be a considerable response attenuation at 0.5 cps or 3.14 rad/sec. Possibly von Békésy's results were dependent upon saccular organs or other senses which may have higher natural frequencies than the utricular otoliths. With frequencies above 0.5 cps, von Békésy found even higher gain ratios, e.g., at 4 cps a 1 mm displacement amplitude yielded an estimate of 2 cm, and he believed these higher gain ratios were attributable to involvement of extralabyrinthine systems. Above 4 cps, observations became impossible because the body no longer vibrated in phase with the stimulus. How the presence or absence of vestibular function influences judgments with the procedures and stimulus frequencies used by VON BÉKÉSY would be of considerable interest, and once this is established, frequency analysis of displacement estimates may provide data relevant to the dynamics of the otolith system.

A measure which has been considered in relation to otolith dynamics is the perception of verticality in relation to directional changes in resultant force vectors on centrifuges, studied by MACH (1875), and by GRAYBIEL (1952) as the "oculogravic illusion".

A lag in the oculogravic effect, noted by GRAYBIEL and BROWN (1951), if explained on the basis of otolith mechanics, would imply a very sluggish response with a time constant of 15–20 sec to a stimulus change. This is long relative to the time constant estimated by MEIRY and YOUNG, which was long relative to that inferred from the observations of DE VRIES and ULRICH.

The 'lag effect' is one of several observations which are perhaps more dependent upon central integration of unusual sensory messages for their dynamic characteristics than upon end-organ mechanics. There are several reactions which may reflect otolith function during constant speed rotation about a tilted or horizontal axis. There is a nystagmus response with several quantifiable characteristics that are probably influenced by otolith dynamics (BARNES, 1971). Also, phase advances in subjective signaling of up-position relative to gravity as well as nystagmus during horizontal linear oscillation (NIVEN et al., 1966) may be related to otolith dynamics (BENSON et al., 1971). During rotation about a horizontal axis, descriptions of the three-dimensional path of body motion and changes in the form of perceived motion as a result of changes in rotation rate may also reflect otolith dynamics (GUEDRY, 1965c; CORREIA and GUEDRY, 1966). In addition, incidence of signs and symptoms of motion sickness has been related to rotation rate about tilted rotation axes (GRAYBIEL and MILLER, 1970). Each of these responses, including the oculogravic lag effect, is probably influenced by the dynamics of otolith function, but each is also influenced by other systems. No single otolith model appears sufficient to account for the variety of stimulus-response relationships observed; for this reason most of these phenomena will be reconsidered in a later section on sensory interactions.

B. Threshold Studies

Threshold stimuli for perceptions presumed related to otolith function have been determined by several methods. In general, four stimulus modes have been used in these studies: 1) controlled oscillation of a linear acceleration vector relative to a given axis of the skull; 2) "sustained" linear acceleration relative to some axis of the head on an earth-horizontal linear track; 3) sustained linear acceleration relative to some axis of the head, as produced by a centrifuge; and 4) sustained gravitational force relative to some axis of the head, as produced by a tilt device.

With stimulus modes 1 and 2, the subjective reports usually obtained have been reports of motion, e.g., direction of linear velocity, whereas with stimulus modes 3 and 4, the reports obtained pertain to perception of "the vertical." From some points of view, stimulus modes 2, 3, and 4 can be considered almost identical, but there are important differences among these stimuli in regard to their dynamics and accompanying accelerative stimuli.

During oscillatory stimulation, a sinusoidal variation in linear acceleration is imposed on the observer. Typically, the direction of imposed motion has been aligned either with gravity or with an earth-horizontal dimension while the observer has been fixed in various orientations relative to the line of motion.[19]

During vertical oscillation, the imposed linear acceleration vectors are aligned with gravity and thus maintain constant orientation relative to the observer. In this case, the magnitude of the instantaneous resultant vector is obtained from the direct algebraic addition of the imposed vector and the gravity vector, and the maximum change in the magnitude of the resultant vector is equal to the maximum magnitude of this imposed vector. Therefore, either the change in resultant magnitude or the imposed acceleration may be specified to indicate stimulus magnitude; the result is the same.

During horizontal linear oscillation, i.e., rectilinear oscillation along an earth-horizontal track, the resultant vector changes in magnitude and orientation relative to the observer because the imposed acceleration is at right angles to gravity. Figure 25 shows this change in orientation of the resultant force when the

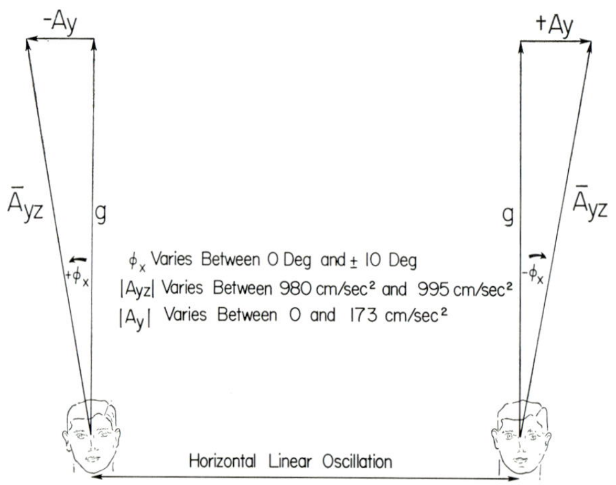

Fig. 25. Changes in postural "tilt" relative to the resultant vector during horizontal linear oscillation. Note: the magnitude of the change in resultant acceleration during horizontal linear oscillation is far less than the magnitude of the horizontal linear acceleration

maximum horizontal linear acceleration within the cycle is 172.8 cm/sec² or 0.1763 g-units. At each end of the excursion, the angular displacement, $\varnothing_x$, of the resultant relative to the man is given by arc tan $\frac{172.8}{980} = 10$ degrees. Thus $\varnothing_x$ varies sinusoidally between ± 10 degrees. The magnitude of the resultant varies between a maximum of $\frac{980}{\cos 10 \text{ deg}} = 995.1$ cm/sec² at the extremes and $\frac{980}{\cos 0} =$

19 Minor curvilinearity is present with a large balance (MACH, 1875), or with a parallel swing, but counterrotation of the carrier practically eliminates angular acceleration stimuli.

980 cm/sec^2 at the midpoint of the excursion. At any one instant, the stimulus to the otolith is the resultant force vector, and in attempting to specify the significant stimulus parameter, one might take the difference between the resultant magnitudes at any two points in time and relate this to changes in perceptual responses. For example, between the midpoint and either end of the excursion, the difference in magnitude amounts to 995–980 cm/sec^2 or 15 cm/sec^2. But with the man oriented as he is in Fig. 25, the otoliths would be exposed to peak shear components at each end of the excursion of almost 172.8 cm/sec^2. Thus it is not reasonable to select the small change-in-resultant magnitude as the relevant aspect of the stimulus when a much larger vector is acting in the plane of maximum sensitivity of the receptor, but this has been done occasionally in "otolith threshold" studies. An additional specification of stimulus conditions is necessary. As mentioned previously, it is possible that the orientation of the macula relative to gravity may alter its dynamic response and so it is necessary to specify not only the maximum imposed acceleration and the frequency, but also the direction of the constant bias due to gravity relative to the macula.

In the order of their apparent sensitivity, subjective indicants dealt with during horizontal linear oscillation have been 1) perception of motion, 2) perception of linear velocity, and 3) perception of "tilt." At a given frequency of oscillation, motion (without discriminable direction) is perceived with very low magnitude stimuli. When stimulus magnitude is increased, linear velocity with a clear direction is perceived (Jongkees and Groen, 1946). With still stronger stimuli, 'tilting' sensations have been reported (Jongkees and Groen, 1946; Lansberg, 1954), although there is fairly clear evidence that the amount of tilt experienced during oscillatory stimuli is far less than the change in the angle $\varnothing$ when head-and-body restraints prevent angular acceleration artifacts (Guedry and Harris, 1963; Guedry, 1965a; Niven et al., 1966).

1. Threshold Determination with Oscillatory Stimulation

Threshold estimates based upon oscillatory stimuli are listed in Table 3. The thresholds determined by Mach (1875) for vertical oscillation along the observer's z-axis are in good agreement with z-axis thresholds determined by Jongkees and Groen (1946), Lansberg (1954), and Walsh (1962) for earth-horizontal linear oscillation. Travis and Dodge (1928) and Gurnee (1934) stated thresholds as average accelerations. In Table 3 these were converted to maximal acceleration values by assuming that average acceleration is 0.636 of the peak acceleration. In both of these studies frequency was varied concomitantly with maximum acceleration (peak displacement was constant), and the threshold was estimated by interpolation to the stimulus value yielding 50% correct response. Thresholds were found that were not too different from other estimates in spite of potential errors from changes in phase shift and response attenuation with different frequencies. This may mean that within the range of stimuli investigated in these two studies, changes in phase and in response attenuation were not very great.*

* However, Walsh (1964) reported considerably less sensitivity (higher thresholds) for low-frequency vertical linear oscillations than for horizontal linear oscillations. This apparent discrepancy with the results of Mach (1875) and Gurnee (1934) indicates a need for further systematic research for situations in which the imposed linear acceleration and gravity are colinear.

Table 3. *Thresholds of detection of linear oscillating stimuli in man*

Author	S	Direction oscillation Rel. to S	Direction oscillation Rel. to earth	Gravity dir. Rel. to S	period	Max accel.	Subjective indicant
Mach (1875)	2	z-axis	vertical	z-axis	7 sec	10–12 cm/sec^2	Linear velocity
Gurnee (1934)	3	z-axis	vertical	z-axis	8–16 sec	2–10 cm/sec^2	Linear velocity
Travis and Dodge (1928)	2	x-axis (S seated)	horizontal	z-axis	2–8 sec	20–25 cm/sec^2	Linear velocity
	2	x-axis (S standing)	horizontal	z-axis	2–8 sec	8 cm/sec^2	Linear velocity
	2	y-axis (S standing)	horizontal	z-axis	2–8 sec	5 cm/sec^2	Linear velocity
Jongkees and Groen (1946)	2	z-axis	horizontal	x-axis	2.5 sec	6–13 cm/sec^2	Linear velocity
Lansberg (1954)		z-axis	horizontal	x-axis	3.8 sec	9 cm/sec^2	Linear velocity
		z-axis	horizontal	x-axis	3.8 sec	15 cm/sec^2	Tilt sensation
		x-axis	horizontal	x-axis	3.8 sec	(>15 cm/sec^2 unreliable)	Tilt sensation
Walsh (1962)	6	z-axis	horizontal	±y-axis[a]	3.0 sec	7 cm/sec^2	Linear velocity
	6	z-axis	horizontal	±y-axis	9.0 sec	9 cm/sec^2	Linear velocity
	6	z-axis	horizontal	±x-axis[a]	3.0 sec	8 cm/sec^2	Linear velocity
	6	z-axis	horizontal	±x-axis	9.0 sec	9 cm/sec^2	Linear velocity
Walsh (1964)	7	x- & y-axes	vertical	x- & y-axes	3.0 sec	3 cm/sec^2	Linear velocity
	7	x- & y-axes	vertical	x- & y-axes	9.0 sec	80 cm/sec^2	Linear velocity

[a] Data for supine (+x) and prone (—x) averaged. Data for right-(+y) and left-(—y) sides down averaged.

2. Threshold Determination by Sustained Horizontal Linear Acceleration

By means of a horizontal linear track, MEIRY (1965) was able to impose different magnitude accelerations and to determine how long such acceleration must be applied to yield 75% correct direction judgments. A maximum travel of 32 feet limited the duration of accelerations. Because the times that low magnitude accelerations could be applied were a little more than twice the obtained mean latency times of signaling linear velocity, the device apparently had sufficient range to permit threshold determinations. Thresholds were reached at imposed acceleration of 10 cm/sec^2 for the supine position (i.e., with the observer's z-axis aligned with the imposed acceleration and his x-axis aligned with gravity) and 6 cm/sec^2 for an upright head position (x-axis aligned with the imposed acceleration and z-axis aligned with gravity). MEIRY reasoned that the difference in threshold values was due to the angle of the imposed acceleration, A, relative to the average utricular shear plane, i.e., in the upright and supine postures, the effective components would be A cos 30 deg and A cos 60 deg, respectively.

As in the case of the semicircular canals, the latency times with accelerations of different magnitudes are threshold determinations; theoretically, response latency is the time required for a given magnitude stimulus to produce threshold deflections of the otoliths. When the latency becomes very long, a threshold magnitude is approached, i.e., a magnitude so low as to be undetectable with very long application.

In addition to the work of MEIRY, thresholds have been roughly estimated by several other investigators by means of devices producing linear motions (BOURDON, 1914; WALSH, 1960; SCHMIDT in MACH, 1875).

3. Thresholds Determined by Centripetal Acceleration on a Centrifuge

The centripetal acceleration vector produced by a centrifuge with an earth-vertical axis is a horizontal linear acceleration of magnitude ω^2r which can be sustained indefinitely in constant direction and magnitude relative to the observer. During constant angular velocity, the resultant vector (of the centripetal and gravity vectors) makes an angle $\varnothing$ relative to gravity, and if the resultant vector is perceived as "the vertical," the observer should feel tilted approximately by the angle $\varnothing$.

JONGKEES and GROEN (1946) measured tilt sensations under three different body orientations on a small centrifuge. All three positions would produce tilting within the observer's xz plane, i.e., about his y-axis. Thus, they were dealing with $\varnothing_y$ tilts. Although not intended to be a rigorous investigation of the "threshold," (results are reported for different observers in different positions), the study was interesting because it introduced two unique experimental procedures. First, the centrifuge was small, so that part of the body was on center while the otoliths were off center and other extremities were across center, antipodal to the position of the otoliths. Second, the observers 'matched' perceived body inclinations experienced on the centrifuge stimulus by using a GRAHE position litter just after the centrifuge stimulus. Attempts to call out tilt angle during centrifugation were apparently considered unsatisfactory. The first point is significant because it introduces a method which affords some control of the ever-present body cues during whole-body tilt; e.g., in some positions the lower part of the body received 'tilt cues' in one direction while the otoliths received cues to tilt in the opposite direction.

In a supine position, apparently with the x-axis aligned with gravity, a centripetal acceleration of 45 cm/sec^2 (directed along the z-axis) was detected as the "faintest sensation of leaning backward" in one observer (J). Another observer (G) in upright position (z-axis aligned with gravity, x-axis aligned with centripetal vector) perceived no tilt when the centripetal acceleration was 22 cm/sec^2, and by interpolation it appears that his threshold was also approximately 45 cm/sec^2. When the same observer (G) assumed a supine position and further rotated his head backward 60 degrees, the threshold was greatly increased and tilt perceptions were considerably less than $\varnothing$. In this position, the resultant vector "acts in the direction of the so-called blind spot of the otolithic organs" (JONGKEES and GROEN, 1946, p. 539; QUIX, 1925). This position of minimal sensitivity to tilt placed the average utricular plane in exact alignment with the centripetal acceleration vector, i.e., in a position to maximize the shear component of the centripetal vector. It was in this position (utricle inverted relative to gravity with the shear component in the plane of the utricle) that WALSH (1960), using perceived subjective linear velocity as an indicant, concluded that the otoliths are in a position of maximum sensitivity. Thus the position of minimal sensitivity with 'subjective tilt' as an indicant may be the position of maximal sensitivity with "subjective linear velocity" as the indicant. There are a number of reasonable alternative explanations to these seemingly paradoxical sets of results. It is possible that the linear velocity perception and the tilt perception in these experiments depend upon differing relative contributions from different sensory systems, e.g., the otolith for the one and somatosensory receptors for the other. However, if sensitivity of these thresholds is primarily dependent upon otolith function, then it is possible that the inverted utricular macula, when the otoliths hang from the hair cells, is more sensitive to dynamic stimuli, as WALSH suggested (1960, p. 356). To use WALSH's analogy, "A bell ..... can be rung by horizontal oscillation easily when in normal position, with difficulty when inverted, and not at all when on its side." Thus an inverted utricle may be in a more sensitive position for horizontal oscillatory stimulation and other stimuli.

Conversely, with static stimuli, the reverse may be true. Consider the two diagrams in Fig. 26. In the diagram to the right, analogous to an inverted utricle during static tilt, deflection will never exceed $\varnothing$ whereas in the diagram to the left, it may exceed $\varnothing$, depending upon the mass, m, and the resistance afforded by the spring system. This figure is presented not in the belief that it is an adequate model of the otolith system, but merely to illustrate the fact that equal shear vectors may well have different effects (i.e., produce different final static displacements of the otolith) depending upon the orientation of the receptor relative to the 'steady state' gravity vector. The magnitude of both the shear and normal (compression or traction) components must be considered, and if the effective stimulus changes as the otolith displacement changes, a certain amount of creeping may occur because a "step-input" shear acceleration is in its effect not a "step-input."

Another factor that cannot be neglected in the third position of JONGKEES and GROEN (1946) is the fact that confusion about 'egocentric' dead-ahead arises when

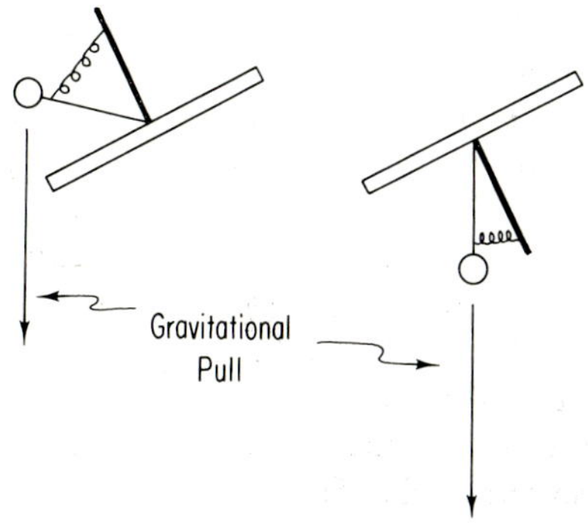

Fig. 26. For a given degree of static tilt relative to gravity, a spring pendulum with the mass above the pivot point (left-hand figure) may be deflected by gravity more than a hanging pendulum (right-hand figure) which would only align itself with gravity. During horizontal oscillation, however, the hanging pendulum might be more responsive to changing horizontal linear acceleration vectors. This crude analogy illustrates the importance of developing models of the otolith organs for assessing results in both static and dynamic situations

the head is rotated backward 60 degrees. Is 'front' in the direction of gaze, or is it determined by the anterior body surface? This additional requirement for central nervous system interpretation could influence dynamic and static responses as manifested by either indicant. This unnatural head and body alignment could therefore introduce confusion as to the direction of linear acceleration. The variation in radial distance of different parts of the body could also influence the perception of tilt because this stimulus during constant velocity was comparable to lying supine across the top of a dome.

Graybiel and Patterson (1955) also used a centrifuge to estimate "thresholds of stimulation of the otolith organs" in three men. The subjective indicant was the perception of tilt as revealed by requiring an observer within a chamber on a centrifuge to set a line of light to apparent vertical. Angular velocity was increased gradually and the observer reported every 5 sec on apparent tilt of the line to the right, to the left (i.e., $\pm \varnothing_X$) or no tilt. Changes in position prior to rotation of the centrifuge were used in efforts to obscure the direction in which tilting would occur. Six body positions were used: 1) seated erect with z-axis aligned with gravity and facing tangentially either forward or backward, 2) upside down with z-axis aligned with gravity and facing tangentially either forward or backward, and 3) lying on side with y-axis aligned with gravity and facing tangentially either forward or backward. In all positions the change of the resultant was in the observer's yz plane, i.e., about his x-axis.

In the seated position, $\varnothing_X$ was increased from 0 to 4 degrees, which means that the centrifuge was accelerated until it reached an angular velocity of 21.6 deg/sec before deceleration commenced. In the other two positions, angular acceleration was maintained to an angular velocity of 36 deg/sec, corresponding to $\varnothing_X = 11$ degrees, and then deceleration commenced. Thresholds were taken as those values of $\varnothing$ which yielded 75% correct responses.

In the erect position, thresholds were found at $\varnothing_X = 1.5$ degrees (ascending) and $\varnothing_X = 1.1$ degrees (descending). A change in $\varnothing_X$ from 0 degrees to 1.5 degrees is accompanied by a change in the resultant force of .00034 g-units, but there is a greater change in the centripetal acceleration, from 0 to 25.7 cm/sec² of .026 g-units. Since the centripetal component represents the greater change and was directed in the utricular shear plane, it is the pertinent component of the total stimulus, even though the lower figure, .00034 g-units, has sometimes been cited as a threshold value from this study.

Thresholds found in side-down positions were considerably higher; $\varnothing_X =$ 8.9 degrees corresponding to a centripetal component of 153.5 cm/sec² or 0.157 g-units was reported as threshold. In this position the centripetal component acted along the z-axis, almost perpendicular to the utricular plane, and hence, utricular shear effects would be very slight relative to the shear already present from the gravity vector (which was aligned with the y-axis), but saccular shear components would be maximized. It is likely that AUBERT (1861) effects complicate threshold determination in this position.

In the inverted position, thresholds were not obtained. Apparently the 11-degree tilt did not yield 75% correct responses. In a subsequent experiment GRAYBIEL and CLARK (1962) did not reach threshold oculogravic tilt with a 12-degree $\varnothing_X$ tilt on the centrifuge.

Again there are interesting comparisons to be made with the data obtained by WALSH (1960, 1962). With a dynamic stimulus and subjective linear velocity as an indicant, he found high sensitivity, threshold 2–12 cm/sec², in side-down orientations, while directing the imposed accelerations along the observer's z-axis (y-axis aligned with gravity). Thus, while the threshold for tilt in this position suggests insensitivity, the threshold for perception of linear velocity indicates a high degree of sensitivity. It is possible that in some of the centrifuge studies, tilt thresholds were elevated by "lag-effects" (GRAYBIEL and BROWN, 1951), but such effects were probably minimized by the procedures used, e.g., low angular accelerations.

4. Thresholds Determined by Tilt Relative to Gravity

Of the many experiments dealing with the perception of the vertical, very few fall into the category of 'threshold studies.' Extensive reviews of this literature are available (CLARK, 1970; HOWARD and TEMPLETON, 1966). Basically, two procedures have been used. A restrained observer is tilted in total darkness relative to gravity by some device, and measurement is made of his accuracy in estimating upright position as the device is returned by either the observer or the experimenter. This has been referred to as measurement of the *postural vertical*. A second procedure involves measurement of the adjustment of a luminous line in a dark field to apparent alignment with gravity from various positions of body tilt. This has been referred to as measurement of the *visual vertical*. In either situation, if very small body tilts are used to find that tilt magnitude which is just sufficient to elicit an adjustment in the correct direction in 75% of the presentations, this value could be taken as a threshold measure comparable to those discussed in the previous section. Similarly, when the observer returns himself repeatedly to upright, a measure of variability about the mean position judged to be vertical gives some estimate of threshold.

As was shown in the previous section, both the estimate of body tilt and the estimate of verticality of a luminous line in a dark room have been used as 'threshold measures' on a centrifuge where the tilt is in reference to the direction of the resultant force. It is reasonable to ask if there is any important difference between the procedures involved in determining thresholds by means of a simple earth-fixed tilt device as opposed to using a human centrifuge, when in either situation we are merely changing the orientation of the observer relative to the existing force field. The most important difference comes from the way in which the tilting is accomplished. Consider a tilt chair in which an observer is tilted about his x-axis. If the tilting is accomplished fairly quickly, then there are appreciable angular accelerations about the x-axis, and these confirm the $\varnothing_X$ change in orientation relative to gravity. Even when the tilting is accomplished very slowly, any bearing, transmission or drive system noise is apt to create torque cues about the x-axis which may be detected by the somatosensory as well as the vestibular system. On the centrifuge with the observer locked in an upright position relative to gravity and facing tangentially, a change in the resultant of gravity and the centripetal vector which is accomplished fairly quickly produces angular accelerations about the observer's z-axis, but the observer eventually achieves a $\varnothing_X$ tilt position. The z-axis semicircular canal stimulus and extraneous torque cues do not confirm (but rather confound) otolith signals concerning a $\varnothing_X$ change in orientation relative to the resultant forces.[20] As noted earlier, 'tilting' without appropriate semicircular canal signals can also be produced by horizontal linear oscillation, but in this case the 'tilt' cannot be sustained as it can be with a tilt chair or a centrifuge because of limited travel on a horizontal track.

These are the primary differences between tilting on the tilt chair and tilting relative to the resultant force on horizontal linear tracks, and on the centrifuge. There is, of course, a change in the magnitude of the resultant force to be considered, but presumably in threshold studies, this magnitude change is of little significance as compared with the change in direction of the resultant vector relative to the receptors. Later, however, it will be shown that magnitude of the resultant is an important consideration at higher levels of stimulation.

4.1. The Postural Vertical

On the earth, the continual presence of gravity means that we are constantly experiencing an above-threshold stimulus to the otoliths. In static tilt studies, the question is: What is our perceived position when the head (and body) are in a given position relative to gravity, and what is the range of positions that will produce this perception with an approximately equivalent probability?

The standard usually selected for judgment has been the vertical upright position, but the following comments apply also to other standard positions such as the horizontal or the inverted position. The mean of the positions one calls vertical in a series of judgments may be highly accurate relative to true gravi-

20 The tangential component, $a_z r$, is not considered here on the assumption that it is of low magnitude. However, even when this vector is included, the a_z canal stimulus does not confirm the change in $\varnothing_X$.

tational vertical, yet the threshold may be quite large. For example, the mean postural vertical in a particular experiment may be 0.5 degrees to the left of true vertical, i.e., $\varnothing_x = 0.5$ degrees, but all positions of $\varnothing_x$ between —5.5 degrees and +4.5 degrees may be perceived as vertical with approximately equal probability. In this case the sensitivity is fairly low, i.e., the threshold is high. Conversely, it is possible to have high sensitivity (low thresholds) when the mean postural vertical is inaccurate. For example, if $\varnothing_y = 10$ degrees is perceived as vertical, the perception is inaccurate, but if $\varnothing_y = 10$ degrees were always reported as upright and if positions ± 0.2 degrees on either side were invariably reported as forward or backward tilt, then the sensitivity would be high. Thus the accuracy of the mean judgment relative to some chosen standard position does not necessarily indicate sensitivity. Most experiments dealing with judgments of verticality have been concerned with accuracy of mean judgments, and have not been designed as threshold studies. For this reason, the variability of judgments has not always been described in a convenient form for threshold estimation.

MANN (1950) reported a mean "arc of uncertainty" (U deg) of 4.4 degrees in judgments of the postural vertical following tilts about the x-axis. This measure of variability was a statistic which encompassed 75% of the judgments of the postural vertical when the observer controlled the return of the chair in giving his estimate of vertical. U deg was calculated from the product of 2 (1.156) σ where σ is the standard deviation of the scores about the mean, which in turn was calculated from the algebraic sum of the signed deviations from true vertical. Judgments of verticality tend to fall in the quadrant of initial tilt, and a convention was adopted in which the signs of errors of estimation were considered plus if the estimate was in the quadrant opposite the initial tilt and minus if the estimate was in the same quadrant as the initial tilt. The reported (MANN and DAUTERIVE, 1949; MANN et al., 1949) mean constant error of —.8 degrees with an arc of uncertainty of 4.4 degrees indicates that the mean estimate of vertical was 0.8 degrees from true vertical biased in the direction of the initial tilt, and 75% of the estimates fell within the limits +1.4 degrees and —3.0 degrees. Presumably, if this bias were eliminated by starting near vertical position, the mean postural vertical would be about 0 degrees, and tilts greater than 2.2 degrees would be correctly identified as tilts with a 0.75 probability.

MANN and DAUTERIVE employed three procedures for estimating the postural vertical from tilts about the x-axis: 1) the observer was tilted to various tilt positions between $\varnothing_x = \pm 5$ degrees and $\varnothing_x = \pm 90$ degrees and returned the chair himself to his estimate of vertical. The results just described were obtained with this method. 2) The subject was rotated from various $\varnothing_x$ tilt positions (between ± 5 degrees and ± 90 degrees) through upright position and attempted to signal as his z-axis was vertical. The rate of rotation was approximately 2.5 deg/sec. 3) The subject was offset to various $\varnothing_x$ positions between ± 0.5 degrees and ± 6.0 degrees and was required to make a three-category decision: right tilt, left tilt, or vertical. An effort was made to move the subject in 'imperceptible steps' to his judgment position. As might be expected, Method 2 yielded slightly greater mean constant errors and standard deviations than Method 1. Results obtained with Method 3 were similar to those found with Method 1, and the $\varnothing_x$ tilts which gave 75% correct response were 2.3 degrees left tilt ($\varnothing_x =$

—2.3 degrees) and 2.1 degrees right tilt ($\varnothing_X = +2.1$ degrees). These two values added together give a threshold zone of 4.4 degrees, the same as the arc of uncertainty calculated in Method 1. The component of gravity acting along the observer's y-axis (i.e., approximately in the plane of the utricle shear plane) is 37.6 cm/sec^2 or .038 g-units when $\varnothing_X$ is 2.2 degrees. This is approximately the same as the value reported by GRAYBIEL and PATTERSON (1955) for "$\varnothing_X$ thresholds" on the centrifuge.

With each of these methods, the arc of uncertainty was increased considerably when the tilt chair was liberally padded with foam rubber. The results referred to in this section were obtained with the unpadded chair.

Several experiments (PASSEY and GUEDRY, 1949; BURTT, 1918; JONES et al., 1947; SHUBERT, 1942; KLEINKNECHT, 1922) indicate that when the upright is approached by motion in the sagittal plane (rotation about the y-axis) the postural vertical is less accurately judged than when the motion is in the lateral plane ($\varnothing_X$). As noted earlier, the difference in accuracy does not necessarily mean a difference in threshold, but it appears that the variability as well as the accuracy is greater when the movement is in the sagittal plane, although CLEGG and DUNFIELD (1954a, b) did not confirm this fairly consistent finding.

Aside from variation related to direction of initial tilt, the judgment of the postural vertical differs depending upon the speed of return to upright (cf. BURTT, 1918; CLEGG and DUNFIELD, 1954a, b; FLEISHMAN, 1953a, b; MANN and RAY, 1956a, b), the magnitude of the initial tilt (MANN and RAY, 1956a; MANN and PASSEY, 1951; MANN et al., 1950; FLEISHMAN, 1953b; CLEGG and DUNFIELD, 1954a, b), the delay time in the initial tilt position (PASSEY and GUEDRY, 1949; MANN et al., 1950; MANN and PASSEY, 1951; MANN and RAY, 1956a, b; CORREIA, 1962), although CLEGG and DUNFIELD (1954a, b) and PEARSON and HAUTY (1960) did not confirm the effects of delay. In many tilt studies, stimuli, e.g., exact head position relative to the tilt device, have not been adequately described. There have been differences in methods of restraint and padding, in methods of tilt control (observer versus experimenter), and in articulation of joints and posture (GESCHEIDER and WRIGHT, 1965; SCHÖNE and UDO DE HAES, 1968, 1971). Despite attention to speed of tilt, delay in tilt, et cetera, limitations in available equipment have introduced uncontrolled higher derivative artifacts and also have severely limited the range of controlled variation with "tilt chairs" of angular acceleration, angular velocity, and stimulus waveform and frequency. All of these factors can contribute to the variability and hence apparent sensitivity in detecting gravitational vertical, and some of these factors undoubtedly influence sensitivity directly. This "sensitivity" is clearly not solely dependent upon otolith function.

4.2. The Visual Vertical

It would seem that the ability of an upright subject to set a line of light to the vertical in an otherwise dark room depends partially upon the person's perception of the vertical as derived from labyrinthine and somatosensory signals and partially upon his ability to place a line in a particular orientation relative to his body. Both of these information sources and curious perceptual interactions between them contribute to variability encountered in the visual vertical (cf. BAUERMEISTER, 1964; BAUERMEISTER et al., 1964). Mean judgments of the visual vertical (where the line tilts about the observer's x-axis and the plane of movement of the line is parallel to the observer's y-z plane) have been found to be accurate to less than 1 degree (CLARK and GRAYBIEL, 1967; see reviews by CLARK, 1970; HOWARD and TEMPLETON, 1966) when the observer is seated upright. MANN et al. (1949) indicate a typical standard deviation of 2.5 degrees which means an arc of uncertainty of 5.8 degrees. Thus 75% of the judgments fell within an arc approximately 2.9 degrees to either side of vertical. From this it can be argued that all line tilts *greater* than 2.9 degrees were correctly identified as tilted on 75% of the judgments and that this is a form of threshold. However, it is not a conventional threshold because 2.9 degrees was not in fact correctly identified as a tilted line on 75% of the judgments. We might ask instead how much deviation from the mean visual vertical would be required to obtain a statistically significant difference. From the variability of the data about the mean, a calculated, just noticeable difference would be on the order of 1 degree.

As with the postural vertical, investigation of the visual vertical (or visual horizontal) with tilt devices has centered on accuracy of judgments. With $\varnothing_X$ body tilts between 20 and 60 degrees, there is a tendency to perceive a truly vertical line as tilted in the direction of body tilt. Thus, in setting a line to apparent vertical, the observer will displace the line in the quadrant opposite to his body tilt (MÜLLER, 1916). This has been called the Müller or E-effect. With larger $\varnothing_X$ body tilts, there is a tendency to perceive a truly vertical line as being tilted in the opposite quadrant, and the visual vertical is therefore displaced in the direction of body tilt (AUBERT, 1861). This has been called the Aubert or A-effect. (See reviews by CLARK, 1970 and by HOWARD and TEMPLETON, 1966.) It increases to a maximum when $\varnothing_X \approx 160$ degrees (BOURDON, 1906; SCHÖNE, 1964). The variability of the visual vertical also changes with different $\varnothing_X$ body tilts (MANN et al., 1949; GRAYBIEL and CLARK, 1962; SCHÖNE, 1964, MILLER et al., 1965a). Variability increases very little with small body tilts, but standard deviations tend to be much larger between 30 degrees and 170 degrees of tilt. At $\varnothing_X = 180$ degrees, inverted position, the standard deviation is reduced, but still apparently is greater than that reported in the upright position (SCHÖNE, 1964; MILLER and GRAYBIEL, 1966a; GRAYBIEL and CLARK, 1962). From the size of these standard deviations, it appears that just noticeable differences (i.e., difference in thresholds) in the visual vertical will be quite different depending upon the particular set of standard positions from which the judgments are made.

C. Effects of Attenuated Vestibular and Nonvestibular Cues on Responses Attributed to Otolith Function

In the interpretation of 'otolith thresholds' as well as perceptual events associated with supraliminal otolith stimulation, it is likely that the results depend upon somatosensory inputs, visual inputs, and memory of changes in orientation, as well as immediate sensory data from the otoliths. Two approaches have been used in attempts to clarify this issue: First, expected mechanical response characteristics during controlled otolith stimulation have been compared with obtained results in an attempt to establish otolith-dependent responses through theoretical inferences. Some of this literature has been reviewed in preceding sections, and it is not conclusive. A second approach involves the modification of sensory inputs. Somatosensory inputs have been altered by a) padded chairs, b) immersion in liquids, c) anesthetizing the buttocks, d) using observers with spinal lesions, and e) changing the force field on the body and head differently. Labyrinthine inputs have been altered by a) using subjects with labyrinthine dysfunction and b) changing the force field on the body and head differently.

1. Perception of Linear Velocity when Selected Sensory Inputs are Attenuated

All of the experiments in this section refer to judgments made without visual reference to an earth-fixed structure. WALSH (1961a) estimated thresholds for perception of linear motion during horizontal linear oscillation with normal observers immersed in water and also in "polycell" cellulose paste. The mean thresholds were elevated slightly to between 4 and 7 cm/sec^2 as compared with mean values between 2 and 5 cm/sec^2 without liquid immersion. Individuals with high spinal lesions gave mean threshold values between 4 and 8 cm/sec^2. This is to be contrasted with results obtained from individuals with complete bilateral labyrinthine loss tested without liquid immersion; mean thresholds ranged between 15 and 26 cm/sec^2. Presumably, if liquid immersion had been used with these labyrinthine-defective (LD) individuals, thresholds would have been elevated even more.

JONGKEES and GROEN (1950) also reported elevation of thresholds for horizontal linear acceleration (acceleration vector along the y-axis) in an observer without labyrinthine function. During sinusoidal stimulation with maximum y-axis acceleration of 16 cm/sec^2, the observer apparently experienced 'tilting' rather than linear velocity; i.e., her sensation was indistinguishable from that produced by tilting. This suggests that the threshold for perception of linear velocity was greater than 16 cm/sec^2 in this observer. In another experiment (GUEDRY and HARRIS, 1963; GUEDRY, 1965a) involving side-to-side oscillation in which the imposed linear acceleration vector acted along the observer's y-axis, much stronger stimuli were used, and yet several men with bilateral labyrinthine loss reported only tilting sensations and no linear velocity. Although not intended as a threshold study, this experiment indicates that the threshold for linear velocity information during oscillation was not reached in some LD subjects with peak accelerations of 280 cm/sec^2 (period 3.6 sec). Under the same circumstances, men with normal vestibular function reported linear velocity and no tilting. Mean estimates of linear displacement during the side-to-side oscillation made by LD observers were about one-fourth of the mean linear extents estimated by normal observers. So, although some LD observers experienced linear velocity, it was apparently of low magnitude (since the displacement estimates were less), and the path of experienced movement was different from that described by normal observers.

By varying head position of individuals with unilateral labyrinthine function, WALSH (1959, 1960) deduced that the utricle is relatively insensitive to vectors normal to its average plane and also to imposed shear vectors when its plane is aligned with gravity. He further inferred that the sensitivity of the saccule to oscillatory shear vectors varies depending upon the direction of gravity, maximum sensitivity to oscillatory shear vectors being achieved when the otoliths 'hang down from the hair cells.'

2. Achievement of Prescribed Postural Positions with Reduced Somatosensory Cues

It has been reported that the constant errors and the variability of positioning the body to apparent vertical increase as somatosensory cues are diminished (Arndts, 1924; Bourdon, 1914; Mann and Dauterive, 1949; Mann et al., 1949; Garten, 1920; Stigler, 1912; Nelson, 1968). In some studies the increased mean constant error is attributable to the method of determining signs of errors. For example, in one convention, an error (relative to true vertical) made to the same side as the initial tilt is given a negative sign while an error made to the opposite quadrant is given a positive sign. Thus, in $\varnothing_X$ tilt, errors in position to the right and to the left of true vertical would be called negative errors if the starting tilt positions were, respectively, to the right and to the left of vertical. With this convention for determining signs of errors, a mean constant error of 3 or 4 degrees when starting positions to right and left of upright were used might be equivalent to a mean error of 0 degrees if signs had been determined by declaring as positive all errors to the right of vertical and as negative all errors to the left of vertical. This latter convention would indicate an error bias relative to gravity, irrespective of starting position, and the effect of starting position could be ascertained by treating the data from different starting positions separately. Under the latter convention, the mean "accuracy" (or error) for pooled data might appear to be the same with and without reduced somatosensory cues, but variability would change significantly. The greater mean constant errors reported by Mann and Berry (1949) with a padded tilt chair as compared with a hard tilt chair were calculated by the first mentioned convention, and since the mean constant error as well as the variability was increased by the padded chair, it appears that the 'arc of uncertainty' calculated by the second convention would be quite large.

If a person completely without position sense were to make a large number of guesses about verticality on a tilt chair preset to various positions between $\varnothing_X = \pm 90$ degrees, the most likely mean constant error would be zero (i.e., upright) because any position would have an equal probability of being chosen, and errors by chance would be symmetrical about the upright position. However, such a person would have a large range of scores, i.e., a large standard deviation. From this point of view, variability of judgments is a more important statistic than mean constant error for making inferences about the 'insensitivity of the position sense.' Variability is sometimes indicated as the *average error* (Mann and Passey, 1951; Passey, 1950), which is the mean (or median) of the unsigned deviations from true vertical, and it is sometimes indicated by the standard deviation around the mean constant error (which may be calculated by either convention) or by the "arc of uncertainty" (U) or by the probable error (PE). The different statistics adopted by different groups of workers for describing results of 'tilt' studies complicate the comparison of experiments.

Arndts (1924) found that anesthetizing the skin produced only a slight effect on the postural judgments and was of the opinion that deep sensibility is important for posture maintenance. Definite reductions in sensitivity (large increases in variability) of the position sense have been produced by padding the restraint system and by water immersion. Thus some part of the somatosensory system makes an important contribution to the judgment of the postural vertical.

In a recent study, NELSON (1968) used an underwater two-axis gimbals system and asked observers to position themselves to one of six positions: head-up, head-down, face-up, face-down, right-ear-up, and left-ear-up.[21] Impressive precautions were used to minimize cues from bubbles, light, buoyancy, et cetera. Observers were given one minute to achieve the designated position by prearranged hand signals to the experimenters.

Because of the two-axis system, a cone of judgments, and of judgment errors, was possible, and this is to be contrasted with one-axis devices in which only a plane of errors is possible. NELSON found a "pitch-forward" bias in the constant errors for the head-up position of 7.5 degrees, for face-down of 23.6 degrees, for head-down of 32.2 degrees, and for face-up of 32.2 degrees. With certain assumptions about the exact position of the head relative to the tilt table, it is interesting to speculate on this pitch-forward bias, which in the face-up and face-down positions would tend to maximize the utricular shear component, whereas in the head-up and head-down positions the bias would tend to minimize the utricular shear component. With these goal positions, the pitch errors were an order of magnitude greater than the roll errors, and it appears that variability was greater in the pitch plane than in the roll plane, although the degrees of freedom of motion complicate this interpretation.

For the left- and right-ear-up goal positions, the mean constant error of positioning the body to earth-horizontal was apparently very small, although there was a significant face-up bias; i.e., the z-axis was horizontal (relative to gravity) but the x- and y-axes were rotated slightly (about 4–8 degrees) so that the face was up. This is important because several authors without using water immersion have indicated that observers lying on their sides at $\varnothing_X$ tilts of 90 degrees felt tilted more than 90 degrees (NAGEL, 1898; MCFARLAND et al., 1962; BAUERMEISTER, 1964); NELSON's results suggest that the head-up bias indicated by these previous workers is attributable to somatosensory inputs which are diminished by water immersion.

Of significance for inferences concerning otolith sensitivity were the large variable errors reported by NELSON for all goal positions. For the head-up position, the probable error in the pitch axis ($\varnothing_Y$) was 17.9 degrees and in the roll axis[22] it was 15.4 degrees. This indicates that 50% of the judgments of head-up fell within an ellipse with a major axis of 35.8 degrees and a minor axis of 30.8 degrees, and 50% fell outside this ellipse. To compare these results with the 'arc of uncertainty' reported by MANN et al., it is necessary to convert the probable error, which is 0.6745 σ degrees to an arc of 1.156 σ degrees and to double this value. Thus the 'ellipse of uncertainty' for the head-up position would be 61 degrees major axis and 53 degrees minor axis. The variable error in the head-up judgments, though

21 Note that although these various positions may be called by different names, i.e., the postural vertical or horizontal, they are all judgments of position relative to true vertical.

22 A position of forward pitch with left-ear-up could be called an error about the x-axis or the z-axis, depending on how the position was attained.

large, was less than the variable error in the head-down judgments, which is consistent with other experiments on the perception of verticality from different positions. However, as NELSON concludes, the data support an otolith model ". . . . in which an initially poor sensitivity in some positions becomes worse in others."

Some of the variability and hence apparent lack of sensitivity in this study may come from the way in which upright position was attained. In response to the observers' hand signals, the experimenters moved the gimbals system "in a best approximation of what was requested, randomly selecting between the alternative axes and/or directions as required." Thus, the change-in-position information did not correspond with the expected change-in-position information, and this probably increased difficulty in making final judgments. The memory of change-in-position sensory data as a contributor to immediate perceptions should not be ignored. It is probably possible for change-in-position information to be negated through inattention or purposeful attention to something else, but the ability of normal subjects and the relative inability of LD observers to retrace a fairly complex path of passive movement (BERITOV, 1959; BARLOW, 1970) suggests the potential importance to present perceptions of the immediate memory of complex vestibular information. Hence, if a fairly weak static position signal is confused by the preceding rate and position information, this could possibly increase variability of judgments.

Nevertheless, if the otoliths were a sensitive and strong indicator of static position, irrespective of preceding *change-in-position* signals, less variability would be expected than NELSON found, and the results seem to justify his conclusion that somatosensory signals must have been quite prominent in those "above-water experiments" which indicate high precision in estimating the postural vertical.

3. Judgment of Postural Position Relative to Gravity with Reduced Vestibular and Somatosensory Cues

Judgments of the postural vertical by LD observers in tilt devices appear to be slightly more variable than judgments made by normal observers. However, the differences in recorded estimates have sometimes been small (GARTEN, 1920; MANN, 1951) and sometimes not statistically significant (CLARK and GRAYBIEL, 1963a).

The effects of delay in a position of tilt prior to estimating the postural vertical were found by CLARK and GRAYBIEL (1964) to increase the differences between normal and LD observers. The fact that adaptation to tilt was found in LD observers indicates that "adaptation effects" of this type are not solely manifestations of vestibular adaptation. Considering the results of water immersion reported by NELSON, the adaptation effects may be a result of a "weak" static contribution from the otoliths to the perception of verticality which is not sufficient to override adaptive changes in somatosensory input.

The orientation ability of blindfolded deaf observers during water immersion has been discussed (JAMES, 1882) and has been studied more recently by PADDEN (1959) in 105 deaf men including some with partial hearing. On the basis of balance tests given prior to water immersion, the deaf observers were further subdivided into those with good balance and those with poor balance. Twenty-four of thirty observers who had lost hearing as a result of meningitis and only four observers whose deafness was attributed to other causes were classified in the poor balance group. None of the normals was so classified, and presumably all of those classified as having good balance also had vestibular function.

Observers in 'tucked position' were dropped into a pool in various entry orientations, and they were scored on the time required to swim to the surface. Immediate swimming was required to reduce buoyancy cues. In the first twenty trials, eyes were open, and in the second twenty trials, a blindfold was used. Time scores for the poor balance group and for the meningitis group differed significantly from all other groups, but this was true both with eyes open and with eyes closed conditions. However, trials were not included in the averages when observers, due to confusion, removed face masks or touched the sides or the bottom of the pool and thus failed to meet the criterion of unaided surfacing. Only observers in the poor-balance group and the meningitis group made these kinds of errors. Note that a person without position sense (or memory for a change in position) would have almost a 50% chance for surfacing, since almost half of all directions would lead to the surface. The least direct route would, of course, take more time, but slight buoyancy cues might permit better than chance performance; and even without buoyancy cues, occasional efficient surfacing should be expected by a person who is totally without orientation sensitivity. It appears from this study that the vestibular system improves spatial orientation during water immersion although other interpretations of the results are possible.

4. Ability to Indicate Vertical from Static Tilt Positions with Somatosensory Cues Attenuated

In experiments described in the two preceding sections, perceptions of verticality were obtained by measuring how the subject positioned his head and body in attempting to achieve prescribed goal positions. In this section, experiments are described in which the body remains fixed in position while the perception of the vertical (or horizontal) is indicated by the positioning of a line on a rod or by hand signals.

Variability of performance is subject to interpretation as an index of sensitivity, especially when this method is used. For example, a person without any sensory basis for detection of position relative to gravity might decide always to incline a line at some angle relative to his body. Consequently when judgments are required in spite of inadequate sensory information, responses may be determined by egocentric orientation ability, limb proprioception, interpretation of instructions, et cetera.

The perception of the vertical during water immersion while in various positions of static tilt has been studied by several investigators (Brown, 1961; Graybiel et al., 1968; Ross et al., 1969; Schöne, 1964; Stigler, 1912). Normal observers (with swimming experience) immersed in water at depths of 18–25 feet were asked to point upward from four positions: head-up, head-down, face-down and face-up (Brown, 1961). Immediately prior to positioning for each judgment, observers were given three to five turns (at a rate of about 180 deg/sec) about an earth-horizontal axis. Errors were greatest with the head-down or face-up, and least with the head-up or face-down. Large errors, roughly between 60 to 180 degrees, were made in the head-down and head-back (face-up) positions, but in all positions, the estimates improved considerably when the observer nodded his head and made a second judgment. Following this, all observers swam efficiently to the surface.

This experiment raises several interesting questions. Following rotation of three to five turns, presumably about the z-axis, the semicircular canals would be left in a stimulating position. The axis of rotation was horizontal, and it has been shown that the subjective rotation aftereffects of rotation about an earth-horizontal axis are very brief (GUEDRY, 1965c). Modulation by the position senses (otolith and somatosensory systems) may be responsible for the reduction of these canal-related responses, but this has not been studied with water-immersed observers. In BROWN's study (1961), the first judgment of *static position* may have occurred while the canals were signaling *change-in-position* and thus canal interference with static position signals from the otoliths (as well as 'past-pointing' errors) was probably involved in these initial judgments. UDO DE HAES and SCHÖNE (1970) have reported that postrotational canal responses can influence perception of vertical even without water immersion. The second judgments in BROWN's study may have been improved by increased information derived from the nodding as well as by the decline in 'after-response' of the canals. However, BROWN's results seem to show once again that in certain positions the static position information available from the otoliths is not very strong, especially in the presence of conflicting sensory information from the canals or at least in the absence of synergistic information from the canals and somatosensory system.

SCHÖNE (1964) studied the visual vertical in three observers positioned under water at various inclinations from 0 through 180 degrees. The long axis of the body was constrained in a horizontal position under water by footstraps attached to a footboard and by a biteboard through which air was supplied. The head was tilted backward relative to the body so that the z-axis of the head was approximately 90 degrees to the trunk. Thus when the body was in a prone position, the head was upright, and when the body was in a supine position, the head was inverted. Under these circumstances, three observers adjusted a line of light to apparent verticality, and these estimates of the 'visual vertical' do not appear very different in regard to mean constant errors or variability from those obtained without water immersion, as shown in Fig. 27. However, this appearance may be deceptive because SCHÖNE indicates that during water immersion, the scatter of the judgments increased gradually as $\varnothing_x$ was increased from 0 to 120 degrees and became very great between 150 degrees and 180 degrees. Some observers apparently reported an occasional inversion phenomenon in 180 degree position; i.e., the upward direction was occasionally perceived in the direction of the top of the head, which was actually directed downward. It is possible that the unnatural position of the head relative to the body, together with the reduced somatosensory cues contributed to these phenomena; but in general, the results seem to agree with several previous indications of a poor position sense when the head is inverted. Comparison of the mean accuracy and variability in the experiments of BROWN and SCHÖNE would be misleading because the scales of measurement were quite different. In BROWN's experiment judgments were tabulated to the nearest

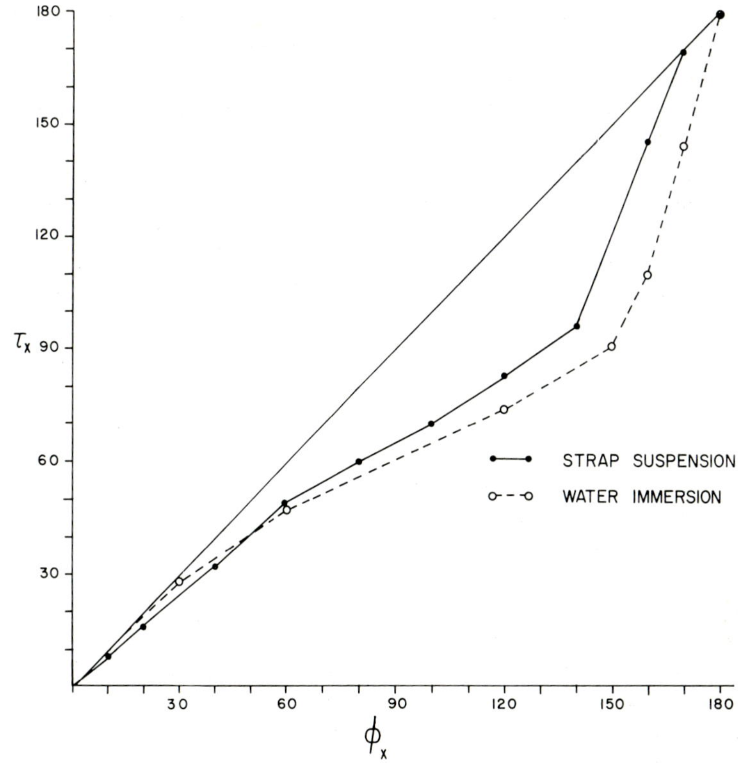

Fig. 27. Comparison of the visual vertical (τ_X) for ($\varnothing_X$) tilts in a normal 1 g field under two conditions: water immersion and suspension by straps without water immersion. Heads of subjects were dorsoflexed almost 90 deg so that rotation of the long axis of body about an earth-horizontal axis rotated the z-axis of the head in the yz plane through $\varnothing_X$ angles between 0 and 180 deg. Adapted from Schöne (1964)

22.5-degree marker, which is greater than the standard errors of measurement indicated by Schöne for most positions. However, both found larger errors and apparently greater variability in the head-down position.

Stigler (1912), in an impressive early study of water-immersed men, concluded that weak orientation information can be disrupted by almost anything including fear or simple distraction.

4.1. *Tilt Devices*

The ability of men without labyrinthine function to adjust a line of light to vertical (or horizontal) in otherwise dark surroundings while seated in various $\varnothing_X$ positions on tilt devices has been studied by a number of investigators (Mann, 1951; Miller and Graybiel, 1963, 1966a; Miller et al., 1966, 1968; Graybiel and Clark, 1965; Feilchenfeld, 1903; Fischer, 1930; Bárány, 1921). The general pattern of results obtained from these observers has been described as qualitatively similar to those yielded by normal observers (Graybiel and Clark, 1965; Miller et al., 1966, 1968). However, it appears that mean constant errors and measures of variability tend to be larger in labyrinthine defective (LD) observers than in normal observers. MILLER et al. (1966) found significant differences in mean settings between normal and LD observers in nine of eighteen different positions of tilt (between $\varnothing_X = \pm 90$ degrees). In many of the remaining positions there were significant differences between the two groups in measures of variability. Because the standard errors of both groups were fairly large in a number of tilt positions, large between-group differences in mean settings would be required for statistical significance. The experiment of MILLER et al. (1966) afforded 36 chances to compare the size of standard deviations of LD and normal observers in 18 positions of tilt (cf. Fig. 2 in MILLER et al., 1966). The standard deviations of the LD observers were larger than those of the normal subjects in 29 of the 36 comparisons.

Much of the discussion of the perception of the visual vertical in LD observers has centered on the presence or absence of Müller or Aubert effects. It is clear that these effects occur in LD observers even though ocular counterrolling is minimal (MILLER and GRAYBIEL, 1971), and there are several indications that the subjective effects may be of greater magnitude in LD than in normal observers (MANN, 1951; MILLER et al., 1966, 1968). Normal observers vary to the extent that they see the Müller and/or Aubert effects, and they differ in the exact $\varnothing_X$ tilt positions at which these effects are present (MILLER et al., 1965a; HOWARD and TEMPLETON, 1966, p. 191f). Nevertheless, the mean pattern in ten normal observers seems fairly consistent as shown in Fig. 28, whereas the mean pattern in ten LD observers was less consistent. Any judgment, other than one which is accurate, will by definition contribute to either a Müller or an Aubert effect, and therefore only statistically significant differences from settings made at zero tilt should be considered. However, LD subjects, while seated on a tilt chair, seem to yield results that may be classified as Müller or Aubert phenomena, and this finding plus indications that conditions other than head tilt influence these phenomena suggests the importance of systems other than the labyrinth (WERNER et al., 1951) to these phenomena. The labyrinth appears to contribute some stability to the judgments at each position and in this way permits a clear manifestation of the shift from the Müller effect to the Aubert effect as $\varnothing_X$ tilt increases.

TEUBER (1960, p. 1631) has summarized several experiments which indicate that the Müller effect is exaggerated in individuals with frontal and frontoparietal lesions. (Also see HOWARD and TEMPLETON, 1966, pp. 211–212.)

4.2. Standing Positions

Results obtained with observers in standing position with various configurations of head relative to trunk and leg tilt have been reported by CLARK and GRAYBIEL (1967, 1968). Under these circumstances the results of five LD and five normal observers were not significantly different in regard to either constant errors or variability of the visual horizontal, and the Müller effect was not manifested by either group. With a maximum of 20 degrees $\varnothing_X$ tilt relative to gravity (CLARK and GRAYBIEL, 1967) or to the resultant vector (CLARK and GRAYBIEL, 1968) a Müller effect was not necessarily to be expected (cf. BAUERMEISTER, 1964; MILLER et al., 1966; SCHÖNE, 1964). The data of CLARK and GRAYBIEL suggest that information from the somatosensory system when the person is in a standing position is sufficient to overcome the occasional differences noted between seated LD and

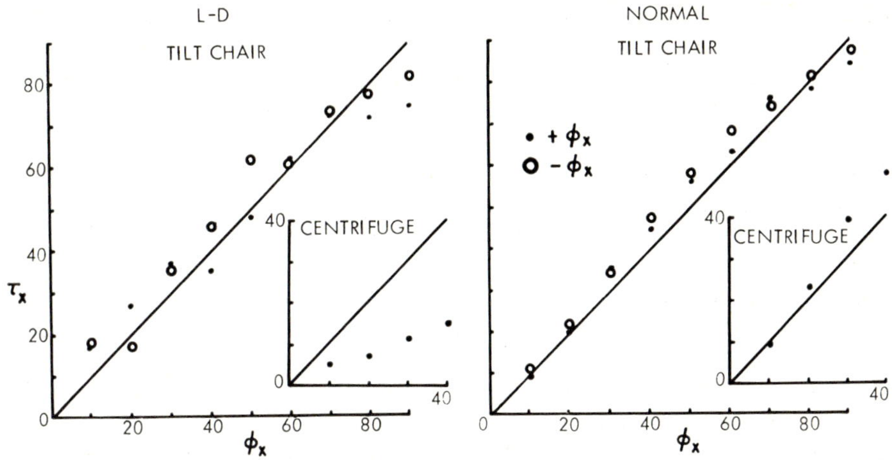

Fig. 28. Comparison of the visual vertical (τ_x) in LD observers, men with little or no vestibular function, and in normal observers when the "tilts" were produced by a tilt chair and by a centrifuge. Adapted from Graybiel and Clark (1965) and from Miller et al. (1966)

normal observers in the judgment of the visual vertical (or horizontal) from positions of 20-degree $\varnothing_x$ tilt, and the findings are in general agreement with other indications that sensory inputs from the limbs and joints are sensitive contributors to postural adjustments relative to gravity (Roberts, 1967; Birren, 1945; Howard and Templeton, 1966).

4.3. Centrifuge Studies

Perception of the apparent visual vertical and horizontal on the human centrifuge, frequently called the oculogravic illusion, has been studied in LD observers. Kreidl (1892; Mach, 1902, p. 159) noted that this "illusion" was not present in about 20% of a group of deaf persons. As was indicated in the previous section, no significant difference was found between LD and normal observers in regard to the oculogravic illusion when observers were in standing position and exposed to steady state $\varnothing_x$ body tilts of 20 degrees. However, with observers seated upright relative to gravity on the centrifuge and $\varnothing_x$ tilts of 0, 10, 20, 30, and 40 degrees relative to the resultant force, Graybiel and Clark (1965) found pronounced differences in the mean settings of nine normal and ten LD observers. The mean inclination of the target line was about 1/3 of the inclination of the resultant vector relative to the body in LD observers, whereas in normal observers, mean settings approximately matched the resultant. Between-subject variability among the LD observers was pronounced, with some LD observers not too different and others differing conspicuously from mean normal data. The standard deviations of individual LD observers for any one condition appeared to be no greater than those of normal observers. Thus LD observers positioned the line fairly consistently relative to the body for each condition, although different LD observers chose different criteria for 'egocentric' positioning of the line relative to the body. In a subsequent experiment comparing four normal and four LD observers during partial water immersion (GRAYBIEL et al., 1968) on a centrifuge, the mean inclination of the line was much less than the $\varnothing_X$ tilts of 10, 20, and 30 degrees relative to the force field in the LD observers.[23] In three of the four normal observers, the mean inclinations of the line closely approximated the $\varnothing_X$ tilt. The odd 'normal' observer gave responses that were not related to the $\varnothing_X$ tilts, and although he had normal caloric responses and ocular counterrolling, his oculogravic response curves resembled those of the LD observers.

Estimates of the visual vertical by LD observers made while tilted relative to gravity and made while tilted relative to the resultant force on a centrifuge appear to be curiously different, as shown in Fig. 28. When LD observers in a chair are tilted between 10 and 40 degrees relative to gravity about the x-axis, they tend to set a luminous line in the opposite quadrant (MANN, 1951; MILLER et al., 1966) in estimating verticality. This error bias is in the direction of the Müller effect. Presumably they feel tilted more than the actual $\varnothing_X$ tilt and thus offset the line more than $\varnothing_X$ degrees from the body. However, when $\varnothing_X$ tilts between 10 and 40 degrees are accomplished by the centrifuge, LD observers tend to set the line between the 'resultant vertical' and the body. This error is in the direction of the Aubert effect. Presumably under these circumstances they feel tilted less than the $\varnothing_X$ tilt and thus offset the line less than $\varnothing_X$ degrees from the body. Such reasoning is open to question because normal observers, when tilted $\varnothing_X$ of 90 degrees relative to gravity without water immersion, feel tilted more than 90 degrees; yet in estimating the visual vertical, they offset the luminous line less than 90 degrees from the body (the Aubert effect). In other words, the line is inclined in the direction of body tilt. Nevertheless, the difference in accuracy of estimation by LD observers of $\varnothing_X$ tilts produced by the tilt chair and by the centrifuge indicates that the change-in-$\varnothing_X$ cues afforded by the tilt chair during the tilting process were fairly accurately assessed by the somatosensory system, whereas the change-in-$\varnothing_X$ cues afforded by the centrifuge were less accurately sensed, and the underestimation by the LD may come from the inadequacy of static tilt cues, once final $\varnothing_X$ position is attained. However, after one hour exposure to $\varnothing_X$ tilt on a centrifuge, the judgments of LD observers are not significantly different from those of normal observers (CLARK and GRAYBIEL, 1966b). Perhaps the static position cues with the higher force field are initially strange but become more useful with experience in the tilt position.

D. Influence of the Magnitude of a Static Force Field on the Perception of Tilt

Experiments in which the magnitude of the force field is varied while its direction is fixed relative to the head permit inferences about the plane of sensitivity of the otoliths.

Most of the experiments relevant to this subject fall under one of two stimulus-response paradigms. In paradigm 2 of Fig. 29, the observer is placed in various positions of $\varnothing_X$ tilt relative to the field, and in each position the force field is varied

23 In the earlier experiment without water immersion, three of these LD observers had shown no "oculogravic effect." However, with subsequent practice, two of them exhibited change toward a 'normal' response.

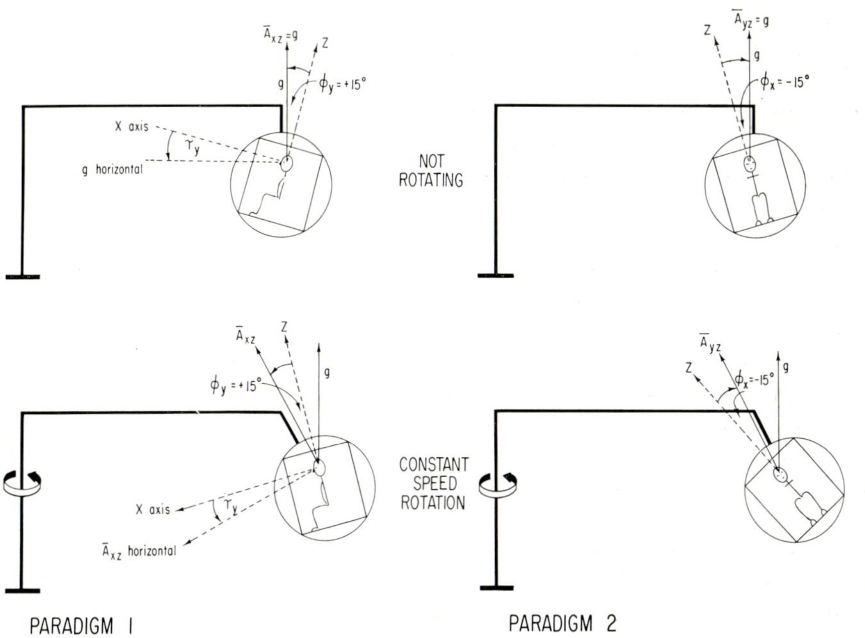

Fig. 29. Illustrating two experimental paradigms used for studying effects of the magnitude of a static force field on perception of the visual vertical (or horizontal) for a given degree of tilt relative to the force field

in magnitude. The perception of lateral tilt in each combination of position and magnitude is measured by having the subject set a line of light to apparent vertical. The symbol, τ_x, is used herein for the angular displacement of the perceptually vertical line from the observer's z-axis. This is the same as the measurement of the visual vertical or the oculogravic illusion described above. These experiments have been carried out on centrifuges with the observer facing in a tangential direction. To achieve different $\varnothing_x$ tilts, the observer is positioned relative to a capsule which is then allowed to swing like a pendulum into alignment with the resultant force.

In paradigm 1 of Fig. 29, the observer is on a centrifuge facing in a radial direction, toward or away from the center of rotation. When facing toward the center, the observer will feel tilted backward about a $\varnothing_y$ axis commensurate with the angular displacement of his z-axis relative to the $\bar{A}_{xz}$ vector, and a spot or line of light fixed in relation to the observer will appear to be displaced upward. If, for example, the light appeared initially at eye level so that the observer believed the line of regard between eyes and light to be approximately horizontal, with the addition of the centripetal acceleration vector, the observer will experience an 'uphill' inclination of the line of regard between the eyes and the light. The symbol used herein for this apparent angular displacement of the light is τ_y, and it has been measured by asking the subject to adjust the position of the light until the line of regard between eyes and light again seems horizontal. The angular displacement between the observer's x-axis and the line of regard from the eyes to the light after the adjustment is τ_y.

1. Magnitude Effects on τ_y Perceptions

In several studies (SCHÖNE, 1964; CORREIA et al., 1965, 1968) involving paradigm 1, it has been found that when the resultant force vector, A_{xz}, was maintained perpendicular to the estimated average plane of the utricle, τ_y did not vary, as the magnitude of $\bar{A}_{xz}$ was increased. This occurred when the z-axis of the head was tilted about 30 degrees forward relative to the resultant force, i.e., $\varnothing_y =$ 30 degrees. Under these circumstances, SCHÖNE (1964) reported an unchanging τ_y tilt of about 24 degrees, and CORREIA et al. (1968) reported an unchanging τ_y tilt of about 30 degrees.[24] However, in other $\varnothing_y$ positions, the apparent tilt τ_y varied as the magnitude changed. In other words, a person tilted backward 15 degrees ($\varnothing_y = +15$ degrees) relative to gravity gave a set of τ_y estimates which differed from those yielded when he was tilted backward 15 degrees ($\varnothing_y =$ 15 degrees) relative to a 1.4 g force field.

One fairly simple explanation of such results assumes that the utricular shear component controls tilt information available from the otoliths and that the saccule may be ignored (cf. VON HOLST, 1950a; SCHÖNE, 1964; MEIRY, 1965). If the average plane of the utricle is 30 degrees above the x-axis of the head and the head and body are inclined forward 30 degrees ($\varnothing_y = -30$ degrees), then the resultant, $\bar{A}_{xz}$, is perpendicular to the utricle, and the utricular shear component, which is given $\bar{A}_{xz} \sin(\varnothing_y + 30$ degrees), will be zero, irrespective of changes in the magnitude of the resultant force, $\bar{A}_{xz}$. Under these circumstances, the observer experiences forward tilt of about 30 degrees, irrespective of the magnitude of $\bar{A}_{xz}$ (cf. SCHÖNE, 1964; CORREIA et al., 1968). However, if the head is tilted forward only 15 degrees so that $\varnothing_y = -15$ degrees, then the shear component, $\bar{A}_{xz} \sin(-15 \text{ deg} + 30 \text{ deg})$, will vary with changes in magnitude of $\bar{A}_{xz}$, as illustrated in Fig. 30. Thus when $\varnothing_y = 15$ deg, a change in the perceived tilt, τ_y, is to be expected with a change in the magnitude of the force field, $\bar{A}_{xz}$. Under these circumstances, SCHÖNE (1964) found that the perceived inclination changes from a forward tilt of about 8 degrees when $\bar{A}_{xz} = 1$ g to a perceived backward tilt of about 7 degrees when $\bar{A}_{xz} = 2$ g.

SCHÖNE reported a linear relationship between τ_y, the perceived inclination, and the magnitude of the utricular-shear components as produced by $\bar{A}_{xz}$ linear acceleration of magnitudes between 1 and 2 g directed between $\varnothing_y = -1$ deg and $\varnothing_y = -35.0$ deg. As the calculated utricular shear component was varied between -0.2 g (forward displaced otoliths) and $+0.9$ g (backward displaced otoliths), there was a directly proportional change in the subjective inclination.[25] Within a comparable range of $\bar{A}_{xz}$ directions and magnitudes, CORREIA et al. (1965, 1968) obtained results similar to those reported by SCHÖNE, as shown in Fig. 30. How-

24 The difference in τ_y when $\varnothing_y = 30$ degrees is probably attributable to instructions and devices for indicating the subjective effects. The fact that τ_y was unchanging at $\varnothing_y = 30$ degrees in both experiments is significant.

25 Indicated directions of the shear components are consistent with those of CORREIA et al. (1968) and opposite those of SCHÖNE, whose vectors show direction of otolith displacement.

ever, the experiment of CORREIA et al. included observations between $\varnothing_y = -30$ deg and $\varnothing_y = +30$ deg, and thus the calculated average shear component was varied between 0 and —1.7 g (backward displaced otoliths). When $\bar{A}_{xz}$ is varied between 1 and 2 g, the calculated shear component varies between 0.7 g and 1.4 g when $\varnothing_y = +15$ deg and between 0.9 g and 1.7 g when $\varnothing_y = +30$ deg. Within these ranges the results obtained by CORREIA et al. exhibit prominent systematic departures from the values predicted by SCHÖNE's equation based upon the magnitude of the utricular shear component.

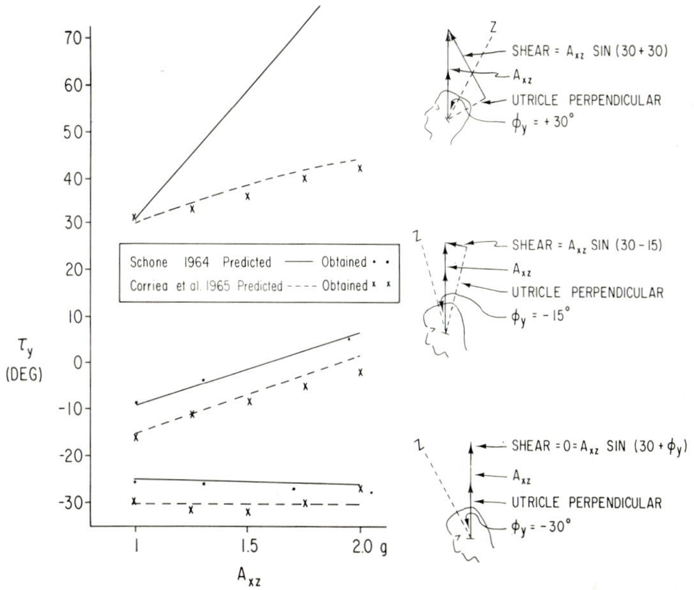

Fig. 30. Effects of change in magnitude of the force field on apparent pitch angle τ_y with the utricle in different positions relative to the force field. Adapted from SCHÖNE (1964) and CORREIA et al. (1965, 1968)

There are many possible explanations for this deviation from the 'utricular-shear' hypothesis. CORREIA et al. suggested that the utricular shear component stimulates the hair cells but that the 'utricular compression component,' which is given by $\bar{A}_{xz} \cos \varnothing_y$, may modify results so that the $\bar{A}_{xz} \tan \varnothing_y$ function yields an empirical fit to the data. Possible mechanisms by which the $\bar{A}_{xz} \cos \varnothing_y$ component might influence the results are through compression effects on the utricle, or shear effects on the anterior portions of the utricle, which slopes upward rather steeply from the posterior part of the utricle, or shear effects on the saccule, or effects on the somatosensory system. Another possibility is that utricular shear components approaching magnitudes of 1 g are approaching a physiological limit (SCHÖNE and PARKER, 1967; SCHÖNE et al., 1967) beyond which tilt signals are not generated in appropriate magnitudes.

2. Magnitude Effects on τ_x Perceptions (Paradigm 2)

There have been a number of studies of magnitude effects on the visual vertical (the oculogravic illusion) in which the observer has been tilted laterally ($\varnothing_x$) relative to the resultant force field (COLENBRANDER, 1963–1964; SCHÖNE, 1964; MILLER and GRAYBIEL, 1966b; CORREIA et al., 1965, 1968; SCHÖNE and PARKER, 1967; SCHÖNE et al., 1967; SCHÖNE and UDO DE HAES, 1971). Several of these studies (MILLER and GRAYBIEL, 1966b; COLENBRANDER, 1963–1964; CORREIA et al., 1968) have shown that the subjective vertical, τ_x, is unchanged by changes in magnitude of $\bar{A}_{yz}$ when $\varnothing_x = 0$. In other words, when the z-axis of the head is aligned with the resultant force vector, $\bar{A}_{yz}$, then a line of light, colinear with $\bar{A}_{yz}$, appears vertical ($\tau_x = 0$) irrespective of changes in the magnitude of $\bar{A}_{yz}$. Under these conditions, the line may appear to be elevated, i.e., there are τ_y changes as noted in the previous section, but it does not appear to tilt laterally ($\tau_x = 0$). From this it has been assumed that man's y-axis is parallel to the average plane of the two utricles and thus, lateral shear would be zero when $\varnothing_x$ is zero, irrespective of the magnitude of $\bar{A}_{yz}$.

When $\varnothing_x \neq 0$, then lateral utricular shear, as calculated by $|\bar{A}_{yz}| \sin \varnothing_x$, changes with differences in magnitude of $\bar{A}_{yz}$, which therefore should influence the subjective vertical, τ_x, even when $\varnothing_x$ is constant.

The fact that τ_x perceptions do change with changes in magnitude of $\bar{A}_{yz}$ when $\varnothing_x$ is constant has been demonstrated by everyone who has studied this situation. SCHÖNE (1964) reported results for various $\varnothing_x$ tilts between 0 and 180 degrees when the $\varnothing_x$ tilts were relative to gravity ($\bar{A}_{yz} = 1$ g) and when the $\varnothing_x$ tilts were relative to a 2 g resultant force. Data obtained when the force field was 2 g ($\bar{A}_{yz} = 2$ g) by several other investigators over a lesser range of $\varnothing_x$ positions [$\varnothing_x = \pm 30$ deg for CORREIA et al. (1968) and $\varnothing_x = \pm 40$ deg for MILLER and GRAYBIEL (1966b)] are in good agreement with SCHÖNE's 2 g results, but they deviate markedly from τ_x values calculated from SCHÖNE's equation, $\tau_x =$ (64 deg/g) $|\bar{A}_{yz}| \sin \varnothing_x$, where $|\bar{A}_{yz}| \sin \varnothing_x$ is the utricular shear component and (64 deg/g) is a constant estimated by SCHÖNE (1964).

Figure 31, adapted from CORREIA et al. (1965), illustrates that in each of several experiments, the τ_x values for a given $\varnothing_x$ tilt increase as $\bar{A}_{yz}$ increases, but the change in τ_x is not linearly related to the change in the utricular shear component; the slope of the relationships between τ_x and $|\bar{A}_{yz}| \sin \varnothing_x$ is progressively less as the magnitude of $\bar{A}_{yz}$ increases. As with the $\varnothing_y/\tau_y$ relationships, CORREIA et al. (1968) have shown that a tangent function affords a better fit to the data than does a sine function. However, for the greater $\varnothing_x$ tilts, the slopes of the response curves appear to be systematically less than the appropriate segment of the tangent curve shown in Fig. 32. Thus the τ_x data do not seem to fit a tangent function as closely as do the τ_y data.[26]

It has been suggested (SCHÖNE et al., 1967; SCHÖNE and PARKER, 1967) that some kind of saturation effect influences the neural input when the shear component exceeds 0.8 g. Under natural conditions of static tilt, the average utricular shear component would range between 0 g, for positions in which A is normal to

26 This is true for the τ_x and τ_y data of CORREIA et al., and the τ_x data of MILLER and GRAYBIEL. However, τ_x data obtained by COLENBRANDER (1963–1964) fit the tangent function fairly well (cf. CORREIA et al., 1968).

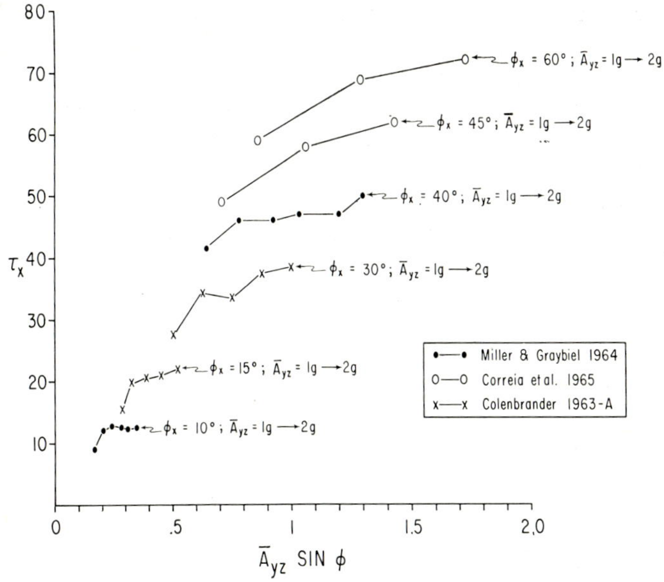

Fig. 31. Effects of variation in force field magnitude between 1 and 2 g on the visual vertical (τ_x) at different positions of lateral tilt relative to the field. The same utricular shear component (A_{yz} sin $\varnothing_x$) can give different results at different $\varnothing_x$ tilts. Adapted from CORREIA et al. (1965, 1968)

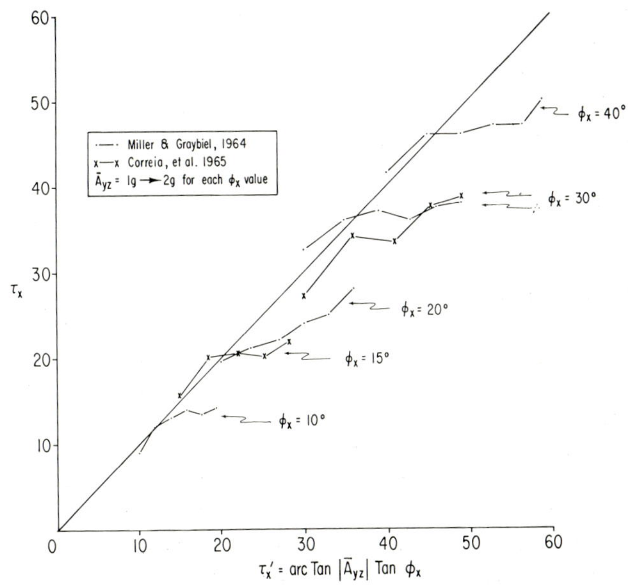

Fig. 32. Relationship between τ_x perceptions and predictions based upon a tangent function. The τ_x data shown here seem to show less conformity with the tangent model than did the τ_y data. Adapted from CORREIA et al. (1965, 1968)

the utricular plane, and 1 g for positions in which A is aligned with the utricular plane. Increasing $\varnothing$ beyond this latter point would not increase the shear component, but rather the shear component would be decreased. It is possible that rates and patterns of neural discharges change as much as they can when the shear component is varied between 0 and 1 g, and any increase in the shear component beyond 1 g has no physiological significance for the perception of tilt. However, even though saturation effects or physiological limits seem reasonable, it does not appear that a saturation effect added to the simple 'utricle shear' hypothesis is sufficient to account for the fact that there are a number of examples in Fig. 31 of equal utricular shear components, produced by different combinations of magnitude and direction of the force field, which yielded different τ_x judgments.

The suggestion that physiological limits are reached at some magnitude of the utricular shear component involves unknowns all the way from utricular and saccular mechanics and the composite pattern of the sensory message they generate to the processing of this message by the central nervous system. However, the work of FLUUR et al. (FLUUR, 1970; FLUUR and MELLSTRÖM, 1970a, b; BRANDT and FLUUR, 1967a, b) suggests both utricular and saccular influence on ocular displacement, and hence both may also be reflected in perceptual judgments. There is a potential difference between τ_x and τ_y perceptions based on the possibility that the saccule plays a role in the perception of tilt. With $\varnothing_x$ tilts, the saccular shear component is approximated by $\bar{A}_{yz}$ cos $\varnothing_x$ whereas the utricular shear component is $\bar{A}_{yz}$ sin $\varnothing_x$. In a natural environment, the increase in $\varnothing_x$ tilt between 0 and 90 degrees would be associated with an increasing utricular shear component, but with a *decreasing* saccular shear component. The observed increase in τ_x when $\bar{A}_{yz}$ is increased while $\varnothing_x$ is constant may be attributable to the increased utricular shear component, but the fact that this increase is less than would be expected on the basis of the utricular shear component may be due to the increased saccular shear component. In other words, the increased utricular shear, which is normally associated with perception of increased $\varnothing_x$ tilt, and the increased saccular shear, which is normally associated with perception of decreased $\varnothing_x$ tilt, yields a compromise perception of slightly increased tilt when the magnitude of the force field is increased. On the other hand, during natural $\varnothing_y$ tilts an increasing utricular shear component would not be accompanied by a simple increase or decrease in the saccular shear signal, but rather by a changing pattern signifying a rotation of the direction shear vector in the saccular plane.

The assumption that saturation is reached when the shear component in the utricle approaches 1 g can also be applied to the saccule. In effect, this assumption implies that the proportionality between the shear component and the tilt information diminishes (due to saturation effects in the end-organ or CNS or both) as the average plane of the otolith macula, utricular or saccular, comes into alignment with gravity. This is tantamount to saying that when the plane of one otolith macula, e.g., the utricle, approaches alignment with gravity, it is the other otolith macula, e.g., the saccule, which serves as the more sensitive vestibular tilt indicator because the latter will be exposed to changes in shear components within its linear range of sensitivity. This system could explain the fact that when $\varnothing_x =$ 10 degrees, τ_x increases fairly sharply as $\bar{A}_{yz}$ is increased from 1 to 2 g. Utricular shear increases approximately in a linear relation to $\bar{A}_{yz}$, but the saccule is in its insensitive range and the increase in saccular shear diminishes τ_x only slightly. For higher values of $\varnothing_x$, the utricle begins to operate out of its linear range as $\bar{A}_{yz}$ is increased, but the saccule begins to operate within its range of maximum sensitivity. Thus the increased saccular shear component becomes more effective in reducing τ_x as $\bar{A}_{yz}$ increases. As SCHÖNE and PARKER (1967) have recently demonstrated, when $\varnothing_x = 75$ degrees, changes in $\bar{A}_{yz}$ between 1 and 2 g do not increase τ_x (τ_x is constant). When $\varnothing_x > 75$ degrees, τ_x actually diminishes as $\bar{A}_{yz}$ is increased between 1 and 1.8 g. The fact that τ_x does not change with changes in $\bar{A}_{yz}$ when $\varnothing_x = 75$ degrees could be interpreted as a point at which utricular shear "saturates," but the utricular shear hypothesis (without reference to the saccule or other external influences) cannot explain the fact that equivalent utricular shear components less than .8 g can yield different τ_x perceptions.

The utricular/saccular shear hypothesis can account for both the flattening of the $\tau_x/\bar{A}_{yz}$ relationship with higher values of $\varnothing_x$ and the discontinuities in the $\tau_x/\bar{A}_{yz} \sin \varnothing_x$ relationship with lower as well as higher values of $\varnothing_x$.

The constancy of τ_x when $\varnothing_x = 75$ degrees, can be interpreted in several ways within the context of the preceding assumption regarding the joint contributions of the saccule and utricle to τ_x perceptions. Considering only one ear, it may be assumed that the saccule is about 15 degrees out of the yz (sagittal) plane. Thus, when $\varnothing_x = 75$ degrees, $\bar{A}_{yz}$ would be normal to the saccular plane, and changes in $\bar{A}_{yz}$ would not change saccular shear. However, the plane of the saccule in the other ear would be 30 degrees angularly displaced from $\bar{A}_{yz}$, but inverted. Perhaps the inverted saccule is of lesser significance to the perception of tilt, a reasonable assumption from some of the threshold studies reviewed above, and from the distinct possibility that an inverted otolith system tilted by a given angle signals less tilt than an upright otolith system tilted by the same angle. The number of assumptions and speculations which are required is large, but it would appear that some of these assumptions could be tested by additional data, especially neurophysiological data in which the 'dynamics' and 'statics' of the stimulus are carefully specified relative to a well-defined anatomical coordinate system.

3. Perception of Vertical when the Effective Force Field is near Zero

There have been a few experiments carried out on ocular counterrolling (MILLER et al., 1965b; KELLOGG, 1971) and perception of verticality (HAMMER, 1962; GRAYBIEL and KELLOGG, 1967) when the resultant total force field has been zero or nearly zero. There have been other experiments in which expected "zero-g" results have been extrapolated from data obtained at several g-levels above 1 g (SCHÖNE, 1964; CORREIA et al., 1965). The "zero-g" experiments have been carried out in parabolic aircraft flights or in orbiting spacecraft (GRAYBIEL et al., 1967). At first glance, it appears that the observers were being asked to report "vertical" or "upright" when there was no such thing for reporting, unless one assumes that EINSTEIN's equivalence principle was being questioned. However, such inquiries do not necessarily constitute a challenge to the equivalence principle because it is not unlikely that many observers retain a perceptual vertical when no vertical from a resultant force field is available. The long history of phylogenetic and ontogenetic development in which vertical is a special dimension may not be as quickly discarded by man as it is by inanimate objects that respond in good conformity to Einstein's equivalence principle. Einstein in his disagreement with Mach referred to man's tendency to consider vertical a special dimension (Schilpp, 1951, p. 29), and of course it is this tendency that influences perception. Thus, Einstein would not really have disagreed with Mach's explanation of the oculogravic or somatogravic illusion. In a zero-g state, there are a number of potential determiners of the perception of upright or verticality that may or may not be used at any one moment by an observer:

1. The upper part of the body, the +z direction could be taken as 'up.'

2. The contact of the buttocks with a seat if the observer is strapped in place could be taken as 'down.'

3. The more prominent straight lines in the visual field and/or dials and other visual data that normally have a cognitive upright could determine perceptual vertical and the memory of this direction could be retained for some time.

4. The direction of last seen movement of an object in the vehicle could be remembered as 'down.'

5. An imagined or remembered orientation of the vehicle relative to the earth could be a determiner of verticality estimates.

It is of interest to find out what man will do in such a circumstance, and the answer seems to be that all men do not do the same thing (Graybiel et al., 1967). Instructions, immediately preceding events, and personality might well be determiners of results in such studies. However, flight personnel and particularly the experienced men who are astronauts have been literally trained in the course of flying to accept intellectual instrument information and to ignore their immediate perceptions of verticality (cf. Cullen and Harper, 1969). Hence, it would seem that such individuals might choose any of the several alternatives more readily than other less trained individuals. The readiness or ability to shift from one perceptual set to another has been of considerable interest to psychologists as a form of personality testing in which individuals are classified as visual field-dependent or visual field-independent. The many possibilities available in the weightless environment point to a number of factors that may enter into judgments of verticality on earth.

IV. The Modulation of Vestibular Responses by Intravestibular and Visual-Vestibular Interactions

Sensory interactions involved in the control of whole-body movement and of head and eye orientation during whole-body movement are complex, and some of these interactions are considered in more detail in other chapters of this volume. However, many of the perceptual and physiological reactions discussed under sections on semicircular canal function or otolith function in this chapter are influenced by complex sensory interactions, and it is the purpose of this section to consider several responses that have been attributed to either canal function or otolith function in the light of sensory interactions that are almost certainly involved in their production.

A. Perceptions during Changing Horizontal Linear Acceleration

There have been a number of indications that the otolith system may provide change-in-orientation information (i.e., angular velocity information) as well as gravity-orientation information, and it is important to consider the potential functional contribution of this dual input to discriminations between different states of motion.

During changing horizontal linear acceleration, or horizontal linear oscillation, the resultant of gravity and the imposed horizontal acceleration is a vector that rotates relative to the observer as though the observer were being tilted relative to gravity, yet he experiences linear velocity, and either greatly underestimates (Schöne and Mortag, 1968) the tilt (relative to the resultant vector) or does not experience tilt at all (Guedry and Harris, 1963).

To imagine how the otolith and canal information might be used to discriminate horizontal linear acceleration from tilt, let us assume that an intelligent operator enclosed in a vehicle has two instruments in front of him. One of these instruments (A), the semicircular canals, responds only to angular acceleration; the other (B), the otoliths, indicates orientation relative to gravity, but it also responds to horizontal linear acceleration. Thus, Instrument B indicates "tilt" during horizontal linear acceleration and also when the vehicle is really tilted. Now, if in addition to the operator, there is an external agent who sees what the vehicle is really doing, and he reports to the operator in the vehicle what happens, then in time the operator would know that Instrument B can give the same reading during horizontal linear acceleration and during change in orientation relative to gravity. However, he would notice that during horizontal linear acceleration, Instrument A does not give readings and that during changes in orientation relative to gravity, both A and B do give readings. Thus, with these two instruments, he has a basis for discriminating horizontal linear acceleration of the vehicle from cases where the vehicle is changing orientation relative to gravity. Note that *during onset* of horizontal linear acceleration, the *absence of indication* from Instrument A is as important as the *presence* of information from Instrument B.

However, if the vehicle has been tilted for a while, Instrument B would show a reading while A would not. This also occurs during a constant horizontal linear acceleration, and thus the discrimination of linear acceleration from tilt would not always be possible. How then is the discrimination ever possible? The temporal sequences of information could be used to make some good guesses about what is happening, but if Instrument B has two dials, one that indicates change in tilt and the other that indicates tilt, then a number of different forms of motion can be immediately discriminated without an analysis of temporal sequences of events. If the change-in-tilt dial of B confirms the angular velocity information from A, then tilting is the conclusion. If A indicates zero angular velocity while the change-in-tilt dial of B gives a reading, then the operator deduces that linear acceleration is underway and that no tilt is taking place. If the change-in-tilt dial of B gives little or no reading while the tilt dial of B gives a reading and A indicates zero angular velocity, then the operator concludes static tilt. In this way, change-in-position information and position information from the otoliths may combine in various patterns with angular velocity information from the canals to permit the immediate discrimination by the central nervous system of static tilt, dynamic tilt, and linear velocity. In this analogy, the external observer can be the visual system that operates separately but synergistically with the vestibular system.

This set of assumptions about the information content of various patterns of vestibular inputs and the neural code for discriminating among different states of motion, angular position relative to the earth, and angular displacement is compatible with a number of experimental results, although further assumptions are necessary to explain some observations.

1. The Underestimation of Tilt and Perception of Linear Velocity during a Changing Horizontal Linear Acceleration

A number of experiments carried out with parallel swings and horizontal accelerators have shown that although the observer may be exposed to a considerable tilt relative to a changing resultant linear acceleration vector, he experiences little or no tilt but rather linear velocity during these dynamic stimuli (Guedry and Harris, 1963; Guedry, 1965a; Schöne and Mortag, 1968; Lansberg, 1954; Niven et al., 1966). The explanation offered here is that change-in-position information from the otoliths accompanied by a zero-angular velocity signal from the semicircular canals is the necessary and sufficient vestibular input for the perception of linear velocity of the head and body, and it is not a sufficient input for the quick assessment of tilt. The stimulus is change in linear acceleration without concomitant angular acceleration. During linear oscillation within frequency ranges yet to be specified, normal observers can integrate the available linear velocity data to make fairly accurate estimates of whole-body displacement relative to the earth (von Békésy, 1940; Guedry and Harris, 1963), whereas individuals without labyrinthine function underestimate displacement and report perception of tilt (Guedry and Harris, 1963).

The findings suggest that in the absence of concomitant semicircular canal signal, the velocity of translation of the utricular otolith mass relative to the underlying hair cells is directly proportional to a linear velocity sensation which can be integrated within time limits into accurate linear displacement estimates.

2. Effects of Attention Shifts on Linear Displacement Estimates: Body Reference Versus Visual Reference during Horizontal Linear Oscillation

The close correspondence between estimated and true displacement in normal observers was changed to a gross underestimation when observers watched a small target light, fixed in the capsule relative to their heads, and estimated its linear displacement in a horizontal plane. Reduced estimates, on shifting attention from a body judgment to a visual target judgment, were present despite the observer's awareness of the fixed relation between the target and the body. Visual afterimages and even imagined visual targets are effective in reducing the estimated displacement. These judgments, either of body or target displacement, are not difficult to make, and they change systematically as the true displacement changes. A shift in attention to different sensory components of the perceptual event apparently controls the shift in magnitude of the perceived displacement (Guedry and Harris, 1963). Figure 33 illustrates the effects of the attention shift in 16 normal observers.

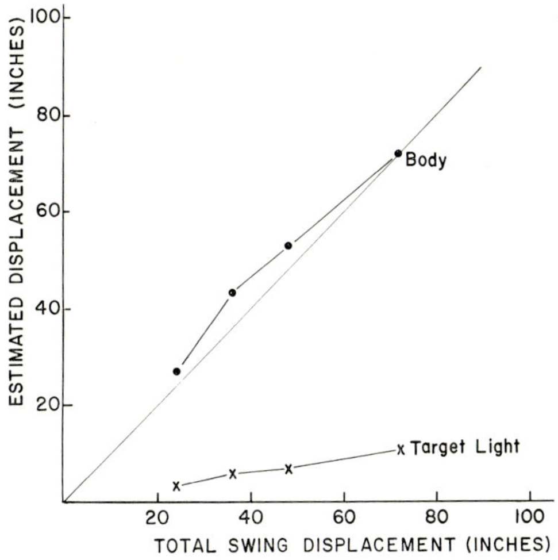

Fig. 33. Estimates of horizontal linear displacement relative to the earth during oscillation (period 3.6 sec) on a parallel swing when the attention was directed toward the body and when the attention was directed toward a line of light fixed relative to the body. Adapted from GUEDRY and HARRIS (1963)

3. The Oculogravic Lag Effect – The Visual Vertical during Intravestibular Conflict

Recent experiments indicate that even with high-magnitude horizontal linear acceleration involving changes (relative to the man) in direction of the resultant force of 77 degrees, observers experience very little tilt (COHEN et al., 1972). These experiments were carried out on a centrifuge with the observer seated upright relative to gravity so that while the resultant linear acceleration vector rotated 77 degrees in the xz plane, there was also a considerable angular acceleration about the z-axis. In this case, the 77-degree change-in-position about the y-axis was not confirmed by synergistic y-axis angular accelerations. Instead of feeling tilted 77 degrees, observers indicated a mean maximum $\varnothing_y$ tilt of less than 7 degrees. Since these studies involved very high-magnitude linear accelerations (more than 4 g-units), the results could not necessarily be estimated by extrapolation from previous studies, but in fact, the results were in good agreement with earlier experiments.

GRAYBIEL and BROWN (1951) and CLARK and GRAYBIEL (1961, 1963b, 1966a) reported a "lag" in oculogravic perceptions of tilt under similar conditions. In these earlier experiments a sustained horizontal linear acceleration was produced by fixing observers upright (z-axis aligned with gravity) on a centrifuge. As centripetal acceleration increased, thereby increasing body tilt relative to the resultant force vector, the observers attempted to set a line of light to apparent vertical (or horizontal). Settings lagged 'far behind' the change in resultant during the 6-sec angular acceleration, and the mean settings approached the resultant tilt of 30 degrees only after about 40–60 sec of constant centripetal acceleration. Such lags in perceived tilt are not present when observers are tilted through

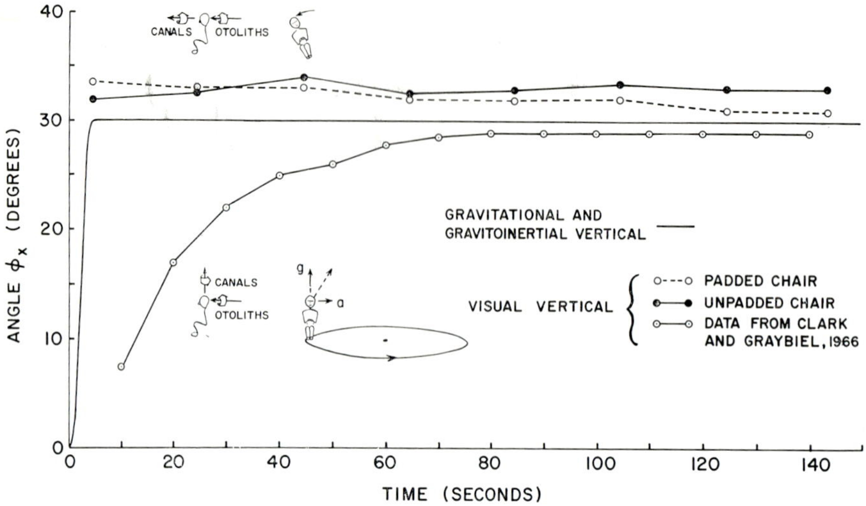

Fig. 34. Comparison of the "lag" in the perception of the visual vertical following tilting in a chair relative to gravity and following tilting relative to the resultant of the centripetal acceleration and gravity vectors on a centrifuge. Adapted from Stockwell and Guedry (1970)

30 degrees in 6 sec about the y-axis with a simple tilt chair (Stockwell and Guedry, 1970) as shown in Fig. 34. Under the latter conditions, semicircular canal data, which can yield accurate angular displacement estimates (Guedry et al., 1971a, b) supplement the otolithic and somatosensory data, and there is no lag in the perception of tilt apparent in the data. However, when tilt was accomplished by rotating the resultant acceleration with the centrifuge, y-axis rate information was generated by the change-in-position of the otoliths while the canals generated conflicting z-axis rate information. This abnormal sensory influx probably accounts for the major part of the initial underestimation. Because the semicircular canal influx decays gradually, it is likely that the gradual increase in the perception of the sustained $\varnothing_y$ tilt is dependent upon the gradual decay of the z-axis angular velocity input from the semicircular canals (Stockwell and Guedry, 1970). Clark and Graybiel (1966a) have shown that visual factors can also contribute some of the perceptual lag, but when the visual contribution is subtracted, there is still a considerable difference between actual and perceived tilt, and the magnitude of the difference follows very closely the time course of the exponential decay of semicircular canal influx as shown in Fig. 35.

It would appear that rate and position information from the otoliths without substantiating canal information can give linear velocity information. Sustained otolith position information attained without initial canal or otolith change-in-position information gives tilt information but only with a slow 'indication' time due to CNS processing. The indication time may be slowed even more if conflicting semicircular canal information is present.

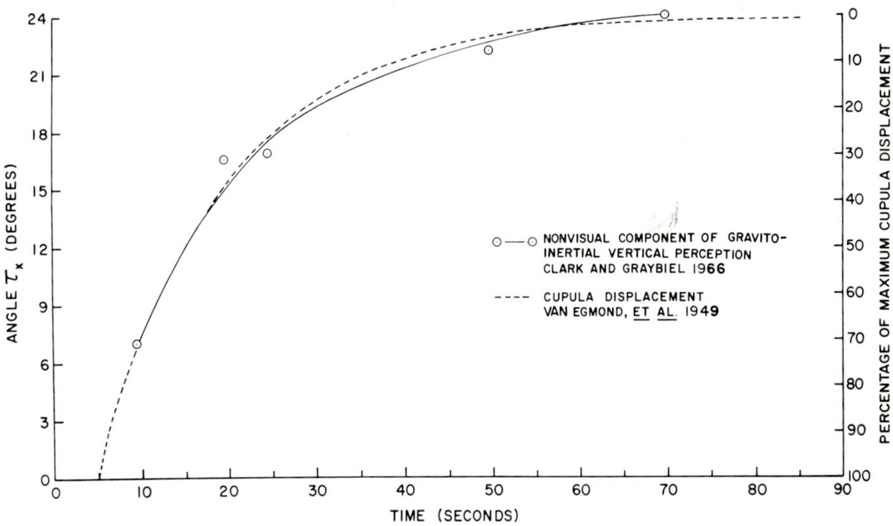

Fig. 35. Illustrating a possible causal relationship between the "lag effect" in the τ_x perception on a centrifuge and the decay in a conflicting $\dot{\psi}_z$ signal from stimulation of the horizontal semicircular canals, assuming a 15-sec long time constant for the horizontal canal response. Adapted from Stockwell and Guedry (1970)

4. Effects of a Visual Frame of Reference – Relation to the Oculogravic Lag Effect

Effects of visual frames on the perception of verticality have been widely studied by having observers set either a line of light (visual vertical) or the body (postural vertical) to upright position while the visible surrounds are tilted (cf. Gibson and Mowrer, 1938). Relatively static conditions have been used in most of these experiments in that either the visual field was stationary while the body was moved slowly to apparent vertical or the visual field and body were stationary while a visible straight line was adjusted to apparent vertical. If a structured visual field is in a tilted position relative to the existing force field, then the mean setting of a line to apparent vertical will lie between the vertical dimensions of the visual display and the direction of the force field. The effect of the visual frame on the visual vertical is dependent upon body tilt position, being least when the body z-axis is upright and greatest when the +z-axis is 150 degrees from upright (Schöne and Udo de Haes, 1971; Udo de Haes and Schöne, 1970). These results coincide with 'accuracy' of visual-vertical settings in different body positions (Schöne, 1964), suggesting that as force field data become less effective, visual field data become more compelling (Young, 1973).

There are large individual differences in the influence of the visual field on visual vertical judgments which may be related to personality (cf. Witkin, 1950; Long, 1972), a possibility which has been vigorously explored under the topic, *field dependence-independence*. In these publications, field dependence means visual-field dependence; i.e., a field-dependent person is one who sets the line more in accord with the visual frame than does the average observer. Some observers seem to be able to shift to any operating mode, e.g., visual field dependent or visual field independent, where the latter can apparently mean force-field-dependent or body-axis-dependent or dependent on the memory of any antecedent event other than the immediate visual field. Dependence on alternatives among non-visual perceptual frames of reference has not been explored extensively, but nevertheless, this general line of work may become a valuable adjunct to the assessment and understanding of personality and its relation to spatial orientation. Results of such studies have been examined for correlation with introversion-extroversion scales and other personality 'dimensions' (REASON and GRAYBIEL, 1972; ANDERSSON et al., 1972; KENNEDY, 1972). It has been claimed that some individuals show a high degree of 'fixity,' suggesting an enduring trait that characterizes their judgments in different situations, in spite of practice and instruction (cf. WITKIN, 1950, 1962; LONG, 1972). However, when the primary interest is examination of average psychophysical relationships, then the magnitude of these individual differences can be reduced by instruction and training on the specific perceptual task (MANN, 1950).

When the force field is tilted relative to both the observer and visual field by use of a centrifuge, then as indicated earlier, there is prolonged lag in the perception of tilt relative to the resultant force. Part of this lag is attributable to the large visual frame which appears less tilted than its angular displacement at the observer's position from the direction of the resultant force. The perceptual property of a large room to appear upright influences the judgments, and it appears from the reactions of people living in tilted buildings (KITAHARA and UNO, 1967) that the property is sustained. The general nature of the effect in centrifuges is probably not different from the effects of other tilt rooms on judgment of the visual vertical. In this case, the centrifuge room is tilted relative to the resultant force field, but it is upright relative to gravity, so it contributes to the "lag effect." The tendency to see the room as upright is thus comparable to the tendency to see other tilted rooms as upright (visual-field dependence), but in this case it may be stronger because of the fact that the process of tilting was accomplished with antisynergistic z-axis semicircular canal stimulation in place of synergistic x-axis stimuli, the increased g-load may reduce somatosensory discrimination of tilt, and moreover, in some experiments, observers have known that the room could not tilt relative to gravity. CLARK and GRAYBIEL (1966a) noted that when the room lights were extinguished, then a luminous line could be seen to drift toward a greater tilt position. Repetitive settings of the luminous line to apparent vertical showed a gradual transition toward alignment of the line with the direction of the resultant force. A similar but smaller "lag effect" occurs when the first setting of the line is made after 1 minute of constant velocity rotation in darkness. However, it should be noted that in this case the first setting is fairly close to the direction of the resultant so that this nonvisual component of the "lag effect," as CLARK and GRAYBIEL refer to it, is small. These experiments considered in relation to the findings of STOCKWELL and GUEDRY (1970) indicate that either 1) the misalignment of a structured visual field with the existing force field, or 2) the misalignment of the axis of rotation signaled by the semicircular canals with change-in-position axis signaled by the otoliths can delay the accurate alignment of a luminous line with the existing force field. It is likely also that memory of how tilt was attained as well as memory of body and room alignment, i.e., memory of dynamic sensory data, also influences judgments.

B. Responses during and after Off-Vertical Rotation

There are a number of ways, other than those described in the immediately preceding sections, in which changes in direction and magnitude of linear acceleration vectors can be introduced without introducing coordinated semicircular canal information (cf. Section F.IV. of this volume by BENSON). For example, stimulus variations of this kind can be produced by counterrotation on a centrifuge (GRAYBIEL and JOHNSON, 1963; BENSON et al., 1970) and by horizontal linear oscillation on a track mounted on a rotating centrifuge (NIVEN et al., 1965). A simpler method involves constant velocity rotation about a tilted or horizontal axis. Once the effects of the initial angular acceleration subside, rotation about an off-vertical axis yields continual reorientation of the head and body relative to gravity, and several responses during this kind of stimulation are noteworthy.

1. Nystagmus, Position-Signaling, and the Perceived Path of Body Movement during Off-Vertical Rotation

During constant angular velocity within certain ranges, nystagmus and the sensation of rotation persist much longer than is expected from theoretical cupula deflection, and from comparison with responses to rotation about a vertical axis (GUEDRY, 1965c; BENSON and BODIN, 1966a). The unidirectional nystagmus persisting beyond the expected response has been referred to as response bias, and the fact that the slow phase velocity fluctuates sinusoidally during each cycle has been referred to as cyclic modulation. During rotation about a horizontal axis, individuals without labyrinthine function do not experience true rotation, but typically report a conical path of body motion but without a sense of turning (like a Ferris wheel), and they do not exhibit a nystagmus response bias (GUEDRY, 1965c). In contrast, individuals with normal vestibular function report true rotation and can render consistent signals of nose-up and nose-down positions (GUEDRY, 1965c; CORREIA and GUEDRY, 1966). According to BENSON (BENSON and BARNES, 1973; BENSON et al., 1971), position signals during constant speed rotation about a tilted axis are phase advanced about 30 degrees relative to true position within a velocity range of 2 deg/sec to 100 deg/sec; otherwise expressed, within the frequency range .005 cps and 0.28 cps, there is a constant 30-degree 'lead effect' instead of a 'lag effect.'

At a higher rotation rate (180 deg/sec or 0.5 cps) about a horizontal axis, the ability to render consistent position signals and the experience of true rotation are present during the initial acceleration, and for about 45 sec afterward, but then the motion experiences become identical to those reported by individuals without labyrinthine function, consistent position signals are no longer given, and this change in experience coincides with the decay of the nystagmus velocity to the zero baseline (CORREIA and GUEDRY, 1966). At 180 deg/sec there appears to be very little nystagmus response bias because nystagmus decays, after the angular acceleration, at a normal rate, but there is an increased cyclic modulation so that with continued rotation beyond 45 sec, there is a clear direction-reversing nystagmus. Thus the subjective response at 180 deg/sec fits fairly well with the idea that rate information from the semicircular canals coordinated with otolith position and change-in-position information is necessary to the quick, nearly veridical perception of orientation relative to the earth, but the results at lower rotation rates appear to be less in accord with this idea.

To explain the persistent rotation experience, consistent position signaling, and nystagmus at lower rates of off-vertical rotation, it was suggested that the semicircular canals might be stimulated by a unique circular pumping action in which differences in specific gravity between endolymph and perilymph created a traveling constriction around the membranous ring (Benson and Bodin, 1966a). This concomitant canal and otolith input would have accounted for the continuous rotation experience and nystagmus, but in spite of biophysical analyses suggesting its feasibility (Steer, 1970), this idea is not well supported by recent empirical evidence (Correia and Money, 1968). If this idea is discarded, then we must still account for the responses during the lower range of constant speed rotation. Moreover, if constant speed rotation about a horizontal axis gives change-in-position information from the otoliths without coordinated canal information, then how is this situation distinguished from linear velocity sensations that we have also attributed to the otolith rate information accompanied by zero canal signal? It may be that temporal patterning of utricular and saccular signals together with patterns of somatosensory signals is sufficient for this discrimination, but a proposed model of otolith dynamics (Benson and Barnes, 1973; Barnes, 1971) offers a more elegant explanation. It was proposed that at certain rates of rotation about a horizontal axis, the utricular otoliths undergo a sustained twist about the macular center while also maintaining a circular orbital motion around the center of underlying cells. The sustained twist accompanied by the continual motion of hairs is presumed to provide a constant signal of angular velocity. The model then presumes that the otoliths are capable of contributing angular velocity information by virtue of an immediate input pattern generated by the twist of the utricular macula. At higher rotation rates, the model predicts lesser twist of the utricular macula so that nystagmus directional bias is lost, and at this time the apparent rotation sensed by normal observers would be approximately like that experienced by individuals without labyrinthine function (cf. Guedry, 1970a), which is approximately what happens. At lower rates the twist provides velocity information, possibly by modulation of canal-dependent units in the vestibular nuclei (Benson et al., 1970), and this velocity information from central canal units would contribute to the sensation of true rotation, the nystagmus, and it would supplement the otolith position information to permit consistent signaling of position, but with a phase advance due to the twist.

Some observations of Stone and Letko (1964) are not entirely consistent with empirical observations on which this theory is based. They reported a Ferris wheel effect during rotation about an earth-horizontal y-axis which changed from a perceived circular path to an elliptical path and finally to vertical linear oscillation as constant rotation rates were increased from 0 to 360 deg/sec. Similar perceptions were reported for the z-axis. These results deviate from other findings in that the Ferris wheel effect was reported at low rotation rates. What caused these different results? The single observer used by Stone and Letko was water-immersed and he was rotated only in one direction about the z-axis and in one direction about the y-axis. In other experiments (GUEDRY, 1965c) not using water immersion, Ferris wheel effects were not described by normal observers at low rates, but were reported consistently by men without vestibular function and by men with spontaneous nystagmus when they were rotated in a direction to oppose their spontaneous nystagmus. These latter observers reported the Ferris wheel effect and had a direction-reversing nystagmus (a cyclic modulation and zero bias) when rotated in one direction, but when rotated in opposite direction, they reported true rotation which was accompanied by a continuous nystagmus. It is apparent that differences in somatosensory cues are not sufficient to account for the presence or absence of the Ferris wheel effects in these various experiments. Possibly the single observer in the STONE and LETKO experiment had spontaneous nystagmus and was rotated in an opposing direction during the z-axis observations, and possibly there is a Ferris wheel effect during low-velocity rotation about an earth-horizontal y-axis. Because there is a difference in vertical nystagmus of opposite directions (BENSON and GUEDRY, 1971), perceptions during rotation in both directions about the y-axis must be investigated. The issue remains unresolved.

2. Detection of Wobble during Constant Speed Off-Vertical Rotation

BENSON et al. (1971) reported that during constant angular velocity, if the rotation axis is gradually tilted, the detection of tilt (or wobble) improves in proportion to the magnitude of constant angular velocity, the range investigated being between 2 deg/sec and 300 deg/sec. During rotation about a tilted axis, the three-dimensional path of body motion perceived may be described approximately as a cone, and the dynamic sensation of motion may be best described as 'wobble.' Recall that the amplitude of the cyclic modulation of nystagmus increases, whereas the nystagmus bias decreases as the magnitude of constant angular velocity is varied within the range of 60 deg/sec to 180 deg/sec. Sensitivity to detection of tilt or wobble reported by BENSON et al. (1971) appears to be correlated with the amplitude of the cyclic modulation of nystagmus, whereas the experience of continuous rotation and the ability to render consistent signals of position during constant speed rotation about a horizontal axis appear to be correlated to the bias component (CORREIA and GUEDRY, 1966).

3. Responses Produced by Deceleration from Off-Vertical Rotation Compared with Caloric Responses

When prolonged rotation about an off-vertical axis stops, the angular deceleration stimulates the semicircular canals in one direction while change-in-position information of opposite sign is generated by the otoliths until the deceleration ends, and then the fixed-position signals and zero rate signals from the otoliths are in conflict with the continuing velocity information from the canals. The conflict involves a number of systems because the sensory message from these two systems normally serves to set up coordinated postural reflexes, but under these conditions the different components of the vestibular sensory message are calling for concomitant postural reflexes in different directions.

During deceleration (e.g., from 60 deg/sec in 3 sec), the ongoing nystagmus (the bias component) stops and reverses direction, and the subjective reaction is unpleasant. The after-sensation of rotating in opposite direction decays very

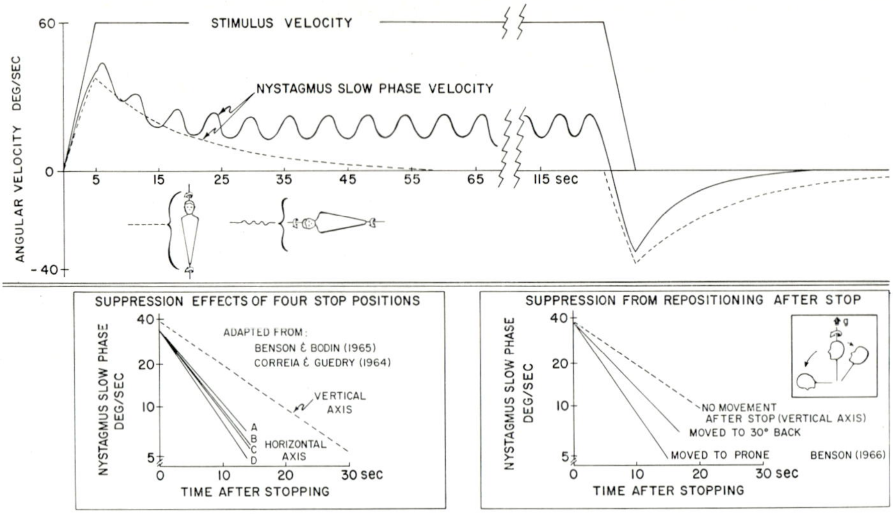

Fig. 36a. Upper Panel: Schematic illustration of pre- and postrotational slow-phase velocity of nystagmus when the axis of rotation is vertical and when it is horizontal. Note cyclic modulation and response bias when the axis is horizontal (solid lines). Lower panels illustrate postrotational suppression effects of different stopping positions. From GUEDRY (1970)

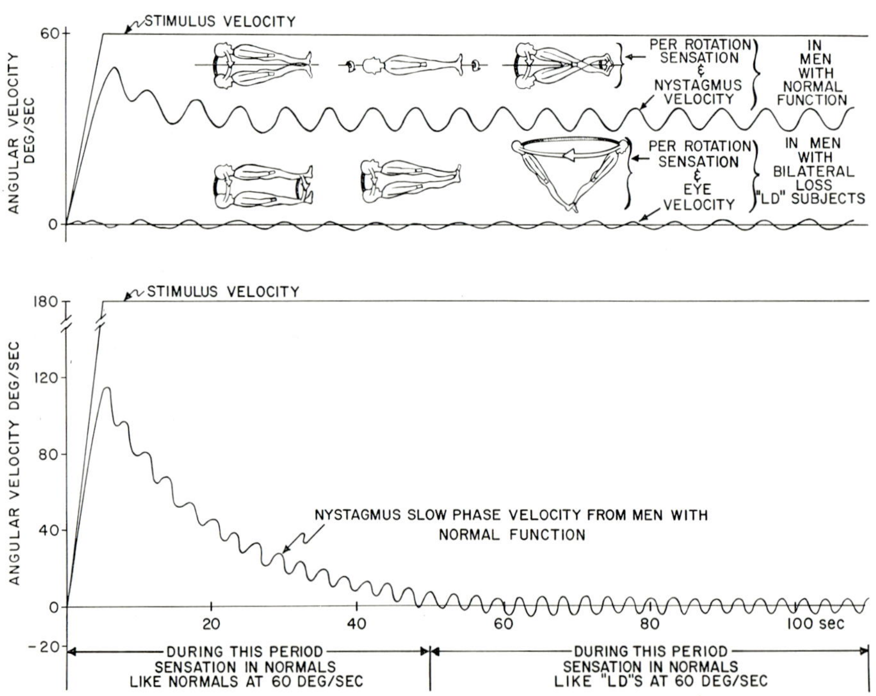

Fig. 36b. Upper Panel: Schematic illustration of nystagmus response bias and perceived motion experiences in men with normal vestibular function and in men without vestibular function (LD subjects) during 60 deg/sec rotation about an earth-horizontal axis. Lower Panel: Schematic illustration of coincidence of nystagmus bias reaching zero and the onset in normal observers of disorientation experiences like those of LD subjects. These effects are found during 180 deg/sec rotation about an earth-horizontal axis. From GUEDRY (1970)

quickly (2 or 3 sec), and postrotational nystagmus also decays rapidly, but not so rapidly as the postrotational sensation of turning (GUEDRY, 1965c; CORREIA and GUEDRY, 1964; BENSON and BODIN, 1966a, b; BENSON, 1966). Some responses during and after rotation are illustrated in Fig. 36a and b.

Caloric irrigation of the ear involves a somewhat similar combination of stimuli, although it is usually restricted to stimulation of a single ear. The position of the head and body during the caloric test is such that the horizontal semicircular canal is stimulated while the otolith presumably signals static tilt, but no change-in-position to correspond with the canal signal. The sensation is confusing, unpleasant and difficult to describe, and a number of patients do not experience rotation (McNALLY and STUART, 1941). COLLINS (1965) reported a variety of rotation experiences: motion through short arcs, sometimes about an apparent earth-vertical axis, floating sensations, tilting and displacement sensations during unilateral and also bilateral caloric stimuli. Considering the magnitude and duration and direction of the nystagmus during caloric testing and the relatively small amounts of turn which are reported, it appears that the otolith and somatosensory systems are suppressing the rotation experience which would otherwise be present in a clear form without the confusion. It is not unlikely that the nystagmus is also suppressed to some degree by these other systems, and hence caloric nystagmus, while dependent upon the functional integrity of the semicircular canals, may be intensified in certain individuals who, for one reason or another, lack the modulating effects of these other systems. The flocculus and nodulus of the cerebellum may be involved in this suppression (inferred from: COHEN and HIGHSTEIN, 1972; WOLFE, 1968; FERNÁNDEZ and FREDRICKSON, 1964; SINGLETON, 1967).

C. Parallel between the Effects of Otolith-Detected and Vision-Detected Earth Reference on Turning Sensation, Malaise, and Nystagmus

It is instructive to consider the close parallel between how nystagmus and the sensation of rotation are influenced in one case by an earth-fixed visual reference, and in the other case by an earth-fixed gravity reference.

During rotation about an earth-vertical axis at constant velocity when the observer is permitted to view earth-fixed surroundings, both nystagmus and the sensation of rotation persist after the angular acceleration much longer than is expected on the basis of cupula mechanics. The persistence of reactions is attributable to "optokinetic" stimulation that sustains the responses during constant velocity rotation. As just noted, similar effects occur during rotation at constant velocity about an earth-horizontal axis when the observer is rotated in darkness; both nystagmus and the sensation of rotation persist after the angular acceleration much longer than is expected on the basis of cupula mechanics. In this second case the continuing reaction is probably attributable to the continual reorientation of the otolith surfaces relative to gravity (GUEDRY, 1970a; BARNES, 1971; cf. BENSON, Section F. IV. this volume).

When rotation about an earth-vertical axis is stopped while the observer is permitted to view external surroundings, the postrotational sensation of turning and the nystagmus are suppressed by the visual information; both decay more rapidly than would be expected on the basis of cupula mechanics (cf. GUEDRY, 1965a, pp. 85–89). During the period of deceleration, while the semicircular canals signal rotation in opposite direction and the visual information still indicates rotation in the initial direction, many individuals are very much disturbed and report nausea primarily from the experience during the deceleration (GUEDRY and AMBLER, 1974). When the stop is achieved, the stationary visual field suppresses the vestibular nystagmus so that it decays with a time constant of about 3 sec (GUEDRY, 1968) as compared with the usual 16 sec decay time constant found in darkness for nystagmus. In the absence of vision, when rotation about an earth-horizontal axis is decelerated to a stop, both the sensation of rotation and the nystagmus decay more rapidly than would be expected on the basis of cupula mechanics. Many observers are very much disturbed by the sensations during deceleration[27] when the semicircular canals signal rotation in opposite direction while change-in-position information from the otoliths is still in the initial direction. In this case, the semicircular canal nystagmus is suppressed by the observer-fixed gravitational field.

The close parallel between these effects should be considered in relation to classical assumptions about the division of function within the labyrinth. According to classical theory of vestibular function, the semicircular canals can locate an angular acceleration vector relative to the head, but cannot locate the orientation of this vector relative to the earth. However, either the visual or the otolith system can locate the head relative to the earth, and either of these other orientation senses can augment or suppress reactions set off by the semicircular canals. The interaction between semicircular canal stimulation and visual information is similar to the interaction between semicircular canal stimulation and otolith function. It is possible that the vestibular nuclei are an early site of neural interaction in both cases. DICHGANS and BRANDT (1972) have reported recording effects of optokinetic stimulation in the vestibular nuclei of the rabbit, and BENSON et al. (1970) have reported results that can be interpreted as an otolithic modulation of canal responses in the vestibular nuclei of the cat. COHEN and TAKEMORI (1973) have shown that visual suppression of caloric nystagmus depends upon the integrity of the flocculus in the cerebellum.

1. The Influence of Visual Information on Apparent Rotation about an Earth-Vertical Axis

The effects of vision on nystagmus and turning sensations are more complicated than the description just given would imply. The information content of the visual surroundings as well as the perceived probability that the visual surroundings can move relative to the earth are complicating factors. When encapsulated in an internally illuminated vertical-axis rotation device, observers frequently report that the device is rotating when it is stationary, before vestibular stimulation from movement of the device has been experienced. The expectation that it can move

27 Observers report nausea during prolonged rotation about a tilted or horizontal axis, but with short periods of rotation of only 30–50 sec, it is the period of deceleration that is the more disturbing.

is apparently sufficient. This is true of large rotatable chambers with diameters of 15 feet to 20 feet, such as the Pensacola Rotating Rooms, as well as smaller chambers like Link trainer cockpits or the Ames MCRP devices (cf. CLARK and STEWART, 1968b). The size and structure of the interior surroundings probably influence the degree of these *autogyral effects*, but this has not been adequately studied. The fact that autogyral effects are not normally experienced in ordinary buildings illustrates the role of expectation in these rotatable chambers. The perceptual property of a large chamber to appear fixed or mobile should be considered in the same light as the perceptual property of a room to appear upright. It is likely that personality and "field dependence" are important here also, and the general problem is probably relevant to predicting perceptual events in space platforms.

When prolonged constant velocity rotation is stopped, the presence of an observer-fixed visual reference will reduce nystagmus, but whether or not it suppresses apparent whole-body rotation depends upon the visual information content. A pinpoint of visible light, an illuminated box outline, and the complex visual structure of a closed Link trainer cockpit all suppress nystagmus considerably, but none of these suppresses the apparent rotation effects appreciably.[28] As a matter of fact, all of the comparisons of OGy with SGy presented earlier show the OGy to be the 'more sensitive' effect. This is probably attributable to the retinal image velocity (or information from the visual suppression of it) which, according to experiments with optokinetic stimuli (DICHGANS and BRANDT, 1972, 1973a, b; DICHGANS and JUNG, 1969; DICHGANS et al., 1969; KÖRNER and DICHGANS, 1967), produce an increased velocity percept, if the observer reduces optokinetic nystagmus (and hence increases image velocity) by purposely gazing through the rotating stripes rather than following them. Despite appropriate arguments by BYFORD (1963), VAN DISHOECK et al. (1954), and MANN et al. (1951) that the OGy is not primarily attributable to retinal image velocity, the experiments of DICHGANS et al. indicate a potential role of image velocity in OGy effects.

However, during postrotational vestibular effects, if a point light source, or an illuminated box, or Link trainer cockpit, or a Stille-Werner frame is viewed against the background of a suddenly illuminated room known to be fixed relative to the earth, then both vestibular nystagmus and the sensation of turning are rapidly suppressed. This sensory suppression is clearly more effective than the intellectual knowledge that rotation is, in fact, nil. The absence of visible relative movement between the body-fixed rotary structure and the external room is sufficient to suppress the sensation of body rotation, and it may be that view of a room known to be earth-fixed or of a very large room alone is sufficient. That immediate visual suppression by a large visual field is not total can be inferred from the subjective experience of MENIERE's patients, but it is substantial. If after a brief period of illumination during postrotational vestibular effects the

28 Again there is insufficient information on the effects of perceived size and structure on the magnitudes and durations of the OGy. Fairly extensive work is available (HOWARD and TEMPLETON, 1966; BISCHOFF and SCHEERER, 1970) on perception of the visual and postural verticals.

room is again darkened, then the nystagmus nearly regains its normal unsuppressed level in about 1 sec; following this it decays at a rate comparable to an uninterrupted response, while the sensation remains suppressed after the room is darkened (GUEDRY et al., 1961). This is analogous to the effects of tilting following rotation about a vertical axis. In this latter case, nystagmus and sensation are suppressed by the earth-fixed gravity reference when the tilt from upright occurs (BENSON, 1966; BENSON and BODIN, 1966b). However, the nystagmus suppression by the gravity reference is less than that produced by a visual reference.

2. Optokinetic Stimulation

DICHGANS and several co-authors have conducted a series of investigations in which a 360-degree visual surrounds could rotate about an earth-vertical axis relative to the observer at center while the observer could rotate independently relative to the earth. Of the many interesting results from these and similar experiments, one is especially relevant to the foregoing discussion; viz., when the surrounds alone rotated, almost all observers soon experienced rotation of the body in a direction opposite to the rotating surrounds which appeared stationary. The effect seems to depend especially upon peripheral as opposed to foveal visual stimulation (DICHGANS and BRANDT, 1972; BRANDT et al., 1973). This finding, along with the autogyral effects mentioned above, seems to show that the absence of any apparent canal stimulus is not alone sufficient to stabilize perceived compass heading of the body relative to earth. It should be noted that the quick onset in most individuals of apparent body rotation (DICHGANS and BRANDT, 1972; BRANDT and DICHGANS, 1972) in these optokinetic experiments is in keeping with the past experience of the individual in that the entire visual field seldom moves uniformly under natural conditions unless the body turns relative to the earth. The fact that the absence of semicircular canal data was not more compelling in the discrimination of body from movement of the surroundings suggests the dominance under these circumstances of visual information in man who, after all, has often traveled in vehicles at relatively constant velocities, a circumstance that produces visual motion information without coordinated vestibular signals. The perception of body rotation with compelling optokinetic stimuli is consistent with the autogyral effects in that both occur without adequate semicircular canal stimuli.

When prolonged optokinetic stimulation is followed by darkness, nystagmus as well as the sensations of rotation persist after the visual stimulus (DICHGANS and BRANDT, 1972), apparently due to a CNS residual effect which decays slowly. If produced by rotation of an observer relative to visible earth-fixed surroundings, these persisting optokinetic effects would be in a direction to suppress post-rotational vestibular nystagmus, a suppression that MOWRER (1937) demonstrated. There is an enhanced vestibular secondary nystagmus when visual stimulation suppresses vestibular primary nystagmus, reported by COLLINS (1968b), which is probably attributable to a similar optokinetic aftereffect; in this case when primary vestibular nystagmus is suppressed by vision, the retinal velocity error signals are in a direction to generate optokinetic nystagmus of opposite sign, the persistence of which enhances the vestibular secondary nystagmus.

3. An Optokinetic Stimulation "Pseudo-Coriolis" Effect Compared with the Purkinje Effect

When the head is tilted during optokinetic aftereffects of a large rotating visual field, the perceptual effects include apparent tilt, dizziness and nausea comparable to vestibular Coriolis cross-coupling effects. This has been called the pseudo-Coriolis effect (BRANDT and DICHGANS, 1972; BRANDT et al., 1971; DICHGANS and BRANDT, 1972), but it is probably more analogous to the PURKINJE (1820) effect which is caused by a head movement during a postrotational semicircular canal response. In the Purkinje effect, a persisting (though diminishing) angular velocity vector is located by the canals relative to the skull, and the position of this vector relative to the earth is signaled by gravity detectors. So, as the head is tilted, the head-fixed canal vector[29] moves with the head; and when gravity-sensing organs locate the vector relative to the earth, tumbling sensations (turning about a tilted axis) occur, but these conflict with the change-in-position information from the gravireceptors. The experience is unpleasant to many people. In the pseudo-Coriolis effect, the optokinetic aftereffects locate an angular velocity relative to the head which moves with the head to produce tumbling sensations and nausea as the gravity sensors locate the vector relative to the earth, but again do not provide synergistic change-in-orientation signals to confirm the persisting head-fixed velocity vector. This experience is also unpleasant. There is evidence that the optokinetic stimuli set off activity in the vestibular nuclei of rabbits (DICHGANS and BRANDT, 1972) and in the peripheral vestibular nerve of goldfish (KLINKE and SCHMIDT, 1970) so that the pseudo-Coriolis phenomenon and the Purkinje phenomenon may share common vestibular as well as oculomotor neural processes (also see COHEN et al., 1973).

Movement of visual surroundings has been used as a means of studying motion sickness (CRAMPTON and YOUNG, 1953). A number of other studies clearly illustrate that movement of 'compelling' visual surroundings can be quite effective in producing symptoms of motion sickness in stationary observers (BENFARI, 1964; KOTTENHOFF and LINDAHL, 1960; MILLER and GOODSON, 1960; DICHGANS and BRANDT, 1972; BRANDT et al., 1971; SINECORI in GUEDRY, 1970b), whereas movement of only a small part, especially the central part, of the visual field does not cause sickness or sense of body rotation (BRANDT et al., 1973). Movement of extensive visual fields about axes which imply tilting also induces sensations of body motion, e.g., the haunted swing illusion, and symptoms of motion sickness (GIBSON and MOWRER, 1938; VON DIRINGSHOFEN, 1940; cf. HOWARD and TEMPLETON, p. 200f, 1966).[30] With flight or automotive simulation devices in which the operator's control moves the visual surrounds while he remains stationary, it has been found on several occasions that experienced pilots or drivers encounter more disturbance than do beginners (BARRETT and THORTON, 1968; MILLER and

29 The vector is not perfectly head-fixed during the head movement because of angular accelerations about the head tilt axis, but these leave zero aftereffects; during and after the head movement, it is the residual postrotational canal response that introduces the anti-synergistic information.

30 Recently it has been demonstrated that a field of random dots, subtending 132 degrees of visual angle, rotated about the observer's x-axis produces a perceived tilt of both the postural and visual verticals of 15 degrees mean angular displacement (DICHGANS et al., 1972).

GOODSON, 1960; REASON and DIAZ, 1971; GUEDRY, 1970b). Apparently associative bonds between control actions and feedback develop with experience in the real vehicle, and the simulator introduces the visual feedback without the expected vestibular and somatosensory signals. In this case it is the absence of motion signals from certain channels that sets off the sickness. PARKER (1971) showed that a visually disorienting film run forward produced signs of motion sickness, whereas run backward, it did not. In many motion situations that induce sickness, there is a discordance either among sensory inputs relevant to orientation and change in orientation or between expected and obtained sensory orientation inputs (cf. REASON and GRAYBIEL, 1972; GUEDRY, 1970b; REASON, 1970; STEELE, 1970).

D. The Coriolis Vestibular Reaction

When the head (or whole body) is rotated about an axis which is itself on a device that is rotating about another axis, there is an instantaneous angular acceleration about a third axis of magnitude $\omega_1 \omega_2 \cos \varnothing$ where ω_2 is the angular velocity about the head-turn axis, ω_1 is the angular velocity of the rotating device and $\varnothing$ is the angle between the ω_1 and ω_2 axes. This $\omega_1 \omega_2$ angular acceleration occurs in addition to the natural sinusoidal angular acceleration/deceleration about the ω_2-axis that would occur during any natural head movement. The natural (ω_2-axis) stimulation leaves almost no aftereffects. However, the $\omega_1 \omega_2 \cos \varnothing$ vector may be conceptualized as lying in the plane of rotation of the device, orthogonal to the ω_1 and ω_2 axes, so that its plane of maximal stimulation is perpendicular to the plane of rotation of the device and also at right angles to the natural head movement stimulus, and it leaves an aftereffect.

This kind of vestibular stimulation was referred to by SCHUBERT (1932) as a Coriolis effect, a name which has gained fairly wide usage, but the appropriateness of this terminology has been questioned (HOWARD and TEMPLETON, 1966). Coriolis acceleration is a linear acceleration, and since the semicircular canals are not stimulated by linear acceleration, it has been indicated that the name implied a misunderstanding of cause and effect. This is an unfortunate confounding of the literature because SCHUBERT and others (BORNSCHEIN and SCHUBERT, 1954, 1958, 1962; MEDA, 1954; GUEDRY and MONTAGUE, 1961; GUEDRY, 1965a; WEAVER, 1965; HIXSON et al., 1966) made it clear that Coriolis acceleration is a linear acceleration and that the canals are stimulated by an inertial torque which develops when the head is turned about one axis while that axis is itself being rotated about an orthogonal axis. The direction and magnitude of the inertial torque (or cross-coupling effect) can be directly derived by integrating the components of the Coriolis acceleration vectors that act in alignment with canal walls at each point around the endolymph ring. Hence, the stimulus in this situation can be derived from analysis of Coriolis accelerations, and the original name was reasonably appropriate. However, the stimulus to the canals can also be derived from calculations of changes in angular momentum (GROEN, 1961c) or from analyses of cross-coupling effects (LANSBERG, 1960), and it would appear that some name like "vestibular Coriolis cross-coupling effects" might serve to identify this particular stimulus and avoid further unnecessary confusion.

If a given canal ring were rotated at constant velocity (ω_2) about an axis lying in its plane and parallel to the plane of a turntable, then the stimulus to the ring would vary sinusoidally according to $\omega_1\ \omega_2 \sin \omega_2 t$ where $\omega_2 t = 0$ is defined as the position where the planes of the canal ring and turntable coincide and ω_1 is the constant angular velocity of the turntable. Another ring in fixed orthogonal relation to the first would be stimulated according to $\omega_1\ \omega_2 \cos \omega_2 t$. However, in natural head movement, rotation of the head through some discrete angle is accomplished fairly quickly, and it is desirable to have an expression for the stimulus for this case. The angular impulse delivered to the canal ring during fairly rapid changes in head position can be calculated by integration of $\omega_1\ \omega_2 \sin \omega_2 t$ over particular arcs of head rotation.

The stimulus can be appreciated by a specific example which will serve to illustrate several points. During counterclockwise rotation of a turntable about an earth-vertical axis at a constant ω_1 velocity of 60 deg/sec, if the head is rotated in about 2 sec from upright to 40 degrees left about an orthogonal x-axis, an angular impulse of magnitude ω_1 sin 40 degrees about the y-axis is delivered to vertical canals; they gain angular momentum in $+\omega_1$ direction proportional to $\omega_1 \sin 40° = \omega_1(.643)$ while the horizontal canals lose angular momentum proportional to $\omega_1(\cos 40°-1) = \omega_1(.234)$. In effect, the canals have been stimulated by the $\omega_1\ \omega_2$ acceleration *vector*, which can be conceptualized as being in the plane of vehicle rotation, but the head has moved relative to the effective vector. The end result is an angular impulse to the vertical canals equivalent to a pitch-up (backward rotation) or y-axis angular impulse of 38.6 deg/sec and an angular impulse[31] to the horizontal canals (or z-axis) of 10.4 deg/sec in the $-\omega_1$ direction. The immediate perception on starting the head movement is a pitch-up sensation, and as the head movement is completed, the plane of motion transitions toward a sensation of $+\omega_1$ rotation, i.e., rotation appears to be up and left.

1. Canal-Otolith Interactions during Coriolis Cross-Coupling

In the example just given, the $+\omega_1$ rotation sensation may seem at variance with the $-\omega_1$ direction of stimulation of the lateral canals, but it is not. At the end of the head movement, the resultant axis of rotation signaled by the three sets of canals is in the yz plane of the head, but it has changed only 20 degrees while the head rotated 40 degrees relative to gravity. The transitional sensation of rotation in the $+\omega_1$ rotation direction refers to rotation of the whole body (and turntable) in a $+\omega_1$ direction relative to the earth. The initial part of the sensation (the pitch-up) is produced by the sudden strong canal stimulus indicating rotation about the y-axis which is approximately earth-horizontal as the stimulus begins, but it is not the canals that locate the orientation of the rotation axis relative to gravity; rather, it is the otoliths and somatosensory system. At the completion of the head movement, the canals indicate an angular velocity *vector* relative to the head in the yz plane pointing 20 degrees below the y-axis (i.e., below the right ear), but located by the otoliths as pointing 20 degrees above the earth-horizontal plane. With the otoliths locating the orientation of the head relative to the earth, the canal signal is projected to an otolith-located earth-vertical axis which yields

31 Angular impulse is used here as used by VAN EGMOND et al. (1949) where a sudden change in constant velocity is implied.

a sensation of rotation diagonally up and to the left ($+\omega$) relative to the earth, as shown in Fig. 37. Note that the nystagmus is up and right relative to the skull, though the nystagmus and sensation are up and left relative to gravity.

Upon return of the head to upright position, the typical sensation is of a forward pitch with only a little transition to a sensation of left rotation. In this case, when the head has achieved upright position, the angular velocity vector signaled by the canals is in the yz plane pointing 20 degrees above the left ear. The sensation in this case is primarily of pitch down with only a little leftward rotation, although the nystagmus is diagonal down and left relative to the skull as expected from the canal stimulus. Apparently with the head upright, the slight tilt of plane of rotation signaled by the canals relative to the skull is overcome by the into-level information from the otoliths and neck. The two situations may be contrasted as follows: With the head tilt away from vertical, the otolith and neck indicate

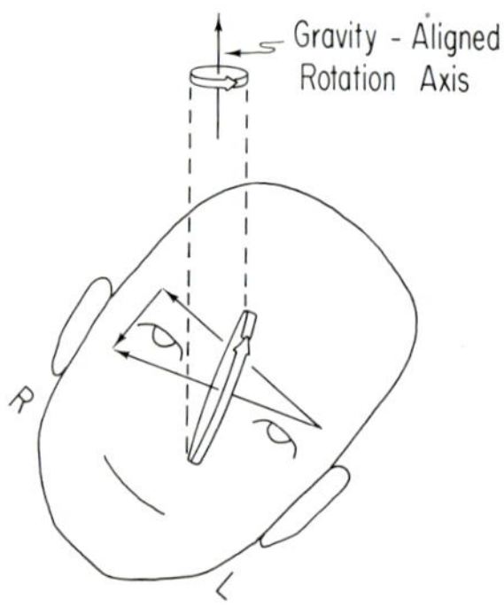

Fig. 37. The residual effect of a 40 deg left lateral head tilt from upright position during whole-body rotation at 60 deg/sec in CCW direction about an earth-vertical axis. The angular impulse delivered to the semicircular canals would be equivalent to a 41 deg/sec velocity-change, with the horizontal canals receiving a 14 deg/sec velocity-change impulse and the vertical canals receiving a 38.6 deg/sec velocity-change impulse. If projected to a gravity reference, the plane of rotation signalled by the canals is pitch-up and yaw-left. If projected to the observer's z-axis, it is pitch-up and yaw-right

40 degree tilt of the head relative to gravity in the same direction as, *but more than*, the canal-generated angular velocity vector is tilted relative to gravity. The plane of perceived rotation is tilted relative to gravity. In the case of the head return, the otoliths indicate no tilt of the head while the resultant canal axis signal is slightly tilted relative to the head and relative to gravity. The sensation is one of almost pure forward pitch with only a little leftward rotation; apparently the into-level position information tends to override the slightly tilted canal axis while the absence of y-axis change-in-position information from the otoliths increases the rate of decay of responses set off by the residual vertical canal signals.

The effects of this stimulus are in some respects quite similar to the effects produced by cessation of rotation about a rotation-axis that is in fixed tilted or horizontal position relative to gravity. This can be clearly demonstrated by selecting stimuli that stimulate the horizontal canals and thus produce nystagmus that is easily recorded. Cessation of rotation about an earth-horizontal axis, when the z-axis is aligned with the rotation axis, stimulates the horizontal canals. As noted above, the sensation of rotation decays very quickly, and the time constant of decay of nystagmus is about one-half that measured when an equivalent z-axis stimulus is delivered when the rotation axis is earth-vertical (BENSON, 1966; BENSON and BODIN, 1966b). The deceleration experience when the axis is tilted (or horizontal) is unpleasant to many observers. The same magnitude stimulus can be delivered to the horizontal canals by a head movement during rotation of a turntable about an earth-vertical axis. When an observer lies supine on a turntable rotating at velocity ω_1 with the head positioned so that the plane of the lateral canals is tipped backward 30 degrees (i.e., 30 degrees tilted in the direction of head inversion), if he then rotates the head about the y-axis 60 degrees forward (ventroflexion) so that a final tilt position of the lateral canals 30 degrees past upright is attained, the lateral canals receive an angular impulse equivalent to a rapid acceleration to ω_1. During the head movement, the vertical canals receive stimulation first in one direction and then in the opposite direction, so that the net residual effect upon completion of the head movement is very nearly zero for the vertical canals. The stimulus thus leaves the cupulae deflected in the lateral canals, but at null position in the vertical canals, and the body and head are still nearly supine. Thus the stimulus just as the head movement is completed is similar to cessation of rotation about a horizontal axis. The time constant of decay of nystagmus and the unpleasant but short after-sensation are quite similar in the two situations (GUEDRY, 1970b). In both cases, the semicircular canals signal rotation about the z-axis while the otoliths signal that the z-axis is tilted relative to gravity and also signal no change in position to supplement the canal signals. The suppression of the canal-dependent responses is dependent upon these otolith and somatosensory signals which indicate 1) a fixed tilt position and 2) no change in position.

The perceptual phenomena associated with the Coriolis cross-coupled stimulus are complex. At first, many observers cannot describe the complex perceptual events clearly and they simply report a confused, unpleasant experience of motion. When the OGy situation is used, many experienced observers report that certain head movements produce incompatible sensations of apparent velocity and displacement of the target light when asked specifically to report on these aspects of the experience.[32] In particular, the velocity of the forward pitch (diving) sensations seems to be too great for the amount of angular displacement experienced and, as shown in Table 4, these same sensations of forward pitch or diving are typically rated as more unpleasant than the climbing sensation (GUEDRY and MONTAGUE, 1961; REASON and GRAYBIEL, 1969a). The confusion and incompatible velocity and displacement sensations are probably a reflection of antisynergistic inputs from the canals, otoliths, and other orientation senses. The displeasure and emotional reactions associated with the diving sensations in particular may be an adult manifestation of the Moro reflex, which is of vestibular origin (PEIPER, 1963). A dive toward the earth typically demands a quicker emergency reaction than a climb away from it (cf. STEELE, 1970).

32 Some individuals are apparently unable to conceptualize independent velocity and displacement sensations and simply report confusion or "dizziness."

Table 4. *Comparison of tilt and return head movements toward the left shoulder and toward the right shoulder in regard to several aspects of the subjective reaction*[a] (GUEDRY and MONTAG, 1961)

Stimulus condition	Direction of reaction	Aspect of reaction: Displacement	Velocity	Disturbance
Rotation right – head tilt right	Climb	7	3	3
Rotation left – head tilt left	Climb	7	3	3
Rotation right – head ret. from right	Dive	7	10	10
Rotation left – head ret. from left	Dive	7	10	10
Rotation right – head tilt left	Dive	3	6	7
Rotation left – head tilt right	Dive	3	6	7
Rotation right – head ret. from left	Climb	10	3[b]	2
Rotation left – head ret. from right	Climb	10	3[b]	2

[a] Numbers presented are not actual ratings but are descriptive of the results of several experiments. Ratings from 0 to 10 designate effects ranging from zero magnitude to greatest magnitude observed.

[b] No more velocity than is derivable from displacement experienced.

Because of the complexity of this reaction, it is difficult to obtain with magnitude estimation the relative intensity of different reactions unless the aspect of the reaction being judged is made very clear by instruction. Moreover, the particular mode of indication of subjective effects and the kind of training given apparently make a considerable difference in the reported magnitude of particular effects (cf. GUEDRY and MONTAGUE, 1961; CLARK and STEWART, 1967; COLLINS, 1968a). The degree of disturbance or unpleasantness of a reaction does not necessarily correlate closely with the apparent angular displacement experienced. However, a few individuals do not find vestibular Coriolis cross-coupling stimuli of this magnitude disturbing, and these particular observers may not agree with the trend in Table 4 on the relative disturbance produced by different stimuli simply because none of the reactions is really unpleasant to them.

Within individuals, there is clearly a positive correlation between intensity of experience and nystagmus produced by Coriolis cross-coupled stimuli of the same direction but different magnitudes (GUEDRY and MONTAGUE, 1961). However, if a given magnitude stimulus is used with different individuals, then there is probably only a low positive correlation between nystagmus intensity and ratings of displeasure (GUEDRY, 1965b). Some individuals with little nystagmus reaction to these stimuli are more disturbed than others with stronger nystagmus reactions, but individuals with little or no vestibular function are typically not disturbed by these stimuli. It is also noticeable in some individuals that the nystagmus reaction does not commence until after the head movement is completed, and it is likely that such long latencies reflect the conflictual nature of the canal and otolithic inputs. During the head movement, the temporal sequence of reactions from sets of canals is unusual, and during as well as after the head movement, the canal and otolith patterns are geometrically conflictual. This unusual input pattern appears to block the nystagmus response during the period of maximal disturbance to these individuals.

In considering the subjective effects of vestibular Coriolis cross-coupling stimuli, it is important to note that fairly strong canal stimuli can introduce dynamic perceptions of tilt which temporarily distort the perception of actual tilt relative to gravity. This is analogous to so-called "lag effect" with the oculogravic illusion where the otoliths may be stimulated as though the tilting were about the x-axis while the canals indicate rotation about the z-axis. Thus the perception of tilt, classically assigned to otolith function, can certainly be modified by semicircular canal stimulation, a result recently further demonstrated by SCHÖNE and UDO DE HAES (1971), whereas perception of angular velocity, classically assigned to the semicircular canals, can be either enhanced or suppressed by otolith stimulation. The recent finding that visual scenes rotating about the observer's x-axis influence the postural as well as the visual vertical (DICHGANS et al., 1972; DICHGANS and BRANDT, 1973b) and that optokinetic nystagmus and optokinetic afternystagmus are strongly influenced by loss of spontaneous vestibular inflow (COHEN et al., 1973) illustrates the intimate interrelation of these systems.

2. Vestibular Coriolis Cross-Coupling Effects and Visual Stimulation

The effects of tilting the head during whole-body rotation can be roughly classified into 1) unexpected perceived changes in body orientation, 2) an immediate startle or fear reaction in some observers, and 3) nausea and sickness in some individuals, though usually several head movements are required to induce vomiting even at fairly high rotation rates (60, 90, 180 deg/sec) of whole-body rotation. These effects are strongest when vision is restricted to internal visual reference or when the eyes are closed (GUEDRY, 1972; REASON and DIAZ, 1970). If external visual reference is permitted during the head movements, then the startle reaction is greatly reduced as is the nausea, though with sufficient exposure the latter may occur without the former. For example, in darkness (or with internal visual reference), a right-lateral head tilt during clockwise rotation produces a climbing sensation (pitch-up relative to earth) and a diagonal vertical nystagmus with slow phase down. The observer expects a sensation of right lateral head tilt and instead experiences an entirely unexpected change in orientation of the head and body relative to the earth. However, with an external view available, it is clear to the observer as soon as he commences the head movement that the lateral head tilt relative to the body "causes" motion of the moving external visual field in a diagonal downward direction relative to the head; moreover, the vestibular nystagmus with slow phase diagonally downward relative to the head is approximately in a direction to aid visual acuity of the moving field. Thus the external visual reference confirms otolith information on orientation relative to gravity, and transforms the egocentric semicircular canal pitch-up sensation into one of veridical clockwise rotation about a vertical axis relative to the earth; the visual information melds the canal and otolith data into adequate perceptual and reflex actions. BRANDT et al. (1971), using an external visual reference that could be rotated independently of the observer, found that the disturbance produced by vestibular Coriolis cross-coupling effects was greatest when the visual and vestibular movement information did not match.

3. Etiology of Individual Differences in Reactions to Discordant Stimuli

There are extreme individual differences in reactions to discordant stimuli of this type, and the fact that brief measures of these differences are predictive of subsequent adjustment to flying suggests that these differences may reflect some enduring traits (Ambler and Guedry, 1971; Guedry and Ambler, 1973; Galle and Emel'ianov, 1967; Lansberg, 1960). It is probable that the limbic system, which is involved in establishing contingencies of relationships among patterns of stimuli and in the production of fear, nausea, sweating, respiratory changes and fainting when stimuli are threatening (Smythies, 1966), is brought into play by discordant orientation data which threaten the individual's control of motion by simultaneously calling for mutually incompatible postural adjustments. Prescott (1971), citing evidence for flocculo-nodular and other paleocerebellar connections with the limbic system and orbital cortex, suggests a major role for the cerebellum in emotional processes. The paleocerebellum is also of primary importance in motion sickness (Money and Wood, 1970). Two-way vestibular-cerebellar connections are well known (Brodal, 1964, 1966). The flocculus is involved in visual suppression of vestibular nystagmus (Cohen and Takemori, 1973), and the flocculo-nodular lobe appears to be important to otolithic modulation of semicircular canal activity (Cohen and Highstein, 1972; Wolfe, 1968; Singleton, 1967; Fernández and Fredericksen, 1964). The cerebellar cortex translates spatial into temporal patterns necessary for rapid "pre-programmed" skilled movement (Kornhuber, 1971) but by disrupting this natural coordinating function, mutually conflictual intralabyrinthine and visual-vestibular inputs may elicit exceptional emotional reactions as well as motion sickness by way of cerebellar-orbital frontal-limbic-reticular circuits suggested by Prescott (1971). That early developmental factors may contribute to these extreme individual differences by influencing different neural structures in the sequence of development (Guedry, 1972; Prescott, 1971; Ornitz, 1970; Peto, 1970) is a possibility with far-reaching practical and theoretical implications.

E. Visual Acuity during Semicircular Canal Stimulation

The visual system has a considerable cortical representation, and much of its function is voluntarily directed so that visual information is *selected* from the environment, but it is also influenced by reflex actions. During voluntary whole-body movement, the visual system provides information on future as well as immediate requirements for changes in orientation of the eyes and body, while the vestibular system operates automatically to provide feedback information and set off oculomotor reflexes appropriate to the immediate state of orientation and motion relative to the earth. Vestibular function can enhance visual acuity for earth-fixed targets during natural movement and during some unnatural passive body movement, but of course it can also degrade visual acuity for either earth-fixed or observer-fixed targets during unnatural states of motion or during the early stages of vestibular/oculomotor pathology.

1. Visual Acuity during Relative Movement between Observer and Target

There have been a number of studies of ability to see during whole-body vibration, but only a few of these permit evaluation of the role of vestibular stimulation in ocular stabilization. BENSON (1972) has recently shown that good dynamic visual acuity for earth-fixed targets is sustained during passive whole-body angular oscillation at frequencies up to 10 Hz, whereas when the head is earth-fixed and the targets are oscillated, then dynamic visual acuity drops off sharply at oscillation frequencies between 0.5 and 1.0 Hz. One observer, whose labyrinths were not functional, lost visual acuity at 1.0 Hz, irrespective of whether the body or the target was oscillated, and thus the visual stabilization during passive body oscillation seems to be attributable to vestibular function.

MELVILL JONES (1966a) recorded nystagmus about the x-, y-, and z-axes of the head when observers were rotated about an earth-vertical axis and viewed an earth-fixed screen containing vertical stripes. By placing the head in various orientations relative to the rotation axis, different amounts of x- (roll), y- (pitch), and z- (yaw) nystagmus were generated by the vestibular stimulus and also by concordant optokinetic stimuli. In the dark, the slow-phase velocity of nystagmus generated by semicircular canal stimulation is usually about 60% of the angular velocity that would be required for stabilization of retinal images. With concordant vestibular and optokinetic stimuli during acceleration to 60 deg/sec and with the head tipped backward 45 degrees, eye velocity in yaw was slightly greater than that required for image stabilization, and it was sustained long after the vestibular component would have dissipated; however, the roll component of the eye movement was less than half that required for image stabilization, and it decayed according to the expected change in cupula deflection. With the head tilted 45 degrees laterally relative to the axis of rotation, yaw and pitch components were similar, both slightly exceeding velocity required for retinal stabilization and decaying slowly during constant velocity rotation.

2. Visual Acuity for Observer-Fixed Targets during Vestibular Nystagmus

The absence of an optokinetic roll component capable of dominating the decaying vestibular input in this experiment is consistent with other visual-vestibular interaction effects in the roll plane. Experiments in which the visual display is fixed relative to the head during semicircular canal stimulation represent the obverse situation in which the visual task requires a near-zero eye velocity while the vestibular system drives the eyes. Such experiments have shown that angular acceleration about the roll-axis interferes much less with visual acuity than does angular acceleration about either the pitch- or yaw-axes (GUEDRY, 1970c). It is probably attributable to the fact that in the roll axis, the foveal image velocity is low because the axis of eye rotation is approximately coincident with the corneo-foveal axis; hence, the tangential linear velocity of the image relative to foveal cells is low because the radius is small. This is in contrast to eye rotation about the y- and z-axes, which are approximately at right angles to the corneo-foveal axis so that any rotation about these other axes generates relatively high foveal image velocities.

2.1. *A Directional Difference in Suppression of Vertical Nystagmus*

This line of experimentation in which a visual task requires the suppression of vestibular nystagmus has introduced several facts about visual-vestibular interplay. There is a pronounced difference in the two directions of vertical nystagmus (y-axis) during visual suppression of the response (BENSON and GUEDRY, 1971). The slow-phase velocity of nystagmus during forward pitch is as much as 10 times the velocity of the response recorded during backward pitch. This is primarily due to differences in visual suppression of the reactions of opposite direction because during sinusoidal oscillation (.04 Hz, ± 60 deg/sec peak velocity) in darkness, the two reactions are roughly equal whereas in the light they are grossly different (GUEDRY and BENSON, 1971). The inability to suppress downbeating vestibular nystagmus is reflected in very poor visual performance during this reaction as compared with performance during either upbeating vestibular nystagmus or nystagmus of either direction in yaw (HIXSON and NIVEN, 1969; GUEDRY and BENSON, 1970; BENSON and GUEDRY, 1971).

There are a number of possible reasons for this directional difference in vertical nystagmus. In man the eye appears to be structured for viewing the lower part of the visual field when the head is in normal upright posture. The eyelid and even eyebrows must be moved to permit a large upward ocular excursion, whereas these structures reflexly follow a downward glance; there is no restriction by the lower lid until the eye has moved downward 10 or 20 degrees from level gaze. Thus the slow-phase downward nystagmus consists of fairly large amplitude nystagmus beats, whereas the slow-phase upward nystagmus is of relatively low amplitude and high frequency (BENSON and GUEDRY, 1971; GUEDRY and BENSON, 1971). If vision is suppressed during and even slightly before the fast-phase saccade, then there is little time for obtaining a good quality visual image during a slow phase of restricted amplitude, even though the vestibular slow-phase velocity signal is no greater than that of the larger amplitude opposite reaction. It is well known that vestibular nystagmus intensifies when visual images are degraded, so it is plausible that the low amplitude and high frequency of this response reduce visual acuity which in turn results in nystagmus of higher slow-phase velocity. It is also possible that there is some natural training in the controlled suppression of slow downward visual tracking arising from the fact that during forward movement, visual fixation of distant objects in the path of movement requires a concomitant suppression of optokinetic stimuli from near objects in the path of movement. This natural practice in the visual control of optokinetically induced slow-phase-down nystagmus may carry over to the visual suppression of vestibular nystagmus.

2.2. Factors Other Than Retinal Velocity Which Influence Vision during Vestibular Nystagmus

Even with horizontal nystagmus, visual acuity is not always the same for a given slow-phase velocity of nystagmus. During each cycle of sinusoidal oscillation of an observer about an earth-vertical rotation axis, nystagmus increases to a maximum and then declines, first in one direction and then the other. As shown in Fig. 38, the visual acuity for three-digit sets, presented 1 set/sec, appears to be superior for a given slow-phase eye velocity when the nystagmus is increasing in slow-phase velocity as opposed to when it was decreasing, and the nystagmus only partially reflects this difference in visual performance. Apparently the ability to perceive sets of targets during the increasing vestibular signals wherein the vision was initially clear is superior to the ability to "clear up" the visual image once vision is blurred. However, the problems of seeing head-fixed targets during

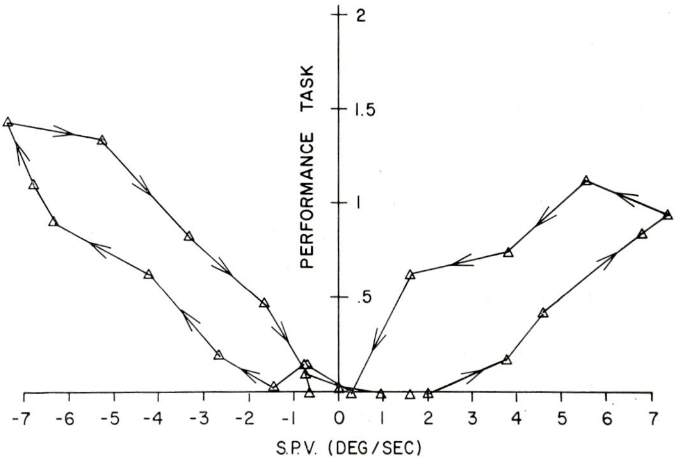

Fig. 38. Mean number of errors (performance task) in identifying digits in 3-digit sets presented 1 set/sec as a function of nystagmus slow-phase velocity (SPV). Nystagmus was generated by sinusoidal oscillation (± 120 deg/sec, .04 Hz) about the z-axis. Arrows on the lines indicate whether nystagmus was increasing or decreasing. Errors and nystagmus shown here were suppressed apparently as a result of 10 min of oscillatory habituation with visual suppression. Adapted from GUEDRY and AMBLER (1973a)

vestibular nystagmus is not solely a matter of acuity nor is it solely a matter of retinal image velocity. During angular acceleration when nystagmus velocity reaches 2–4 deg/sec, individual sets of three digits appear to move slowly in the direction of rotation relative to apparent "dead ahead," but the digits do not necessarily appear blurred even though there is a recordable low retinal image velocity at this time. With higher image velocity, the digits become blurred, but the image velocity at which blurring occurs seems to be different for different people, and some individuals appear to have much better visual acuity than others at a given image velocity.[33] In some individuals there appears to be a directional difference in dynamic vision which is not necessarily matched by a directional difference in nystagmus. During sinusoidal oscillation (± 120 deg/sec, .04 Hz) about the z-axis, visual performance may be superior in one direction, even though nystagmus slow-phase velocity in that direction is greater than the reaction of opposite direction (GUEDRY and AMBLER, 1973a). Thus, it appears in some few individuals that the visual system is differentially capable of producing good quality images depending upon whether images are moving right or left. Because these conclusions are based on mean eye velocities measured by the corneoretinal potential method, a finer examination of eye movement characteristics and visual acuity is desirable. There are a number of neurological deficits that can cause a differential ability to make horizontal eye movements of opposite directions (cf. COHEN, Section D.IV. this volume), but it is possible that some of these effects are dependent on central processing of visual information. Possibly

33 Observers were flight students who had passed through flight physical examinations, but more detailed visual examinations are desirable for these special cases.

the vestibular system sends corollary signals to prepare the visual system for directions of retinal image velocity at the same time that it sends messages to oculomotor centers. Experiments suggest corollary vestibular influences on lateral geniculate neurons (cf. Montandon and Monnier, 1964; Horn and Hill, 1969; Meshman, 1970, 1968; Teuber, 1960; Marchiafava and Pompeiano, 1966; Morrison and Pompeiano, 1966). Recent indications that cerebral lateralization of thought processes can influence the direction of eye and head turning (Kinsbourne, 1972) suggest the potential complexity of differential ability to see during right- and left-beating vestibular nystagmus.

With a horizontal visual display of 7 or 9 digits (Guedry and Holmes, 1972), when the observer is required to report the middle 2 or 3 digits during horizontal nystagmus, the visual problem changes from blurred vision to one of identifying the specified set in the specified ordinal sequence. Errors are made in set selection as well as ordinal sequence while vision is still relatively unblurred. The problem of locate-and-see requires control of visual scanning superimposed on vestibular nystagmus, and the vestibular reflex control introduces errors in perceived spatio-temporal sequences. With more complex visual displays, the vestibular interference with the visual task increases the incidence of 'motion' sickness (Guedry and Ambler, 1973). The problem of seeing during eye movement has been widely studied as a visual problem (Miller and Ludvigh, 1962; Duffy and Lombrose, 1968), but seeing during vestibular stimulation is a problem involving two naturally interacting systems which needs the concerted attention of visual and vestibular researchers.

2.3. Effects of Alcohol and Effects of Practice on Dynamic Visual Acuity

Mild alcohol intoxication greatly reduces the visual control of vestibular nystagmus, and it produces concomitant reduction in visual performance during vestibular stimulation (Collins et al., 1971; Collins et al., 1973; Gilson et al., 1972). These effects have been noted with both z- and y-axis stimuli (Schroeder et al., 1973). Apparently the alcohol reduces the control by the higher-order visual system of the more primitive and automatic vestibular-oculomotor reflex system because alcohol does not increase the nystagmus reaction or turning sensation to angular acceleration about an earth-vertical axis in darkness (Collins et al., 1973).

There are surprising improvements in visual performance as a result of practice during visual-vestibular interaction for oculomotor control. A mean improvement of 57% was found in visual acuity for 3-digit sets of numbers presented tachistoscopically as a result of 10 min of intervening practice on a psychomotor task requiring visibility of a dial during vestibular nystagmus (Guedry and Ambler, 1973). There was also a reduction of nystagmus during the visual task which seems to reflect increased visual control of the vestibular oculomotor reflex.

F. Effects of Sensory Interactions on Vestibular Habituation

Experiments involving fairly extensive repetitive exposure to alternately presented equal and opposite angular acceleration have shown that visual suppression of only one direction of nystagmus results in a directional preponderance of vestibular nystagmus habituation (Guedry, 1964, 1965a). Although some studies of brief habituation schedules with visual suppression have not indicated a nystagmus habituation which carries over to subsequent testing in darkness (BROWN and CRAMPTON, 1966), other studies have demonstrated some modification of nystagmus after only short habituation schedules, especially when visual stimuli were present during the criterion trials as well as during the habituation schedule (MARSHALL and BROWN, 1967; GUEDRY and AMBLER, 1973; GILSON et al., 1973a). It is likely that the visual task, the magnitude of vestibular stimuli, and the amount of training are relevant considerations. Tasks which do not demand visual control even though vision is permitted, and vestibular reactions which are so strong that vision is ineffective in suppressing nystagmus, are conditions which probably do not especially enhance the development of exceptional visual control over vestibular nystagmus.

One of the most interesting experiments on this topic has been carried out by GONSHOR and MELVILL JONES (1971) and MELVILL JONES and GONSHOR (1972) who showed that prolonged sinusoidal oscillation did not produce nystagmus habituation as long as mental arousal was sustained by arithmetic computation. However, when observers wore right-left reversing prisms throughout the day and were tested from time to time by 2-min periods of passive sinusoidal oscillation in darkness during mental computation, nystagmus was reduced, and there were marked changes in phase relations (almost 180 degrees) between nystagmus reversal and chair reversal; i.e., the ocular response to vestibular signals was phase shifted to accomplish a functional coordination of the visual and vestibular inputs. Thus the normal coordination between visual, vestibular, and proprioceptive inputs was rearranged by active voluntary movement while the observers wore right-left reversing lenses, and evidence of this adaptive rearrangement was obtained from vestibular nystagmus recorded during *passive* angular oscillation in darkness. In this study, the "habituation schedule" involved only natural vestibular stimuli produced by *voluntary* movement (MELVILL JONES and GONSHOR, 1972).

With repeated exposure to vestibular Coriolis cross-coupling effects, there is typically a reduction in the perceived orientation change, in the unpleasant sensations, and in the nystagmus induced by voluntary head movements on a rotating platform with only internal visual reference. A number of experiments have been carried out in which men lived on enclosed rotating platforms for hours and days (GRAYBIEL et al., 1960; GUEDRY and GRAYBIEL, 1962; GUEDRY et al., 1964; GUEDRY, 1965b; BERGSTEDT, 1965; REASON and GRAYBIEL, 1970). After prolonged exposure to such conditions, many observers adjust so that the unpleasantness, the fear reaction, the nausea and vomiting are eliminated and the functionally inefficient perceptual effects and vestibular oculomotor responses are replaced by functionally efficient responses. This functional change involves neurophysiological recoding which is revealed by head movements made in a normal static environment after the adjustment to the rotating environment has occurred; head movements in a natural static environment now yield perceptual and reflex reactions in a geometric plane which is approximately orthogonal to that of normal reactions (GUEDRY and GRAYBIEL, 1962; GUEDRY, 1965b). Nystagmus and the sensations of motion are valuable signs of the kind of neurophysiological recoding which can take place during exposure to this kind of situation, as shown schematic-

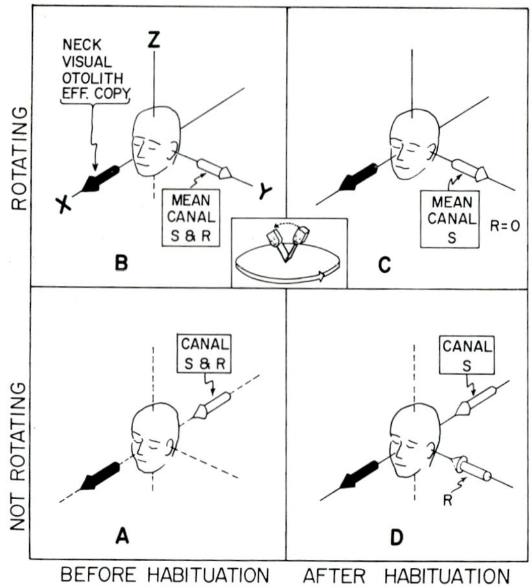

Fig. 39. Canal stimuli (S) and responses (R) during head tilts in normal and in rotating environments before and after habituation

ally in Fig. 39. In a natural environment, head rotation about the x-axis from a left lateral position to a right lateral position produces a counterrolling eye movement about the x-axis and a sensation of x-axis head tilt (A). As the head movement stops, the sensation stops and the eye velocity stops. In the enclosed rotating environment, however, the same head movement about the x-axis produces eye movement and rotary sensation about a changing axis intermediate between the x-, y-, and z-axes and an after-response of almost pure y-axis nystagmus which in darkness requires 10 or 15 sec to dissipate (B). During habituation with active movement and visual suppression, these discordant canal responses diminish (C). About 1 hour after stopping rotation, testing in darkness with head movements in the natural nonrotating environment reveals eye movements and sensations opposite in direction to those which had occurred in the rotation condition; this represents a new sensory-motor relationship in which a particular sensory input in a natural environment produces a sensation and nystagmus in a plane which differs by almost 90 degrees (D) from the plane of the original response in the natural environment. At this time, a head movement while the subject is standing unsupported and with eyes closed causes him to fall in a direction compensatory to the recoded message. A recoding or reorganization of sensory-motor and sensory-perceptual relations has occurred (cf. GUEDRY, 1965b; GUEDRY and GRAYBIEL, 1962).

Experiments have shown that the rate of perceptual and nystagmus modification is influenced by visual-vestibular interaction (GUEDRY, 1964; REASON and DIAZ, 1970). It is influenced also by other sensory interactions (GUEDRY, 1965b; GUEDRY et al., 1964; COLLINS, 1969). In this connection it is relevant that after several days of adjustment to a rotating environment, the oculomotor responses during rotation are diminished, as illustrated schematically in Fig. 39, but when head movements are made during rotation in opposite direction, nystagmus and sensation are as great as responses which occurred before the habituation schedule. This is an important point because nystagmus in almost the same plane and direction relative to the head can be produced during platform rotation in either direction (cf. Fig. 7 in GUEDRY, 1965b), but the accompanying information is different 1) from the otoliths, 2) from the natural canal stimulus about the head-tilt axis, 3) from the neck proprioceptors, and 4) from preparatory actions for voluntary movement, because the head movement was different. For example, during counterclockwise platform rotation, head return from left lateral position produces approximately the same nystagmus plane as does head tilt to left lateral position during clockwise platform rotation. The information which precedes and accompanies the Coriolis torque stimulus is sufficient to set off a counteracting reaction in the practiced rotation direction, but when this counteracting reaction is set off by the same head movement relative to gravity and the body in the unpracticed direction of platform rotation, the conditioned reaction augments the Coriolis cross-coupled semicircular canal stimulus so that the reaction is not suppressed, but in some cases it is increased.

These maladaptive reactions which may include nausea and vomiting in a natural static environment and which are manifest during opposite direction of platform rotation illustrate that this form of adaptation or habituation which involves a reordering of sensory-motor and sensory-perceptual relations is not an efficient form of adjustment unless the organism is to remain in the changed conditions. It is a form of adjustment which is forced on the organism, and it would not be functionally efficient if it developed quickly and was retained very long because such changes would be maladaptive for other more likely states, such as movement in a natural environment. Forty-eight hours after 12 days of living in a rotating environment, the directional specificity of the oculomotor and perceptual evidence of adaptation disappears, reactions are diminished for head movements made during rotation in either direction of platform rotation, and normal responses to head movements in a static environment replace the geometrically rearranged responses[34] (GUEDRY, 1965a, b). The diminished vestibular Coriolis cross-coupled reaction for the unpracticed rotation direction after 48 hours of recovery may indicate that an over-all suppression of Coriolis vestibular reaction developed during the 12-day habituation schedule, but was partially masked in the 1-hour posthabituation tests by the geometrically reordered response which added to the adequate Coriolis cross-coupled canal stimulus when rotation was in the unpracticed direction. It is also possible that the recovery process in the natural environment is tantamount to a degree of habituation to control of movement during rotation in opposite sense (REASON and GRAYBIEL, 1969b). Three weeks after the habituation schedule, nystagmus was still somewhat suppressed; but whereas the vertiginous sensations from Coriolis cross-coupling had returned in some observers, no discomfort or nausea was produced by 2 hours of voluntary movement within the practiced rotating environment. Moreover, the

34 The recovery to normal from the 'rearranged nystagmus responses' probably occurs much sooner than 48 hours, but tests were not administered within the 2–48 hour interval.

protracted habituation schedule had little apparent effect on nystagmus produced by simple angular acceleration at any time in the experiment (GUEDRY, 1965b). This and similar kinds of findings (for a complete review of vestibular habituation, see COLLINS, Sections F.VI.,VII. this volume) may be conceptualized as failures of habituation of transfer from one condition to another, but from another point of view there is an adaptive efficiency in the reduction of only those stimulus patterns that have set off perceptual and motor reactions which are inefficient in relation to the voluntary control of movement.

These experiments and those of GONSHOR are closely analogous to a whole class of experiments involving what has been referred to as "geometric displacement" or "sensory rearrangement" (cf. SMITH and SMITH, 1962; HABER, 1968; HELD, 1965, 1961; HELD and HEIN, 1958, 1963). Typically, observers have worn optical devices such as prisms or mirrors, which displace, tilt, invert, or reverse the visual field (cf. KOHLER in HABER, 474f, 1968). Unfortunately, measures of vestibular reflexes such as nystagmus and ocular counterrolling have not been measured in most of these experiments. Quantitative performance measures have usually involved some kind of eye-hand coordination test or walking test during and after the period of sensory rearrangement. These studies have usually shown a considerable improvement in performance during the exposure period, impressive aftereffects when the distorted visual input was removed, and pronounced individual differences in the initial effects and in rate of adjustment to distorted input. In general, HELD's work (1965) has demonstrated that sensory-motor adjustments are more readily learned when the observers made active (voluntary) movements during the sensory rearrangement, although this is subject to some debate (cf. FREEDMAN, Ed., 1968). The work of TAUB and BERMAN (1968), however, suggests that volition contributes to the learning process, as indicated by the demonstration of learning after deafferentation of limbs. There is evidence of phylogenetic differences in the rearrangement experiments (TAUB, 1968), and there is probably variation among species in the extent to which various mechanisms of adjustment are used.

V. Mechanisms of Vestibular Habituation

In describing nystagmus and turning sensations during and after unusually long or repetitive stimuli, a number of changes in responses have been referred to as signs of adaptation, adjustment, accommodation or habituation in preceding sections of this chapter. The fact that these changes occur at different rates under different combinations of sensory stimulation and task assignments suggests that several mechanisms of response alteration are involved (cf. GRAYBIEL et al., 1965). The following speculations are presented to conceptualize how several adaptive mechanisms might operate to provide more efficient adjustments to changing conditions than any one alone would accomplish.

1. First, it is assumed that control of eye, head and body movements during changing visual and vestibular inputs contributes to survival of species and that efficiency in adjusting to temporary and persistent environmental changes is a necessary characteristic of surviving species. Fish and tree-dwelling monkeys

must adjust to passive motion, and all species experience passive motion in infancy. It is likely that early exposure to passive motion is necessary to development and that adjustment to it is a necessary part of normal maturation.

2. It is proposed that there are several interrelated mechanisms involved in habituation to unnatural semicircular canal stimuli and unnatural patterns of sensory input from the various spatial orientation senses. Two lower-order processes serve to reduce responses without introducing a learned sensory motor rearrangement. One is a suppressing mechanism and the other a switching mechanism. The first may be more prominent in lower animals than in man (cf. TAUB, 1968; COLLINS and GUEDRY, 1967; GUEDRY and COLLINS, 1968), and both serve for adjustment to motion when a simple short-term reduction of response is required for efficient behavior. The effects of the suppressive process are approximately described by the adaptation model in an earlier section. This short-term adaptive change occurs independently of arousal state, although arousal may have some influence on the rate of change. Any sustained change in level of vestibular sensory input initiates counter processes to return the effects of the sensory inflow toward zero response output (cf. SHARPLESS, 1964). This process operates irrespective of cognitive assessment of stimulus significance. The second mechanism, the switching mechanism, may be referred to as attention habituation, whereby repeated stimuli become classified as familiar and inconsequential, leading to reaction reduction. This process involves more complex systems than those involved in the short-term adaptive change in that pattern recognition or matching is involved. The functional value is that attention and energies are not expended unnecessarily on unnecessary actions, and attention can be switched to other environmental changes. However, heightened mental arousal through such activities as mental arithmetic can reinstitute the vestibular reflex actions which have been lost through attention habituation. The fact that arousal sources other than attention to vestibular messages can re-elicit the response is attributable to the fact that the vestibular system normally functions when the attention is directed to sensory inputs other than the incoming vestibular signals; i.e., vestibular information seldom reaches cognitive awareness during natural coordinated movement in adult life. These mechanisms are present in the course of natural ontogenetic development. A third mechanism of adaptation is brought into play when performance requirements under unusual conditions of sensory stimulation require a rearrangement of sensory-perceptual and sensory-motor relations for effective control of motion. The organism is required to adjust to a new and different environment. Since the process of growth involves sensory-motor rearrangements (cf. HELD, 1965), this form of adjustment is required in normal development. It is akin to a learning process and is facilitated by pairing stimuli which elicit involuntary reflex actions with stimuli to other senses that also influence the same reflex, especially through voluntary control mechanisms (cf. KIMBLE and PERLMUTER, 1970). Thus the pairing of visual and vestibular stimulation involves voluntary control of eye movements in attempts to fixate visual targets and also involuntary vestibular control of eye movements. Repeated prolonged exposure to such stimulation where a change in the sensory response contributes to the efficiency of control of motion results in the establishment of new sensory-motor—sensory-perceptual relations.

3. The two lower-order mechanisms permit rapid adjustment of behavior to novel sensory inputs. It is proposed that they also serve to prevent rapid development of the third process, i.e., sensory-motor and sensory-perceptual rearrangements that would be maladaptive in most natural circumstances. It is assumed, therefore, that attention habituation (switching mechanism) and the short-term adaptation process (suppressing mechanism) serve to prevent learning of rearrangements except when this additional stage of adjustment is demanded by the individual's task in an unnatural motion environment.

4. Individual differences in habituation to unnatural motions are probably influenced by early conditioning of emotional reactivity related to the innate fear of falling and also by differences in amount of sensory stimulation associated with and elicited by whole-body movement in the parent-child relationship.

References

ADRIAN, E.D.: Discharges from vestibular receptors in the cat. J. Physiol. (Lond.) **101**, 389–407 (1943).

AMBLER, R.K., GUEDRY, F.E.: Reliability and validity of the Brief Vestibular Disorientation procedure compared under 10 rpm and 15 rpm conditions. Aerospace Med. **42**, 186–189 (1971).

ANDERSSON, S., GERNANDT, B.: Cortical projection of vestibular nerve in cat. Acta oto-laryng. (Stockh.), Suppl. **116** (1954).

ANDERSSON, S., NILSSON, A., RUUTH, E., SMITH, G.: Visual aftereffects and the individual as an adaptive system. CWK Gleerup, Lund, Sweden 1972.

ARNDTS, F.: Zur Frage nach der Lagewahrnehmung dienenden Sinnesfunctionen. Pflügers Arch. ges. Physiol. **204**, 539–540 (1924).

ARNOULT, M.: Postrotatory localization of sound. Amer. J. Psychol. **63**, 229–236 (1950).

ASCHAN, G., BERGSTEDT, M.: The genesis of secondary nystagmus induced by vestibular stimuli. Acta Soc. Med. upsalien. **60**, 113–122 (1965).

ASCHAN, G., NYLÉN, C.O., STAHLE, J., WERSÄLL, R.: The rotation test. Cupulometric data from 320 normals. Acta oto-laryng. (Stockh.) **42**, 451–459 (1952).

ARSLAN, M., MOLINARI, J.A.: Modification of the activity of the vestibular nuclei in the cat following stimulation in the temporal lobe. Acta oto-laryng. (Stockh.) **59**, 338–343 (1965).

AUBERT, H.: Eine scheinbare bedeutende Drehung von Objekten bei Neigung des Kopfes nach rechts oder links. Virchows Arch. **20**, 381–393 (1861).

BÁRÁNY, R.: Physiologie und Pathologie des Bogengangsapparates beim Menschen. Vienna: Deuticke 1907.

BÁRÁNY, R.: Zur Klinik und Theorie des Eisenbahn-Nystagmus. Arch. Augenheilk. **87**, 139–142 (1921).

BARLOW, J.S.: Inertial navigation as a basis for animal navigation. J. theor. Biol. **6**, 76–117 (1964).

BARLOW, J.S.: Vestibular and non-dominant and parietal lobe disorders. Dis. nerv. Syst. **31**, 624–679 (1970).

BARNES, G.R.: A theoretical model of the utricular otolith and its response to angular motion with respect to an acceleration in shear. IAM Report 506. Farnborough, England: RAF Institute of Aviation Medicine 1971.

BARRETT, G.V., THORTON, C.L.: Relationship between perceptual style and simulator sickness. J. appl. Psychol. **52**, 304–308 (1968).

BAUERMEISTER, M.: Effect of body tilt on apparent verticality, apparent body position, and their relation. J. exp. Psychol. **67**, 142–147 (1964).

BAUERMEISTER, M., WERNER, H., WAPNER, S.: The effect of body tilt on tactual-kinesthetic perception of verticality. Amer. J. Psychol. **77**, 451–456 (1964).

BECHINGER, D., KONGEHL, G., KORNHUBER, H.H.: Dependence of human sensory information transmission on distribution of stimuli. Naturwissenschaften **56** (8), 419 (1969).

BELANGER, F., MAYNE, R.: The dynamics of the semicircular canals. GERA-1085. Litchfield Park, Ariz.: Goodyear Aerospace Corp. 1965.

BENFARI, R.C.: Perceptual vertigo: A dimensional study. Percept. Mot. Skills **18**, 633–639 (1964).

BENSON, A.J.: Modification of per- and post-rotational responses by the concomitant linear acceleration. NASA SP-115. Washington, D.C.: U.S. Government Printing Office 1966.

BENSON, A.J.: Postrotational sensation and nystagmus as indicants of semicircular canal function. NASA SP-152. Washington, D.C.: U.S. Government Printing Office 1968a.

BENSON, A.J.: Personal communication 1968b.

BENSON, A.J.: Interactions between semicircular canals and gravireceptors. In: Recent advances in aerospace medicine. Dordrecht, Holland: Reidel 1970.

BENSON, A.J.: Effect of angular oscillation in yaw on vision. Proc. Aerospace Med. Assn. Annual Meeting, Miami 1972.

BENSON, A.J., BARNES, G.R.: Responses to rotating linear acceleration vectors considered in relation to a model of the otolith organs. NASA SP-314. Washington, D.C.: U.S. Government Printing Office 1973.

BENSON, A.J., BODIN, M.: Interaction of linear and angular accelerations on vestibular receptors in man. Aerospace Med. **37**, 144–154 (1966a).

BENSON, A.J., BODIN, M.: Comparison of the effect of the direction of the gravitational acceleration on post-rotational responses in yaw, pitch and roll. Aerospace Med. **37**, 889–897 (1966b).

BENSON, A.J., BRAND, J.L.: Some effects of l-hyoscine hydrobromin on post-rotatory sensation and nystagmus in man. IAM Report 378. Farnborough, England: RAF Institute of Aviation Medicine 1966.

BENSON, A.J., GUEDRY, F.E.: Comparison of tracking-task performance and nystagmus during sinusoidal oscillation in yaw and pitch. Aerospace Med. **42**, 593–601 (1971).

BENSON, A.J., DIAZ, E., FARRUGIA, P.: The perception of body orientation relative to a rotating linear acceleration vector. Personal communication 1971.

BENSON, A.J., GUEDRY, F.E., MELVILL JONES, G.: Response of the semicircular canal dependent units in the vestibular nuclei to rotation of a linear acceleration vector without angular acceleration. J. Physiol. (Lond.) **210**, 475–494 (1970).

BENSON, A.J., GOORNEY, A.B., REASON, J.T.: The effect of instruction upon post-rotational sensations and nystagmus. Acta oto-laryng. (Stockh.) **62**, 442–452 (1966).

BERGSTEDT, M.: Stepwise adaptation to a velocity of 10 rpm in the Pensacola Slow Rotation Room. NASA SP-77. Washington, D.C.: U.S. Government Printing Office 1965.

BERITOV, I.S.: The mechanism of spatial orientation in man. Pavlov J. higher nerv. Activ. **9** (1), 1–11 (1959). Translated from the Russian and published by National Institute of Health, U.S. Public Health Service, and U.S. Department of Health, Education and Welfare. Translation S.A. CORSON, Ed. New Haven, Conn.: Yale University.

BIRREN, J.E.: Static equilibrium and vestibular function. J. exp. Psychol. **35**, 127–133 (1945).

BISCHOFF, N., SCHEERER, E.: Systemanalyse der optisch-vestibulären Interaktion bei der Wahrnehmung der Vertikalen. Psychol. Forsch. **34**, 99–181 (1970).

BORNSCHEIN, V.H., SCHUBERT, G.: Objektivierung und Analyse des vestibulären Coriolis-Effektes. Z. Biol. **107**, 95–107 (1954).

BORNSCHEIN, V.H., SCHUBERT, G.: Die Reizparameter des vestibulären Coriolis-Effektes. Z. Biol. **110**, 269–275 (1958).

BORNSCHEIN, V. H., SCHUBERT, G.: Die Richtung des vestibulären Coriolis-Effektes. Z. Biol. **113**, 145–160 (1962).

BOURDON, B.: Sur le rôle de la tête dans perception de l'espace. Rev. Philos. **61**, 526–529 (1906).

BOURDON, B.: Reserches sur la perception des movements rectilignes de tout le corps. L'année Psychol. **20**, 1–16 (1914).

Brandt, Th., Dichgans, J.: Circularvektion, optische Pseudocoriolis-Effekte und optokinetischer Nachnystagmus. Albrecht v. Graefes Arch. klin. exp. Ophthal. **184**, 42–57 (1972).

Brandt, Th., Dichgans, J., Koenig, E.: Differential effects of central versus peripheral vision on egocentric and exocentric motion perception. Submitted to Exp. Brain Res. **16**, 476–491 (1973).

Brandt, Th., Wist, E., Dichgans, J.: Optisch induzierte Pseudocoriolis-Effekte und Circularvektion. Arch. Psychiat. Nervenkr. **214**, 365–389 (1971).

Brandt, U., Fluur, E.: Postural perceptions and eye displacements produced by a resultant vector acting in the medial sagittal plane of the head. I. Responses along three axes by stepwise increasing phi with the subject heading centripetally in an erect and tilted position. Acta oto-laryng. (Stockh.) **63**, 489–502 (1967a).

Brandt, U., Fluur, E.: Postural perceptions and eye displacements produced by a resultant vector acting in the median sagittal plane of the head. II. Continuous responses along the Y axis with the subject in a vertical position, heading centripetally and centrifugally. Acta oto-laryng. (Stockh.) **63**, 564–578 (1967b).

Brodal, A.: Anatomical observations on the vestibular nuclei, with special reference to their relations to the spinal cord and the cerebellum. Acta oto-laryng. (Stockh.), Suppl. **192** (1964).

Brodal, A.: Anatomical aspects on functional organization of the vestibular nuclei. NASA SP-115. Washington, D.C.: U.S. Government Printing Office 1966.

Brown, J. H.: Magnitude estimation of angular velocity during passive rotation. J. exp. Psychol. **72** (2), 169–172 (1966).

Brown, J. H.: Cross-modal estimation of angular velocity. Percept. Psychophysics **3**, 115–117 (1968).

Brown, J. H., Crampton, G. H.: Quantification of the human nystagmic response to angular acceleration. Prediction formulae and nomograph. Acta oto-laryng. (Stockh.) **58**, 555–564 (1964).

Brown, J. H., Crampton, G. H.: Concomitant visual stimulation does not alter habituation of nystagmic, oculogyral or psychophysical responses to angular acceleration. Acta oto-laryng. (Stockh.) **61**, 80–91 (1966).

Brown, J. H., Wolfe, J. W.: Adaptation to prolonged constant angular acceleration. Acta oto-laryng. (Stockh.) **67**, 389–398 (1969).

Brown, J. L.: Orientation to the vertical during water immersion. Aerospace Med. **32**, 209–217 (1961).

Brown, R. H., Imus, H., Niven, J. I., Graybiel, A.: The relationship between apparent displacement and motion in the oculogyral illusion. NSAM-460. Pensacola, Florida: Naval School of Aviation Medicine 1949.

Burtt, N. E.: The perception of slight changes of equilibrium with special reference to the problems of aviation. J. appl. Psychol. **2**, 101–115 (1918).

Buys, E.: Contribution à l'étude du nystagmus oculaire de la rotation chez l'homme. Rev. Oto-Neuro-Ouil. **2**, 641–659, 721–749 (1924).

Byford, G. H.: Eye movements and the optogyral illusion. Aerospace Med. **34**, 119–123 (1963).

Cappel, K.: Determination of physical constants of semicircular canals from measurement of single neural unit activity under constant angular acceleration. NASA SP-115. Washington, D.C.: U.S. Government Printing Office 1966.

Carlstrom, D.: A crystallogravic study of vertebrate otoliths. Biol. Bull. **125**, 441 (1963).

Cawthorne, T., Dix, M., Hallpike, C., Hood, J.: The investigation of vestibular function. Brit. med. Bull. **12** (2), 131–142 (1956).

Christian, P.: Über unbewusste Vestibulariswirkung. Z. für Neurol. und Psychiat. **165**, 214–219 (1939).

Clark, B.: Thresholds for the perception of angular acceleration in man. Aerospace Med. **38**, 443–450 (1967).

Clark, B.: The vestibular system. Ann. Rev. Psychol. **21**, 273–306 (1970).

Clark, B., Graybiel, A.: The effect of angular acceleration on sound localization: The audiogyral illusion. J. Psychol. (Provincetown) **28**, 235–244 (1949).

Clark, B., Graybiel, A.: The duration of the oculogyral illusion as a function of the interval between positive and negative acceleration. J. appl. Physiol. **5**, 147–152 (1952).

Clark, B., Graybiel, A.: Antecedent visual frame of reference as a contributing factor in the perception of the oculogravic illusion. NSAM-457. Pensacola, Fla.: Naval School of Aviation Medicine 1961.

Clark, B., Graybiel, A.: Visual perception of the horizontal during prolonged exposure to radial acceleration on a centrifuge. J. exp. Psychol. **63**, 294–302 (1962).

Clark, B., Graybiel, A.: Perception of the postural vertical in normals and subjects with labyrinthine defects. J. exp. Psychol. **65**, 490–494 (1963a).

Clark, B., Graybiel, A.: Contributing factors in the perception of the oculogravic illusion. Amer. J. Psychol. **76**, 18–27 (1963b).

Clark, B., Graybiel, A.: Perception of the postural vertical following prolonged bodily tilt in normals and subjects with labyrinthine defects. Acta oto-laryng. (Stockh.) **58**, 143–148 (1964).

Clark, B., Graybiel, A.: Factors contributing to the delay in the perception of the oculogravic illusion. Amer. J. Psychol. **79**, 377–388 (1966a).

Clark, B., Graybiel, A.: Perception of the visual horizontal in normal and labyrinthine defective subjects during prolonged rotation. Amer. J. Psychol. **79**, 608–612 (1966b).

Clark, B., Graybiel, A.: Egocentric localization of the visual horizontal in normal and labyrinthine defective observers as a function of head and body tilt. Percept. Psychophysics **2**, 609–611 (1967).

Clark, B., Graybiel, A.: Influence of contact on the perception of the oculogravic illusion. Acta oto-laryng. (Stockh.) **65**, 373–380 (1968).

Clark, B., Stewart, J.D.: Perception of angular acceleration about the yaw axis of a flight simulation: Thresholds and reaction latency for research pilots. Aerospace Med. **33**, 1426–1432 (1962).

Clark, B., Stewart, J.D.: Vestibular and nonvestibular information in judgments of attitude and Coriolis motion in a piloted flight simulator. Aerospace Med. **38**, 936–940 (1967).

Clark, B., Stewart, J.D.: Comparison of three methods to determine thresholds for the perception of passive bodily acceleration. Amer. J. Psychol. **81**, 207–216 (1968a).

Clark, B., Stewart, J.D.: Comparison of sensitivity for the perception of bodily rotation and the oculogyral illusion. Percept. Psychophysics **3**, 253–256 (1968b).

Clark, B., Stewart, J.D.: Magnitude estimates of rotational velocity during and following prolonged increasing, constant, and zero acceleration. J. exp. Psychol. **78**, 329–339 (1968c).

Clark, B., Stewart, J.D.: Effects of angular acceleration on man: Thresholds for the perception of rotation and the oculogyral illusion. Aerospace Med. **40**, 952–956 (1969).

Clark, B., Stewart, J.D.: The power law for the perception of rotation by airline pilots. Percept. Psychophysics **11**, 433–436 (1972a).

Clark, B., Stewart, J.D.: Comparison of the sensitivity to rotation of pilots and nonpilots. Aerospace Med. **43**, 8–12 (1972b).

Clark, B., Graybiel, A., MacCorquodale, K.: The illusory perception of movement caused by angular acceleration and centrifugal force during flight. II. Visually perceived motion of a fixed target during turns. J. exp. Psychol. **38**, 298–309 (1948).

Clegg, W.C., Dunfield, N.M.: Non-visual perception of the postural vertical. I. Sagittal plane. Canadian J. Psychol. **8**, 1–8 (1954a).

Clegg, W.C., Dunfield, N.M.: Non-visual perception of the postural vertical. II. Lateral plane. Canadian J. Psychol. **8**, 80–86 (1954b).

Cohen, B., Highstein, S.M.: Cerebellar control of vestibular pathways to oculomotor neurons. In: Progress in Brain Research, Vol. 37, Basic aspects of central vestibular mechanisms. Amsterdam: Elsevier 1972.

Cohen, B., Takemori, S.: Visual inhibition of nystagmus by the flocculus. Fed. Proc. (in press 1973).

Cohen, B., Takemori, S., Uemura, T.: Visual-vestibular interaction: The role of the labyrinth in the production of optokinetic nystagmus and optokinetic afternystagmus. AGARD-CPP-128. London: Technical Editing and Reproduction Ltd. 1973.

Cohen, M.M., Crosbie, R.J., Blackburn, L.H.: Disorienting effects of air-craft catapult launchings. AGARD-CP-95-Part I. London: Technical Editing and Reproduction Ltd. 1972.

Colenbrander, A.: Eye and otoliths. Aeromed. Acta (Soesterberg) **9**, 45–92 (1963–1964).

Collins, W.E.: Task control of arousal and the effects of repeated unidirectional angular acceleration on human vestibular responses. Acta oto-laryng. (Stockh.) Suppl. **190** (1964).

Collins, W.E.: Subjective responses and nystagmus following repeated unilateral caloric stimulation. Ann. Otol. (St. Louis) **74**, 1034–1055 (1965).

Collins, W.E.: Coriolis vestibular stimulation and the influence of different visual surrounds. Aerospace Med. **39**, 125–130 (1968a).

Collins, W.E.: Special effects of brief periods of visual fixation on nystagmus and sensations of turning. Aerospace Med. **39**, 257–266 (1968b).

Collins, W.E.: Influence of head position on the habituation of vertical vestibular nystagmus in the cat. J. comp. physiol. Psychol. **67**, 156–159 (1969).

Collins, W.E., Guedry, F.E.: Arousal effects and nystagmus during prolonged constant acceleration. Acta oto-laryng. (Stockh.) **54**, 349–362 (1962).

Collins, W.E., Guedry, F.E.: Duration of angular acceleration and ocular nystagmus from cat and man. I. Responses from the lateral and the vertical canals to two stimulus durations. Acta oto-laryng. (Stockh.) **64**, 373–387 (1967).

Collins, W.E., Schroeder, D.J., Hill, R.J.: Some effects of alcohol on vestibular responses. Advanc. oto-rhino-laryng. **19**, 295–303 (1973).

Collins, W.E., Schroeder, D.J., Gilson, R.D., Guedry, F.E.: Effects of alcohol ingestion on tracking performance during angular acceleration. J. appl. Psychol. **55**, 559–563 (1971).

Correia, M.J.: An empirical and theoretical consideration of anchoring effects in the judgment of verticality. Thesis. University, Alabama: University of Alabama 1962.

Correia, M.J., Guedry, F.E.: Influence of labyrinth orientation relative to gravity on responses elicited by stimulation of the horizontal semicircular canals. NSAM-905. Pensacola, Fla.: Naval School of Aviation Medicine 1964.

Correia, M.J., Guedry, F.E.: Modification of vestibular responses as a function of rate of rotation about an Earth-horizontal axis. Acta oto-laryng. (Stockh.) **62**, 297–308 (1966).

Correia, M.J., Money, K.E.: The effect of blockage of all six semicircular canal ducts on nystagmus produced by dynamic linear acceleration in the cat. DRET Report 728. Toronto: Defence Research Establishment, Defence Research Board 1968.

Correia, M.J., Hixson, W.C., Niven, J.I.: Otolith shear and the visual perception of force direction: Discrepancies and a proposed resolution. NAMI-951. Pensacola, Fla.: Naval Aerospace Medical Institute 1965.

Correia, M.J., Hixson, W.C., Niven, J.I.: On predictive equations for subjective judgments of vertical and horizon in a force field. Acta oto-laryng. (Stockh.) Suppl. **230** (1968).

Corso, J.I.: A theoretico-historical review of the threshold concept. Psychol. Bull. **60**, 356–370 (1963).

Corvera, J., Hallpike, C.S., Schuster, E.H.J.: A new method for the anatomical reconstruction of the human macular planes. Acta oto-laryng. (Stockh.) **49**, 4–16 (1958).

Cramer, R.L.: Subjective responses to oscillation in yaw. Aerospace Med. **38**, 457–458 (1964).

Crampton, G.H., Gall, K.: Responses of single cells within the cat medulla during prolonged constant angular acceleration. Tech. Report EATR 4505. Edgewood Arsenal, Maryland: Dept. of the Army, Edgewood Arsenal Research Laboratories 1971.

Crampton, G.H., Young, F.A.: The differential effects of a rotatory visual field on susceptibles and non-susceptibles to motion sickness. J. comp. physiol. Psychol. **46**, 451–453 (1953).

CRITCHLEY, M.: The Parietal Lobes. London: Arnold 1953.

CROSBY, E.C., HUMPHREY, T., LAUER, E.W.: Correlative Anatomy of the Nervous System. New York: MacMillan 1962.

CULLEN, J.F., HARPER, C.R.: Perceptual differences of airline pilots and engineers. Aerospace Med. **40**, 407–408 (1969).

DAY, R., WADE, N.: Visual spatial aftereffect from prolonged head tilt. Science **154**, 1201–1202 (1966).

DE VRIES, HL.: The minimum perceptible angular acceleration under various conditions. Acta oto-laryng. (Stockh.) **37**, 218–229 (1949).

DE VRIES, HL.: The mechanics of the labyrinth otoliths. Acta oto-laryng. (Stockh.) **38**, 263–273 (1950).

DE VRIES, HL., SCHIERBEEK, P.: The minimum perceptible velocity under various conditions. Pract. oto-rhino-laryng. (Basel) **15**, 65–72 (1953).

DICHGANS, J., BRANDT, TH.: Visual-vestibular interaction and motion perception. In: Cerebral control of eye movements and motion perception. Basel/New York: S. Karger 1972.

DICHGANS, J., BRANDT, TH.: The psychophysics of visually induced perception of self-motion and tilt. In: F.O. SCHMITT and F.G. WORDEN (Eds.): The Neurosciences, Cambridge, Mass.: MIT Press 1974.

DICHGANS, J., BRANDT, TH.: Self-motion-sensation, pseudo-Coriolis effects and motion sickness induced by optokinetic stimuli. AGARD-CPP-128. London: Technical Editing and Reproduction Ltd. 1973b.

DICHGANS, J., JUNG, R.: Attention, eye movements and motion detection: Facilitation and selection in optokinetic nystagmus and railway nystagmus. In: Attention in Neurophysiology. London: Butterworth and Co. 1969.

DICHGANS, J., KÖRNER, F., VOIGT, K.: Vergleichende Skalierung des afferenten und efferenten Bewegungssehens beim Menschen: Lineare Funktionen mit verschiedener Anstiegssteilheit. Psychol. Forsch. **32**, 277–295 (1969).

DICHGANS, J., HELD, R., YOUNG, L., BRANDT, TH.: Moving visual scenes influence the apparent direction of gravity. Science **178**, 1217–1219 (1972).

DOBIE, T.B.: Evaluation of subjective cupulometry as a selection technique with potential aircrews. Presented at 40th Aerospace Medical Assn. Annual Meeting, San Francisco 1969.

DOCKSTADER, S.L.: Comparison of cupulometric and psychophysical thresholds for perception of rotation and the oculogyral illusion. Percept. Psychophysics **9**, 299–302 (1971).

DODGE, R.: Habituation to rotation; thresholds of rotation. J. exp. Psychol. **6**, 1–35, 107–137 (1923).

DOTY, R.L.: Effect of duration of stimulus presentation on the angular acceleration threshold. J. exp. Psychol. **80**, 317–321 (1969).

DUENSING, F., SCHAEFER, K.P.: Über die Konvergenz verschiedener labyrinthärer Afferenzen auf einzelne Neurone des Vestibularis-Kerngebietes. Arch. Psychiat. Nervenkr. **199**, 345–371 (1959).

DUFFY, F.H., LOMBROSE, C.T.: Electrophysiological evidence of visual suppression prior to the onset of a voluntary saccadic eye movement. Nature (Lond.) **218**, 1074–1075 (1968).

EK, J., JONGKEES, L.B.W., KLIJN, J.: The threshold of the vestibular organ. Acta oto-laryng. (Stockh.) **50**, 292–299 (1959).

EK, J., JONGKEES, L.B.W., KLIJN, J.: On the effect of continuous acceleration. Acta oto-laryng. (Stockh.) **51**, 416–419 (1960).

ELSNER, W.: The power laws for the perception of rotation and the oculogyral illusion. Percept. Psychophysics **9**, 418–420 (1971).

ENGEN, T., ROSS, B.M.: Effect of reference number on magnitude estimation. Percept. Psychophysics **1**, 74–76 (1966).

ENGSTRÖM, H., WERSÄLL, J.: Structure and innervation of the inner ear sensory epithelia. Int. Rev. Cytol. **7**, 535–585 (1958).

Engström, H., Lindeman, H.H., Ades, H.W.: Anatomical features of the auricular sensory organs. NASA SP-115. Washington, D.C.: U.S. Government Printing Office 1966.

Feilchenfeld, H.: Zur Lageschätzung bei seitlichen Kopfneigungen. Z. Psychol. Physiol. Sinnesorg. **31**, 127–150 (1903).

Fernández, C., Fredrickson, J.M.: Experimental cerebellar lesions and their effect on vestibular function. Acta oto-laryng. (Stockh.) Suppl. **192** (1964).

Fernández, C., Goldberg, J.M.: Physiology of peripheral neurons innervating the semicircular canals of the squirrel monkey. The response to sinusoidal stimulation and dynamics of the peripheral vestibular system. J. Neurophysiol. **34**, 661–675 (1971).

Fischer, M.H.: Messende Untersuchungen über die Gegenrollung der Augen und die Lokalisation der scheinbaren Vertikalen bei seitlicher Neigung des Körpers, Kopfes und Stammes: III. Mitteilung. Untersuchungen an einem Ertaubten mit Functionsuntüchtigkeit beider Vestibularapparate und einem einseitig Labyrinthlosen. Albrecht v. Graefes Arch. klin. exp. Ophthal. **123**, 509–531 (1930).

Fleishman, E.A.: The perception of body position-effect of speed, magnitude, and direction of displacement on accuracy of adjustment to an upright position. Human Resources Research Center Bulletin, 53–61 (1953a).

Fleishman, E.A.: Perception of body position in the absence of visual cues. J. exp. Psychol. **46**, 261–270 (1953b).

Fluur, E.: The interaction between the utricle and saccule. Acta oto-laryng. (Stockh.) **69**, 17–24 (1970).

Fluur, E., Mellström, A.: Utricular stimulation and oculomotor reactions. Laryngoscope (St. Louis) **80**, 1701–1712 (1970a).

Fluur, E., Mellström, A.: Saccular stimulation and oculomotor reactions. Laryngoscope (St. Louis) **80**, 1713–1721 (1970b).

Fredrickson, J.M., Schwarz, D.: Multisensory influence upon single units in the vestibular nucleus. NASA SP-187. Washington, D.C.: U.S. Government Printing Office 1970.

Fredrickson, J., Figge, U., Scheid, P., Kornhuber, H.H.: Vestibular nerve projection to the cerebral cortex of the Rhesus monkey. Exp. Brain Res. **2**, 318–327 (1966).

Freedman, S.J.: The Neuropsychology of Spatially Oriented Behavior. Homewood, Illinois: Dorsey Press 1968.

Galebsky, A.: Vestibular nystagmus in new-born infants. Acta oto-laryng. (Stockh.) **11**, 409–423 (1927).

Galle, R.R., Emel'ianov, M.D.: Results of physiological studies performed in a slow rotation chamber. Space Biol. Med. **1**, 108–118 (1967).

Garner, W.R.: Uncertainty and Structure as Psychological Concepts. New York: Wiley 1962.

Garner, W.R., Hake, H.W.: The amount of information in absolute judgments. Psychol. Rev. **58**, 446–459 (1951).

Garten, S.: Über die Grundlagen unserer Orientierung im Raume. Abh. Sachs. ges. (Akad.) Wiss. **26**, 433–510 (1920).

Geldard, F.A.: The Human Senses. Second Edition. New York/London/Sydney/Toronto: John Wiley and Sons, Inc. 1972.

Gernandt, B.E.: Vestibular influence upon spinal reflex activity. CIBA Symposium on myotatic, kinesthetic and vestibular mechanisms (1967).

Gescheider, G.A., Wright, J.H.: Effects of body position on judgments of postural vertical. Percept. Mot. Skills **21**, 783–786 (1965).

Gibson, J.J., Mowrer, O.H.: Determinants of the perceived vertical and horizontal. Psychol. Rev. **45**, 300–323 (1938).

Gilson, R.D., Guedry, F.E., Stockwell, C.W.: Conditioned suppression of vestibular nystagmus with visual stimuli. Presented at 44th Annual Aerospace Medical Assn. Meeting, Las Vegas, Nevada 1973a.

Gilson, R.D., Stockwell, C.W., Guedry, F.E.: Nystagmus responses during triangular waveforms of angular velocity about the y- and z-axes. Acta oto-laryng. (Stockh.) **75**, 21–26 (1973b).

Gilson, R.D., Schroeder, D.J., Collins, W.E., Guedry, F.E.: Effects of different alcohol dosages and display luminance on tracking performance during vestibular stimulation. Aerospace Med. **43**, 656–660 (1972).

GOLDBERG, J.M., FERNÁNDEZ, C.: Physiology of peripheral neurons innervating the semicircular canals of the squirrel monkey. I and III. J. Neurophysiol. **34**, 636–660, 676–684 (1971).

GONSHOR, A., MELVILL JONES, G.: Vestibular habituation induced by mirror vision: An optimising process. Presented at 42d Annual Aerospace Medical Assn. Meeting, Houston, Texas 1971.

GRAYBIEL, A.: Oculogravic illusion. AMA Arch. Ophthal. **48**, 605–615 (1952).

GRAYBIEL, A., BROWN, R.H.: The delay in visual reorientation following exposure to a change in direction of resultant force on a human centrifuge. J. genet. Psychol. **45**, 143–150 (1951).

GRAYBIEL, A., CLARK, B.: Perception of the horizontal or vertical with the head upright, on the side, and inverted under static conditions, and during exposure to centripetal force. Aerospace Med. **33**, 147–155 (1962).

GRAYBIEL, A., CLARK, B.: The validity of the oculogravic illusion as a specific indicator of otolith function. Aerospace Med. **36**, 1173–1181 (1965).

GRAYBIEL, A., HUPP, D.I.: The oculogyral illusion: A form of apparent motion which may be observed following stimulation of the semicircular canals. J. Aviat. Med. **3**, 1–12 (1946).

GRAYBIEL, A., JOHNSON, W.H.: A comparison of symptomatology experienced by healthy persons and subjects with loss of labyrinthine function when exposed to unusual patterns of centripetal force in counter-rotating room. Ann. Otol. (St. Louis) **72**, 357–373 (1963).

GRAYBIEL, A., KELLOGG, R.S.: The inversion illusion in parabolic flight: Its probable dependence on otolith function. Aerospace Med. **38**, 1099–1102 (1967).

GRAYBIEL, A., MILLER, E.F.: The otolith organs as a primary etiological factor in motion sickness: With a note on "off-vertical" rotation. NASA SP-187. Washington, D.C.: U.S. Government Printing Office 1970.

GRAYBIEL, A., PATTERSON, J.L.: Thresholds of stimulation of the otolith organs as indicated by the oculogravic illusion. J. appl. Psychol. **7**, 666–670 (1955).

GRAYBIEL, A., CLARK, B., ZARRIELLO, J.J.: Observations on human subjects living in a "slow rotation room" for periods of two days. AMA Arch. Neurol. **3**, 55–73 (1960).

GRAYBIEL, A., CLARK, B., MACCORQUODALE, K., HUPP, D.: The role of vestibular nystagmus in the visual perception of a moving target in the dark. Amer. J. Psychol. **59**, 259–266 (1946).

GRAYBIEL, A., KERR, W., HUPP, D., BARTLEY, S.: Threshold of stimulation of the horizontal semicircular canals in man with particular reference to the first derivative of angular acceleration as a stimulus. Amer. J. Psychol. **61**, 21–36 (1948).

GRAYBIEL, A., MILLER, E.F., NEWSOM, B., KENNEDY, R.: The effect of water immersion on perception of the oculogravic illusion in normal and labyrinthine-defective subjects. Acta oto-laryng. (Stockh.) **65**, 599–610 (1968).

GRAYBIEL, A., MILLER, E.F., BILLINGHAM, J., WAITE, R., BERRY, C.A., DEITLEIN, L.F.: Vestibular experiments in Gemini flights V and VII. Aerospace Med. **38**, 360–370 (1967).

GRAYBIEL, A., KENNEDY, R.S., KNOBLOCK, E.C., GUEDRY, F.E., MERTZ, W., MCLEOD, M.E., COLEHOUR, J.K., MILLER, E.F., FREGLY, A.R.: The effects of exposure to a rotating environment (10 rpm) on four aviators for a period of 12 days. Aerospace Med. **36**, 733–754 (1965).

GROEN, J.J.: The semicircular canal system of the organs of equilibrium II. Phys. in Med. Biol. **1**, 225–242 (1956–1957).

GROEN, J.J.: Adaptation. Pract. oto-rhino-laryng. (Basel) **19**, 524–530 (1957).

GROEN, J.J.: Vestibular stimulation and its effects from the point of view of theoretical physics. Confin. neurol. (Basel) **21**, 380–389 (1961a).

GROEN, J.J.: Problems of the semicircular canals from a mechanico-physiological point of view. Acta oto-laryng. (Stockh.) Suppl. **163** (1961b).

GROEN, J.J.: The problems of the spinning top applied to the semicircular canals. Confin. neurol. (Basel) **21**, 454–455 (1961c).

Groen, J.J.: Postnatal changes in vestibular reactions. Acta oto-laryng. (Stockh.) **56**, 390–396 (1963).

Groen, J.J.: Central regulation of the vestibular system. Acta oto-laryng. (Stockh.) **59**, 211–216 (1965).

Groen, J.J.: Central regulations of vestibular function. In: Recent advances in aerospace medicine. Dordrecht, Holland: Reidel 1970.

Groen, J.J., Jongkees, L.B.W.: The threshold of angular acceleration perception. J. Physiol. (Lond.) **107**, 1–7 (1948a).

Groen, J.J., Jongkees, L.B.W.: The turning test with small regulable stimuli. IV. The cupulogram obtained by subject angle estimation. J. Laryng. **62**, 236–240 (1948b).

Groen, J.J., Lowenstein, O., Vendrick, A.J.H.: The mechanical analysis of the responses from the end organs of the horizontal semicircular canal in the isolated elasmobranch labyrinth. J. Physiol. (Lond.) **117**, 329–346 (1952).

Guedry, F.E.: Some effects of interacting vestibular stimuli. USAMRL Report 261. Ft. Knox, Kentucky: U.S. Army Medical Research Laboratory 1957.

Guedry, F.E.: Visual control of habituation to complex vestibular stimulation in man. Acta oto-laryng. (Stockh.) **58**, 377–389 (1964).

Guedry, F.E.: Psychophysiological studies of vestibular function. In: Contributions to sensory physiology. New York: Academic Press 1965a.

Guedry, F.E.: Habituation to complex vestibular stimulation in man: Transfer and retention of effects from twelve days of rotation at 10 rpm. Percept. Mot. Skills Monogr. Suppl. 1–V21 (1965b).

Guedry, F.E.: Orientation of the rotation-axis relative to gravity: Its influence on nystagmus and the sensation of rotation. Acta oto-laryng. (Stockh.) **60**, 30–48 (1965c).

Guedry, F.E.: Relations between vestibular nystagmus and visual performance. Aerospace Med. **39**, 570–579 (1968).

Guedry, F.E.: Effects of concomitant stimulation of the semicircular canals and otoliths by "barbecue spit" rotation, rotation about a tilted axis, and other forms of stimulation. Excerpta Med. Int. Cong. Ser. 206. Amsterdam 1970a.

Guedry, F.E.: Conflicting sensory orientation cues as a factor in motion sickness. NASA SP-187. Washington, D.C.: U.S. Government Printing Office 1970b.

Guedry, F.E.: Vision during angular acceleration considered in relation to aerospace operations. In: Vestibular function on earth and in space. Oxford and New York: Pergamon Press 1970c.

Guedry, F.E.: Theory of development of reactions to whole-body motion considered in relation to selection, assignment and training of flight personnel. AGARD-CP-95-Part I. London: Technical Editing and Reproduction Ltd. 1972.

Guedry, F.E., Ambler, R.K.: Assessment of reactions to vestibular disorientation stress for purposes of aircrew selection. AGARD-CP-109. London: Technical Editing and Reproduction Ltd. 1973a.

Guedry, F.E., Ambler, R.K.: The subjective disturbance introduced by simple angular acceleration when visual and vestibular inputs are synergistic and when they are anti-synergistic. In preparation (1973b).

Guedry, F.E., Benson, A.J.: Tracking performance during sinusoidal stimulation of the vertical and horizontal semicircular canals. In: Recent advances in aerospace medicine. Dordrecht, Holland: Reidel 1970.

Guedry, F.E., Benson, A.J.: Nystagmus and visual performance during sinusoidal stimulation of the vertical semicircular canals. NAMRL-1131. Pensacola, Fla.: Naval Aerospace Medical Research Laboratory 1971.

Guedry, F.E., Ceran, S.J.: Derivation of subjective velocity from angular displacement estimates made during prolonged angular acceleration: Adaptation effects. USAMRL Report 376. Ft. Knox, Kentucky: U.S. Army Medical Research Laboratory 1958.

Guedry, F.E., Collins, W.E.: Duration of angular acceleration and ocular nystagmus from cat and man. Acta oto-laryng (Stockh.) **65**, 257–269 (1968).

Guedry, F.E., Graybiel, A.: Compensatory nystagmus conditioned during adaptation to living in a rotating room. J. appl. Physiol. **17**, 398–404 (1962).

GUEDRY, F.E., HARRIS, C.S.: Labyrinthine function related to experiments on the parallel swing. NSAM-874. Pensacola, Fla.: Naval School of Aviation Medicine 1963.

GUEDRY, F.E., HOLMES, J.T.: Personal observation (1972).

GUEDRY, F.E., LAUVER, L.S.: Vestibular reactions during prolonged constant angular acceleration. J. appl. Physiol. **16**, 215–220 (1961).

GUEDRY, F.E., MONTAGUE, E.K.: Quantitative evaluation of the vestibular Coriolis reaction. Aerospace Med. **32**, 487–500 (1961).

GUEDRY, F.E., RICHMOND, G.: Differences in response latency with different magnitude angular acceleration. USAMRL Report 301. Ft. Knox, Kentucky: U.S. Army Medical Research Laboratory 1957.

GUEDRY, F.E., COLLINS, W.E., GRAYBIEL, A.: Vestibular habituation during repetitive complex stimulation: A study of transfer effects. J. appl. Physiol. **19**, 1005–1015 (1964).

GUEDRY, F.E., COLLINS, W.E., SHEFFEY, P.L.: Perceptual and oculomotor reactions to interacting visual and vestibular stimulation. Percept. Mot. Skills **12**, 307–324 (1961).

GUEDRY, F.E., CRAMER, R.L., KOELLA, W.P.: Experiments on the rate of development and rate of recovery of apparent adaptation effects in the vestibular system. USAMRL Report 338. Ft. Knox, Kentucky: U.S. Army Medical Research Laboratory 1958.

GUEDRY, F.E., OWENS, G.G., NORMAN, J.W.: Assessment of semicircular canal function. I. Measurements of subjective effects produced by triangular waveforms of angular velocity. NAMI-1073. Pensacola, Fla.: Naval Aerospace Medical Institute 1969.

GUEDRY, F.E., STOCKWELL, C.W., GILSON, R.D.: Comparison of subjective responses to semicircular canal stimulation produced by rotation about different axes. Acta oto-laryng. (Stockh.) **72**, 101–106 (1971b).

GUEDRY, F.E., OWENS, G.G., CUMMINGS, M., NORMAN, J.W.: Unpublished observations 1968.

GUEDRY, F.E., STOCKWELL, C.W., NORMAN, J.W., OWENS, G.G.: Use of triangular waveforms of angular velocity in the study of vestibular function. Acta oto-laryng. (Stockh.) **71**, 439–448 (1971a).

GURNEE, H.: Thresholds of vertical movement of the body. J. exp. Psychol. **17**, 270–285 (1934).

HABER, R.N.: Contemporary Theory and Research in Visual Perception. New York/San Francisco/London: Holt, Rinehart, and Winston 1968.

HALLPIKE, C.S., HOOD, J.D.: The speed of the slow component of ocular nystagmus induced by angular acceleration of the head: Its experimental determination and application to the physical theory of the cupula mechanism. Proc. roy. Soc. B **141**, 216–230 (1953a).

HALLPIKE, C.S., HOOD, J.D.: Fatigue and adaptation of the cupular mechanism of the human horizontal semicircular canal: An experimental investigation. Proc. roy. Soc. B **141**, 542–561 (1953b).

HALLPIKE, C.S., HOOD, J., BYFORD, G.: The design, construction and performance of a new type revolving chair. Acta oto-laryng. (Stockh.) **42**, 511–538 (1952).

HAMMER, L.R.: Perception of the visual vertical under reduced gravity. MRL-TDC-62-55. Wright-Patterson AFB, Ohio: AMRL 1962.

HEBB, D.O.: The Organization of Behavior. New York: Wiley 1949.

HELD, R.: Exposure history as a factor in maintaining stability of perception and coordination. J. nerv. ment. Dis. **132**, 26–32 (1961).

HELD, R.: Plasticity in sensory motor systems. Sci. Amer. (Nov. 1965).

HELD, R., HEIN, A.: Adaptation and disarranged hand-eye coordination contingent upon reafferent stimulation. Percept. Mot. Skills **8**, 87–90 (1958).

HELD, R., HEIN, A.: Movement-produced stimulation in the development of visually guided behavior. J. comp. physiol. Psychol. **56**, 872–876 (1963).

HENRIKSSON, N.G., LUNDGREN, A., TIBBLING, L., NILSSON, A., ANDERSON, A.: Tests of canal function with special reference to central vestibular pathways. NASA SP-152. Washington, D.C.: U.S. Government Printing Office 1968.

HERNÁNDEZ-PÉON, R., DONOSO, M.: Subcortical photically evoked activity in the human waking brain. Excerpta Med., p. 155 (1957).

HERNÁNDEZ-PÉON, R., DONOSO, M.: Influence of attention and suggestion upon subcortical evoked electric activity in the human brain. The First Int'l. Cong. of Neurological Sciences, Bruxelles, Vol. III. New York: MacMillan (Pergamon) 1959.

HILDING, A.C.: Studies on the otic labyrinth. III. On the threshold of minimum perceptible angular acceleration. Ann. Otol. (St. Louis) **62**, 5–14 (1953).

HIXSON, W.C.: Personal communication (1969).

HIXSON, W.C., NIVEN, J.I.: Frequency response of the human semicircular canals. II. Nystagmus phase shift as a measure of nonlinearities. NSAM-830. Pensacola, Fla.: Naval School of Aviation Medicine 1962.

HIXSON, W.C., NIVEN, J.I.: Directional differences in visual acuity during vertical nystagmus. NAMI-1079. Pensacola, Fla.: Naval Aerospace Medical Institute 1969.

HIXSON, W.C., NIVEN, J.I., CORREIA, M.J.: Kinematics nomenclature for psychological accelerations. Monograph 14. Pensacola, Fla.: Naval Aerospace Medical Institute 1966.

HORN, G., HILL, R.M.: Modifications of receptive fields of cells in the visual cortex occurring spontaneously and associated with bodily tilt. Nature (Lond.) **221**, 186–188 (1969).

HOWARD, I.P., TEMPLETON, W.B.: Human Spatial Orientation. New York: John Wiley and Sons 1966.

HULK, J., JONGKEES, L.B.W.: The turning test with small regulable stimuli. II. The normal cupulogram. J. Laryng. **62**, 70–75 (1948).

IGARASHI, M.: Dimensional study of the vestibular end organ apparatus. NASA SP-115. Washington, D.C.: U.S. Government Printing Office 1966.

JAMES, W.: The sense of dizziness in deaf-mutes. Amer. J. Otol. **4**, 239–254 (1882).

JONES, R.E., MILTON, J.L., FITTS, P.M.: An investigation of errors made by pilots in judging the attitude of an aircraft without the aid of vision. TSSAA 694-13. Wright Patterson AFB, Ohio: Aerospace Medical Laboratory, Engineering Division 1947.

JONGKEES, L.B.W.: On the function of the saccule. Acta oto-laryng. (Stockh.) **38**, 18–26 (1950).

JONGKEES, L.B.W.: On the otoliths: Their function and the way to test them. NASA SP-152. Washington, D.C.: U.S. Government Printing Office 1968.

JONGKEES, L.B.W.: Role of the otolith organ in the study of nystagmus. Rev. Laryng. **90**, 493–501 (1969).

JONGKEES, L.B.W., GROEN, J.J.: The nature of the vestibular stimulus. J. Laryng. **61**, 529–541 (1946).

JONGKEES, L.B.W., GROEN, J.J.: A quantitative analysis of the reactions of a person after loss of the function of both inner ears. J. Laryng. **64**, 135–140 (1950).

KELLOGG, R.S.: Vestibular influences on orientation in zero gravity produced by parabolic flight. Ann. N.Y. Acad. Sci. **188**, 217–223 (1971).

KEMPINSKY, W.H.: Cortical projection of the vestibular and facial nerves in the cat. J. Neurophysiol. **14**, 203–210 (1951).

KENNEDY, R.S.: The relationship between habituation to vestibular stimulation and vigilance: Individual differences and subsidiary problems. Thesis. Rochester, New York: The University of Rochester 1972.

KIMBLE, G.A., PERLMUTER, L.C.: The problem of volition. Psychol. Rev. **77**, 361–384 (1970).

KINSBOURNE, M.: Eye and head-turning indicates cerebral lateralization. Science (May 5) 539–541 (1972).

KITAHARA, M., UNO, R.: Equilibrium and vertigo in a tilting environment. Ann. Otol. (St. Louis) **76**, 166–178 (1967).

KLEINKNECHT, F.: Ein weiterer Beitrag zur Frage des Übungseinflusses und der Übungsfestigkeit am Neigungsstuhl. Z. Biol. **77**, 11–28 (1922).

KLINKE, R., SCHMIDT, C.L.: Efferent influence on the vestibular organ during active movement of the body. Pflügers Arch. **318**, 325–332 (1970).

KÖRNER, F., DICHGANS, J.: Bewegungswahrnehmung, optokinetischer Nystagmus und retinale Bildwanderung. Der Einfluß visueller Aufmerksamkeit auf zwei Mechanismen des Bewegungssehens. Albrecht v. Graefes Arch. klin. exp. Ophthal. **174**, 34–48 (1967).

KONGEHL, G., KORNHUBER, H.H.: Die Kanalkapazität des vestibulären Systems für Wahrnehmung von Drehbeschleunigungen. Pflügers Arch. **307**, 129–130 (1969).

KONGEHL, G., KORNHUBER, H.H.: Information transmission in the human vestibular system for perception of angular acceleration and angular displacement in the horizontal plane. Proc. Bárány Soc., 1st Extraord-Meeting Amsterdam, p. 179–183, 1970.

KORNHUBER, H.H.: Motor functions of cerebellum and basal ganglia: The cerebello-cortical saccadic (ballistic) clock, the cerebello nuclear hold regulator, and the basal ganglia ramp (voluntary speed smooth movement) generator. Kybernetik **8**, 157–162 (1971).

KOTTENHOFF, H., LINDAHL, L.: Laboratory studies on the psychology of motion sickness. Acta psychol. (Amst.) **17**, 89–112 (1960).

KREIDL, A.: Beiträge zur Physiologie des Ohrlabyrinths auf Grund von Versuchen an Taubstummen. Pflügers Arch. ges. Physiol. **51**, 119–150 (1892).

LANSBERG, M.P.: Some considerations and investigations in the field of labyrinthine functioning. Aeromed. Acta (Soesterberg) **3**, 209–267 (1954).

LANSBERG, M.P.: A Primer of Space Medicine. Amsterdam/New York: Elsevier 1960.

LEDOUX, A.: Activité électrique des nerfs des canaux semi-circulaires, du saccule et de l'utricle chez la grenouille. Acta oto-rhino-laryng. belg. **3**, 335–349 (1949).

LEDOUX, A.: Les canaux semicirculaires. Acta oto-rhino-laryng. belg. **12**, 109–348 (1958).

LEDOUX, A.: L'adaptation du systeme vestibulaire périphérique. Acta oto-laryng. (Stockh.) **53**, 307–315 (1961).

LICKLIDER, J.C.R.: Three auditory theories. In: Psychology: A study of science. New York: McGraw-Hill 1959.

LINDEMAN, H.H.: Studies on the morphology of the sensory regions of the vestibular apparatus. In: Advances in Anatomy Embryology. Berlin-Heidelberg-New York: Springer 42, 1–113, 1969.

LONG, G.M.: Field dependency-independency. A review of the literature. Monograph 19. Pensacola, Fla.: Naval Aerospace Medical Research Laboratory 1972.

LOWENSTEIN, O.: The effect of galvanic polarization on the impulse discharge from sense endings in the isolated labyrinth of the thornback ray (Raja Clavata). J. Physiol. (Lond.) **127**, 104–117 (1955).

LOWENSTEIN, O.: Peripheral mechanisms of equilibrium. Brit. med. Bull. **12**, 114–118 (1956).

LOWENSTEIN, O., ROBERTS, T.D.M.: The equilibrium function of the otolith organs of the Thornback Ray. J. Physiol. (Lond.) **110**, 392–415 (1949).

LOWENSTEIN, O., ROBERTS, T.D.M.: The localization and analysis of the responses to vibration from the isolated elasmobranch labyrinth. J. Physiol. (Lond.) **114**, 471–489 (1951).

MACCORQUODALE, K.: Effects of angular acceleration and centrifugal force on nonvisual space orientation during flight. J. Aviat. Med. **19**, 146–157 (1948).

MACH, E.: Grundlinien der Lehre von den Bewegungsempfindungen. Verlag von Wilhelm Englemann 1875.

MACH, E.: The Analysis of Sensations. Republication of fifth edition (1959). Tr. by C.M. Williams 1902. New York: Dover 1902.

MAGNUS, R.: The experimental basis for theories on vestibular function. Roy. Soc. Med. Sect. Laryng. Otol., 11–17 (1924).

MALCOLM, R., MELVILL JONES, G.: A quantitative study of vestibular adaptation in humans. Acta oto-laryng. (Stockh.) **70**, 126–135 (1970).

MANN, C.W.: Studies in space perception. NSAM-477. Pensacola, Fla.: Naval School of Aviation Medicine 1950.

MANN, C.W.: The effects of auditory-vestibular nerve pathology on space perception. J. exp. Psychol. **42**, 450–456 (1951).

MANN, C.W., BERRY, N.: The perception of the postural vertical. II. Visual factors. NSAM-464. Pensacola, Fla.: Naval School of Aviation Medicine 1949.

MANN, C.W., CANELLA, C.J.: An examination of the technique of cupulometry. NSAM-501. Pensacola, Fla.: Naval School of Aviation Medicine 1956.

MANN, C.W., DAUTERIVE, H.J.: The perception of the vertical. I. The modification of non-labyrinthine cues. J. exp. Psychol. **39**, 700–707 (1949).

MANN, C.W., PASSEY, G.E.: The perception of the vertical. V. Adjustment to the postural vertical as a function of the magnitude of postural tilt and duration of exposure. J. exp. Psychol. **41**, 108–113 (1951).

MANN, C.W., RAY, J.T.: The perception of the vertical. An investigation of quadrant differences. NSAM-498. Pensacola, Fla.: Naval School of Aviation Medicine 1956a.

Mann, C.W., Ray, J.T.: The perception of the vertical. The effect of rate of movement on the judgment of the vertical. NSAM-499. Pensacola, Fla.: Naval School of Aviation Medicine 1956b.

Mann, C.W., Ray, J.T.: Absolute thresholds of perception of direction of angular acceleration. NSAM-500. Pensacola, Fla.: Naval School of Aviation Medicine 1956c.

Mann, C.W., Berthelow-Berry, N.H., Dauterive, H.J.: The perception of the vertical. I. Visual and non-labyrinthine cues. J. exp. Psychol. **39**, 538–547 (1949).

Mann, C.W., Guedry, F.E., Ray, J.T.: Postrotational perception of apparent bodily rotation. J. exp. Psychol. **41**, 114–120 (1951).

Mann, C.W., Passey, G.E., Ambler, R.K.: The perception of the vertical. VII. Effect of varying intervals of delay in a tilted position upon perception of the postural vertical. NSAM-471. Pensacola, Fla.: Naval School of Aviation Medicine 1950.

Marchiafava, P.L., Pompeiano, O.: Enhanced excitability of intrageniculate optic tract endings produced by vestibular volleys. Arch. ital. Biol. **104**, 459–479 (1966).

Marshall, J.E., Brown, J.H.: Visual-arousal interaction and specificity of nystagmus habituation. Aerospace Med. **38**, 597–599 (1967).

Mayne, R.: The dynamic characteristics of the semicircular canals. J. comp. physiol. Psychol. **43**, 309–319 (1950a).

Mayne, R.: The operating principle of the vestibular mechanisms. In: Psychophysiological factors in spatial orientation. ONR Symposium. NAVEXOS P-966, 1950b.

Mayne, R.: Some engineering aspects of the mechanism of body control. Electrical Engineering AIEE, March 1951.

Mayne, R.: The audiogyral illusion and the mechanism of spatial representation. Bull. Math. Biophysics **14**, 27–34 (1952).

Mayne, R.: The match of the semicircular canals to the dynamics requirements of various species. NASA SP-77. Washington, D.C.: U.S. Government Printing Office 1965.

Mayne, R.: The biological inertial system. Proc. IEEE Conf. IEEE Cat. No. 69, C 12, Reg. 6, IEEE, Phoenix, Ariz. 1969.

McFarland, J.H., Wapner, S., Werner, H.: Relation between perceived location of objects and perceived location of one's own body. Percept. Mot. Skills. **15**, 331–341 (1962).

McNally, W.J.: Some facts and fancies about the utricle. Ann. Otol. (St. Louis) **64**, 355–363 (1955).

McNally, W.J., Stuart, E.A.: Vertigo from the standpoint of the otolaryngologist. Trans. Amer. Acad. Ophthal. Otolaryng. **46**, 33–37 (1941).

McNally, W.J., Stuart, E.A.: Physiology of the labyrinth reviewed in relation to seasickness and other forms of motion sickness. War Med. (Chic.) **2**, 683–771 (1942).

McNally, W.J., Stuart, E.A.: Physiology of the Labyrinth. A manual prepared for graduates in Medicine, American Academy of Ophthalmology and Otolaryngology. Montreal: McGill University and Royal Victoria Hospital 1967.

Meda, E.: A research on the threshold for the Coriolis and Purkinje phenomena of excitation of the semicircular canals. Arch. Fisiol. **52** (1952). Tr. by E.R. Hope. Defense Scientific Information Service DRB Canada T 171, 1954.

Meiry, J.L.: The Vestibular System and Human Dynamic Space Orientation. Thesis. Cambridge, Mass.: Massachusetts Institute of Technology 1965.

Melvill Jones, G.: Interactions between optokinetic and vestibulo-ocular responses during head rotation in various planes. Aerospace Med. **37**, 172–177 (1966a).

Melvill Jones, G.: Vestibular inaptitude in the environment of flight and space. J. Laryng. **53**, 207–221 (1966b).

Melvill Jones, G.: Neural reflections of vestibular mechanics. NASA SP-152. Washington, D.C.: U.S. Government Printing Office 1967.

Melvill Jones, G., Gonshor, A.: Extreme vestibular habituation to long-term reversal of vision during natural head movements. Presented at 43d Annual Aerospace Medical Assn. Meeting, Miami 1972.

Melvill Jones, G., Milsum, J.H.: Spatial and dynamic aspects of visual fixation. IEEE Trans. Biomed. Eng. BME **12**, 54–62 (1965).

Melvill Jones, G., Milsum, J.H.: Relations between neural and mechanical responses of the semicircular canals. Presented at 38th Annual Aerospace Medical Assn. Meeting, Washington 1967.

Melvill Jones, G., Spells, K.E.: A theoretical and comparative study of the functional dependence of the semicircular canal upon its physical dimensions. Proc. roy. Soc. B **157**, 403–419 (1963).

Melvill Jones, G., Barry, W., Kowalsky, N.: Dynamics of the semicircular canals compared in yaw, pitch and roll. Aerospace Med. **35**, 984–989 (1964).

Meshman, V.F.: Changes in general electrical activity and primary response to light induced by stimulation of the vestibular apparatus of the cat. Zh. vyssh. nerv. Deyat. Pavlova **18**, 525–527 (1968).

Meshman, V.F.: Change of the bioelectric activity in the visual system and the anterior ectosylvian gyrus during vestibular stimulation. Fiziol. Zh. (Mosk.) **56**, 1570–1578 (1970).

Mickle, W., Ades, H.: A composite sensory projection area in the cerebral cortex of the cat. J. Neurophysiol. **170**, 682–689 (1952).

Miller, E.F., Graybiel, A.: Role of the otolith organs in the perception of horizontality. NSAM-851. Pensacola, Fla.: Naval School of Aviation Medicine 1963.

Miller, E.F., Graybiel, A.: Role of the otolith organs in the perception of horizontality. Amer. J. Psychol. **79**, 24–37 (1966a).

Miller, E.F., Graybiel, A.: Magnitude of gravito inertial force, an independent variable in egocentric visual localization of the horizontal. J. exp. Psychol. **71**, 452–460 (1966b).

Miller, E.F., Graybiel, A.: Effect of gravito inertial force on ocular counterrolling. J. appl. Physiol. **31**, 697–700 (1971).

Miller, E.F., Fregly, A.R., Graybiel, A.: Visual horizontal perception in relation to otolith function. NAMI-989. Pensacola, Fla.: Naval Aerospace Medical Institute 1966.

Miller, E.F., Fregly, A.R., Graybiel, A.: Visual horizontal perception in relation to otolith function. Amer. J. Psychol. **81**, 488–496 (1968).

Miller, E.F., Graybiel, A., Kellogg, R.S.: Otolith organ activity within earth standard, one-half standard and zero gravity environment. Aerospace Med. **37**, 399–403 (1965b).

Miller, E.F., Fregly, A.R., van den Brink, G., Graybiel, A.: Visual localization of the horizontal as a function of body tilt up to $\pm 90°$ from gravitational vertical. NAMI-942. Pensacola, Fla.: Naval Aerospace Medical Institute 1965a.

Miller, G.A.: The magical number seven, plus or minus two: Some Limits on our capacity for processing information. Psychol. Rev. **63**, 81–97 (1956).

Miller, J.W., Goodson, J.E.: Motion sickness in a helicopter simulator. Aerospace Med. **31**, 204–211 (1960).

Miller, J.W., Ludvigh, E.: The effect of relative motion on visual acuity. Surv. Ophthal. **7**, 83–116 (1962).

Money, K.E., Wood, J.D.: Neural mechanisms underlying the symptomatology of motion sickness. NASA SP-187. Washington, D.C.: U.S. Government Printing Office 1970.

Montandon, P., Monnier, M.: Correlations of the diencephalic nystagmogenic area with the bulbo-vestibular nystagmogenic area. Brain **87**, 673–690 (1964).

Montandon, A., Russbach, A.: Etude de quelques syndromes vestibulaires par l'épreuve gératoire luminaire. Acta oto-laryng. (Stockh.) **46**, 264–276 (1956).

Morrison, A.R., Pompeiano, O.: Vestibular influences during sleep. IV. Functional relations between vestibular nuclei and lateral geniculate nucleus during desynchronized sleep. Arch. ital. Biol. **104**, 425–458 (1966).

Mowrer, O.H.: Nystagmus response of pigeons to constant acceleration at liminal and supraliminal intensities. J. comp. Psychol. **19**, 177–193 (1935).

Mowrer, O.H.: Influence of vision during bodily rotation upon the duration of post-rotational vestibular nystagmus. Acta oto-laryng. (Stockh.) **25**, 351–364 (1937).

Mulder, W.: Quantitatieve betrekking tusschen prikkel en effect bij het statisch organ. Dissertation. Rijks University of Utrecht (1908). NASA Technical Translation F-11, 489, 1968.

Müller, G.E.: Über das Aubertsche Phänomen. Z. Sinnesphysiol. **49**, 109–244 (1916).

Mygind, S.H.: Static function of the labyrinth attempt at synthesis. Acta oto-laryng. (Stockh.) Suppl. **70** (1948).

Nagel, W.A.: Über kompensatorische Raddrehungen der Augen. Z. Psychol. Physiol. Sinnesorg. **12**, 331–354 (1896).

Nagel, W.A.: Über das Aubertsche Phänomen und verwandte Täuschungen über die vertikale Richtung. Z. Psychol. Physiol. Sinnesorg. **16**, 373–398 (1898).

Neal, M.: Vestibular stimulation and developmental behavior of the small premature infant. In: Nursing Research Report, 3, 1–4. New York: American Nurses Foundation 1968.

Nelson, J.G.: Effect of water immersion and body position upon perception of the gravitational vertical. Aerospace Med. **39**, 806–811 (1968).

Nilsson, A., Henriksson, N.G.: The oculogyral illusion — a form of rotation after-effect — and its relation to spiral after-effect in repeated trials. Psych. Res. Bull. **7**, 5 (1967). Lund, Sweden: Lund University.

Niven, J.I., Hixson, W.C.: Frequency response of the human semicircular canals. I. Steady-state ocular nystagmus response to high level, sinusoidal angular rotations. NSAM-459. Pensacola, Fla.: Naval School of Aviation Medicine 1961.

Niven, J.I., Hixson, W.C., Correia, M.J.: An experimental approach to the dynamics of the vestibular mechanisms. NASA SP-77. Washington, D.C.: U.S. Government Printing Office 1965.

Niven, J.I., Hixson, W.C., Correia, M.J.: Elicitation of horizontal nystagmus by periodic linear acceleration. Acta oto-laryng. (Stockh.) **62**, 429–441 (1966).

Ornitz, E.M.: Vestibular dysfunction in schizophrenia and childhood autism. Comprehens. Psychiat. **11**, 159–173 (1970).

Outerbridge, J.S.: Experimental and theoretical investigation of vestibularly-driven head and eye movement. Thesis. Montreal: McGill University 1969.

Padden, D.A.: Ability of deaf swimmers to orient themselves when submerged in water. Res. Quart. V**30**, 214–226 (1959).

Parker, D.M.: A psychophysiological test for motion sickness susceptibility. J. genet. Psychol. **85**, 87–92 (1971).

Parsons, R.D.: Magnitude estimates of the oculogyral illusion during and following angular acceleration. J. exp. Psychol. **84**, 230–238 (1970).

Passey, G.E.: The perception of the vertical. IV. Adjustment to the vertical with normal and tilted visual frames of reference. J. exp. Psychol. **40**, 738–745 (1950).

Passey, G.E., Guedry, F.E.: The perception of the vertical. II. Adaptation effects in four planes. J. exp. Psychol. **39**, 700–707 (1949).

Pearson, R.G., Hauty, G.T.: Role of postural experiences in proprioceptive perception of verticality. J. exp. Psychol. **59**, 425–428 (1960).

Peiper, A.: Cerebral Function in Infancy and Childhood. New York: Consultants' Bureau 1963.

Penfield, W.: Vestibular sensation and the cerebral cortex. Ann. Otol. (St. Louis) **66**, 691–698 (1957).

Peto, A.: To Cast Away — A vestibular forerunner of the superego. Psychoanal. Stud. Child **25**, 401–416 (1970).

Poulton, E.C.: The new psychophysics: Six models for magnitude estimation. Psychol. Bull. **69**, 1–19 (1968).

Prescott, J.W.: Early somatosensory deprivation as an ontogenetic process in the abnormal development of the brain and behavior. In: Medical primatology. Basel/New York: S. Karger 1971.

Price, R.H.: Signal detection methods in personality and perception. Psychol. Bull. **66**, 55–62 (1966).

Purkinje, J.E.: Beiträge zur näheren Kenntnis des Schwindels aus heautognostischen Daten. Med. Jb. (Österreich) **6**, 79–125 (1820).

Quix, F.H.: L'Examen clinique de la fonction des Otolithes. Ann. Mal. Oreil. Larynx **42**, 261–286 (1923).

Quix, F.H.: The function of the vestibular organ and the clinical examination of the otolithic apparatus. J. Laryng. **40**, 425–443 (1925).

Reason, J.T.: Individual differences in motion sickness susceptibility: A further test of the receptivity "hypothesis." Brit. J. Psychol. **60**, 321–328 (1969).

Reason, J.T.: Motion sickness: A special case of sensory rearrangement. Advanc. Sci. **26**, 386–393 (1970).

Reason, J.T., Benson, A.J.: Individual differences in the reported persistence of visual and labyrinthine after-sensations, and of exponentially decaying visual and auditory signals. Brit. J. Psychol. **59**, 167–172 (1968).

Reason, J.T., Diaz, E.: The effects of visual reference on adaptation to Coriolis acceleration. FPRC Report 1303. London: Ministry of Defence (Air Force Dept.) 1970.

Reason, J.T., Diaz, E.: Simulator sickness in passive observers. FPRC Psychological Sub-Committee paper, April 1971.

Reason, J.T., Graybiel, A.: Magnitude estimation of Coriolis sensations. NAMI-1082. Pensacola, Fla.: Naval Aerospace Medical Institute 1969a.

Reason, J.T., Graybiel, A.: Adaptation to Coriolis accelerations. Its transfer to the opposite direction of rotation as a function of intervening activity at zero velocity. NAMI-1086. Pensacola, Fla.: Naval Aerospace Medical Institute 1969b.

Reason, J.T., Graybiel, A.: Progressive adaptation to Coriolis accelerations associated with 1 rpm increments in the velocity of the Slow Rotation Room. Aerospace Med. **41**, 73–79 (1970).

Reason, J.T., Graybiel, A.: Predictability of motion sickness in the selection of pilots. AGARD CP-109. London: Technical Editing and Reproduction Ltd. 1972.

Roberts, T.D.M.: Neurophysiology of Postural Mechanisms. New York: Plenum Press 1967.

Roggeveen, L.J., Nijhoff, P.: The normal and pathological threshold of the perception of angular accelerations for the optogyral illusion and the turning sensation. Acta oto-laryng. (Stockh.) **46**, 533–541 (1956).

Rohrer, F.: Zur Theorie der Drehreizung des Bogengangsapparates. Schweiz. med. Wschr. **3**, 669–674 (1922).

Ross, H.E., Crickmar, S.D., Sills, N.V., Owen, E.P.: Orientation to the vertical in free divers. Aerospace Med. **40**, 728–732 (1969).

Sadoff, M., Matheson, F.A., Havill, C.D.: A method for evaluating the loads and controllability aspects of the pitchup problem. NACA RMA 55 DO6, 1955.

Schilder, P.: The vestibular apparatus in neurosis and psychosis. J. nerv. ment. Dis. **78**, 1–23, 137–164 (1933).

Schilpp, P.A.: Albert Einstein: Philosopher-Scientist. Second Edition. New York: Tudor Publishing Co. 1951.

Schöne, H.: On the role of gravity in human spatial orientation. Aerospace Med. **35**, 764–772 (1964).

Schöne, H., Mortag, H.-G.: Variation of the subjective vertical on the parallel swing at different body positions. Psychol. Forsch. **32**, 124–134 (1968).

Schöne, H., Parker, D.E.: Inversion of the effect of increased gravity on the subjective vertical. Die Naturw. Heft 11, 288–289, 54. Jahrgang, 1967.

Schöne, H., Udo de Haes, H.: Perception of gravity — vertical as a function of head and trunk position. Z. vergl. Physiol. **60**, 440–444 (1968).

Schöne, H., Udo de Haes, H.: Space orientation in humans with special reference to the interaction of vestibular, somesthetic, and visual inputs. In: Biokybernetik 3, Materialen des II. Internationalen Symposiums "Biokybernetik" Leipzig 1969. Jena: Gustav Fischer Verlag 1971.

Schöne, H., Parker, D.E., Mortag, H.-G.: Subjective vertical as a function of body position and gravity magnitude. Naturwissenschaften **54**, 288 (1967).

Schoen, L.: Mikroableitungen einzelner zentraler Vestibularisneurone von Knochenfischen bei Statolithenreizen. Z. vergl. Physiol. **39**, 399–417 (1957).

Schroeder, D.J., Gilson, R.D., Guedry, F.E., Collins, W.E.: Alcohol and disorientation-related responses. VI. Effects of alcohol on eye movements and tracking performance during laboratory angular accelerations about the y and z axes. Aerospace Med. **44**, 477–483 (1973).

Schubert, G.: Die physiologischen Auswirkungen der Coriolisbeschleunigungen bei Flugzeugsteuerung. Arch. Ohr.-, Nas.-, u. Kehlk.-Heilk. **30**, 595–604 (1932).

Semmes, J., Winestein, S., Ghent, L., Teuber, H.L.: Spatial orientation in man after cerebral injury. J. Psychol. (Provincetown) **39**, 227–244 (1955).

SHAMES, I.H.: Engineering Mechanics, Statics and Dynamics. Englewood Cliffs, N.J.: Prentice-Hall, Inc. 1960.

SHARPLESS, S.K.: Reorganization of function in the nervous system — use and disuse. Ann. Rev. Physiol. **26**, 357–380 (1964).

SHIMAZU, H., PRECHT, W.: Tonic and kinetic responses of cat's vestibular neurones to horizontal angular acceleration. J. Neurophysiol. **27**, 991–1013 (1965).

SHUBERT, E.: Perception of body tilt. Proc. Iowa Acad. Sci. **49**, 450 (1942).

SINGLETON, G.T.: Relationships of cerebellar nodulus to vestibular function: A study of the effects of nodulectomy on habituation. Laryngoscope (St. Louis) **77**, 1579–1620 (1967).

SMITH, K.U., SMITH, W.M.: Perception and Motion. Philadelphia/London: W.B. Saunders Co. 1962.

SMYTHIES, J.R.: The Neurological Foundations of Psychiatry. New York: Academic Press 1966.

SPIEGEL, E.A., EGYED, J., SZEKELY, E.: Cortical responses to rotation. II. Responses recorded at the onset of rotation from the second somatic sensory and posterior areas. Acta oto-laryng. (Stockh.) **66**, 261–272 (1968b).

SPIEGEL, E.A., SZEKELY, E.G., MOFFET, R.: Cortical responses to rotation. I. Responses recorded after cessation of rotation. Acta oto-laryng. (Stockh.) **66**, 81–88 (1968a).

SPOENDLIN, H.H.: Ultrastructure of the vestibular sense organ. In: The vestibular system and its diseases. Philadelphia: Univ. of Pennsylvania Press 1966.

STEELE, J.E.: The symptomatology of motion sickness. NASA SP-187. Washington, D.C.: U.S. Government Printing Office 1970.

STEER, R.W.: Progress in vestibular modeling. Part I: Response of semicircular canals to constant speed rotation on a linear acceleration field. NASA SP-187. Washington, D.C.: U.S. Government Printing Office 1970.

STEINHAUSEN, W.: Über die Beobachtung der Cupula in den Bogengangsampullen des Labyrinthes des lebenden Hechts. Pflügers Arch. ges. Physiol. **232**, 500–512 (1933).

STEINHAUSEN, W.: Über die durch die Otolithen ausgelösten Kräfte. Pflügers Arch. ges. Physiol. **235**, 538–544 (1934–1935).

STEVENS, S.S.: The psychophysics of sensory function. Amer. Sci. **48**, 226–253 (1960).

STEVENS, S.S.: A metric for the social concensus. Science **151**, 530–541 (1966).

STIGLER, R.: Experiments dealing with the participation of the sensation of gravity in the orientation of man in space. Arch. ges. Physiol. **148**, 573–584 (1912). Tr. by Mrs. A. Woke NMRI, 1972.

STOCKWELL, C.W., GUEDRY, F.E.: The effect of semicircular canal stimulation during tilting on the subsequent perception of the visual vertical. Acta oto-laryng. (Stockh.) **70**, 170–175 (1970).

STOCKWELL, C.W., GILSON, R.D., GUEDRY, F.E.: Adaptation of horizontal semicircular canal responses. Acta oto-laryng. (Stockh.) **75**, 471–476 (1973).

STONE, R.W., LETKO, W.: Some observations during weightlessness simulation with subject immersed in a rotating water tank. NASA Technical Note NASA TN D-2195. Washington, D.C.: National Aeronautics and Space Administration 1964.

SWETS, J.A.: Detection theory and psychophysics. A review. Psychometrika **26**, 49–63 (1961).

SZENTÁGOTHAI, J.: Die Rolle der einzelnen Labyrinthreceptoren bei der Orientation von Augen und Kopf im Raume. Akad. Kiade (Budapest) 1952.

TAUB, E.: Prism compensation as a learning phenomenon: A phylogenetic perspective. In: The neuropsychology of spatially oriented behavior. Homewood, Ill.: Dorsey Press 1968.

TAUB, E., BERMAN, A.J.: Movement and learning in the absence of sensory feedback. In: The neuropsychology of spatially oriented behavior. Homewood, Ill.: Dorsey Press 1968.

TEN KATE, J.H.: The oculo-vestibular reflex of the growing pike. A biophysical study. Thesis. Groningen: Rijksuniversitet te Groningen 1969.

TEUBER, H.L.: Perception. In: Handbook of Neurophysiology, Vol. 3. Washington, D.C.: American Physiol. Soc. 1960.

TEUBER, H.L.: Space perception and its disturbances after brain injury in man. Neurophysiologia **1**, 47–57 (1963).

TEUBER, H.L., MISHKIN, M.: Judgment of visual and postural vertical in man after brain injury. J. Psychol. (Provincetown) **38**, 161–175 (1954).

TIBBLING, L.: The rotatory nystagmus response in children. Acta oto-laryng. (Stockh.) **68**, 459–467 (1969).

TRAVIS, R.C., DODGE, R.: Experimental analysis of the sensorimotor consequences of passive oscillation — rotary and rectilinear. Psych. Mon. **38**, 1–96 (1928).

TRINCKER, D.: Neuere Untersuchungen zur Elektrophysiologie des Vestibular-Apparates. Naturwissenschaften **46**, 344 (1959).

TRINCKER, D.: Transformation of mechanical stimulus into nervous excitation. Soc. Exp. Biol. Symp. **16**, 289–316 (1962).

TUMARKIN, I.A.: Some observation on the function of the labyrinth. J. Laryng. **52**, 438–451 (1937).

UDO DE HAES, H., SCHÖNE, H.: Interaction between statolith organs and semicircular canals on apparent vertical and nystagmus. Acta oto-laryng. (Stockh.) **69**, 25–31 (1970).

ULRICH, H.: Die Function des Otolithen, geprüft durch direkte mechanische Beeinflussung des Utriculusotolithen am lebenden Hecht. Arch. ges. Physiol. **235**, 545–553 (1934–1935).

VAN DISHOECK, H.A.E., SPOOR, A., NIJHOFF, P.: The opto-gyral illusion and its relation to the nystagmus of the eyes. Acta oto-laryng. (Stockh.) **44**, 597–607 (1954).

VAN EGMOND, A.A.J., GROEN, J.J., JONGKEES, L.B.W.: The mechanics of the semicircular canals. J. Physiol. (Lond.) **110**, 1–17 (1949).

VILSTRUP, G., VILSTRUP, T.: Does the utricular otolithic membrane move on postural changes of the head? Ann. Otol. (St. Louis) **61**, 189–197 (1952).

VON BÉKÉSY, G.: Über die Stärke der Vibrationsempfindung und ihre objektive Messung. Sonderdruck aus "Akustische Zeits." **5**, 113–124 (1940).

VON BÉKÉSY, G.: Subjective cupulometry. AMA Arch. Otol. **61**, 16–28 (1955).

VON BÉKÉSY, G.: Pressure and shearing forces as stimuli of labyrinthine epithelium. Arch. Otolaryng. **84**, 26–130 (1966).

VON DIRINGSHOFEN, H.: In: Medical Guide for Flying Personnel. Toronto: Univ. of Toronto Press 1940.

VON DIRINGSHOFEN, H., KESSEL, G., OSYPKA, P.: Thresholds for the perception of linearly increasing angular accelerations. Aerospace Med. **35**, 775–778 (1964).

VON HOLST, E.: Die Arbeitsweise des Statolithenapparates bei Fischen. Z. vergl. Physiol. **32**, 60–120 (1950a).

VON HOLST, E.: Die Tätigkeit des Statolithenapparats im Wirbeltierlabyrinth. Naturwissenschaften **37**, 265–272 (1950b).

WADE, N.J.: The interaction of postural systems in visual orientation. Percept. Psychophysics **6**, 309–310 (1969).

WADE, N.J., DAY, R.H.: Development and dissipation of a visual spatial aftereffect from prolonged head tilt. J. exp. Psychol. **76**, 439–443 (1968).

WALSH, E.G.: Sensibility of patients to linear acceleration after unilateral labyrinthectomy. J. Physiol. (Lond.) **149**, 33P–34P (1959).

WALSH, E.G.: Perception of linear motion following unilateral labyrinthectomy: Variation of threshold according to the orientation of the head. J. Physiol. (Lond.) **153**, 350–357 (1960).

WALSH, E.G.: Role of the vestibular apparatus in the perception of motion on a parallel swing. J. Physiol. (Lond.) **155**, 506–513 (1961a).

WALSH, E.G.: Sensations aroused by rhythmically repeated linear motion-phase relationships. J. Physiol. (Lond.) **155**, 53P–54P (1961b).

WALSH, E.G.: The perception of rhythmically repeated linear motion in the horizontal plane. Brit. J. Psychol. **53**, 439–445 (1962).

WALSH, E.G.: The perception of rhythmically repeated linear motion in the vertical plane. Quart. J. exp. Physiol. **49**, 58–65 (1964).

WALZL, E., MOUNTCASTLE, V.: Projection of vestibular nerve to cerebral cortex of the cat. Amer. J. Physiol. **159**, 594 (1949).

WAPNER, S., WERNER, H., MARANT, R.B.: Experiments of sensori-tonic field theory of perception. III. Effect of body rotation on the visual perception of vertical. J. exp. Psychol. **42**, 351–357 (1951).

WEAVER, R.S.: Theoretical aspects of the role of angular acceleration in vestibular stimulation. Acta oto-laryng. (Stockh.) Suppl. **205** (1965).

WENDT, G.R.: Vestibular functions. In: Handbook of Experimental Psychology. New York: Wiley 1951.

WERNER, H., WAPNER, S., CHANDLER, K.A.: Experiments on sensory-tonic field theory of perception. II. Effect of supported and unsupported tilt of the body on the visual perception of verticality. J. exp. Psychol. **42**, 346–350 (1951).

WHITE, H.E.: Classical and Modern Physics. New York: Doran Nostrand Co., Inc. 1940.

WHITESIDE, T.D.M., GRAYBIEL, A., NIVEN, J.I.: Visual illusions of motion. NSAM-877. Pensacola, Fla.: Naval School of Aviation Medicine 1963.

WHITESIDE, T.D.M., GRAYBIEL, A., NIVEN, J.I.: Visual illusions of movement. Brain **88**, 193–210 (1965).

WITKIN, H.A.: Orientation to visual and postural vertical. Individual differences in mode of space orientation. In: Psychophysiological factors in spatial orientation. ONR Symp. NAVEXOS P-966. Pensacola, Fla. 1950.

WITKIN, H.A.: Origins of cognitive style. In: Cognition: Theory, research, promise. New York: Harper Row 1962.

WOLFE, J.W.: Evidence for control of nystagmic habituation by folium-tuber vermis and fastigial nuclei. Acta oto-laryng. (Stockh.) Suppl. **231** (1968).

YOUNG, L.R.: On visual-vestibular interaction. NASA SP-314. Washington, D.C.: U.S. Government Printing Office 1973.

YOUNG, L., MEIRY, J.: A revised dynamic otolith model. NASA SP-152. Washington, D.C.: U.S. Government Printing Office 1968.

YOUNG, L., OMAN, C.M.: Model for vestibular adaptation to horizontal rotation. Aerospace Med. **40**, 1076–1080 (1969).

Chapter II.

Optic-Vestibular Orientation to the Vertical

By

N. Bischof, Pasadena, Calif. (USA)

With 12 Figures

Contents

I. Introduction: On Orientation

By "orientation" we mean the proper arrangement of an object within a frame of reference.

Using the term "proper" takes account of a connotation of value attached to the concept of orientation in common language. It may be understood either in a merely *formal* sense, referring to aspects of symmetry, equilibrium, and the like, or *functionally*: we may call an animal "well" or "poorly" oriented if it is able or unable to find its way home after having been displaced; or, generally speaking, if its "arrangement within a frame of reference" is such as to optimize the animal's (or its species') chances of survival.

In humans, the "arrangement" may be understood to occur in the realm either of body activity or of perceptual organization, the "object" and the "frame of reference" beeing defined physically in the former case, and psychophysically in the latter. We therefore distinguish between *body orientation* and *perceptual orientation*.

We speak of *spatial orientation* if the frame of reference is a spatial one. Within spatial orientation two general groups can be distinguished, with the frame of reference being the essentially horizontal *map of life space*, on one hand, and the vertical *pull of gravity*, on the other. The former group, including, for instance, the problem of homing and route perception, will not be discussed here, although both the eye (as in sun-orientation, cf. Braemer, 1960) and the vestibular organ (Beritoff, 1962, 1963) seem to play an important part in these performances, too. Instead, we shall restrict discussion to orientation to the vertical where, as we shall see, optic and vestibular sense are substantially involved.

Applying the dichotomy of "body" and "perceptual" orientation to this case, we may distinguish between

(1) *postural equilibrium responses*, i.e., motor activity serving to stabilize the intended posture of the body in the field of gravity (e.g., vestibular righting responses), and

(2) *perceptual space transformations*, i.e., physiological processes monitoring the constancy of space perception in the presence of factors changing the position of sense organs.

Perceptual space transformations will be called "*external*" if non-nervous processes like muscular mechanics are involved (as in the case of eye-movements), and "*internal*" if they are confined to pure nervous system activity (for further detail, see below, pp. 159 f.).

Postural equilibrium responses and perceptual space transformations are by no means independent of each other; instead, it is commonly felt that there is one and the same system producing both. In man, to be sure, much more sophistication has been invested in the study of the latter, at least in healthy subjects. The following chapter will therefore deal mostly with problems of perceptual orientation.

This report shall be organized with a *functional* viewpoint. In a field of research where the data available are clustered on two widely different levels of complexity — reports of perceptual phenomena on one hand, and records of neuronal discharges on the other — a functional approach seems to be most promising to bridge the gap. It might, moreover, provide us with heuristic strategies for further research both in neurophysiology and in psychophysics.

Three functional principles, i.e. three major types of information processing involved in orientational achievements, shall be distinguished below under the names of "compensation", "reconstruction", and "correction". Each of these principles has been introduced and discussed by a different group of authors: Compensation processes were first postulated by K. Bühler (1922) and form the core of the famous, though originally not quite consistently defined "reafference principle" of von Holst and Mittelstaedt (1950); the importance of reconstruction processes has been stressed by Gibson (1950, 1966) and MacKay (1966); correction processes play an outstanding role in the perceptual theory of E. Bruns-

WIK (1934, 1956). A synopsis of these three principles has, connected with partial re-formulation, first been attempted by BISCHOF (1966b, p. 357–399). They will serve as a frame of classification of the following report.

II. Directional Constancy and the Compensation Principle

A. On Vertical Constancy

When exposed to a laterally tiltable, fronto-parallel luminous line in a dark room, a normal subject is able to estimate the slope of the line with quite satisfactory approximation: the inclination of the perceived contour to the apparent vertical nearly corresponds to the inclination of the physical contour with respect to the field of gravity. The sensory datum referred to by the brain in this estimation apparently consists in the slant of the line's retinal image or, more precisely, in the angle between the retinal projection of the line and a given reference axis fixed to the retina. This retinal image (the so-called *proximal stimulus*) serves, as it were, as the causal bridge connecting the object of interest, namely the luminous line outside in the dark room (the *distal stimulus*), and the perceived inclination (the *phenomenon*). Moreover, unless the subject contacts the distal object via an additional sensory channel (e.g., by touching), it is the *only* causal bridge of this kind.

Considering the latter we ought to be surprised that the relation between the retinal image and the distal object is by no means unique. Any particular inclination of the proximal stimulus contour within the retinal frame of reference may occur in the presence of a given slope of the distal stimulus line, because of the interference of a further independent variable, namely, the head tilt. When, for instance, the head is laterally inclined, the picture of a vertical line will appear on a retinal meridian different from the one upon which it is projected with upright head position. If the brain, in anthropomorphic terms, were to "rely" solely upon the information conveyed to it via the optic channel, it would be entirely unable to distinguish this situation from one in which the body remained upright but the line was tilted. The fact is, however, that the central-nervous perceptive mechanism is quite capable of making this distinction. This performance is usually referred to as "vertical constancy". The analysis of vertical constancy, then, has to start from the fundamental biological problem common to all constancy performances (others being, e.g., color, brightness, size and shape constancy): How can a veridical correspondence between the perceptual phenomenon and the distal object be established despite the fact that the only causal bridge intervening between them, i.e., the proximal stimulus, is disturbed unpredictably by the interference of a further variable?

B. The Compensation Principle

The solution of this general constancy problem was found, after preparatory work by HELMHOLTZ, HERING, MACH, and others, by K. BÜHLER and L. KARDOS (BÜHLER, 1922; KARDOS, 1928, 1929; BRUNSWIK and KARDOS, 1929) and later restated by VON HOLST and MITTELSTAEDT (1950). The basic idea is this: the organism neutralizes the interference *by repeating it with reversed sign.* Since a process of this kind may aptly be called "compensatory", BISCHOF (1966b) has proposed the term *compensation principle* to characterize this form of biological information processing.

The compensation principle is illustrated by the flow diagram Fig. 1a. The sensory channel S (generally the eye) is affected by a proximal stimulus, the latter

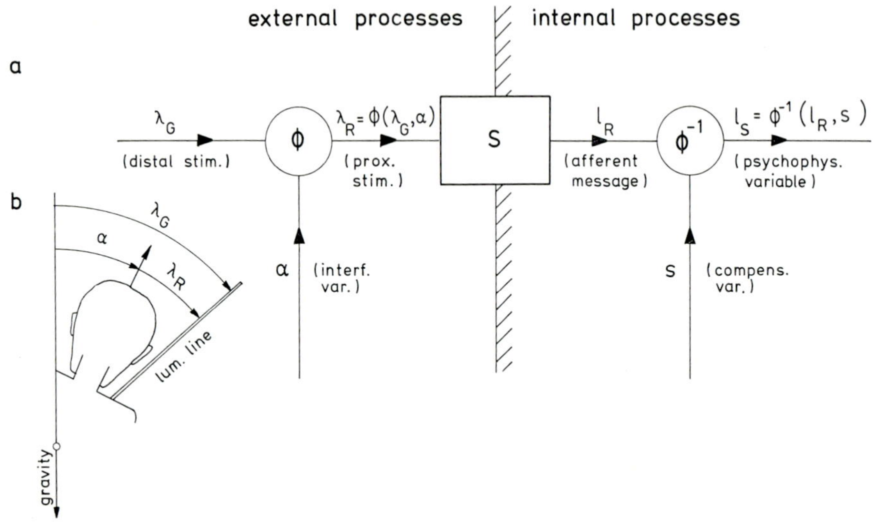

Fig. 1. a) Control diagram of the compensation principle. Here and in all subsequent block diagrams arrows represent variables, and boxes represent operators. Orientation of arrows denotes direction of causal influence. Φ = interference function, Φ^{-1} = compensatory function, S = mapping function of sensory channel. b) Interference function in the perception of verticality. Distal stimulus (λ_G) equals the *sum* of interfering variable (a) and proximal stimulus (λ_R), if orientation of angles is uniformly defined (here: clockwise inclinations positive, when viewed from Subject)

depending upon a distal stimulus and an "interfering variable", according to an "interference function" Φ. In our case, the interfering variable is the angle of head tilt (a), while the inclination λ of the luminous line relative to *gravity* (subscript G) is the distal stimulus. The slant of the line measured within the *retinal* coordinate system (subscript R) can serve as a representative of the proximal stimulus. The interference function has the form of a simple subtraction, as shown in Fig. 1b:

$$\lambda_R = \lambda_G - a.$$

The proximal stimulus is reported to higher central-nervous centers by means of afferent messages (l_R). Making use of this information, now, the organism has to arrive at a psychophysical variable[1] (l_S) representing veridically the distal

1 By the expression "a psychophysical variable" we denote a hypothetical central-nervous process thought directly to underly a consciously experienced phenomenon (cf. also BISCHOF, 1966a).

stimulus. This is done by means of a compensatory process consisting of the following two operations:

(1) The organism ascertains in a suitable way a representation of the interfering variable, the "compensatory variable" (s).

(2) This compensatory variable is fed into the afferent information flow in such a way as to compensate for the influence of the interfering variable ("compensatory function").

In Fig. 1a the compensatory function is denoted by Φ^{-1}, since it can easily be seen that *in the ideal case* it would have to be exactly the inverse of the interference function. In our case, consequently, the ideal compensatory function would be an addition:

$$l_S = l_R + s.$$

In connection with the compensation principle three main questions arise: (1) Where is the compensatory process performed? (2) How should the flow diagram be modified to take account of the compensatory errors recorded under experimental conditions and in every-day life? (3) Where does the organism obtain the information about the interfering variable needed to determine the compensatory variable? These problems will be discussed successively in the following sections, with respect to the special case of vertical constancy.

C. External and Internal Compensation

As far as localization is concerned, two possible types of compensation are conceivable: (1) "external" compensation outside the boundary of neurophysiological processes, and (2) "internal" compensation within the central nervous system. Only the second possibility is taken into account in Fig. 1. The first is more obvious and easier to analyse. It consists in the so-called *ocular countertorsion* (rolling of the eyeballs around their sagittal axes). In the ideal case the amount of countertorsion should exactly equal the degree of lateral head tilt, thus leading to complete constancy of the retinal stimulus pattern. This, however, is never attained in any vertebrate species. In man, particularly, the countertorsion response can only be called vestigial (Fischer, 1927, 1930a; Woellner and Graybiel, 1959; Schöne, 1962; Miller, 1962; Miller and Graybiel, 1963; Colenbrander, 1964; Kellogg, 1965; Brandt and Fluur, 1966, 1967; Udo de Haes, 1970; Bischof and Scheerer, 1970). When plotted against head tilt, ocular countertorsion shows a sinusoidal curve with extreme values ocurring at tilts of about 60°. Even at its extremes, the response seldom exceeds values of 6–8°, being, therefore, far too small to account for the compensatory achievements actually observed.

Consequently, there remains only the alternative of assuming an "internal" compensation, i.e., a central-nervous processing of the optical afference according to Fig. 1. Formally, such a process could be conceived as a rotatory transformation of a functional coordinate system, the latter being the physiological correlate of phenomenal space. The anatomical localization of these processes is still open to speculation, although recent neurophysiological findings (cf. chapter Fredrickson,

Kornhuber and Schwarz, this volume), contradicting the earlier opinion that no vestibular afferences reach the cerebral cortex, may turn out to be a first step towards answering this obscure question.

D. Allowance for Compensatory Errors

The argumentation in favor of the compensation principle (see above pp. 158 f.) may sound somewhat artificial, as it starts from the fictitious presupposition of exact veridicality of directional perception. This presupposition is, indeed, only approximately fulfilled in every-day life, and even larger deviations occur under experimental conditions.

If the optical stimulus field is reduced to a single luminous rod in a dark room, a subject's apparent vertical (as indicated by his setting of the rod) will exhibit systematic deviations from the physical plumbline, especially if the body is in a tilted position (cf. Fig. 2). Large amounts of lateral body tilt are undercompensated (Aubert, 1861), i.e., the apparent vertical deviates towards body axis, whereas moderate amounts of tilt are sometimes overcompensated (Müller, 1916), i.e., the apparent vertical deviates in the opposite direction (A and E phenomenon, respectively: Udo de Haes, 1970; Schöne and Udo de Haes, 1971; for a review of earlier investigations, see Bischof, 1966c, pp. 474f.). Errors of the same order of magnitude occur with forward-backward body tilt (Brecher and Schubert, 1934; Schöne, 1962, 1964; Correia et al., 1965). Considerable deviations are also observed when the subject is presented with an optical stimulus pattern containing one or more distinct main axes besides the luminous rod, provided that none of the main axes coincides with the pull of gravity. This phenomenon has been called "Richtungsinduktion" (directional induction) by Kleint (1936). It obtains with such stimulus configurations as a field of parallel stripes (Hofmann and Bielschowsky, 1909; Gibson and Radner, 1937; Bischof and Scheerer, 1970), a grid pattern (Boring, 1952; Mann, 1952), or a luminous frame (Witkin and Asch, 1948; Witkin, 1949b; Passey, 1950; Young, 1959; Naylor, 1963, 1965; Bertini, 1964; Morant and Aronoff, 1966). Under such conditions the subject's apparent vertical, as shown by his settings of the luminous rod, is "attracted" to a certain degree by the axes of the stimulus pattern. Directional induction effects are strongest with stimulus patterns that are closely similar to natural environments except for their slanted bearing. Such situations are created when the subject observes a natural scene through a suitable mirror system (Wertheimer, 1912; Gibson and Mowrer, 1938; Asch and Witkin, 1948a) or through prism spectacles (Kohler, 1951; Ohwaki, 1961; Witkin and Asch, 1948b; Witkin, 1949a), or if the natural scene is tilted as a whole, e.g., in a rotatable dummy room ("haunted swing", Wood, 1895; Kleint, 1936; Asch and Witkin, 1948b; Mann, 1952); see also Howard and Templeton (1966).

In the flow diagram (Fig. 1), three possible sources for deviations of this kind are conceivable: (i) the afference l_R may be a distorted image of the proximal stimulus configuration λ_R. (ii) The compensatory variable s may be an inaccurate representation of the interfering variable a. (iii) The compensatory function Φ^{-1} may differ from a mathematically exact summation process.

In this connection the three variables l_R, l_S, and s merit further consideration[2]. First, these quantities are to be regarded as "hypothetical constructs" in the sense of the terminological differentiation proposed by McCorquodale and Meehl (1948); i.e., they are meant to be not directly observable, but nevertheless physically existing, links of an innerorganismic causal chain. Simultaneously, however, they are "intervening variables" in the stricter sense defined by the authors — viz., they are conceived as products of a mere mental abstraction drawn out of (unknown) physiological entities likely to be in fact much more complex. The same holds for the above-mentioned compensatory operation Φ^{-1}.

2 For more detailed discussion, see Bischof and Scheerer (1970).

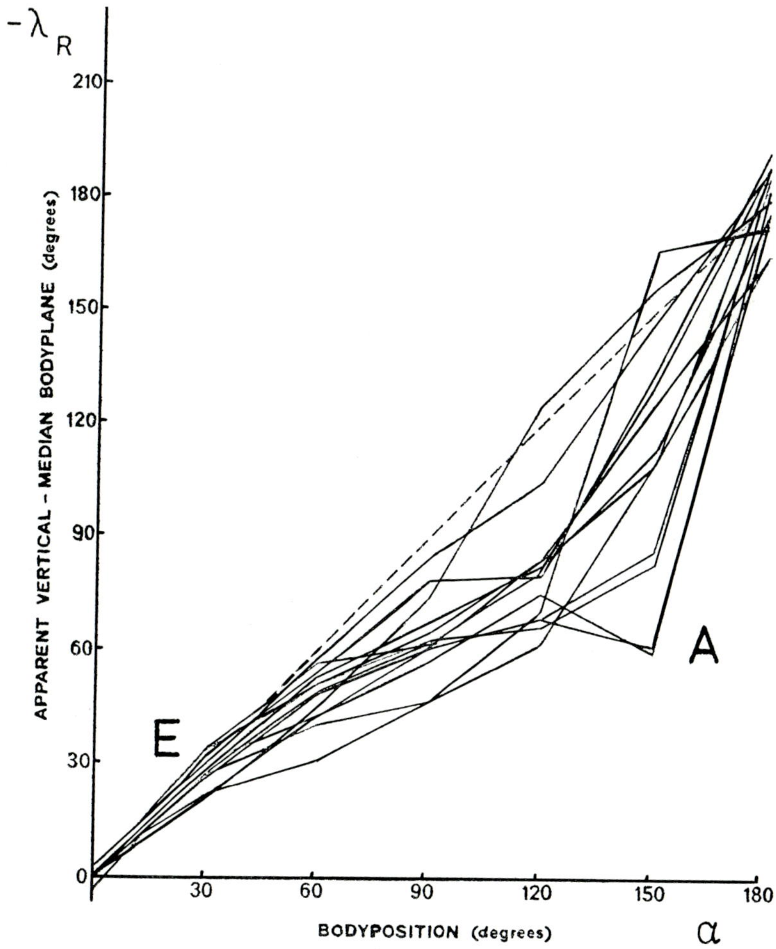

Fig. 2. Apparent vertical as a function of lateral body tilt for 13 Ss (according to UDO DE HAES 1970). Abscissa: Clockwise body tilt. Ordinate: Inclination of a luminous rod, set to Ss apparent vertical, measured in retinal coordinates with inverted sign (for explanation, see below, p. 162). Dotted line indicates ideal veridicality of directional perception. E- (MÜLLER) Phenomenon: measured value *above* dotted line (as shown in some Ss with body tilt of 30°), A- (AUBERT) phenomenon: measured value *below* dotted line (most marked in the majority of Ss under body tilt of 150°)

With regard to the three alternatives listed above, BISCHOF and SCHEERER (1970) arrive at the following proposition: If deviations from ideal veridicality in directional perception consist merely in rigid orthogonal rotations of phenomenal space without angular distortions occurring, they can be due solely to inaccuracy of the compensatory variable (alternative ii accepted), whereas the input-output characteristics of the optic channel and the compensatory summation process must be linear (i and iii rejected).

In this case, an indirect measure for the compensatory variable s could be derived from the setting of a luminous rod to the apparent vertical: If (i) $\lambda_R = l_R$, and (iii) $l_S = l_R + s$, and if further the apparent inclination l_S of the rod is zero (= vertical), then we should arrive at $\lambda_R = l_R = l_S - s = -s$. Thus the proximal stimulus λ_R with reversed sign, as plotted in Fig. 2, could serve as an operational measure for s.

As to the premise of this proposition, GIBSON and RADNER (1937, p. 464) state that the apparent vertical and horizontal "behave as if they were aspects of a single system for visual orientation"; the authors add, however, that both axes nevertheless "are not rigidly linked together; there is, as it were, a certain amount of 'play' or 'lost motion' between them". This angular distortion phenomenon was observed as an after-effect of prolonged exposure of an optical stimulus pattern containing (or consisting of) one predominating axis. Under these conditions, two factors seem to be involved in direction perception. They generate, respectively, (a) a so-called "*normalization effect*", which amounts to a rigid transformation of the phenomenal frame of reference as a whole (GIBSON, 1937a, b; GIBSON and RADNER, 1937), and (b) a "*satiation effect*", which only occurs in the vicinity of the stimulus axis, thus indeed impairing the orthogonality of space perception (KÖHLER and WALLACH, 1944). The latter phenomenon can probably be accounted for in terms of adaptation or inhibition of orientation detectors in the visual channel S of Fig. 1 (SUTHERLAND, 1961; COLTHEART, 1971; cf. also CARPENTER and BLAKEMORE, 1974). Thus, possibility (i), as listed above, cannot be ruled out entirely. However, satiation seems to be a second order effect. By factoring out the normalization effect be means of a "split-field technique", a magnitude of maximally 1.5° has been found for the satiation phenomenon (MORANT and MISTOVICH, 1960; MORANT and HARRIS, 1965).

These studies, to be sure, have only been performed with upright body posture. In a survey of the literature, unfortunately, no investigation dealing with the influence of body *tilt* on the orthogonality of space perception could be found. This leaves alternative (iii) undecided. Actually, some authors did record the apparent vertical and horizontal alternately in the same subjects as a function of head tilt, body tilt, or centrifuging, both with and without optical direction cues presented (GIBSON and MOWRER, 1938; ASCH and WITKIN, 1948a, b; WITKIN and ASCH, 1948a, b; BITTERMAN and WORCHEL, 1953, GRAYBIEL and CLARK, 1962). However, these experiments yield no answer to our problem since they are not sufficiently precise for that aim or, as in the studies of the WITKIN group, because of some peculiarities in the data analysis performed by the investigators. Nevertheless, the authors do not seem to have encountered a conspicuous decay of perceptual space orthogonality. Generally, one may presume that if body tilt and the like did produce startling angular distortions, this would have attracted the attention of some of the numerous investigators of vertical constancy during the past century, especially since under *pathological* conditions (cerebral lesions) or with *inadequate stimulation* (e.g., by electric currents) considerable distortions of the space coordinates have been repeatedly observed and reported under the name of *metamorphosia* or *dysmorphosia* by GELB (1926), BENDER and JUNG (1948), HALPERN (1949), DERWORT (1953) and others.

E. Postural Direction Cues

For the time being we may therefore assume that the errors of directional perception observed under physiological conditions are due virtually alone to the compensatory quantity s not precisely coinciding with the head inclination a. Thus the third problem stated above (see p. 159), namely, where the organism obtains a representation of a, becomes crucial. Clearly, the sources of pertinent information have to be looked for in the realm of stimulus parameters that are correlated with head and/or body tilt. Such parameters are hereafter referred to as "direction cues".

The sensory systems thought to be capable of providing direction cues are usually classified into (1) *optical* and (2) *postural* groups. The postural group may be subdivided into (a) *tactile*, (b) *kinesthetic*, and (c) *vestibular* cues.

(a) The *distribution of pressure* on the body surface may well be taken into account as a direction cue, as its maximum corresponds to the physical "down" unless, to be sure, the support at the surface of contact is in a slanted position (Gibson, 1966). The functional effectiveness of this factor at least for the "posture reflexes" has been demonstrated by Magnus (1924), its relevance for verticality perception follows from experiments of Schöne and Udo de Haes (1968, 1971).

(b) Coping with gravitation necessitates a continuous tonic innervation of the whole skeletal musculature, the pattern of which has to reflect in fine gradations the distribution of forces acting upon the body. Therefore the combined messages of *tension* and *position receptors* in muscles, tendons and joints (see Bischof, 1966c) may well be used as a source of information about the arrangement of trunk, head, and limbs with respect to gravity. The importance of these factors is underlined by the fact that asymmetric body tonus brought about, for example, by means of additional weights is accompanied by changes of the apparent vertical (Kleint, 1937; Schneider and Bartley, 1962; Klix, 1962; Werner et al., 1951).

(c) Whereas the two aforementioned sensory systems are primarily concerned with tasks apart from the perception of body posture in the gravito-inertial field, the vestibular apparatus appears to be constructed directly to serve this purpose.

Among the vestibular cues, both *ampullar* and *macular* messages can be shown to contribute to human perception of verticality. In the maculae, *phasic* and *tonic* responses may be distinguished, according to Lowenstein and Roberts (1950). There are few pertinent investigations deliberately involving stimulation of all vestibular portions mentioned (e.g., von Holst and Griesebach, 1951; Udo de Haes and Schöne, 1970). In experiments with parallel swings (Jongkees, 1952; Walsh, 1960, 1961; Schöne et al., 1967) the semicircular canals remain essentially unexcited. Devices providing steady-state head tilt, as employed by most investigators, additionally rule out phasic receptor activity in the maculae. This restricts stimulation to the tonic (non-adaptive) receptor system in the otolith apparatus, which may be considered the basic issue in postural control of vertical constancy, at least as far as the *external* compensatory mechanism (eye countertorsion, see above, p. 159) is concerned (Fischer, 1930a; Miller, 1962; Schöne, 1962; Fluur and Mellström, 1970a, b).

F. The Significance of Vestibular Direction Cues

The question as to whether vestibular afference has a direct access also to the *internal* mechanisms of perceptual space transformation is comparatively more intricate.

The significance and even preponderance of the vestibular apparatus in this respect has been maintained by investigators like Jongkees (1952), but denied by some earlier authors (Alexander and Barany, 1904; Beck, 1912; Stigler, 1912; Garten, 1920); partly, perhaps, since the latter expected (and failed) to encounter particular "postural sensations", reported by their subjects. These authors did not realize that a sense organ might well have the function of solely controlling perceptual *coordinate systems* rather than contributing new *qualities* to the perceptual world.

There is, of course, great difficulty in assessing the relative importance of each of the three postural systems mentioned above, since they convey information about one and the same stimulus parameter and may mutually substitute for each other. Thus, it is in no way conclusive if, in the case of deficiency of one of them, the performance in question does not substantially decrease — especially if the subjects have been allowed to adapt to the loss.

When, e.g., Garten (1920) and Arndts (1924) could demonstrate that the ability of subjects to judge the vertical position of their bodies remains unimpaired with *tactile information* being cut off by local anaesthesia, this finding nevertheless cannot disprove the possible participation of tactile direction cues in the same performance under normal conditions or after labyrinth loss.

On the other hand the same holds true for findings according to which patients with bilateral loss of *labyrinth function*, when tilted laterally, are still able to set a luminous rod in a dark surround in rather good alignment with the physical vertical, or even surpass the achievement of subjects without labyrinth malfunction (cf. Fischer, 1930b; Girotti and Bordogna, 1963; Girotti, 1963; Miller and Graybiel, 1966; Clark and Graybiel, 1966a; Graybiel et al., 1968). These experiments show that the activity of the vestibular apparatus may be substituted by other postural factors, if necessary. But they do not tell us anything about the error one is likely to commit if, as a first approximation, one ignores the latter when working with healthy subjects, and interprets the results obtained in the absence of optical cues as attributable mainly to the vestibular apparatus.

There seems to be only one consistent method for determining whether in the postural system vestibular cues are of prior importance in the perception of verticality: one has to play the vestibular information off against other conflicting postural direction cues. Experiments with this particular aim show that there is little extra-otolith postural influence on verticality perception with body tilt up to 90°, whereas in body positions unlikely to occur in normal life, somesthetic factors do play a role which is, however, not very marked (Schöne, 1962; Schöne and Udo de Haes, 1968, 1971; Correia et al., 1965).

Unfortunately, it is still an open question as to how the organism gathers information about the direction of gravitational force from the excitation patterns of *utricle* and *saccule*, separately.

Within the framework of his "bicomponent theory", Mittelstaedt (1964, 1966) has called attention to the fact that the formula for rotatory transformation of a Cartesian coordinate system requires information about the sine and the cosine of the angle of rotation, and that the utricle and saccule, respectively, could well be understood to supply this information.

Actually, there is evidence that earlier views, according to which only the utricle, but not the saccule, has a static function at all (e.g., MAXWELL, 1923; VERSTEEGH, 1927; MCNALLY, 1929; TAIT, 1932) are untenable at least for birds and mammals and also for some fishes (BENJAMINS and HUIZINGA, 1927; HASEGAWA, 1935; PERLMAN, 1940; ADRIAN, 1942; JONGKEES, 1950; LOWENSTEIN, 1950; SZENTÁGOTHAI, 1952; HUIZINGA, 1955; MEYER ZUM GOTTESBERGE and PLESTER, 1965; FLUUR and MELLSTRÖM, 1970b). Whether, however, in the perception of verticality saccular and utricular information is computed in the elegant way proposed by the bicomponent theory, remains to be investigated. (For pertinent theoretical considerations, see SCHÖNE, 1962; CORREIA et al., 1965; YOUNG and MEIRY, 1968; SCHÖNE and UDO DE HAES, 1970). The main difficulty with a bicomponent transformation of perceptual-space coordinates is that it could in principle be independent of otolith weight. When, however, the amount of gravito-inertial force is actually changed by means of applying *centrifugal forces* (SCHÖNE, 1962, 1964; CORREIA et al., 1965; MILLER and GRAYBIEL, 1966; SCHÖNE et al., 1967; SCHÖNE and PARKER, 1967; SCHÖNE and UDO DE HAES, 1970) marked changes of the apparent vertical do occur, showing that the aforementioned independence does not exist[3].

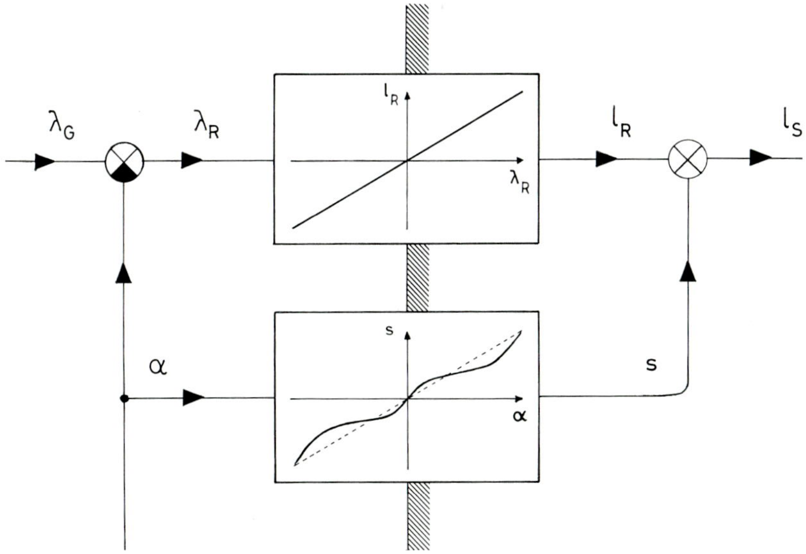

Fig. 3. Vestibular heterocompensation. Crossed circles: Operational symbols for addition. If a quadrant is black, the respective input variable is subtracted rather than added. Upper box: Visual system with linear input-output characteristics. Lower box: Otolith system with nonlinear characteristics according to Fig. 2

3 We are, of course, not referring here to changes of the apparent vertical due to changes in the *direction* (rather than the amount) of mechanical force during centrifugation. This effect is a physical triviality which never needed to be authenticated by psychophysicists, and which certainly did not deserve any pretentious labelling ("oculogravic illusion"). For a criticism of pertinent experiments designed by the GRAYBIEL and WITKIN groups, see HOWARD and TEMPLETON (1966, pp. 197ff.) and BISCHOF (1966c, p. 481).

While leaving this question to further analysis, we are free to characterize the function of the otolith apparatus in vertical constancy by the control diagram Fig. 3. In this diagram the A and E deviations result from the input-output characteristics of a single black-box labeled "otolith system", leaving aside intra-vestibular differentiations for the time being.

The particular type of network presented in Fig. 3, in which the compensatory variable is provided via a sensory channel separate from the one conveying information about the proximal stimulus, will be referred to hereafter as "hetero-compensation" (Bischof, 1966b). A possible alternative, called "autocompensation" of the optic message, shall be introduced in the next section.

III. Visual Direction Cues and the Reconstruction Principle

A. The Concept of Perceptual Reconstruction

The idea that the eye itself should be able to mediate perceptual information about the position of the head with respect to gravity not only seems to contradict our statements above, concerning the independence of retinal and distal coordinates (see p. 157); it also does not fit into the theoretical framework of classical sensory psychology. For the latter it was a matter of trivial self-evidence that a distal object could be immediately perceived (rather than inferred by logical reasoning) only in the presence of a proximal stimulus-pattern which to a sufficient degree "looks like" the distal object or, as Gibson (1950) characterized this view, which can serve as a "facsimile" of the object. Since, now, neither the subject's own head nor the field of gravity is portrayed on the retina, perceptual information about these features cannot be conveyed via the optic system, according to classical understanding.

Modern perceptional psychology (cf. Gibson, 1950, 1966; Attneave, 1954; Kohler, 1961; Metzger, 1968) has abandoned this unreflected conception and arrived at the following principle: Although it makes sense to conceive of the perceptual phenomena as "images" of *distal* objects, it is entirely misleading to expect them to portray the *proximal* stimulus-configurations as well; a particular percept may be established on the basis of any sensory process whatsoever, provided only that the proximal stimulus concerned is at least *correlated* to the distal object. In terms of information theory, the principle maintains that the perceptual system takes advantage of the *redundancy* within its physical surroundings in a manner that could be compared to the way one reconstructs the text of an abbreviated or distorted telegram. Therefore, Bischof (1966b) has proposed the term "*reconstruction processes*" for this kind of stimulus elaboration.

B. Visual Direction Cues

Put in anthropomorphic terms the reconstruction principle states, in essence, that the organismic perceptual system "relies" on certain regularities "expected" in its physical surroundings (Lorenz, 1959).

Such "redundancy expectations" may be very concrete. It can be expected, for instance, that cigarette smoke rises opposite to the pull of gravity. One can show that such data, accumulated apparently in the course of individual life-experience, influence spatial perception without any noticeable intervention of higher cognitive processes (cf. KOHLER, 1951, 1953; KLOPP, 1956).

In addition to these, however, there are redundancy expectations of a far more generalized and abstract nature. For these is would be difficult to determine whether they have been acquired in an individual learning process or whether they are part of the phylogenetically preadapted organization of the perceptual system. This question, to be sure, is rather irrelevant in the present connection. With regard to vertical constancy two general redundancy expectations are of particular significance.

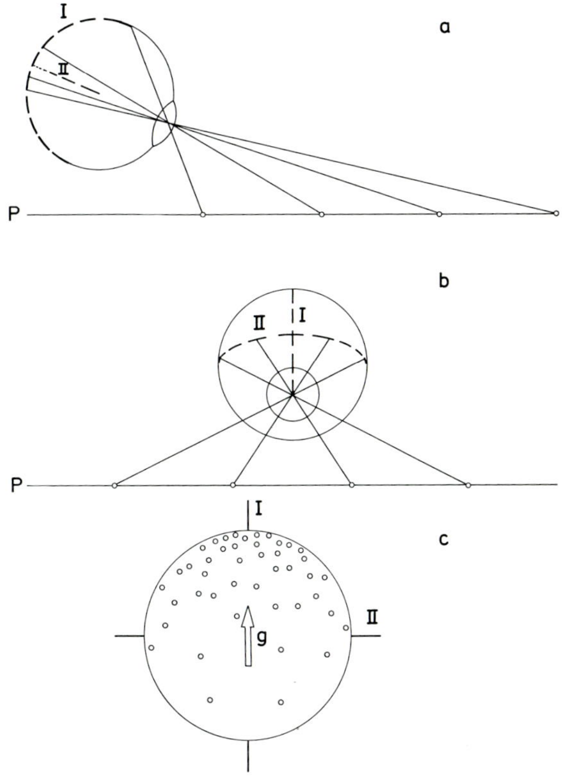

Fig. 4. Natural redundancy: Texture gradients. Equidistant marks on a plane surface (P) project on the retina in such a way that (a) the pairwise distance between proximal stimuli decreases monotonically in a retinal meridian (I) perpendicular to P, but (b) decreases symmetrically in a meridian (II) orthogonal to the former. If the marks are not equidistant but distributed in random fashion, as they are in most of the natural surface textures, the above statements would still hold true for the local average density of proximal stimulus distribution (Fig. 4c). Thus the *gradient* (g) of proximal-stimulus texture (i.e., the vector defining maximal change of stimulus density) should coincide with the physical vertical, providing that the surface regarded is horizontal

(1) The clarification of the first one has been pioneered by Gibson (1950). It consists of two mutually independent assumptions: (a) in a natural environment the texture of large surfaces is generally homogeneous, and (b) an approximately plain surface, filling large portions of the visual field, is likely to be of horizontal extension. From these two premises the following conclusion can be drawn: the mean gradient of retinal texture density, i.e., the direction in which retinal stimulation exhibits maximal average compression of its microstructure, will usually correspond to the projection of the physical vertical upon the frontal head plane (for explanation, see Fig. 4).

(2) The second redundancy expectation, the biological utilization of which has been substantiated by many authors (like, e.g., Koffka, 1935), assumes that under natural conditions equilibrium-states are encountered with a probability higher than that of any other comparable states. Consequently, objects of elongated shape should be likely either to stand upright (labile equilibrium), to hang down (stable equilibrium), or to lie horizontally on the ground (indifferent equilibrium), rather than to have any other *preferential* bearing. It can be shown by means of projective

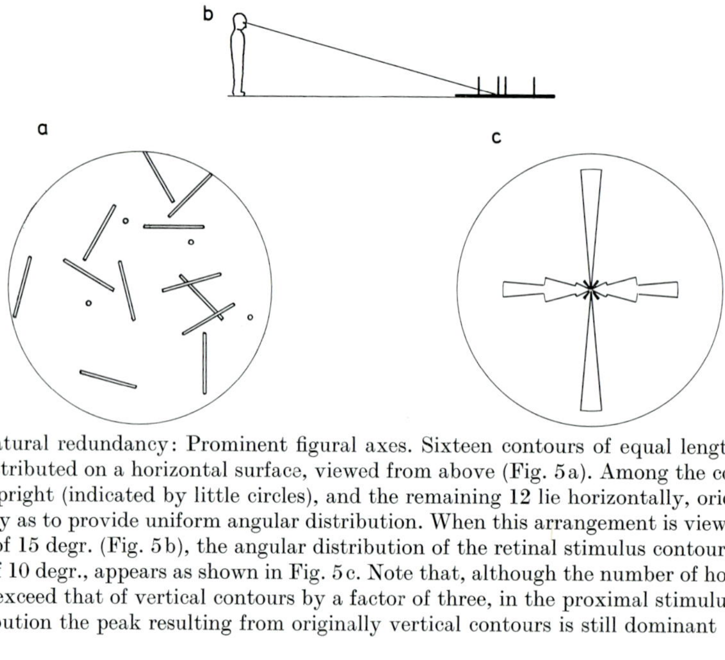

Fig. 5. Natural redundancy: Prominent figural axes. Sixteen contours of equal length, arbitrarily distributed on a horizontal surface, viewed from above (Fig. 5a). Among the contours, 4 stand upright (indicated by little circles), and the remaining 12 lie horizontally, oriented in such a way as to provide uniform angular distribution. When this arrangement is viewed from an angle of 15 degr. (Fig. 5b), the angular distribution of the retinal stimulus contours, taken in steps of 10 degr., appears as shown in Fig. 5c. Note that, although the number of horizontal contours exceed that of vertical contours by a factor of three, in the proximal stimulus distribution the peak resulting from originally vertical contours is still dominant

geometry that the outlines of such objects, when projected on the retina, form a stimulus pattern containing two prominent figural axes perpendicular to each other, and that one of these axes again corresponds to the projection of the physical vertical upon the fronto-parallel plane (see Fig. 5).

Whenever, therefore, the stimulus pattern impinging upon the retina contains a marked figural axis (particularly if the prominence of this axis is due to many single contours being parallel to each other), this axis tends to be accepted as a cue for either verticality or horizontality. It should be noted that the directional cue thus provided may be ambiguous. At least it can easily be rendered so by proper experimental device. If exposed, for instance, to a striped field or a square frame, the optical system is left in absolute doubt as to (a) which of the two prominent axes is vertical, and (b) which end of the vertical axis is the upper.

Experiments carried out by BISCHOF and SCHEERER (1970) illustrate how the organism copes with this fourfold ambiguity. The authors investigated three (female) subjects who were tilted by means of a chair rotatable around the sagittal head axis. The subjects looked towards a stimulus pattern consisting of a circular field of twenty-five parallel stripes on a dark ground. Shining on to the surface of the striped field from a pivot at its center, was a narrow light beam, which was to be set continuously to the subject's apparent vertical. The striped field was automatically rotated with a constant angular velocity of no more than 0.5 degrees per second either clockwise or counterclockwise. In each trial, the field made one full revolution of 360 degrees (taking a time of 12 min), while body-tilt was held constant at one of seven values (0, 30, 60, 90, 120, 150, 180 degrees clockwise). The subject's settings of the luminous beam were automatically recorded on a time scale.

The responses of one of the subjects are plotted in Fig. 6; they show that the apparent vertical is indeed entrained by both the direction of the stripes (referred to as the "primary axis" by the authors) and the axis perpendicular to the stripes ("secondary axis"). Each end of both axes, alternately, behaves as the upper one. Incidently, it can be seen that the "attractive power" of the primary axis exceeds that of the secondary axis to a noticeable degree. Applying a FOURIER-analysis to the curves shows that the primary axis is also dominant for body inclinations of $a = 150$ and 180 degrees, although this is not easily recognizable in the raw material, due to noise.

These results are in substantial agreement with earlier findings of GIBSON (1937a, b) and GIBSON and RADNER (1937), who observed that in the presence of a single tilted line the apparent vertical deviates towards the line if the latter's tilt is moderate, but away from it if its inclination is nearing the horizontal (cf. also CULBERT, 1954; MORANT and BELLER, 1965).

C. Visual Auto-Compensation

When outlining in his 1966 publication what is basically the reconstruction principle, GIBSON contrasts this idea with the compensation principle in the form proposed by VON HOLST and MITTELSTAEDT (1950). According to GIBSON, the optical feed-back produced by displacement of the body is substantially different from an optical stimulation caused by changes in the distal environment. Thus the visual afference is not really "disturbed" by the body activity (a), and consequently no compensatory process is required. This consideration is felt to dispense with the concept of "a brain that copies, stores, compares, matches, and decides" (*loc.cit.*, p. 39). This remark, however, is misleading. What really turns out to be dispensable from this point of view is what we have called "hetero-compensation" (see p. 166). The need for a compensatory process as such still

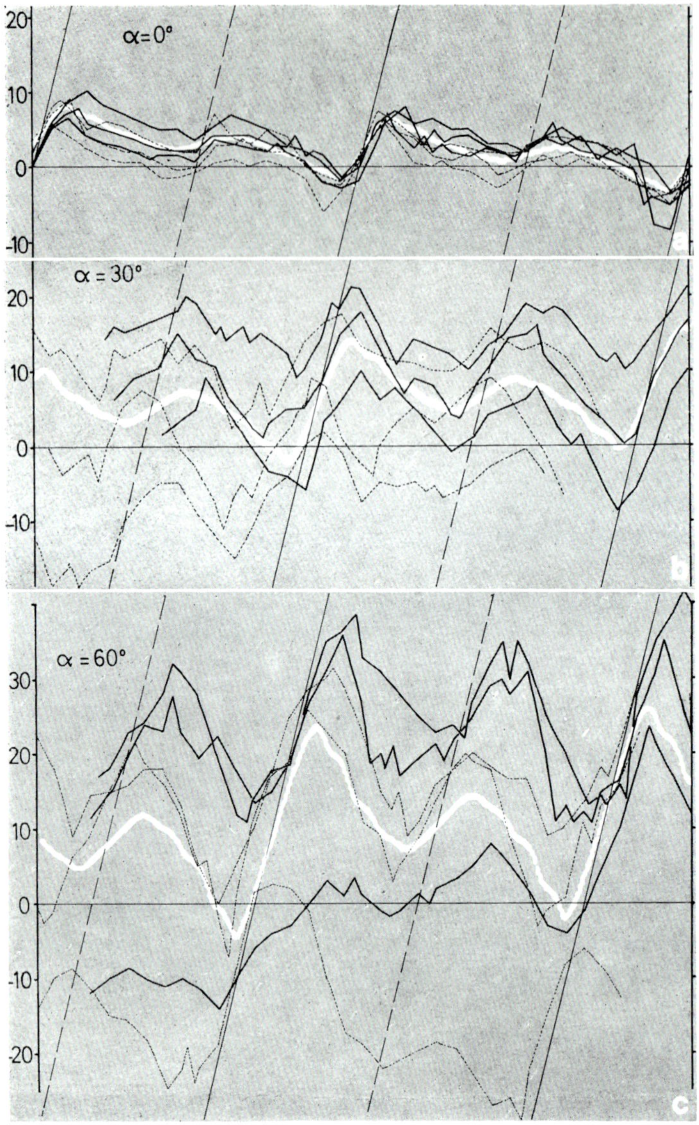

Fig. 6. Raw data of one S in the experiments of Bischof and Scheerer (1970). Each single diagram (a–g) comprises about 6 measurements of the apparent vertical in one particular body position (α), the latter being specified in the upper left corners. Half of the curves are from clockwise (solid lines), half from counter-clockwise rotation of the striped field (dotted lines). *Ordinate:* Angle (λ_G) between gravity and light beam set contineously to S's apparent vertical. *Abscissa:* Angle (β_G) between gravity and primary axis of background striped field. Full length of abscissa = 360 degrees = one revolution of the striped field. Since the latter rotates with constant velocity, the abscissa may also be understood as a time scale (full length = 12 min). In this case, the abscissa reads from left to right for the solid curves, but from right to left for the dotted ones. Recordings in most cases begin about 1 min after the striped field starts to rotate, in order to eliminate onset transients. *Diagonals* indicate the position of the striped field's primary axis (solid diagonals) or secondary axis (broken diagonals). The underlying white curves are simulations computed from the model Fig. 12 (see below, p. 184)

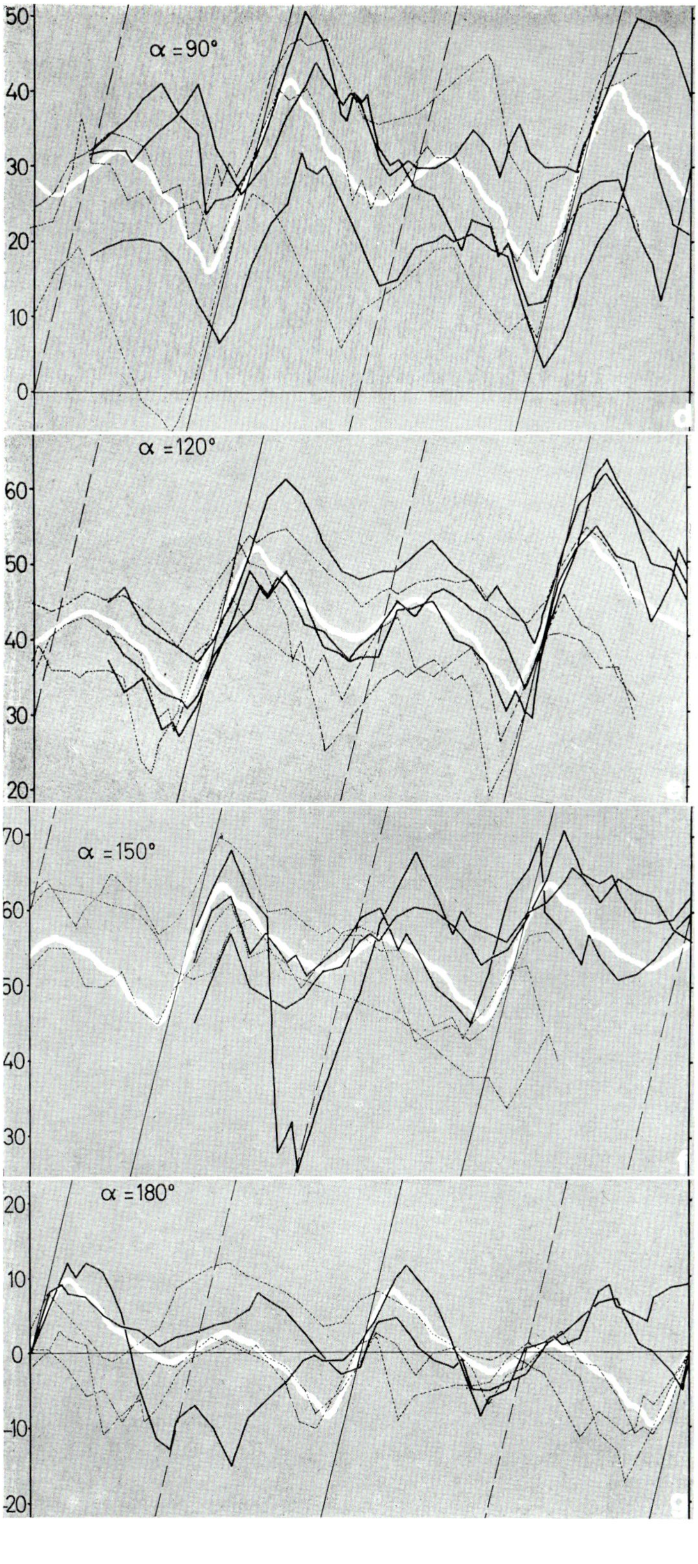

α = 90°
α = 120°
α = 150°
α = 180°

remains. It may now be, however, of a different type, namely, what could be termed "auto-compensation".

The essentials of auto-compensation are most easily understood in the case of *motion constancy*. Looking down at an ant-heap, e.g., causes a great deal of stimulus movement on the retina. Suppose, now, that the central nervous system would simply average the messages of all the retinal motion detectors, thus computing the vector sum of the velocities of all proximal stimulus elements. Since these elementary vectors are virtually independent of each other, the outcome of the calculation would more or less equal zero. If, however, the reafferent stimulation of smooth eye movement — caused, e.g., by pursuing one particular ant — were superimposed on the retinal stimulus-processes, then the average taken would equal with considerable exactness the eye velocity (with reversed sign, to be sure) and thus be fit to function as a compensatory variable for motion constancy. This procedure evidently is followed, erroneously, in cases of so-called "induced movement" (swimming up-stream with the bridge, etc).

Speaking generally, in auto-compensation the compensatory variable is derived directly from the afferent (in our case visual) message contaminated by the interfering variable. It presupposes the existence of a *filter mechanism* that selects, utilizing redundancy-expectations, the reafferent component (a) out of the retinal message itself (cf. Fig. 7).

How the filtering process is performed in the case of vertical constancy remains unknown. Presumably contour detection as described by Hubel and Wiesel (1959) is involved, with subsequent averaging to compute the predominant

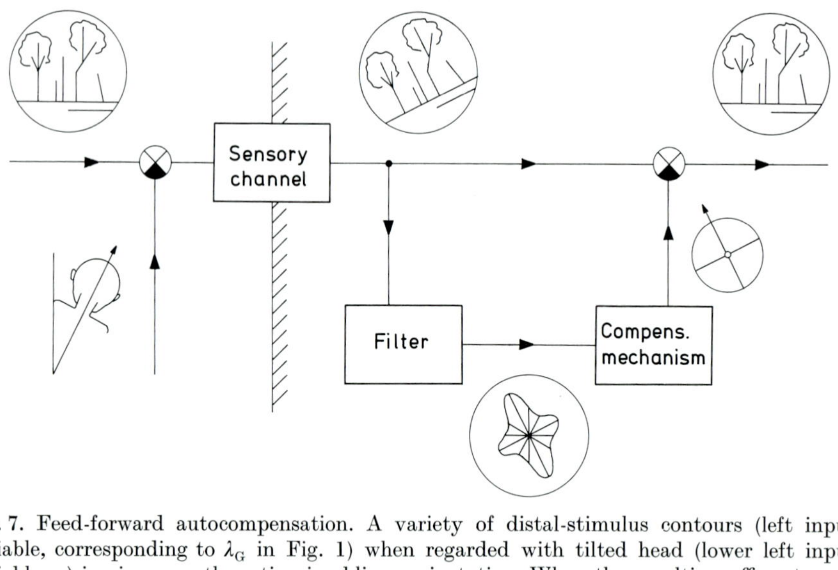

Fig. 7. Feed-forward autocompensation. A variety of distal-stimulus contours (left input variable, corresponding to λ_G in Fig. 1) when regarded with tilted head (lower left input variable, a) impinges on the retina in oblique orientation. When the resulting afferent message (l_R) is "filtered" in such a way as to compute the angular distribution of contour directions (according to Fig. 5c), the resulting main axis of retinal contour elements should, with sufficiently high probability, equal head inclination (with reversed sign). Consequently, it could be used as a compensatory variable (s, symbolized by a coordinate frame). When referred to these coordinates, the retinal afference should indeed be transformed in such a way as to render a sufficiently veridical perceptive representation (right output, l_S) of distal stimuli

proximal-stimulus axis, but for a definitive answer one must await further neurophysiological evidence. In this connection, moreover, neurophysiologists should also look for detectors sensitive to GIBSON texture-gradients (cf. p. 168).

Auto-compensation by a filter-mechanism can in some degree be compared to an *adaptive* process. The crucial difference between it and a genuine local adaptation is, however, that in the latter every site of the sensory field tends independently of the others to approach the zero-level of excitation; whereas in auto-compensation the zero-level of the entire stimulus field shifts uniquely, which has the important consequence that the differences appearing within the proximal stimulus pattern are preserved (cf. also METZGER, 1968, p. 167ff.). In the special case of verticality perception, adaptation and auto-compensation are exemplified, respectively, by the "satiation" and "normalization" effects mentioned earlier (see p. 162).

D. Feed-Forward and Feed-Back Compensation

In all cases of auto-compensation two fundamentally different ways of feeding the compensatory variable into the optic afference are available: the compensatory variable may enter *after* the branching point to the filter (*feed-forward compensation*, Fig. 7), or *before* it (*feed-back compensation*, Fig. 8). In terms of control theory the first model has been called a "mesh", the second one a "loop" (MITTELSTAEDT, 1960).

In feed-forward compensation, provided that the filter can reconstruct the head inclination without error, the compensatory variable has to equal the filter output in order to establish ideal space constancy. In feed-back compensation, on the other hand, veridicality requires that the compensatory variable

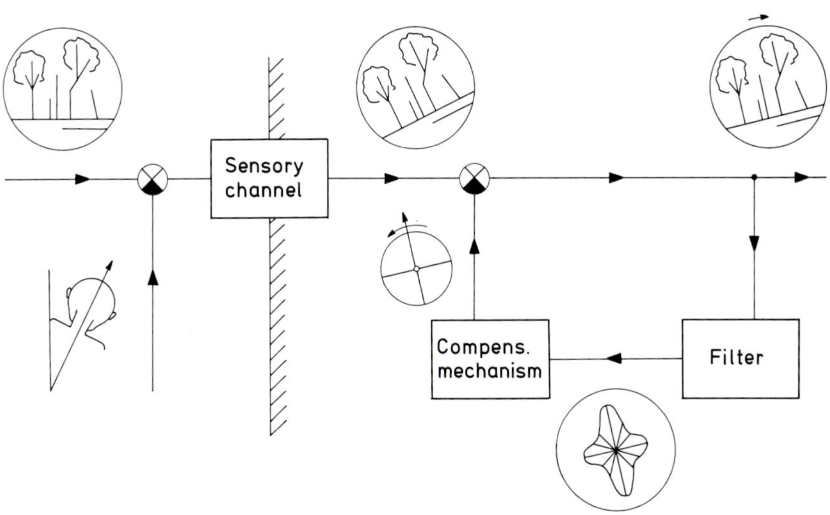

Fig. 8. Feed-back autocompensation. Differing from the system of Fig. 7 in that the perceptual output (l_S) itself undergoes the "filtering" procedure, and that the compensatory coordinate frame (s) is *rotated* as long as the inclination of the main axis of apparent contour distribution differs from zero

equal the time integral of the filter output. In the latter case, the magnitude of the compensatory variable will *change* as long as the filter output is different from zero; obviously, this process cannot come to rest with a steady value of s until the filter output has vanished, i.e., until the main axis of the perceptual field has turned *apparently* vertical. For a broader discussion see BISCHOF and SCHEERER (1970).

Which of the two possibilities is actually realized in the organism can be readily answered in the case of "external" compensation (cf. p. 159). Here, by definition, the compensation takes place outside the boundary of neurophysiological] processes, whereas the compensatory variable comes from the filter that lies within this boundary. Thus, the ocular countertorsion and, incidentally, also all optokinetic reactions including nystagm, are examples for feed-back auto-compensation.

Much more difficulty arises when we try to answer the same question in the field of "internal" compensation, since here the entire network is hidden within the brain, inaccessible to direct analysis. However, BISCHOF and SCHEERER (1970) could develop a method that allowed them to solve the problem in an indirect way. We can only outline their argumentation here; for a more thorough presentation, see the publication cited.

Regarding the oscillations in Fig. 6, which are schematized in Fig. 9, it is easy to see that for each particular curve the abscissa could be partitioned into sections extending, respectively, between two successive extreme values of the oscillation of the apparent vertical. In Fig. 9a, one half of such a section is labeled as B. Each of these sections would then mark a range of stripe inclinations which have in common a particular dominance relation between the four main directions of the striped field. The abscissa of each extreme value denotes the critical inclination of the field at which one of its main directions starts or ceases to predominate over the other three in determining the apparent vertical. What, now, causes the dominance to shift from one main direction to the next? Evidently, in the course of field rotation each particular main direction is alternately perceived to be more and more, and then less and less, likely to be a valid representative of the physical vertical. This, however, presupposes a *standard* reference with which the perceptual system may decide about accepting a given optical main direction as a cue for verticality (cf. also DAY and WADE, 1969). Presumably, the additional information required for this decision is supplied by the postural senses. However, this information appears in crucially different forms in feed-forward and feed-back compensation, respectively.

(1) *In feed-forward compensation* (Fig. 7) the standard determining the dominance relations within the set of optical main directions would consist essentially[4] of the vestibular compensatory variable (the "vestibular vertical") established according to Fig. 3. Thus, the inclination of a particular optical main direction with respect to the *vestibular vertical* decides about the acceptance of this direction as an optic cue for verticality. The vestibular vertical, however, depending as it does upon postural stimuli that are kept constant during each trial, should be expected to show limited systematic shifting at most, even when one allows for

4 Possible other postural cues (non-vestibular, non-optic) are being neglected here; this, however, is not relevant in the line of argument.

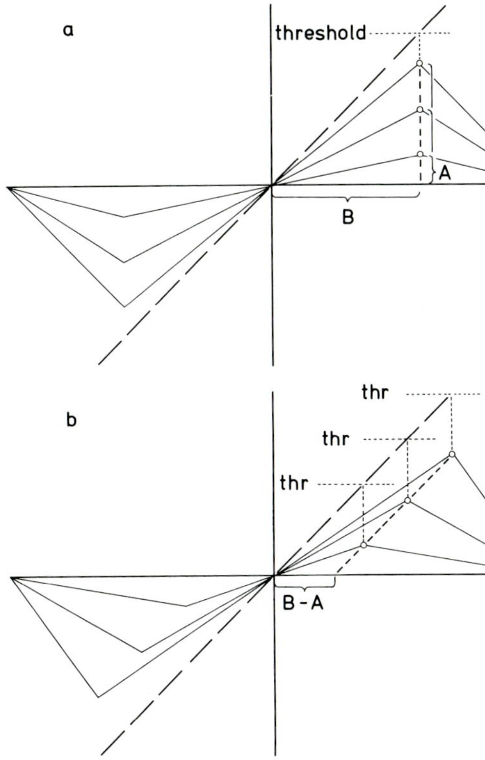

Fig. 9. Comparison of alternative compensatory mechanisms. Oscillations of an apparently vertical light beam. Ordinate: Angular inclination of light beam with respect to the DC component of oscillation (the latter representing the vestibular standard). Abscissa: Time; solid lines: settings of light beam for different body inclinations. Broken diagonals: Position of one particular main axis of the striped field. a) *Feed-forward compensation.* When the striped field axis has deviated far enough from the vestibular standard and reached a threshold (horizontal dotted line), the dominance will be taken over by the next axis. Hence the light beam would cease following the first axis and turn back to meet the next one. The curves should therefore show extreme values at this point. Since this process ought to be independent of body tilt, the maxima should all occur at the same time (B) in the cycle, irrespective of the amount (A) of oscillation. b) *Feed-back compensation.* If, however, the dominance of the striped field axis depends upon its deviation from the apparent vertical, i.e., from the respective light-beam curves, the threshold (dotted lines) *will* vary with the amplitude of oscillation. Thus all extreme values should now have a position such that their distance to the broken diagonal is constant. This distance ought to be the difference between the abscissa value (B) and the ordinate value (A) for every extremum

moderate changes due to system dynamics (transfer characteristics and the like) of the sensory systems concerned (cf. MÜLLER, 1916; MILLER and GRAYBIEL, 1963; GEISSLER, 1965; MCFARLAND and CLARKSON, 1966; CLARK and GRAYBIEL, 1966b; SCHÖNE and UDO DE HAES, 1968; UDO DE HAES and SCHÖNE, 1969). Hence the ranges of influence of the four main directions in the striped field are distributed according to a standard reference direction that remains virtually fixed during any given trial. To be sure, the reference direction will change from trial to trial, owing to there being different head inclinations, but within each of these it will remain essentially constant. This means, however, that we should find the sections of the abscissa apportioned by one and the same ratio regardless of head inclination, as indicated in Fig. 9a.

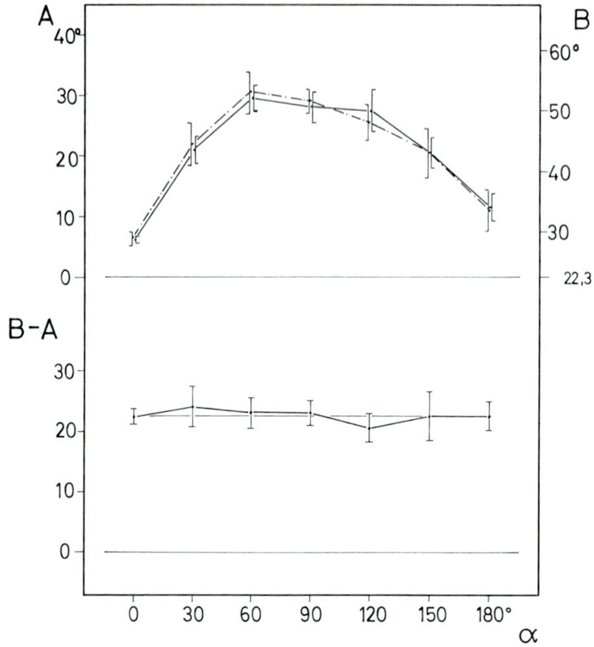

Fig. 10. Experimental support of feed-back autocompensation hypothesis in the perception of verticality (from Bischof and Scheerer, 1970). Comparison of ordinate (A: solid lines) and abscissa (B: broken lines) for extreme values of apparent vertical (cf. Fig. 9). Mean values of three subjects, with average variance of means shown by bars. B scale shifted so as to accomplish maximal coincidence of curves. Evidently, B is dependent on head inclination (abscissa), whereas B–A is not

(2) Hypothesizing *feed-back compensation* (Fig. 8) yields quite different predictions. In this case the optic messages do not reach the filter mechanism before having undergone the (combined optic-vestibular) compensatory process that transforms them into the final coordinate system of apparent space. It is thus the *apparent* inclination of the four optical main directions (rather than their inclination with respect to a postural standard) that determines the partitioning of their spheres of influence. In other words, with feed-back compensation the apparent vertical, as represented by the luminous beam controlled by the subject, serves as the reference required for the validation of the optical main directions. Defined in this fashion, however, the reference is no longer invariant during a trial, and it varies, moreover, in a different way with different head inclinations. With feed-

back compensation, consequently, the abscissa sections between extreme values in Fig. 6 would not be apportioned independent of head inclination. Only if we refer the stripe inclination at every moment to the position of the apparent vertical, i.e., if we project the extreme values, as in Fig. 9b, parallel to the diagonal broken lines, rather than perpendicularly, should we obtain an invariant partitioning of the abscissa.

Bischof and Scheerer (*loc. cit.*) could show, that, with this latter transformation carried out, the partitioning of ranges of influence among the four optical main directions in fact becomes invariant relative to head inclination (see Fig. 10). This indicates that the internal auto-compensatory system of visual perception of verticality is of the feed-back type.

IV. Optic-Vestibular Interaction and the Correction Principle

A. The Utilization of "Convergent Detection"

The simultaneous occurrence of both (optical) auto- and (vestibular) hetero-compensation in human vertical constancy sheds light on another peculiarity of perceptual information processing. Apparently, compensatory achievments are confined within the limits of precision of the mechanisms that provide the compensatory variable s. When, owing to possible shortcomings in information conveyance or computation, the compensatory variable does not exactly correspond to the interfering variable a, then s is unable to balance the effect of a exactly, and the interference is under- or overcompensated. The A and E phenomena described above (see Fig. 2) are examples of this.

In order to minimize such errors, the organism often seeks to provide information about an interesting distal item by using, in parallel, a plurality of sensory channels which are susceptible to different kinds of disturbing effects. Thus, the probability of error can be reduced by "convergent detection", as it were, a possibility that has been repeatedly discussed in psychological literature (cf. especially Brunswik, 1934, 1940, 1956). For reasons that will be explained later (see p. 180), Bischof (1966b) has proposed the term "correction principle" for this method of perceptual information processing.

B. Optic-Vestibular Equivalence

Separate sensory data which provide information about one and the same distal issue, and which are, accordingly, exchangeable with respect to their biological significance to the organism, will be referred to in the following as "*equivalent signals*". In this respect, a remarkably close relationship exists between optical and vestibular messages: for every particular output of the vestibular organs there exists an equivalent optical signal-parameter; likewise, every motor or perceptual effect known to be controlled by vestibular inputs can also be elicited by proper optical excitation.

More particularly, stimulation of the *semi-circular canals* is equivalent to visual excitation produced by uniform movement of the entire stimulus field. The perceptual results of the latter are usually referred to as "*induced movement*"

(Duncker, 1929; Linschoten, 1952; cf. also Gibson, 1950, 1954); the corresponding motor reactions are known under the name of "*optokinetic responses*". The optical counterparts of stimulation of the *otolith organs* have been discussed in an earlier section (see pp. 166 ff.); their perceptual effect, viz., their influence on the apparent vertical, has been termed "*directional induction*" by Kleint (1936), with obvious reference to Duncker. In labeling the corresponding motor reactions, it might be convenient to speak of "*optostatic responses*" in analogy to "optokinetics". The impairment of body balance while observing a slightly but uniformly slanted mountain meadow is an optostatic effect, as is the "dorsal light reaction" in fishes (von Holst, 1950). The occurrence of optostatic eye countertorsion in man has been reported by Greenberg (1960) (cf. however Howard and Templeton, 1964b).

Note that optic and vestibular signals are *not* equivalent with respect to information concerning straight body movements. Here only the eye is able to convey reliable information (Gibson, 1954), and not the vestibular apparatus, contrary to repeated speculations (e.g., by Magnus, 1924). Whether and how messages of the latter may yet play some role in this connection, will not be discussed here (cf. Bischof, 1966c, p. 483f).

C. Incongruity of Equivalent Signals

Like reconstruction processes, the method of convergent detection is also based on the utilization of redundancy — not, to be sure, within the domain of distal objects, but rather on the level of sensory messages referring to these objects: the organism tries to keep on the safe side by seeking information from different "warrantors". But what if those warrantors are at odds with each other; i.e., what if equivalent messages exhibit *incongruity*? In general there are three possible organismic reactions in such a situation; all three do also appear in the special case of optic-vestibular incongruity.

1. "Compromise" Solution

The most usual organic reaction encountered with optic-vestibular incongruity is the calculation of a weighted average of the competing messages. The weight factors involved in this type of information processing will be discussed below (see pp. 180ff.). Evidently, the results of the experiments of Bischof and Scheerer (1970), as depicted in Fig. 6, can be understood as compromise solutions of this type. Von Holst (1950) and Braemer (1957) obtained comparable results with fishes.

2. "Alternative" Solution

A second possibility is that the organism takes account of only one of the competing signals while entirely blocking the others. The dominance may or may not flip-flop between the signals concerned. Here, again, weight factors are likely to play a role. Effects of this kind may be encountered if very suggestive optic direction cues, for instance a (tilted) dummy room, are viewed in upright body position. Some subjects of Kleint (1936) reported that under these circumstances the dummy room appeared to them alternately tilted and upright.

3. "Simultaneity" Solution

Whereas the two previous solutions to the incongruity problem will always provide an unequivocal basis of orientation, there are cases in which the incompatible signals reach conscious perception simultaneously, without mutual suppression. It may be questioned, of course, whether we can speak of a "solution" here, as the resulting perceptual phenomenon is over-determined in a paradoxical way, unfit for being reacted to. If, for example, a subject remains stationary, surrounded by a dummy room that rotates slowly around a horizontal axis, he generally experiences his body at first to be somewhat tilted in the opposite direction; subsequently he feels that his body keeps rotating, yet that its position no longer changes: the experience of motion ("I am rotating with constant angular velocity") and the experience of position ("I never reach the head-down posture") break apart (KLEINT, 1937; cf. also DUNCKER, 1929; OPPENHEIMER, 1935; METZGER, 1940, 1954, p. 150). — Even in the absence of visual information, some subjects experience two possibilities of setting a luminous line to apparent verticality simultaneously under body tilt of about 150°. This would indicate a conflict within the postural cue system (FISCHER, 1930; UDO DE HAES and SCHÖNE, 1969; GRAYBIEL and CLARK, 1962; MILLER and GRAYBIEL, 1966; cf. also below, p. 182).

D. Error Detection and Error Correction

The practice of obtaining information about the same item through parallel channels is in some measure analogous to that of modern communication technique, which uses, for conveying a message over a single channel, a number of symbols that exceeds the theoretically required minimum. Both methods utilize signal redundancy, and both do so for the sake of the advantage that in case of error the receiver is supplied with at least (1) a warning that an error is present, but perhaps also (2) with cues for its correction.

1. Error Detection

The receiving system can tell from certain irregularities in the signals received — in the case in point, from the incongruity of equivalent messages — at least *that* an error has occurred, although it may have no idea at which particular place. There is indication that the sensory systems react to this kind of "alarm" by forwarding only in a restricted form (with a proviso, as it were) the message likely to be erroneous. The corresponding phenomenal quality is often referred to by the subject with terms like "uncertain", "vague", "feeble", "faint", "unconvincing", "unreal", and the like (cf. METZGER, 1954, pp. 109f.). From experiments with the "haunted swing", for example, it is known that under conditions of strong optic-vestibular ambiguity a weakening, even a loss, of phenomenal verticality may result; in the extreme case, the subject may become unable to assign the terms "up" and "down" to *any* direction of his phenomenal space (KLEINT, 1936, 1940).

A particularly vigorous reaction of the organism to error warnings due to incongruities within the optic-vestibular domain consists, according to many authors, in the phenomenon of *vertigo*. Indeed, certain distinct features of this response, like anxiety and release of primitive security reflexes (clinging), may well be understood as emergency measures in the face of threatening decomposition of space orientation. For more details, see the chapters F.VIII; IX; G.I. in this volume.

2. Error Correction

In certain communication systems the receiver may not only be informed, by inconsistencies in the message, that an error has occurred, but also where it is probably sited and what the original text most likely was. We have reason to believe that the method of convergent ascertainment in the perceptual system also works as an error-correcting routine in this sense. That is why we have proposed the term "correction principle" here.

Above (see p. 178) we introduced the notion of "*weight factors*" that control the relative power available to equivalent sensory messages when they compete with each other in the case of incongruity (cf. KLEINT, 1936). The evidence obtained up to now allows us to conjecture that those weight factors tend to be computed according to the following rule: The less a signal is likely to convey an erroneous message (i.e., the more and the better cues speak in favor of its reliability) the higher is it weighted in competition with contradicting equivalent signals (BRUNSWIK, 1956; KLIX, 1962). Thus we may tentatively summarize the *correction principle* as follows: The organism reduces the probability of error in the perceptual processes by providing for equivalent messages through different sensory channels and then "relying" exclusively or preferably upon those whose validity is supported by the better cues.

E. Determinants of the Optic-Vestibular Weight Ratio

In his classical investigations on the equilibrium responses of fish during conflicting optic and vestibular stimulation, VON HOLST (1950) coined the term "statisch-optische Verhältniszahl" (translatable as "vestibular-optic weight ratio") to refer to a specific parameter that expresses the degree to which the vestibular righting-response prevails over a conflicting dorsal light reaction (cf. also BRAEMER, 1957). VON HOLST defined this coefficient as the cotangent of the angle between the dorso-ventral axis of the fish and the plumb line, recorded under conditions of horizontal light incidence. For the results to be interpretable the angle had to be measured when the fish was in a state of physiological equilibrium, i.e., after possible postural reflexes had ceased. Because of the latter condition VON HOLST's definition of the "vestibular-optic weight ratio" is suitable only for experimental situations in which the subject senses his body to be vertical. For perceptual experiments in which, by body fixation, every possible feed-back of the apparent vertical on body posture is blocked and in which, therefore, body inclination and apparent vertical do not necessarily correspond, a different way of defining the weight ratio is advisable. For reasons to be elucidated below (see p. 182), BISCHOF and SCHEERER (1970) suggest taking the *average range of oscillation* of the apparent vertical, under conditions of steady rotation of the optical pattern around the visual axis, as an index of the weight ratio discussed.

In distinction to VON HOLST's term, we feel it would be better to speak of an "*optic-vestibular* weight ratio" here, since the value of the coefficient — the mean amplitude of oscillation in Fig. 6 — increases monotonically with optic predominance.

The factors governing the optic-vestibular weight ratio (however defined) have not yet been thoroughly investigated, partly because for years authors have engaged in a fruitless debate as to which of the two sensory channels, the optical or the vestibular, is "prior" or "more basic" to the perception of the vertical, instead of taking for granted that *both* are important and simply asking how they interact (for a critical review of this discussion, see GIBSON, 1952).

1. As far as the *optical* determinants of the optic-vestibular weight ratio are concerned, we know this much: with labyrinthine stimulation constant, the induction of the apparent vertical by a striped field rises with the size of the latter and with the number of parallel contours within it; when patterns of higher complexity are used, the induction effect is enhanced according to the degree of their similarity to natural scenes (for references, see above, p. 160). These findings harmonize well with the correction principle, since each of the factors mentioned apparently makes it more probable — outside the laboratory situation — that the main direction of the retinal stimulus field coincides with the direction of gravity.

2. Less transparent is the biological advantage of certain *intra-organismic* factors influencing optic-vestibular competition. Between different fish species, for instance, considerable variation in the vestibular-optic weight ratio has been found by VON HOLST (1950) and BRAEMER (1957). In man, typological differences are asserted to occur: women and children give comparably more weight to visual stimuli than adult males, according to WITKIN et al. (1954). It is difficult to see what all this should have to do with the "reliability" of optical or vestibular cues. Actual needs, moods, attention and the like can also influence the perceptual response in optic-vestibular conflict situations. VON HOLST (1948) could demonstrate that the body inclination of laterally illuminated fishes is markedly enhanced when objects of high motivational valence (e.g., food) are presented. The animal, as it were, becomes "all eyes" and consequently rates the light source as a directional cue comparatively higher than he otherwise would, although the light source is not his object of attention at all and certainly has not become any more "reliable." The effect of light intensity upon the weight of optical directional cues (CURRAN and LANE, 1962) may be mentioned in this connection. Findings like these suggest that the correction principle should not be understood as a general postulate, but rather as a heuristic principle.

3. The *vestibular-somesthetic* influences upon the optic-vestibular weight ratio are, again, interpretable in "reliability" terms. According to observations of VON HOLST (1950), shaking the water in an aquarium, simulating surf, is apt to enhance considerably the optical component with some fish species. In this experiment, the laterally illuminated animals inclined their bodies more and more towards the light source, only gradually returning to the previous position after the water movement had stopped. VON HOLST also noted that an increase in hydrostatic pressure tends to augment the weight of the vestibular component. This, too, can be understood teleonomically, since water pressure normally rises with depth and is thus positively correlated with the calmness of the water layer and, consequently, with the reliability of the vestibular positional messages.

The most important problem concerning vestibular control of the optic-vestibular weight ratio is the dependence of the latter upon *body inclination*.

Information about this dependence has been provided for head tilts up to 40° by earlier authors (Hofmann, 1910; Vernon, 1935; Witkin and Asch, 1948; Witkin, 1949) and extended to 180° by Bischof and Scheerer (1970) and Schöne and Udo de Haes (1971). According to the correction principle, the visual induction of the apparent vertical should be minimum in upright position, since with slight or no body tilt the precision of the statolith apparatus is maximal. This expectation was confirmed in all investigations cited. Additionally, however, one would predict a maximal visual induction effect in a body position of 150–180°, since in this range the A-deviation, the variance of the apparent vertical, the subjective uncertainty, and also the influence of various other directional cues, are all known to be maximal (cf. Quix and Eijsvogel, 1929; Brown, 1961; Correia and Guedry, 1964; Schöne, 1964; Guedry, 1965; Benson and Bodin, 1966; Schöne and Udo de Haes, 1968, 1971; Udo de Haes and Schöne, 1969; Udo de Haes, 1970).

Actually, the results of Schöne and Udo de Haes (1971) seem to confirm this expectancy. They exposed to their subjects a stimulus pattern consisting of a single line and a striped field, both rigidly connected so that the stripes formed a fixed angle of either plus or minus 15 degrees with the line. The subject, that is, when adjusting the single line to his apparent vertical, had to move the striped field as well, which therefore kept appearing to him inclined by 15 degrees in clockwise, or counterclockwise direction. In both conditions, the settings for the apparent vertical differed, due to directional induction, and the angle between both settings turned out to be greatest with a body tilt of 150 degrees.

However, the authors call attention to their method being rather susceptible to the well-known effect (cf. p. 179) that the vestibular vertical can be equivocal with extreme body tilt. If, say, with $a = 150°$ the vestibular vertical has two different possible positions, it is difficult to tell from the data obtained by Schöne and Udo de Haes whether the visual induction of the apparent vertical was due to a flip-flop kind of effect, or to a greater tolerance of any *one* of both possible states against continuous deflection. This distinction can easier be made using the method of Bischof and Scheerer (1970). Actually, Fig. 6f (cf. p. 171) shows one case (lowest unbroken line) in which a temporary shift between two possible DC-states of the apparent-vertical might have occurred. Normally, however, there were no such shifts, and the optic-vestibular weight ratio, defined as the average range of oscillation, was most marked with body inclinations between 60 and 90 degrees (cf. Fig. 6). Surprisingly enough, the optic-vestibular weight ratio, when plotted against body tilt, rendered a curve that was highly correlated with the counter-torsion characteristic of the subject's eye (cf. Fig. 11).

Fig. 11. Mean range of oscillation of luminous beam setting (ψ = filled dots and solid lines) and ocular countertorsion (ρ = empty dots and broken lines), plotted against body tilt (a) for three Ss. Raw data and mean values (from Bischof and Scheerer, 1970). Ordinate scale ratio $\psi : \rho = 1.48$ calculated such as to minimize square difference of means over all three Ss. Note that there is not only a satisfactory proportionality between ψ and ρ but that even the factor of proportionality can be taken to be the same in all three subjects: the S with the highest amount of eye countertorsion (Vp H) also shows the widest oscillations of the apparent vertical in the presence of a rotating striped field. Considering the small number of Ss, the latter effect, of course, should not be generalized at the moment

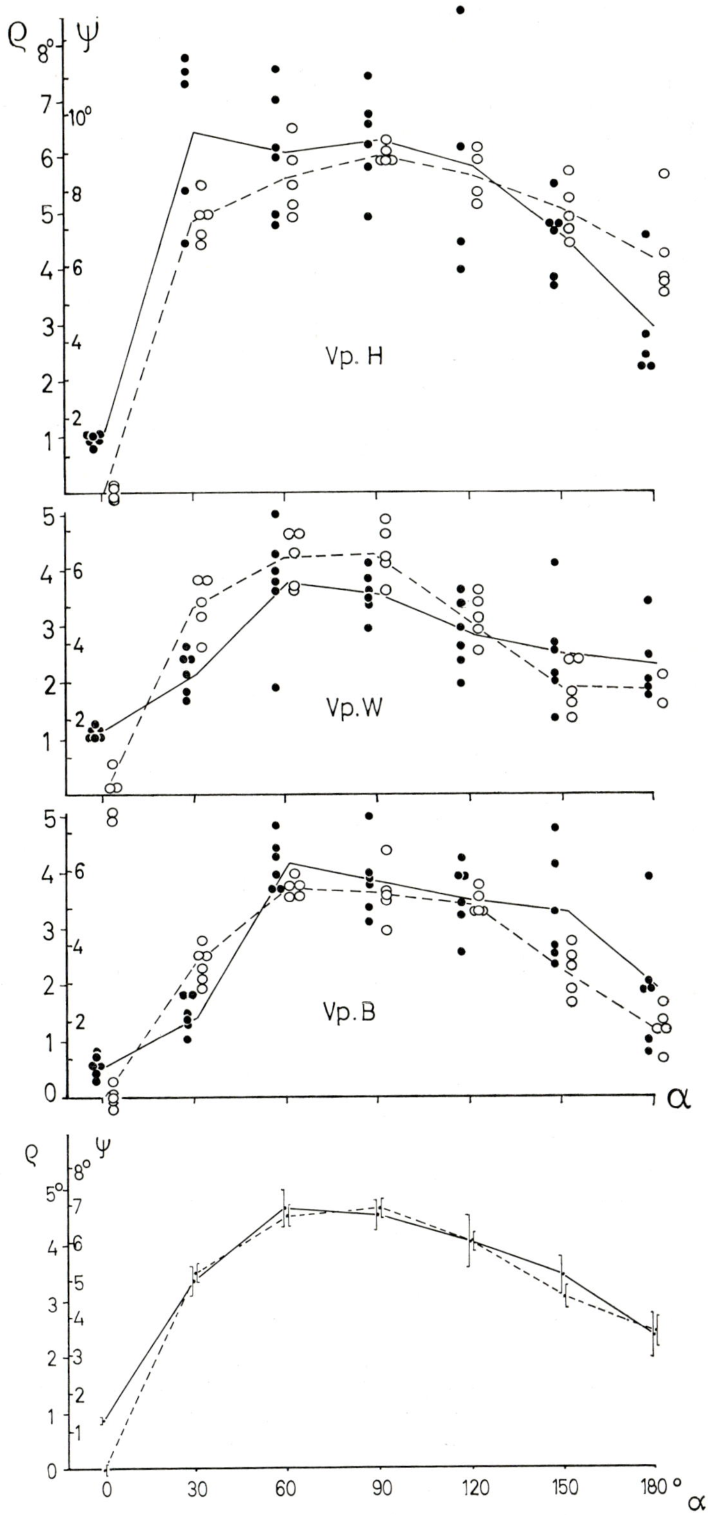

Fig. 11

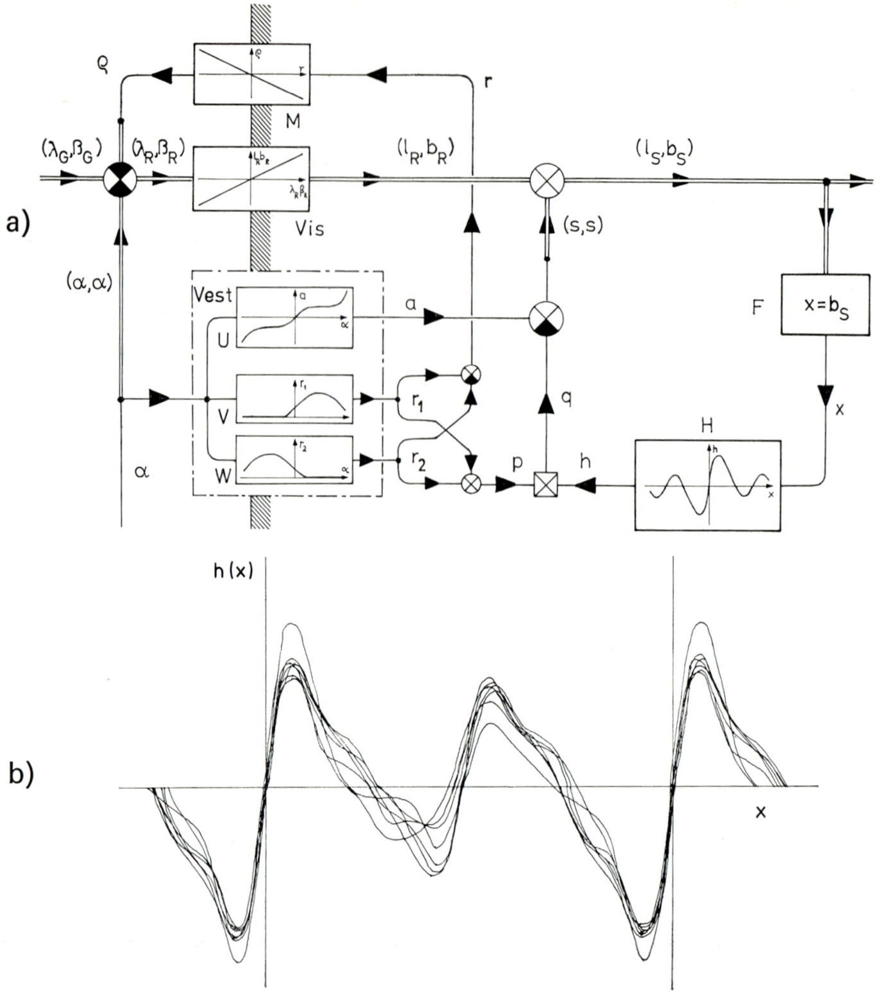

Fig. 12. a) Model of optic-vestibular orientation to the vertical. From BISCHOF and SCHEERER (1970). Double arrows represent two-component variables. Crossed square is multiplication symbol. For the remaining graphic symbols see the legends of Figs. 1 and 3. M: oculomotor system; Vis: visual system; Vest: vestibular system, split up into three subsystems U, V and W, which can be distinguished functionally but must not necessarily be anatomically different. (λ_G, β_G): distal stimulus field, described by the inclination of light beam (λ) and of primary axis of the striped field (β) with respect to gravity (subscript G). (λ_R, β_R): corresponding proximal stimulus field in retinal coordinates (subscript R), resulting from (λ_G, β_G) by componentwise subtraction of head inclination (a) and eye countertorsion (ρ). (l_R, b_R): corresponding visual afference, operationally defined as a linear mapping of (λ_R, β_R). (l_S, b_S): apparent inclination of light beam and striped field, issuing from (l_R, b_R) by componentwise addition of a compensatory variable (s, s). The latter can also be understood to act like a subjective frame of reference (subscript S) into which (l_R, b_R) is mapped to yield apparent contour inclinations. According to the model, s results from *arithmetic* averaging of vestibular and optic direction cues, i.e., from a linear superposition of the vestibular tilt signal a (equivalent to s in Fig. 3) and a quantity q which itself is a product of a vestibular weight factor p and an optical induction component h. The factor p is operationally measured by the average range of oscillation ψ as plotted in Fig. 11. It derives from the *addition* of two vestibular outputs r_1 and r_2, each of which reacts sinusoidally to head tilt to one side. The *difference* of r_1 and r_2 results in a command (r) for eye countertorsion (ρ). The apparent inclinations (l_S, b_S) of the contours in the optic field are "filtered" by a mechanism F producing a quantity x which

The authors take this correlation as an indication that the optic-vestibular weight ratio as defined by them might be more than an arbitrary construction, and might refer to an actually existing physiological variable.[5]

Only in the upright position ($a = 0°$) is there a significant difference between the two curves in Fig. 11, the countertorsion being zero in this case (and changing sign for negative abscissa values), whereas the mean range of oscillation does not vanish entirely (and remains positive when the body is inclined counterclockwise). This discrepancy is accounted for by BISCHOF and SCHEERER (*loc. cit.*) as being the effect of the subtraction or addition, respectively, of two separate otolith output components, one of which signals clockwise, the other counterclockwise head inclinations (for this distinction, cf. also MILLER, 1962, 1966, 1970; TERINS, 1971).

Relying upon these assumptions and on systems-analytic elaborations previously cited, BISCHOF and SCHEERER summarize their theory about optic-vestibular interaction in human perception of verticality in the flow diagram of Fig. 12. Because obtained from the investigation of only a limited number of subjects, this model can only claim the status of a preliminary hypothesis, the confirmation or refinement of which must be left to further research.

References

ADRIAN, E.D.: Discharges from vestibular receptors in the cat. J. Physiol. (Lond.) **101**, 389 (1942).

ALEXANDER, G., BARANY, R.: Psychophysiologische Untersuchungen über die Bedeutung des Statolithenapparates für die Orientierung im Raume an Normalen und Taubstummen, nebst Beiträgen zur Orientierung mittels taktiler und optischer Empfindungen. Z. Psychol. **37**, 312–362; 414–456 (1904).

ARNDTS, F.: Zur Frage nach der Lagewahrnehmung dienenden Sinnesfunktionen. Pflügers Arch. ges. Physiol. **204**, 539–540 (1924).

ASCH, S.E., WITKIN, H.A.: Studies in space orientation. I. Perception of the upright with displaced visual fields. J. exp. Psychol. **38**, 325 (1948a).

ASCH, S.E., WITKIN, H.A.: Studies in space orientation. II. Perception of the upright with displaced visual fields and with body tilted. J. exp. Psychol. **38**, 455 (1948b).

ATTNEAVE, F.: Some informational aspects of visual perception. Psychol. Rev. **61**, 183–193 (1954).

AUBERT, H.: Eine scheinbare bedeutende Drehung von Objekten bei Neigung des Kopfes nach rechts oder links. Virchows Arch. **20**, 381–393 (1861).

BECK, K.: Untersuchungen über den statischen Apparat von Gesunden und Taubstummen. Z. Psychol. **46**, 362–378 (1912).

BENDER, M.B., JUNG, R.: Abweichungen der subjektiven optischen Vertikalen bei Gesunden und Hirnverletzten. Arch. Psychiat. Nervenkr. **181**, 193–212 (1948).

BENJAMINS, C.E., HUIZINGA, E.: Untersuchungen über die Funktion des Vestibularapparates bei der Taube. Pflügers Arch. ges. Physiol. **217**, 105 (1927).

5 Interpretable perhaps as the output of the utricles, which, due to their anatomical site, should yield afferent messages roughly proportional to the sine of head tilt (cf. VON HOLST, 1950).

equals the apparent inclination of the striped field's primary axis. The optical induction quantity h, then, is a periodic function of x. b) The model predicts that *one single* function $h(x)$ may be calculated from *any* given curve in Fig. 6 (see p. 170—171) by: 1. reassigning the ordinate values to the oblique co-ordinate system consisting of the diagonals and the abscissa in Fig. 6; 2. normalizing the transformed curve to the mean oscillation level; 3. dividing the resulting curve through its mean range of oscillation. Fig. 12b shows that this prediction is valid. Drawn are 6 curves calculated as described above from the mean-value curves for one Subject at 6 different body tilts. As is apparent, one single empirical curve $h(x)$ results. When $h(x)$ is inserted in block H in Fig. 12a, theoretical λ_G-values yielding a permanent $l_S = 0$ can be computed; they are shown in white in Fig. 6

Benson, A.J., Bodin, M.A.: Effect of orientation to the gravitational vertical on nystagmus following rotation about a horizontal axis. Acta oto-laryng. (Stockh.) **61**, 517 (1966).

Beritoff, J.S.: Spatial orientation of man and animals. 22. Int. Kongr. Physiol. Sci. Excerpta Med. Int. Congr. Ser. **47**, 3 (1962).

Beritoff, J.S.: Les mechanism nerveux de l'orientation spatiale chez l'homme. Neuropsychologia **1**, 233 (1963).

Bertini, M.: Studio sulla natura dell'effeto "frame" nella percezione della verticale. Riv. Psicologia **58**, 1–35 (1964).

Bischof, N.: Erkenntnistheoretische Grundlagenprobleme der Wahrnehmungspsychologie. In: Handbuch der Psychologie, Bd. 1/I, Bewußtsein und Wahrnehmung. W. Metzger and H. Erke, Eds. pp. 21–78. Göttingen: Verlag f. Psychologie 1966a.

Bischof, N.: Psychophysik der Raumwahrnehmung. Ibid. P. 307–408, 1966b.

Bischof, N.: Stellungs-, Spannungs- und Lagewahrnehmung. Ibid. P. 409–497, 1966c.

Bischof, N., Scheerer, E.: Systemanalyse der optisch-vestibulären Interaktion bei der Wahrnehmung der Vertikalen. Psychol. Forsch. **34**, 99–181 (1970).

Bittermann, M.E., Worchel, P.: The phenomenological vertical and horizontal in blind and sighted subjects. Amer. J. Psychol. **66**, 588 (1953).

Boring, E.G.: Visual perception as invariance. Psychol. Rev. **59**, 141. The Gibsonian visual field. Psychol. Rev. **59**, 246 (1952).

Braemer, W.: Verhaltensphysiologische Untersuchungen am optischen Apparat bei Fischen. Z. vergl. Physiol. **39**, 374–398 (1957).

Braemer, W.: A critical review of the sun-azimuth hypothesis. Cold Spr. Harb. Symp. quant. Biol. **15**, 413 (1960).

Brandt, U., Fluur, E.: Postural perceptions and compensatory displacements of the eye in respect to a presented force field. Acta oto-laryng. (Stockh.) **62**, 252–264 (1966).

Brandt, U., Fluur, E.: Postural perceptions and eye displacements during the variation of a force field acting in the midfrontal plane. Acta oto-laryng. (Stockh.) **63**, 49–64 (1967).

Brecher, G.A., Schubert, G.: Über optische Lokalisation und Augenstellung bei Vor-Rückwärtsneigung oder exzentrischer Rotation des Körpers. Z. Sinnesphysiol. **65**, 1 (1934).

Brown, L.: Orientation to the vertical during water immersion. Aerospace Med. **32**, 209–217 (1961).

Brunswik, E.: Wahrnehmung und Gegenstandswelt. Leipzig, Wien: Deuticke 1934.

Brunswik, E.: Thing constancy as measured by correlation coefficients. Psychol. Rev. **47**, 68 (1940).

Brunswik, E.: Perception and the representative design of psychological experiments. Berkeley: University of California Press 1956.

Brunswik, E., Kardos, L.: Das Duplizitätsprinzip in der Theorie der Farbenwahrnehmung. Z. Psychol. **111**, 315 (1929).

Bühler, K.: Die Erscheinungsweisen der Farben. Jena: 1922.

Carpenter, R.H.S., Blakemore, C.: Interactions between orientations in human vision. Exp. Brain Res. **18**, 287—303 (1973).

Clark, B., Graybiel, A.: Perception of the visual horizontal in normal and labyrinthine defective subjects during prolonged rotation. Amer. J. Psychol. **79**, 608–612 (1966a).

Clark, B., Graybiel, A.: Factors contributing to the delay in the perception of the oculogravic illusion. Amer. J. Psychol. **79**, 377–388 (1966b).

Colenbrander, A.: Eye and otoliths: A centrifuge study on the ocular response to otolith stimulation. Aeromed. Acta (Soesterberg) **9**, 45–91 (1963–1964).

Coltheart, M.: Visual feature-analyzers and after-effects of tilt and curvature. Psychol. Rev. **78**, 114—121 (1971).

Correia, M.J., Guedry, F.E.: Influence of labyrinth orientation relative to gravity on responses elicited by stimulation of the horizontal semicircular canals. U.S. Naval School of Aviat. Med. N.A.S.A. joint report, Pensacola, Fla., 1964.

Correia, M.J., Hixson, W.C., Niven, J.: Otolith shear and the visual perception of force direction. Discrepancies and a proposed resolution. Nami-951, Nasa Order R-93. Pensacola, Fla: Naval Aerospace Med. Inst., 1965.

Culbert, S.S.: Directional after-effects following systematic distortion of the visual field. J. Psychol. (Provincetown) **37**, 81–93 (1954).

CURRAN, C.R., LANE, H.L.: On the relation of some factors that contribute to estimates of verticality. J. exp. Psychol. **64**, 295 (1962).

DAY, R.H., WADE, N.J.: The reference for visual normalization. Amer. J. Psychol. **82**, 191–267 (1969).

DERWORT, A.: Über vestibulär induzierte Dysmorphopsien. Dtsch. Z. Nervenheilk. **170**, 295–325 (1953).

DUNCKER, K.: Über induzierte Bewegung. Psychol. Forsch. **12**, 180 (1929).

FISCHER, M.H.: Messende Untersuchungen über die Gegenrollung des Auges und die Lokalisation der scheinbaren Vertikalen bei seitlicher Neigung des Kopfes, des Stammes und des Gesamtkörpers. I. Neigungen bis zu 40°. Graefes Archiv **118**, 633–680 (1927).

FISCHER, M.H.: Messende Untersuchungen über die Gegenrollung der Augen und die Lokalisation der scheinbaren Vertikalen bei seitlicher Neigung des Gesamtkörpers bis zu 360°. II. Untersuchungen an Normalen. Graefes Archiv **123**, 476–508 (1930a).

FISCHER, M.H.: III. Untersuchungen an einem Ertaubten mit Funktionsuntüchtigkeit beider Vestibularapparate und einem einseitig Labyrinthlosen. Graefes Archiv **123**, 509–531 (1930b).

FLUUR, E., MELLSTRÖM, A.: Utricular stimulation and oculomotor reactions. Laryngoscope (St. Louis) **53**, 1701–1712 (1970a).

FLUUR, E., MELLSTRÖM, A.: Saccular stimulation and oculomotor reactions. Laryngoscope (St. Louis) **53**, 1713–1721 (1970b).

GARTEN, S.: Über die Grundlagen unserer Orientierung im Raum. Abh. Math. Phy. Klasse, Sächs. Akad. **36**, 431 (1920).

GEISSLER, H.G.: Zur Analyse adaptiver Prozesse bei der Orientierung im Raum. Z. Psychol. **171**, (1965).

GELB, A.: Die psychologische Bedeutung pathologischer Störungen der Raumwahrnehmungen. Ber. 9. Kongr. f. exp. Psychol. München. Jena 23–80, 1926.

GIBSON, J.J.: Adaptation, after-effect, and contrast in the perception of tilted lines. II. Simultaneous contrasts and the areal restriction of the after-effect. J. exp. Psychol. **20**, 553–569 (1937a).

GIBSON, J.J.: Adaptation with negative after-effects. Psychol. Rev. **44**, 222–244 (1937b).

GIBSON, J.J.: The perspective of the visual world. Boston: Houghton Mifflin Comp. 1950.

GIBSON, J.J.: The relation between visual and postural determinants of the phenomenal vertical. Psychol. Rev. **59**, 370–375 (1952).

GIBSON, J.J.: The visual perception of objective motion and subjective movement. Psychol. Rev. **61**, 304 (1954).

GIBSON, J.J.: The senses considered as perceptual systems. Boston: Houghton Mifflin Comp. 1966.

GIBSON, J.J., MOWRER, O.H.: Determinants of the perceived vertical and horizontal. Psychol. Rev. **45**, 300 (1938).

GIBSON, J.J., RADNER, M.: Adaptation, after-effect and contrast in the perception of tilted lines. J. exp. Psychol. **20**, 452–467; 553–569 (1937).

GIROTTI, G.: La percezione dello spazio in rapporto alla neuropatologia. I. Determinazione della verticale visiva e del vertice acustico. Arch. Psicol. Neurol. Psichiat. **24**, 175–336 (1963).

GIROTTI, G., BORDOGNA, A.: La determinazione della verticale e del piano mediano visivi nelle compressioni vestibulari. Riv. Psicologia **57**, 301–339 (1963).

GRAYBIEL, A., CLARK, B.: Perception of the horizontal or vertical with head upright, on the side, and inverted under static conditions, and during exposure to centripetal force. Aerospace Med. **33**, 147–155 (1962).

GRAYBIEL, A., MILLER, E.F.II, NEWSOM, B.D., KENNEDY, R.S.: The effect of water immersion on perception of the oculogravic illusion in normal and labyrinthine-defective subjects. Acta oto-laryng. (Stockh.) **65**, 599–610 (1968).

GREENBERG, G.: Visual induction of eye torsion, as measured with an after-image technique, in relation to visual perception of the vertical. Ph.D. Diss. Duke Univ., 1960.

GUEDRY, F.E.: Orientation of the rotation-axis relative to gravity: its influence on nystagmus and the sensation of rotation. Acta oto-laryng. (Stockh.) **60**, 30 (1965).

HALPERN, L.: Sensorimotor induction in disturbed equilibrium. Arch. Neurol. Psychiat. (Chic.) **62**, 330–354 (1949).

Hasegawa, T.: Labyrinthreflexe nach Abschleuderung der Otolithenmembranen. Pflügers Arch. ges. Physiol. **236**, 589 (1935).

Hofmann, F.B.: Über den Einfluß schräger Konturen auf die optische Lokalisation bei seitlicher Kopfneigung. Pflügers Arch. ges. Physiol. **136**, (1910).

Hofmann, F.B., Bielschowsky, A.: Über die Einstellung der scheinbaren Horizontalen und Vertikalen bei Betrachtung eines von schrägen Konturen erfüllten Gesichtsfeldes. Pflügers Arch. ges. Physiol. **126**, 453–475 (1909).

Holst, E. von: Quantitative Untersuchungen über Umstimmungsvorgänge im Zentralnervensystem. I. Der Einfluß des "Appetits" auf das Gleichgewichtsverhalten bei Pterophyllum. Z. vergl. Physiol. **31**, 134 (1948).

Holst, E. von: Die Arbeitsweise des Statolithenapparates bei Fischen. Z. vergl. Physiol. **32**, 60–120 (1950).

Holst, E. von, Griesebach, E.: Einfluß des Bogengangssystems auf die "subjektive Lotrechte" beim Menschen. Naturwissenschaften **38**, 67–68 (1951).

Holst, E. von, Mittelstaedt, H.: Das Reafferenzprinzip. Naturwissenschaften **37**, 464 (1950).

Howard, I.P., Templeton, W.B.: The effect of steady fixation on the judgement of relative depth. J. exp. Psychol. **16**, 193–203 (1964a).

Howard, I.P., Templeton, W.B.: Visually-induced eye torsion and tilt adaptation. Vision Res. **4**, 433–437 (1964b).

Howard, I.P., Templeton, W.B.: Human spatial orientation. New York: Wiley 1966.

Hubel, D.H., Wiesel, T.N.: Receptor fields of single neurons in the cat's striate cortex. J. Physiol. (Lond.) **148**, 574 (1959).

Huizinga, E.: The physiological and clinical importance of experimental work on the pigeon's labyrinth. J. Laryng. **69**, 260 (1955).

Jongkees, L.B.W.: On the function of the sacule. Acta oto-laryng. (Stockh.) **38**, 18–26 (1950).

Jongkees, L.B.W.: Some remarks on the function of the vestibular organ. Reports of the Institute of Laryng. Otol. **2**, 1 (1952).

Kardos, L.: Dingfarbenwahrnehmung und Duplizitätstheorie. Z. Psychol. **108**, 240 (1928).

Kardos, L.: Die "Konstanz" phänomenaler Dingmomente. In: E. Brunswik Ed. Beiträge zur Problemgeschichte der Psychologie (Bühler-Festschrift). Jena: 1929.

Kellogg, R.S.: Dynamic counterrolling of the eye in normal subjects and in persons with bilateral labyrinthine defects. NASA Sp-**77**, 195–202 (1965).

Kleint, H.: Versuche über die Wahrnehmung. Z. Psychol. **138**, 1 (1936); **140**, 109 (1937); **141**, 9 (1937); **142**, 259 (1938); **143**, 299 (1938); **148**, 145 (1940); **149**, 31 (1940).

Klix, F.: Elementaranalysen zur Psychophysik der Raumwahrnehmung. VEB Dtsch. Verlag d. Wissensch., Berlin, 1962.

Klopp, H.W.: Über die Entwicklung und den Abbau des aufrechten Bildes. Fortschr. Neurol. Psychiat. **24**, 27 (1956).

Köhler, W., Wallach, H.: Figural after-effects. Proc. Amer. Phil. Sci. **88**, 269–357 (1944).

Koffka, K.: Principles of Gestalt Psychology. Routledge and Kegan Paul: London, 1935.

Kohler, I.: Über Aufbau und Wandlungen der Wahrnehmungswelt. Sitzber. Österr. Akad. Wiss. **227**, Wien, 1951.

Kohler, I.: Umgewöhnung im Wahrnehmungsbereich. Die Pyramide **3**, 92 (1953).

Kohler, I.: Interne und externe Organisation in der Wahrnehmung. Psychol. Beitr. **6**, 426 (1961).

Linschoten, J.: Experimentelle Untersuchung der sogenannten induzierten Bewegung. Psychol. Forsch. **24**, 34–92 (1952).

Lowenstein, O.: Labyrinth and equilibrium. In: Physiol. Mechanisms in Animal Behav. Soc. exp. Biol. Symp. IV. Cambridge: Univ. Press 1950.

Lowenstein, O., Roberts, T.D.M.: The equilibrium function of the otolith organs of the Thornback Ray (Raja clavata). J. Physiol. (Lond.) **110**, 392 (1950).

Lorenz, K.: Gestaltwahrnehmung als Quelle wissenschaftlicher Erkenntnis. Z. exp. angew. Psychol. **6**, 118 (1959).

MacCorquodale, K., Meehl, P.E.: On a distinction between hypothetical constructs and intervening variables. Psychol. Rev. **55**, 95–107 (1948).

McFarland, J.H., Clarkson, F.: Perception of orientation: Adaptation to lateral body-tilt. Amer. J. Psychol. **79**, 265–271 (1966).

MacKay, D.M.: Cerebral organization and the conscious control of action. In: Brain and conscious experience. J.C. Eccles, Ed. pp. 422–445, Berlin-Heidelberg-New York: Springer 1966.

McNally, W.J.: Five lectures on the physiology of the ear. Ann. Otol. **38**, 1180 (1929).

Magnus, R.: Körperstellung. Berlin: Springer 1924.

Mann, C.W.: Visual factors in the perception of verticality. J. exp. Psychol. **44**, 460–464 (1952a).

Mann, C.W.: An analysis of the oculogyral effect. J. Aviat. Med. **23**, 246–253 (1952b).

Maxwell, S.S.: Labyrinth and Equilibrium. Philadelphia-London: 1923.

Metzger, W.: Zur anschaulichen Repräsentation von Rotationsvorgängen und ihre Deutung durch Gestaltkreislehre und Gestalttheorie. Z. Sinnesphysiol. **68**, 261 (1940).

Metzger, W.: Psychologie. Darmstadt: Steinkopff 1954[2]; 1968[3].

Meyer zum Gottesberge, A., Plester, D.: Nachweis der statischen Funktion des Sacculus beim Menschen. Arch. Ohr.-, Nas.-, u. Kehlk.-Heilk. **185**, 254–258 (1965).

Miller, E.F.II.: Counter-rolling of the human eyes produced by head tilt with respect to gravity. Acta oto-laryng. (Stockh.) **54**, 479–501 (1962).

Miller, E.F.II.: Ocular counter-rolling. In: R.J. Wolfson, Ed. The vestibular system and its diseases. Philadelphia: Univ. of Pennsylvania Press, 229–241, 1966.

Miller, E.F.II.: Evaluation of otolith organ function by means of ocular counter-rolling measurements. In: J. Stahle, Ed. Vestibular function on earth and in space. Oxford: Pergamon Press, 97–111, 1970.

Miller, E.F.II., Graybiel, A.: A comparison of ocular counter-rolling movements between normal persons and deaf subjects with bilateral labyrinthine defects. Ann. oto-rhino-laryng. **72**, 885 (1963).

Miller, E.F.II., Graybiel, A.: Role of the otolith organs in the perception of horizontality. Amer. J. Psychol. **79**, 24–37 (1966).

Mittelstaedt, H.: The analysis of behavior in terms of control systems. In: B. Schaffner, Ed. Group Processes. Transactions of the 5. Conf. of the J. Macy Found. New York 45, 1960.

Mittelstaedt, H.: Basic solutions to a problem of angular orientation. In: R.F. Reiss, Ed. Neural Theory and Modeling, 259–272. Stanford Univ. Press 1964.

Mittelstaedt, H.: Grundprobleme der Analyse von Orientierungsleistungen. Jahrb. d. Max-Planck-Ges. p. 121, 1966.

Morant, R.B., Aronoff, J.C.: Starting position, adaptation, and visual framework as influencing the perception of verticality. J. exp. Psychol. **71**, 684–686 (1966).

Morant, R.B., Beller, H.K.: Adaptation to prismatically rotated visual fields. Science **148**, 530 (1965).

Morant, R.B., Harris, J.: Two different aftereffects of disposure to visual tilts. Amer. J. Psychol. **78**, 218–226 (1965).

Morant, R.B., Mistovich, M.: Tilt after-effects between the vertical and horizontal axes. Percept. Mot. Skills **10**, 75–81 (1960).

Müller, G.E.: Übeт das Aubertsche Phänomen. Z. Sinnesphysiol. **49**, 109–246 (1916).

Naylor, G.F.: Effects of stress on the perception of direction. Australian J. Psychol. **15**, 17–28 (1963).

Naylor, G.F.K.: Subjective judgements of the vertical: An estimate of their nature and consistency. Australian J. Psychol. **17**, 188–192 (1965).

Ohwaki, S.: An investigation of figural adaptation: a study within the framework of sensory-tonic field theory. Amer. J. Psychol. **74**, 3–16 (1961).

Oppenheimer, E.: Optische Versuche über Ruhe und Bewegung. Psychol. Forsch. **20**, 1–46 (1935).

Passey, G.E.: The perception of the vertical. IV. Adjustment to the vertical with normal and tilted visual frames of references. J. exp. Psychol. **40**, 738–745 (1950).

Perlman, H.B.: The saccule, observations from a differentiated reinforced area of the saccular wall in man. Acta oto-laryngol. (Stockh.) **32**, 678 (1940).

Quix, F.H., Eijsvogel, M.H.: Experimente über die Funktion des Otolithenapparates beim Menschen. Z. Hals-, Nas.- u. Ohrenheilk. **23**, 68–96 (1929).

Schöne, H.: Über den Einfluß der Schwerkraft auf die Augenrollung und auf die Wahrnehmung der Lage im Raum. Z. vergl. Physiol. **46**, 57–87 (1962).

Schöne, H.: On the Role of gravity in human spatial orientation. Aerospace Med. **35**, 764 (1964).

Schöne, H., Parker, D.E.: Inversion of the effect of increased gravity on the subjective vertical. Naturwissenschaften **54**, 288–289 (1967).

Schöne, H., Parker, D.E., Mortag, H.G.: Subjective vertical as a function of body position and gravity magnitude. Naturwissenschaften **54**, 288 (1967).

Schöne, H., Udo de Haes, H.: Perception of gravity-vertical as a function of head and trunk position. Z. vergl. Physiol. **60**, 440–444 (1968).

Schöne, H., Udo de Haes, H.: Space orientation in humans with special reference to the interaction of vestibular, somaesthetic and visual inputs. Biokybernetik **3**, 172–191 (1971).

Schneider, C.W., Bartley, S.H.: A study of the effects of mechanically induced tension of the neck muscles on the perception of verticality. J. Psychol. (Provincetown) **54**, 245–248 (1962).

Stigler, R.: Versuche über die Beteiligung der Schwereempfindung an der Orientierung des Menschen im Raume. Pflügers Arch. ges. Physiol. **148**, 573–584 (1912).

Sutherland, N.S.: Figural after-effects and apparent size. Quart. J. exp. Psychol. **13**, 222–228 (1961).

Szentágothai, J.: Die Rolle der einzelnen Labyrinthreceptoren bei der Orientation von Augen und Kopf im Raume. Budapest: Akadémiai Kiado 1952.

Tait, J.: Is all hearing cochlear. Ann. Otol. (St. Louis) **41**, 681 (1932).

Terins, J.: Counter-rolling of the eyes in some unilateral vestibular disorders. In: J. Stahle, Ed. Vestibular function on earth and in space. Oxford: Pergamon Press, 109–113, 1971.

Udo de Haes, H.: Stability of apparent vertical and ocular coutertorsion as a function of lateral tilt. Perception & Psychophysics **8**, 137–142 (1970).

Udo de Haes, H., Schöne, H.: Interaction between statolith organs and semicircular canals on apparent vertical and nystagmus. Acta oto-laryng. (Stockh.) **69**, 25–31 (1970).

Vernon, M.D.: The perception of inclined lines. Brit. J. Psychol. **25**, 186 (1935).

Versteegh, L.: Ergebnisse partieller Labyrinthexstirpation bei Kaninchen. Acta oto-laryng. (Stockh.) **11**, 393 (1927).

Walsh, E.G.: Perception of linear motion following unilateral labyrinth ectomy: variation of threshold according to the orientation of the head. J. Physiol. (Lond.) **153**, 350 (1960).

Walsh, E.G.: Role of the vestibular apparatus in the perception of motion on a parallel swing. J. Physiol. (Lond.) **155**, 506 (1961).

Werner, H., Wapner, S., Chandler, K.A.: Experiments on sensory-tonic field theory of perception. II. Effect of supported and unsupported tilt of the body on the visual perception of verticality. J. exp. Psychol. **42**, 346 (1951).

Wertheimer, M.: Experimentelle Studien über das Sehen von Bewegung. Z. Psychol. **61**, 161–265 (1912).

Witkin, H.A.: The nature and importance of individual differences in perception. J. Personality **18**, 145 (1949a).

Witkin, H.A.: Sex differences in perception. Trans. N.Y. Acad. Soc. **12**, 22 (1949b).

Witkin, H.A., Asch, S.E.: Studies in space orientation. III. Perception of the upright in the absence of a visual field. J. exp. Psychol. **38**, 603 (1948a).

Witkin, H.A., Asch, S.E.: Studies in space orientation. IV. Further experiments on perception of the upright with displaced visual fields. J. exp. Psychol. **38**, 762 (1948b).

Witkin, H.A., Lewis, H.B., Hertzman, M., Machover, K., Meissner, P.B., Wapner, S.: Personality through perception. New York: Haper 1954.

Woellner, R.C., Graybiel, A.: Counterrolling of the eyes and its dependence on the magnitude of gravitational or inertial force acting laterally on the body. J. appl. Physiol. **14**, 632–634 (1959).

Wood, R.W.: The "haunted-swing" illusion. Psychol. Rev. **2**, 277–278 (1895).

Young, H.H.: Personality test correlates of orientation to the vertical: A test of Witkin's Field dependency hypothesis. J. abnorm. soc. Psychol. **59**, 188–192 (1959).

Young, H.H., Meiri, J.L.: A revised dynamic otolith model. Aerospace Med. **39**, 606–608 (1968).

F. Applied Aspects

Chapter I.

Nystagmus and Related Phenomena in Man: An Outline of Otoneurology*

By

H. H. KORNHUBER, Ulm

With 16 Figures

Contents

* In memory of HERMANN FRENZEL.

I. Introduction: The Function of the Vestibular System and the Nature of Vestibular Symptoms

Besides its contribution to conscious orientation in space, the vestibular system is essentially an apparatus for automatic holding or stabilization of the position of the body and eyes. Correspondingly — and contrary to some other parts of the motor system — vestibularly induced movements are automatic, involuntary, forced movements, independent of voluntary action, dependent only on wakefulness. They include movements like the vestibular nystagmus of the eyes or the tilting reflexes of the limbs.

II. Clinical History of Vertigo and Related Symptoms

A good clinical history and knowledge of typical symptoms and syndromes is usually more important for diagnosis than nystagmography. The term vertigo is often used to describe extravestibular symptoms such as blurring of vision, faintness, unsteadiness of gait, dizziness, etc. Typical vestibular vertigo is a "systemic" sensation with a feeling of being turned or tilted; it is often associated with apparent motion of the environment. In some languages, e.g. German, fear of heights (an instinct whose function is to prevent falling) is also termed vertigo ("Höhenschwindel").

There are *three main types of vestibular vertigo*: continuous (long-lasting) vertigo, attacks of vertigo, and positional vertigo.

A. Continuous (Long-Lasting) Vertigo

may be due to peripheral labyrinthine or central lesions, especially those of the vestibular nuclei. It is the type of vertigo seen after traumatic lesions of the statoacoustic nerve. In the initial state continuous vertigo is often connected with vegetative symptoms (vomiting) and with inability to stand or walk. Later, when the intensity of the vertigo has declined, it may vary depending on head motions, head position and state of alertness. Continuous vertigo of peripheral origin may occur with or without hearing loss. If it occurs without hearing loss (vestibular "neuronitis", or better, neuritis, because a neuron cannot be affected by inflammation), it may be due either to a vascular lesion of the inner ear or to viral neuritis of the vestibular nerve (Kornhuber and Waldecker, 1958).

B. Attacks of Vertigo

that are independent of movement or different positions of the head and may occur at any time of the day, can be due to Menière's disease, cerebro-vascular (vertebro-basilar) insufficiency, or convulsive disorders.

1. Menière's Disease

In Menière's disease vertigo is sooner or later associated with tinnitus and hearing impairment, but the first attacks may occur without any cochlear symptoms. The violent Menière's vertigo usually lasts only 15 min or so, but in rare cases it may last 1 min or several hours; however, less severe vertigo is often experienced for the rest of the day. At the beginning of the attack, the spontaneous nystagmus is usually directed towards the side of the affected ear; at the point of reversal there may be a direction-changing positional nystagmus; at the end of the attack the spontaneous nystagmus usually reverses towards the contralateral side (Günther, 1961). This rule is, however, not reliable enough to diagnose the affected side. Usually there is no impairment of consciousness during the attack but in rare cases the concomitant vegetative symptoms may induce vascular collapse and unconsciousness.

2. Vertebro-Basilar Insufficiency

In vertebro-basilar insufficiency vertigo is the most common symptom, but it is often accompanied by drop-attacks, occipital headache, double vision, blurred vision, or other symptoms caused by insufficiency of the vertebral, basilar and posterior cerebral arteries and their branches; tinnitus and hearing loss are uncommon. All of these symptoms occur most often with backward tilting and or turning of the head (due to compression of the vertebral artery), but may also occur spontaneously as in Menière's disease. Therefore, in all cases of attacks of vertigo the blood pressure should be measured on both brachial arteries (because of the possibility of a subclavian steal syndrome), and careful auscultation for bruit over the carotid artery should be performed, since in many cases of vertebro-basilar insufficiency the vertigo starts only after additional carotid obstruction. A systolic difference between right and left brachial blood pressure of more than 30 mm of mercury is pathologic.

3. Epileptic Vertigo

Although the cortical projection of the vestibular nerve is not situated in the temporal lobe, patients with temporal-lobe epilepsy sometimes report vertigo (though not true vestibular whirling or tilting sensations) as one of the symptoms of their attacks, in addition to sudden anxiety, abdominal or thoracic sensations of pressure, and clouding of consciousness. More rarely, the petit mal attacks of pyknolepsia are experienced by the patient as a kind of vertigo. Epileptic vertigo is always of very short duration. Two items are essential for diagnosis: an objective history taken from family members, friends or fellow workers, and an EEG. If the normal EEG does not show any paroxysmal symptoms, an EEG recording, made as the patient falls asleep after one night of sleep deprivation, shows epileptic discharge much more often than does the usual EEG (Bechinger et al., 1973).

C. Positional Vertigo

should be distinguished from head-turning vertigo, which is due to compression of the vertebral artery. There are two types of positional vertigo (1) long-lasting positional vertigo, accompanied by positional nystagmus of the central, long-lasting type (due to central lesions or intoxications); (2) positioning vertigo, which is also called paroxysmal positional vertigo. It is accompanied by positional nystagmus of the peripheral, benign type (also called positioning nystagmus).

D. Vertigo: General Criteria

The general criteria for the analysis of vertigo are: circumstances of occurrence, duration, concomitant symptoms, changes in consciousness, and nystagmus. Regarding circumstances of occurrence, attacks of Menière's disease and epileptic vertigo occur without any obvious trigger, while positional vertigo and head-turning vertigo in vertebro-basilar insufficiency have characteristic triggers. The duration of vertigo is very brief in epilepsy, several seconds in the benign paroxysmal positioning vertigo of peripheral origin, about 15 min in Menière's disease, and much longer in massive lesions of the labyrinths, vestibular nerve or brain stem. Concomitant symptoms characteristic of vertebro-basilar insufficiency are drop attacks, double vision, and blurred vision. The chief symptom in epileptic vertigo is unconsciousness, and in vertigo of labyrinthine origin it is tinnitus and hearing loss. The combination of vertigo and nystagmus is rather constant (and proportional in intensity) in the case of peripheral lesions, while in central lesions vertigo does not always parallel nystagmus. In cases of gaze nystagmus and fixation nystagmus, there is usually no vertigo. Intensive nystagmus without vertigo is always of central origin. On the other hand, in cases of slow loss of labyrinthine function without vertigo an acoustic neuroma should be suspected.

E. Vertigo, Apparent Motion of the Environment, and Visual Space Constancy

Bilateral loss of labyrinthine function (which may occur almost without vertigo, e.g. in the case of streptomycin intoxication) induces apparent motion of visual objects during fast head movements, at least in the acute stage. A typical complaint of the patient is that he must stand still in order to read a clock on the wall. This is because the optokinetic regulation of eye position is slower than the vestibular regulation. The reader can demonstrate this to himself by a simple test: if he moves his finger back and forth at a frequency of 4 Hz through an angle of about 20 degrees, the finger is blurred; but if he turns his head at the same frequency and angle but holds the finger still, he sees it clearly because vestibular regulation is faster.

In cases of spontaneous or experimental vestibular nystagmus there is apparent motion of the visual objects in the opposite direction to the slow phase of nystagmus, but not to the rapid phases. This is not simply because of faster eye movement in the rapid phases since in the slow nystagmus phases it may be as fast as 100° per sec. Small rapid phases or saccades, on the other hand, with an average eye velocity of 4° per sec do not result in apparent motion. The reason is that during active eye movements and the fast phases of vestibular and optokinetic nystagmus there is central inhibition of visual motion perception, while during involuntary eye movements, including slow phases of vestibular and optokinetic nystagmus, the visual system interprets the environment as though the eyes were not moving. Although I admire the opposing arguments put forward by DONALD MACKAY in this Handbook (Vol. VII/3A p. 322), it seems to me that this phenomenon is not suppression of visual brightness perception or mislocation, but inhibition of visual motion perception; the visual system has separate channels for location and motion (KORNHUBER, 1971).

F. Clinical History: General Rules

The physician must himself see and hear the patient. Information transmitted through other media (personal or impersonal) loses something in the process. First, the patient must express his memories and feelings, but often this is not enough. Usually the physician must help the patient to remember by offering typical alternative possibilities. From the first case history a diagnostic hypothesis is developed and is later tested by the general examination and special tests. It will often be necessary to add to the history or to re-evaluate specific points. Therefore, all available information should be considered before the patient leaves the office or clinic.

III. Spontaneous Nystagmus and Other Involuntary Eye Movements

As pointed out in the introduction, it is essential for the vestibular system to evoke involuntary reflex counter-movements in order to stabilize eye position during head movements. Because of the spontaneous discharge of the vestibular receptors, this regulation occurs very easily during the waking state, almost without threshold. In consequence of this arrangement, however, lesions of the vestibular system result in spontaneous, forced eye movements of constant direction — the slow phase of a spontaneous nystagmus. The rapid phases that bring the eyes back are of central, extravestibular origin.

A. Three Kinds of Pathologic Nystagmus

It is not enough to state that a patient has spontaneous nystagmus and to record the degree of its intensity: first degree — nystagmus only when gazing in the direction of the rapid phases; second degree — nystagmus also when gazing straight ahead; and third degree — nystagmus even when gazing in the direction of the slow phases. Vestibular regulation is not the only regulation of eye position, and there are other kinds of nystagmus which should be distinguished from vestibular nystagmus.

Spontaneous nystagmus in the narrower sense, gaze nystagmus and fixation nystagmus (Frenzel, 1955; Kornhuber, 1966). There are three different types of pathologic nystagmus, caused by lesions of three different regulatory mechanisms of eye position:

1. Spontaneous Nystagmus in the Narrower Sense

is a forced movement that depends on wakefulness alone, not on eccentric positions of eye fixation. Therefore, it can be seen or recorded with the eyes closed or open, gazing straight ahead in darkness, or with Frenzel's glasses. Spontaneous

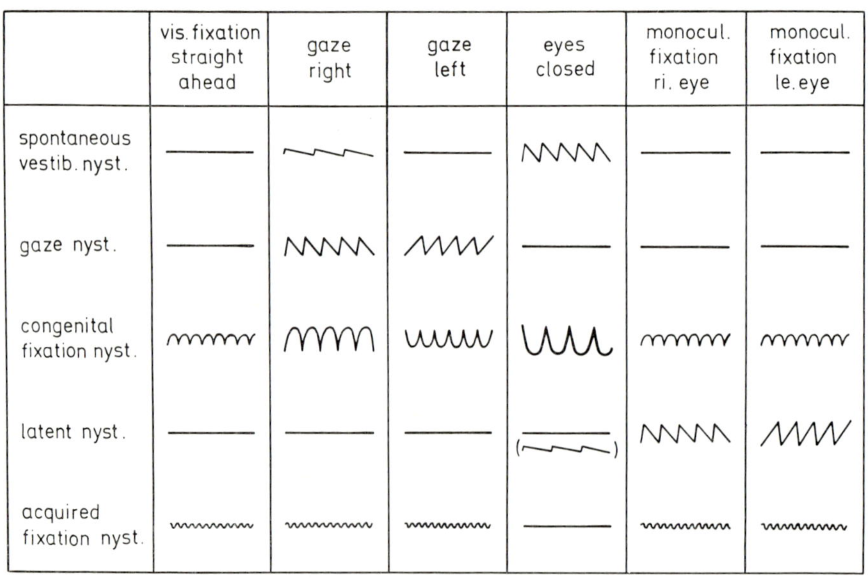

Fig. 1. Differences in behavior of spontaneous nystagmus in the narrower sense (vestibular nystagmus of peripheral or central origin), gaze nystagmus (gaze deviation nystagmus), congenital fixation nystagmus (arc type), latent nystagmus upon monocular fixation, and acquired pendular nystagmus in multiple sclerosis under different conditions of investigation

nystagmus in the narrower sense may be identical with spontaneous vestibular nystagmus; in any case, spontaneous vestibular nystagmus of peripheral or central origin is always a spontaneous nystagmus in this narrower sense.

2. Gaze Nystagmus

(also called gaze deviation nystagmus) depends on voluntary eccentric eye positions and is not caused by lesions of the vestibular system, but by lesions of the neural apparatus that holds the eyes in eccentric positions. A spontaneous visual regulation exists for this purpose. In darkness, a normal man is not able to sustain an eccentric gaze position; instead, the eyes drift slowly to the midposition and jump back toward the eccentric point; thus, in darkness, a normal man can show gaze nystagmus. The velocity of the drift toward the midposition is a function of the eccentricity (Becker and Klein, 1973). The regulation mechanism for holding eccentric gaze positions is probably identical with the mechanism for optokinetic regulation of smooth pursuit eye movements at slow speeds, because there is usually a combination of gaze nystagmus and disturbance of smooth pursuit eye movements. The neural mechanism of this holding regulation includes the cerebellar nuclei since lesions of the nuclei result in gaze nystagmus.

Both spontaneous nystagmus in the narrower sense and gaze nystagmus have a jerky form, but it is important not to confuse them because their diagnostic significance is quite different. Spontaneous vestibular nystagmus may be of either central or peripheral origin, while gaze nystagmus is always of central origin (lesion or intoxication). The distinction can easily be made with the use of Frenzel's glasses or by nystagmography (with the eyes closed or with the eyes open in darkness): these circumstances provoke only spontaneous nystagmus in the narrower sense and not gaze nystagmus.

3. Fixation Nystagmus

depends on visual fixation; it disappears or changes its direction or form after eye closure. It is a holding tremor similar to the intention tremor of the arm following lesions of the dentate nucleus. There are cases of fixation nystagmus in which the nystagmus is quite independent of the direction of gaze. Fixation nystagmus may be congenital or acquired. It has been shown that acquired fixation nystagmus is due to lesions of the cerebellar nuclei or their fiber connections with the brainstem (Aschoff et al., 1974). The fact that gaze nystagmus and fixation nystagmus occur independently points toward different visual regulatory mechanisms for fixation and for lateral gaze and smooth pursuit eye movements, respectively.

B. Physiological Spontaneous Nystagmus

By the term physiological spontaneous nystagmus I do not mean very small drifts of changing direction and the corresponding microsaccades of the eyes when fixating a point straight ahead. Both are important for normal vision in order to overcome the local adaptation of the retina, but both of them can only be recorded with high precision methods, not by the normal electrooculogram (Ratliff and Riggs, 1950). Nor do I mean the slow, pendular deviations with closed eyes that are especially liable to occur when the subject is drowsy. By the term physiological spontaneous nystagmus I mean a nystagmus with slow and rapid phases of constant direction and with amplitudes which can easily be seen in the electrooculogram or with Frenzel's glasses. FRENZEL (1955) correctly emphasized that the search for spontaneous nystagmus is the most important part of an otoneurological investigation; using his glasses (Leuchtbrille), he found that there is no such nystagmus in normal subjects. Once electronystagmography was widely used, it became obvious that Frenzel's glasses somewhat reduce the intensity of spontaneous nystagmus. It was therefore supposed that nystagmography with the eyes closed was a better method than the use of Frenzel's glasses (ASCHAN et al., 1956). Although this matter was never thoroughly investigated, it was tacitly assumed that Frezel's statement (no spontaneous nystagmus in normal subjects with his glasses) could be extended to nystagmography with the eyes closed. However, various investigators have found spontaneous nystagmus in normal subjects when recording with the eyes closed, in 30 to 40% of cases in a vertical direction, and in 13 to 22% in a horizontal direction (FLUUR and ERIKSSON, 1961; VISSER, 1963; MILOJEVIC, 1967; KAMEI and KORNHUBER, 1974).

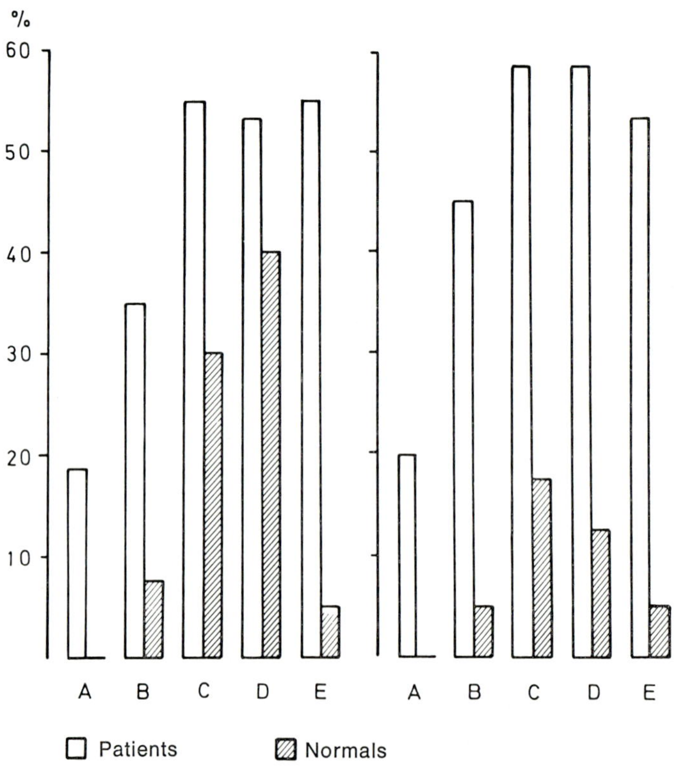

Fig. 2. Occurrence of spontaneous nystagmus in the narrower sense in 60 patients with central lesions and 40 normal persons. A: Eyes open, fixation of a point straight ahead. B: Eyes open, gaze straight ahead with Frenzel's glasses in a dark room. C: Eyes open, gaze straight ahead in darkness. D: Eyes closed. E: Head-shaking test with eyes open with Frenzel's glasses in darkness (From KAMEI and KORNHUBER, Canad. J. Otolaryng. 1974)

In addition, positional nystagmus with the eyes closed has been found in 92 out of 112 normal persons (Barber and Wright, 1973). Obviously, the vestibular system cannot completely stabilize eye position when vision is excluded. This is not surprising from a system engineering point of view, since double integration is necessary between the cupula and the eye muscles; technically, it is very difficult to stabilize a system with double integration without some constant drift.

1. What is the Best Way to Distinguish Physiologic from Pathologic Spontaneous Nystagmus?

Nystagmus intensity has been used to distinguish physiologic from pathologic horizontal spontaneous nystagmus with the eyes closed (Visser, 1963). The normal limit of slow phase velocity was said to be 5° per sec. This intensity method, however, yields poor results for two reasons: first, like experimental vestibular nystagmus, spontaneous vestibular nystagmus varies in intensity depending on wakefulness, psychic excitement, or drowsiness. Spontaneous nystagmus is reduced when the patient is tired and it disappears during sleep. Any delimitation of the normal range on the basis of nystagmus intensity must therefore depend on the time of day, meals, drugs taken, the social situation, etc. Visser cited 5° per sec as the normal limit, but the investigations of Kamei and Kornhuber would set the normal limit at 2° per sec. Moreover, intensity criteria cause many false-negative classifications. Thus, only about 10% of the patients of Kamei and Kornhuber would have been classified as pathologic when using an intensity criterion. Investigation of spontaneous nystagmus with the eyes open in darkness (without Frenzel's glasses) offers no advantage for it yields the same results as closed eyes.

Fixation is not a good method either, since it completely inhibits pathologic spontaneous nystagmus in most patients. The best method known at present for distinguishing between physiologic and pathologic spontaneous nystagmus is the use of Frenzel's glasses in a totally dark room, combined with the head-shaking test and the positional test. Frenzel's glasses greatly inhibit physiologic spontaneous nystagmus but only slightly inhibit pathologic spontaneous nystagmus (Kamei and Kornhuber, 1974).

2. Partial Visual Inhibition of Vestibular Eye Movements as the Basis of Action of Frenzel's Glasses

For the distinction between physiologic and pathologic spontaneous nystagmus by means of Frenzel's glasses partial visual inhibition of the vestibular eye movements obviously plays a major role. Frenzel's glasses work, not by totally excluding vision, but rather by excluding the stimuli in the central visual field while stimuli in the peripheral field can still be seen, but grossly out of focus. It seems that pathologic spontaneous vestibular nystagmus is less inhibited by vision. In 20% of the patients of Kamei and Kornhuber with central lesions spontaneous nystagmus occurred despite visual fixation (without Frenzel's glasses, eyes open, gaze straight ahead); in other words, the spontaneous nystagmus was not inhibited even by visual stimuli in the central field.

3. Does Spontaneous Nystagmus in the Narrower Sense Occur with Frenzel's Glasses in Normal Subjects?

In healthy persons spontaneous nystagmus with Frenzel's glasses has been found in 1% (KNAPP, 1950) and in 0.4% of cases, respectively (YOUNGERMANN, 1933). In apparently healthy persons an occurrence is to be expected of at least this order of magnitude of brainstem damage due to birth trauma, undiagnosed fixation nystagmus of jerky type, and long-lasting spontaneous nystagmus following inner ear disease. Furthermore, after-effects of alcohol and other drugs can rarely be excluded with certainty. Therefore, we fully support Frenzel's teaching that any spontaneous nystagmus in persons wearing his glasses (including nystagmus in the positional and head-shaking tests) must be regarded as a pathologic phenomenon that calls for further investigation.

4. Further Advantages of Frenzel's Glasses

In central lesions spontaneous and caloric nystagmus may disappear when the eyes are closed, while it is present with Frenzel's glasses; probably this is due to deficient facilitation of the rapid phases with the eyes closed, caused by certain brainstem lesions. Rotatory eye movements that cannot be recorded by the electrooculogram are seen with Frenzel's glasses. Caloric nystagmus is more regular and therefore easier to evaluate with Frenzel's glasses than with the eyes closed. Finally, the investigation with Frenzel's glasses is simple and quick. Since it is done by the physician himself, it contributes more to otoneurologic experience than does nystagmography. This is not said to denigrate nystagmography in general. Nystagmography allows documentation of the nystagmus and makes evaluation of induced nystagmus easier. It also has further advantages, e.g. in some cases of congenital nystagmus diagnosis can only be made by comparison of the nystagmus with the eyes open and the eyes closed. It should, however, be used in addition to Frenzel's glasses and not instead of them.

C. Significance of the Direction of Spontaneous Nystagmus in the Narrower Sense

Because of the functional density of the peripheral labyrinthine structures including the vestibular nerve, which represent all three planes of space, peripheral lesions cause spontaneous nystagmus of mixed direction. This peripheral spontaneous nystagmus is predominantly horizontal with some rotatory and/or vertical components, especially if the nystagmus has existed for a long time. Only positioning nystagmus of peripheral origin, which is probably due to a mechanical disturbance of a semicircular canal, is of purely rotatory or vertical or horizontal direction, but it lasts only up to 30 sec. Unlike the mixed but predominantly horizontal direction of long-lasting spontaneous nystagmus of peripheral origin, the long-lasting central nystagmus caused by lesions of the brainstem is often of a purely horizontal, vertical, or rotatory direction. Rotating nystagmus, that is to say, a nystagmus of the jerking type with the eyes rotating around their optical axes, is pathognomonic for lesions of the medulla oblongata (region of the vestibular nuclei). It occurs most often in syringobulbia or in Wallenberg's syndrome (ischemic infarction of the dorsolateral medulla caused by blocking of the posterior inferior cerebellar artery, usually due to thrombosis of the vertebral artery). Rotating nystagmus of the pendular type, which is often connected with a seesaw movement of both eyes is, however, most often due to diencephalic tumor. It is probably a release phenomenon of the mesencephalic premotor apparatus for eye rotation. Purely horizontal nystagmus occurs as a consequence of lesions in the vestibular nuclei or pontine tegmentum, while purely vertical nystagmus of the jerking type (spontaneous in the narrower sense) may be due to lesions between the vestibular nuclei and the mesencephalon. Whereas destruction of the vestibular nerve causes spontaneous nystagmus to the contralateral side, lesions of the vestibular nuclei may produce spontaneous nystagmus and postural changes to either the ipsi- or contralateral side (UEMURA and COHEN, 1972). The same has been observed in Wallenberg's syndrome. The direction of the slow phases of spontaneous nystagmus is the same as the direction of the change in body posture.

D. Recovery Nystagmus

In case of permanent destruction of one labyrinth or vestibular nerve, the direction of the nystagmus (which is by convention the direction of the quick phase) is contralateral to the affected ear. However, after transitory damage to one labyrinth or vestibular nerve (for instance, in head trauma or viral neuritis) there is often some recovery of peripheral function. If function recovers after several days or weeks, when partical central compensation of the peripheral defect has occurred, the spontaneous nystagmus reverses direction from contralateral

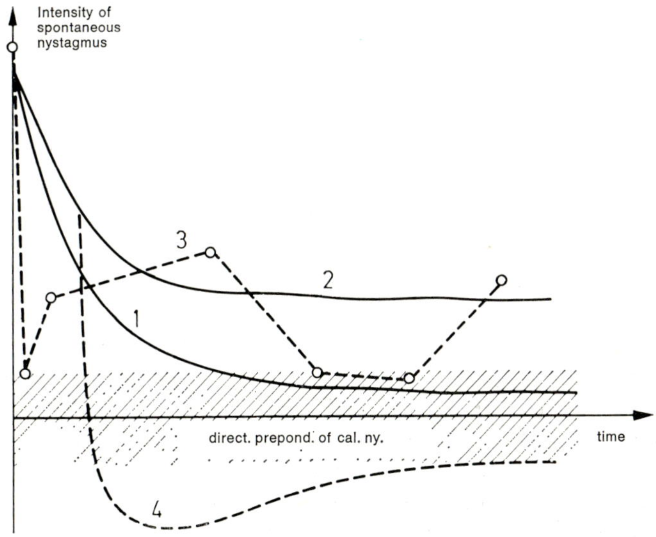

Fig. 3. Different types of time course of spontaneous nystagmus following traumatic lesions of the labyrinths. Type 1: Complete disappearance of spontaneous nystagmus. Type 2: Persisting spontaneous nystagmus. Type 3: Possible nystagmus findings in a type-2 course; the intensity of the spontaneous nystagmus changes with drowsiness and alertness. Type 4: Recovery nystagmus (From KORNHUBER, Arch. Ohrenheilk. **194**, 1969)

to ipsilateral, i.e. to the side of the affected ear (STENGER, 1959). In cases of recovery nystagmus, the affected labyrinth gives nearly normal caloric responses. For this and other reasons, the presence of normal caloric nystagmus should never lead to the conclusion that spontaneous nystagmus must be of central origin when the spontaneous nystagmus is of a type which could also be of peripheral origin. Therefore, when evaluating spontaneous nystagmus and caloric responses, the case history should always be considered.

E. The Course of Spontaneous Nystagmus Following Head Trauma

Head trauma often causes spontaneous or positional nystagmus, irrespective of whether there was cerebral contusion or only concussion. Most of these vestibular symptoms are due to peripheral lesions (LANGE and KORNHUBER, 1962). Several days or weeks after a partial peripheral lesion a recovery nystagmus may appear, beating towards the side of the labyrinthine lesion. On the other hand, spontaneous nystagmus after unilateral loss of peripheral function may last for decades. Depending on alertness and fatigue, the intensity of spontaneous nystagmus changes, so that sometimes one finds only a directional preponderance of caloric nystagmus and later, in the same case, spontaneous nystagmus.

F. Head-Shaking Nystagmus

Head-shaking nystagmus is a latent spontaneous vestibular nystagmus. It is provoked in a seated patient by rapid passive head shaking around a vertical axis. With Frenzel's glasses in a dark room there is no spontaneous nystagmus after head shaking in normal man. In patients with peripheral and central vestibular lesions, however, passive head shaking is a powerful means to activate spontaneous nystagmus. In the series of KAMEI and KORNHUBER (1974) 25% of the patients with central lesions showed head-shaking nystagmus with Frenzel's glasses as the only spontaneous nystagmus. After peripheral vestibular lesions, head-shaking nystagmus often persists over many years, even if all other spontaneous nystagmus has disappeared. Head-shaking nystagmus usually has the same direction as spontaneous nystagmus provoked by other means. The only exception is recovery nystagmus: in patients with recovery nystagmus to the side of the lesion, the head-shaking nystagmus may still be directed to the contralateral side. The head-shaking test is a very useful and simple test which should be performed routinely in every otoneurologic investigation.

G. Positional Nystagmus

Positional nystagmus (NYLÉN, 1931; FRENZEL, 1961) is a nystagmus of the spontaneous vestibular type, provoked by certain head positions other than vertical, especially the right and left lateral positions, the supine position and the head hanging position. The latter is usually investigated in the following way: head hyperextended backward with the body in the supine position. If there is nystagmus in any of these positions, one must be sure that it is really due to head position and not to neck torsion, for neck-torsion nystagmus has a different origin: it is due to ischemia of the brainstem caused by compression of the vertebral artery when there is insufficient collateral circulation (SANDSTRÖM, 1961), usually because of arteriosclerotic lesions in other arteries such as both carotids or the circle of Willis. Furthermore, positional nystagmus should not be confused with spontaneous nystagmus activated by other means, such as head shaking, psychic excitement, or mental arithmetic. Very often the intensity of spontaneous nystagmus is influenced by different head positions; this also should not be regarded as positional nystagmus. Keeping this in mind, it will be apparent that there are only two clear types of positional nystagmus: first, positional nystagmus in the narrower sense or positional nystagmus of the central type, and second, positioning nystagmus or positional nystagmus of peripheral origin, also called benign paroxysmal positional nystagmus.

1. Positional Nystagmus of the Central Type

may be due to lesions in the posterior fossa, especially lesions of the cerebellar nodulus (FERNÁNDEZ, 1960; GRANT et al., 1964) or the vestibular nuclei (UEMURA and COHEN, 1972), or to intoxication by alcohol, barbiturates, diphenylhydantoin, etc. When caused by intoxication it usually shows a regular pattern in the lateral body positions, either divergent, i.e. geotropic with both eyes beating towards the lower ear, or convergent, i.e. antigeotropic with the eyes beating towards the upper ear. On the other hand, positional nystagmus due to tumor often shows some asymmetry or combination with spontaneous nystagmus in the upright sitting position. There are, however, exceptions to this rule; during intoxication, in addition to a regular direction-changing pattern in the lateral body positions, there might also be a vertical or rotatory spontaneous nystagmus in the upright sitting position.

2. Positioning Nystagmus of Peripheral Origin

This nystagmus is not due to particular positions per se but to rapid changes in position (positioning), i.e. when changing from a sitting to a supine position with the head hanging over the edge of the examination table simultaneously with head rotation to right or left. The criteria for differentiating between central positional and peripheral positioning nystagmus are given in Table 1.

Table 1 (after KORNHUBER, 1969)

	Positioning nystagmus of peripheral origin	Positional nystagmus of central origin
Repetition of the positional test	nystagmus inconstant	nystagmus constant
Duration	usually less than 30 sec	more than 30 sec
Direction	often rotating towards the lower ear	often vertical or horizontal to upper ear
Vertigo	strong	sometimes lacking

Vertigo is always strongly present in the peripheral positioning nystagmus while it may be present or absent in central positional nystagmus. In cases of peripheral positioning nystagmus the direction of nystagmus is often rotatory towards the lower ear, while in the central positional nystagmus it is more often horizontal towards the upper ear, or vertical. However, there are many exceptions to this rule, and duration is also not a very reliable criterion. The duration of positioning nystagmus is usually less than 30 sec, while positional nystagmus lasts longer. However, positional nystagmus of central origin can adapt and disappear earlier or later, depending on the wakefulness of the patient. The most important criterion is the constancy of occurrence of the nystagmus with repetition of the positioning tests: while positional nystagmus of central origin always occurs with repetition of the test, positioning nystagmus of peripheral origin does not usually occur with every repetition. Therefore, after taking the history, the first test in cases of positional vertigo should always be the search for positioning nystagmus with Frenzel's glasses in a dark room, after the patient has been instructed not to close his eyes if vertigo occurs.

Inconstancy of occurrence also sheds light on the pathogenesis of positioning nystagmus of peripheral origin because it is compatible with the assumption of a mechanical disturbance in a semicircular canal (blood clot or conglomerate of desquamated cells in the endolymph or perilymph). Positioning nystagmus can be caused by traumatic lesions of a labyrinth. Experimentally, it has been shown that a small amount of blood in the perilymph can cause this type of nystagmus (MIEHLKE, 1955). Contrary to the statement of DIX and HALLPIKE (1952), it cannot be caused by lesions of the otoliths since stimulation and lesions of the otolith apparatus produce little or no nystagmus, and certainly not the rotatory type seen in many cases of positioning nystagmus in man.

In cases of positioning nystagmus there is often transient nystagmus in reversed direction when a normal sitting position is resumed. Nystagmus similar to traumatic or cryptogenic positioning nystagmus of peripheral origin may be caused by a labyrinthine fistula (STENGER, 1955). This should be checked by the pressure test.

3. Is there Positional Nystagmus of Cervical Proprioceptive Origin?

It has been claimed in recent years that vertigo and positional or positioning nystagmus may be of proprioceptive cervical origin. However, neck reflexes, while important for body equilibrium, are unimportant for eye stabilization, since the labyrinths in the head are in the right place to measure head movements but cannot sense body position without taking neck afferents into account (for details, see KORNHUBER, 1966, 1971; and this volume, Chapt. G II.). The neck contribution to eye stabilization is very small (MEIRY, 1971) and there is no spontaneous nystagmus after section of upper dorsal cervical roots (L. A. COHEN, 1961). It has been shown by DE JONG (1967, 1973) that cutting the upper dorsal cervical roots in the rabbit or cat may sometimes result in positional nystagmus if recorded without vision. However, since this effect is not constant (unlike the severe disturbance of body posture and gait), and since most normal persons show positional nystagmus when vision is excluded (BARBER and WRIGHT, 1973), it seems doubtful whether this finding has any pathologic significance. In any case, proprioceptive cervical mechanisms cannot account for typical positioning nystagmus of peripheral origin since this nystagmus is not abolished by visual fixation and is not associated with cervical root lesions, osteochondrosis, or disk protrusion (KORNHUBER, 1965). On the other hand, occipital headache and vertigo are common signs of vertebrobasilar artery insufficiency. Especially when vertigo or nystagmus is evoked by neck torsion or head reclination, one should first of all consider sclerotic lesions in several cranial arteries and compression of a vertebral artery by disk protrusion (Sandström, 1961) rather than a dorsal root lesion.

H. Latent Nystagmus (Nystagmus upon Monocular Fixation)

This type of nystagmus, which occurs with monocular fixation, is a special form of congenital fixation nystagmus. In most cases it is obviously a hereditary disorder since it occurs together with strabismus in certain families (Kornhuber, 1960). No latent nystagmus has been found associated with central lesions resulting

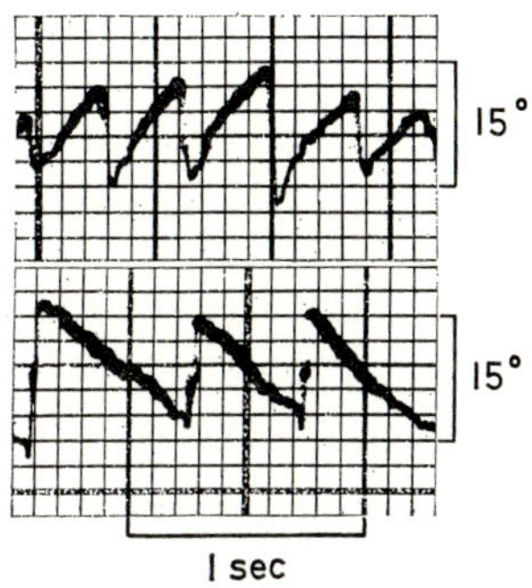

Fig. 4. Latent nystagmus upon monocular fixation is a jerk nystagmus although it is congenital. Upper trace: Left eye fixates point straight ahead, right eye closed: nystagmus to the left. Lower trace: Spontaneous nystagmus to the right in the same case when both eyes are closed

from multiple sclerosis, tumor, etc. The sibling of some probands with latent nystagmus also show horizontal pendular nystagmus. Mild cases of latent nystagmus are more frequent than is usually assumed and are often overlooked. Mild latent nystagmus can easily be detected with the Thorner opthalmoscope or by investigation of optokinetic nystagmus with monocular stimulation. Most cases of latent nystagmus also have strabismus, and latent nystagmus is the most common abnormal oculomotor symptom associated with strabismus. Since about 15 to 20% of cases with concomitant squint have latent nystagmus, and since some 2 to 3% of the normal population have strabismus, latent nystagmus occurs in approximately 0.3 to 0.6% of the population.

Latent nystagmus is part of a characteristic syndrome (Kornhuber, 1960) together with squint, alternating hyperphoria (in about half of the cases), jerking nystagmus even with both eyes closed, inconstant pendular rotating nystagmus with both eyes open, and latent rotating gaze deviation of both eyes when one eye is covered (about 15% of cases). Latent nystagmus is a jerking nystagmus of both eyes with the quick phases in the direction of the fixating eye. Asymmetry of the latent nystagmus during monocular fixation occurs often and is important for determination of the squinting eye in unilateral strabismus (the other factor is anisometropia). The direction of spontaneous nystagmus with both eyes closed is independent of the side where the latent nystagmus is more prominent. The rotatory component in the syndrome of latent nystagmus and spontaneous nystagmus with both eyes closed cannot be explained by an anomaly of foveal vision in early life, previously considered to be the cause of latent nystagmus.

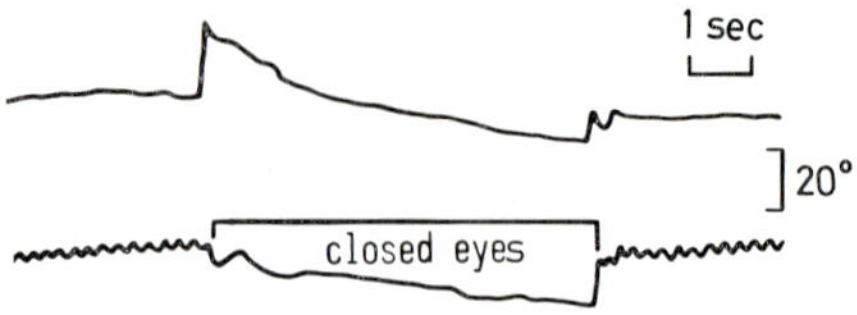

Fig. 5. Acquired pendular fixation nystagmus in a case of multiple sclerosis. Horizontal leads from both eyes: upper trace right eye, lower trace left eye. The nystagmus disappears when the eyes are closed. In this case only the left eye shows nystagmus

I. Fixation Nystagmus: Congenital or Acquired?

It has often been said that fixation nystagmus is pendular in form and that pendular nystagmus is congenital in origin. Pendular and congenital nystagmus, however, are not equivalent, because congenital nystagmus is frequently not pendular, and pendular nystagmus may be acquired, for instance, miner's nystagmus or pendular nystagmus in multiple sclerosis, which occurs in about 4% of cases (Aschoff et al., 1974).

Table 2

	Fixation nystagmus acquired	congenital
oscillopsia	often	never [a]
form of nystagmus	purely sinusoidal	jerk, arc, sinus, saddle etc.
differences in nystagmus direction and amplitude between the eyes	often, even monocular nystagmus	very rare
direction of nystagmus	all directions	mostly horizontal or rotatory, rarely vertical
inversion of optokinetic nystagmus	never	often
other neurologic symptoms (except nystagmus and head tremor)	in most cases	never, except for concomitant squint in latent nystagmus

[a] Except for latent nystagmus in which oscillopsia often occurs if one eye is covered or closed; furthermore, vision may be blurred, especially in the autosomal hereditary type of pendular nystagmus with a marked vertical component (Dichgans and Kornhuber, 1964).

Differences between acquired and congenital fixation nystagmus are listed in Table 2. In addition, some cases of congenital nystagmus show cycloid forms (arc, sinus, spike) or saddle-shaped forms with both eyes closed, sometimes with large amplitudes. In acquired pendular nystagmus, however, the nystagmus initially

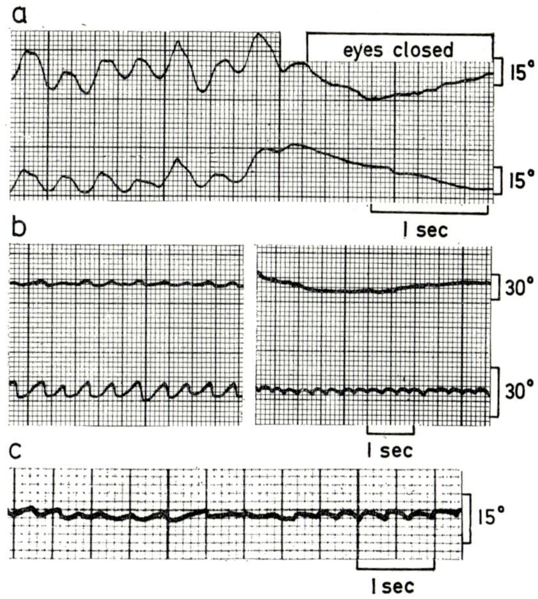

Fig. 6. Different types of congenital fixation nystagmus. a: Disappearance of pendular fixation nystagmus after eye closure (right half of figure); horizontal leads from both eyes. b: Changed direction of nystagmus after lid closure; upper trace: vertical, lower trace: horizontal component of movement; in this case the nystagmus shows a jerky form when the eyes are open (left part of b) and arc forms when the eyes are closed. c: Spontaneous change of direction during steady fixation of a point straight ahead; horizontal lead (a and b from KORNHUBER, Arch. Ohrenheilk. **194**, 1969; c from KORNHUBER, Hals-Nasen-Ohrenheilkunde, Handbuch, Stuttgart: Thieme, 1966)

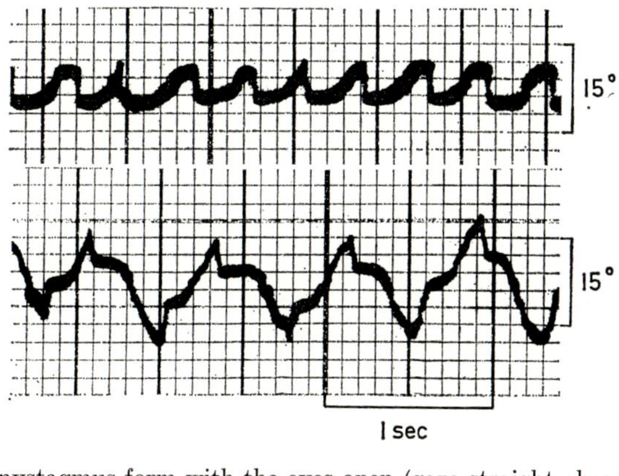

Fig. 7. Change of nystagmus form with the eyes open (gaze straight ahead, upper trace) and closed (lower trace) in a case of congenital fixation nystagmus. Horizontal leads. The nystagmus is jerky, but shows a saddle-like deformation of the slow phase (From KORNHUBER, Arch. Ohrenheilk. **194**, 1969)

disappears after closure of both eyes and may in some cases reappear after a few seconds in sinusoidal form with small amplitudes. In case of a combination of acquired pendular nystagmus with spontaneous jerk nystagmus of central vestibular origin, pure jerk nystagmus occurs after eye closure, without cycloid or saddle forms.

The general characteristic of fixation nystagmus is the change caused by closing both eyes, which is different from the change in vestibular nystagmus: it either disappears or changes direction or form. Another important characteristic of many cases of fixation nystagmus is the form per se: very often there are deviations from the pure jerk form with its slow and rapid phases: pendular nystagmus, cycloid forms, abnormalities of the slow phase with saddle form. However, congenital nystagmus may have a pure jerk form; this is usually the case in latent nystagmus upon monocular fixation.

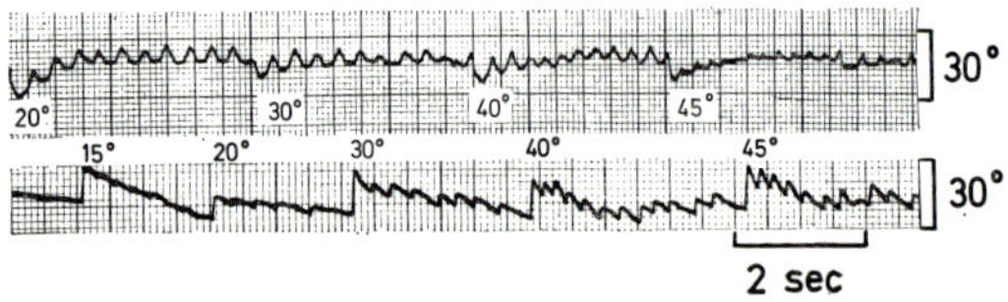

Fig. 8. Possible differences in behavior of congenital pendular nystagmus and acquired gaze nystagmus at different angles of horizontal gaze deviation. Upper trace: In this case of congenital pendular nystagmus, increasing gaze deviation to the left (20° to 45° from midposition) causes decrease of nystagmus amplitude. (This is not so in all cases of congenital nystagmus; see also Fig. 1). Lower trace: Increasing gaze deviation to the right causes increase of the amplitude and frequency of acquired gaze nystagmus in a case of multiple sclerosis (From Kornhuber, Hals-Nasen-Ohrenheilkunde, Handbuch, Stuttgart: Thieme, 1966)

K. Miner's Nystagmus

This type of nystagmus is very similar to the acquired pendular nystagmus in multiple sclerosis. Often it is a purely pendular nystagmus with different amplitudes and directions in the two eyes. The vertical and rotatory directions are most common. The frequency (usually 3.5 to 6 Hz; Ohm, 1954) is in the range of acquired pendular nystagmus in multiple sclerosis, and there is no inversion of optokinetic nystagmus. Furthermore, like pendular nystagmus in multiple sclerosis but unlike congenital nystagmus, miner's nystagmus shows oscillopsia. Although it has often been assumed that miner's nystagmus is caused by poor illumination, after the results with pendular nystagmus in multiple sclerosis (Aschoff et al., 1974) it seems more likely to be due to intoxication of the cerebellar nuclei. In support of this, miner's nystagmus occurs almost exclusively in coal mining but not in ore mining; and it has now disappeared not only in consequence of improved illumination but also of better ventilation in the mines.

L. Involuntary Spontaneous Eye Movements in Blindness

Persons blind since birth often have spontaneous wandering or fluttering eye movements, slow pendular deviations, sometimes mixed with pendular or jerky nystagmus, the jerks being (contrary to gaze nystagmus) often opposite to the momentary eye deviation. These movements are predominantly horizontal and are usually associated, i.e. in both eyes, but can often be of different amplitude. They disappear during sleep. Few blind people can perform voluntary eye movements on command (BARTELS, 1928).

Animals raised in total darkness from birth develop spontaneous nystagmus; in dogs and cats this is pendular with a frequency of 3–6.5 Hz, in chimpanzees, it may be jerky and irregular (CHOW et al., 1957; RIESEN, 1960). This nystagmus is independent of the labyrinths (DE KLEYN and VERSTEEGH, 1920) but seems to depend on some retinal afferents, since it disappears after section of the optic nerves (BARTELS, 1924; SATTLER and BLOHMKE, 1925).

M. Nystagmus in Achromatopsia

In most cases of congenital nystagmus there is no evidence of any impairment of foveal function; instead, there is evidence of impaired central regulation of fixation (and sometimes also of the regulation of head position: holding tremor). Even in total color blindness it seems doubtful whether the nystagmus is simply due to the retinal defect, since in many such individuals the fixation nystagmus is purely horizontal in direction and is associated with defects of the horizontal but not the vertical optokinetic responses. Nystagmus in achromatopsia is not uniform; some cases show high-frequency pendular nystagmus while others show latent nystagmus upon monocular fixation.

N. Heredity of Nystagmus

There are several different kinds of hereditary nystagmus (DICHGANS and KORNHUBER, 1964) (1) the frequently occurring fixation nystagmus of horizontal direction and with disturbance of only the horizontal optokinetic nystagmus; genetic transmission is recessive or incompletely dominant and sex-linked; (2) latent nystagmus upon monocular fixation; inheritance is certainly not X-chromosomal, it is probably autosomal recessive or irregularly dominant; (3) the rarely occurring hereditary nystagmus with a marked vertical component and disturbance of vertical and horizontal optokinetic nystagmus; transmission is autosomal dominant with strong penetrance; (4) Nystagmus in total color blindness; transmission is probably autosomal recessive; (5) the latent nystagmus in Åland eye disease; transmission is X-chromosomal and either dominant with decreased penetrance in female carriers or recessive (VAN VLIET et al., 1973).

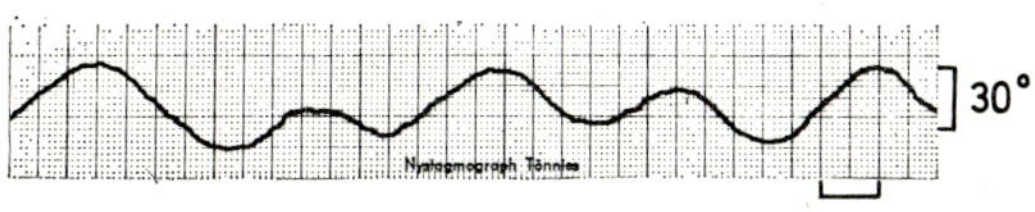

Fig. 9. Slow pendular eye deviations after lid closure, during near-threshold angular acceleration: a sign of drowsiness. Horizontal lead. Typical frequency, about 0.3 Hz (From KORNHUBER, Hals-Nasen-Ohrenheilkunde, Handbuch, Stuttgart: Thieme, 1966)

O. Slow, Rhythmic Pendular Eye Deviations

that occur with closed eyes usually have a frequency of about 0.3 per sec and amplitudes of up to 60°. These nonnystagmic spontaneous eye movements are associated with diminished vestibular excitability, and both symptoms are signs of drowsiness. Therefore, in the presence of these slow rhythmic pendular eye deviations, one cannot trust the magnitude of the induced (caloric or rotatory) vestibular nystagmus.

P. Square-Wave Jerks

on the other hand, with a rate of up to 3 per sec (corresponding to 5 to 6 small saccades) are signs of alertness. They should not be confused with nystagmus since the first characteristic of vestibular and optokinetic nystagmus is the alternation of slow and fast phases. Square-wave jerks of moderate amplitude (about 6°) with Frenzel's glasses or with the eyes closed are a normal phenomenon.

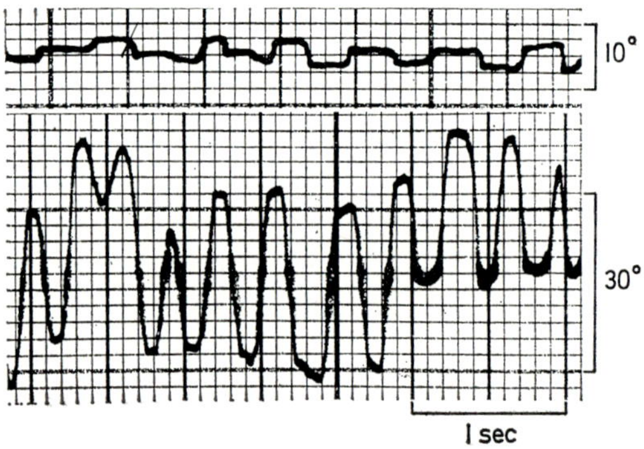

Fig. 10. Square-wave jerks with the eyes closed, horizontal leads. Upper trace: Normal square-wave jerks of a healthy person, a sign of alertness. Lower trace: released square-wave jerks of large amplitude in a patient after encephalitis (From KORNHUBER, Arch. Ohrenheilk. **194**, 1969)

Continuous release of square-wave jerks with amplitudes up to 30° with closed or open eyes is a rare consequence of brainstem or cerebellar disease (JUNG and KORNHUBER, 1964), called "Kippdeviationen" in the German literature.

The occurrence of coarse fixation jerks while fixating a steady point without Frenzel's glasses (best seen with the Thorner ophthalmoscope) is a pathologic sign often seen in multiple sclerosis; it is due to dysmetria of saccadic eye movements. The cause is either impaired central vision or a lesion of the cerebellum.

Q. Ocular Myoclonus or Opsoclonus

consists of rapid to-and-fro coordinated jerks of both eyes in rapid succession, mostly occurring in series at irregular intervals. They may also appear with eyes open, but are in some cases triggered by lid closure. The predominant direction

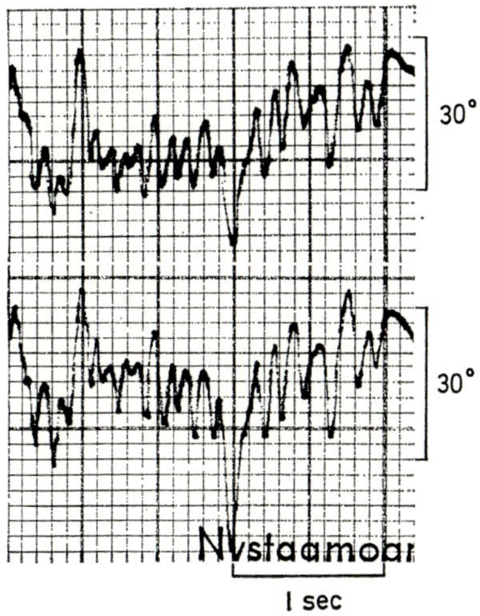

Fig. 11. Ocular myoclonus in a case of viral encephalitis. Monocular leads in the horizontal plane. Upper trace: right eye, lower trace: left eye. Eyes open, gaze straight ahead (From KORNHUBER, Arch. Ohrenheilk. **194**, 1969)

is horizontal, but rotatory or vertical jerks are also observed. The frequency is up to 13 to-and-fro movements per sec, which is much higher than can be voluntarily produced (only 3 per sec). In the course of the disease ocular myoclonus is accompanied in some cases by myoclonus of skeletal muscles. The 6 cases of ocular myoclonus investigated by the author were all caused by encephalitits with signs of brainstem and cerebellar involvement. However, ocular myoclonus also occurs as a paraneoplastic (nonmetastatic) consequence of a remote neoplasm. In such cases demyelination around the dentate nuclei has been found (ALESSI, 1940). In children a special association of paraneoplastic cerebellar encephalopathy with thoracic neuroblastoma can exist. When the neuroblastoma is removed, ocular myoclonus may disappear (SOLOMON and CHUTORIAN, 1968; BRAY et al., 1969).

R. Spontaneous Eye Movements Associated with Palatal Myorhythmia

Myorhythmia consists of regular rhythmic movements of the soft palate, sometimes also involving facial muscles, tongue, pharynx, and diaphragm. The rate is much slower than in opsoclonus, usually around 2 per sec. In some cases, eye movements are associated with palatal myorhythmia; they may be either jerky or more pendular in form, often with a vertical component. The underlying lesion is usually in the dentate nucleus or the inferior olive. Sometimes palatal myoclonus develops after operation on a pontine-angle tumor with compression of the brainstem. Anatomically, the characteristic finding is a pseudohypertrophy of the inferior olive.

S. Voluntary Nystagmus

is a normal phenomenon, although it can be produced by only a few people. The ability to produce voluntary nystagmus is hereditary. Voluntary nystagmus is often associated with slight convergence of the eyes. It lasts only a few seconds, rarely more than 30 sec; during this time the eyes usually converge more and more. The subject has apparent motion of visual objects during this time. Voluntary nystagmus is pendular, of small amplitude and high frequency. In some cases, both eyes move in a conjugate way, in other cases there is a convergence — divergence nystagmus. The direction is usually horizontal. In most cases in which voluntary nystagmus was recorded the frequency was between 15 and 25 Hz, with a mode of 17 to 18 Hz (KORNHUBER, 1966).

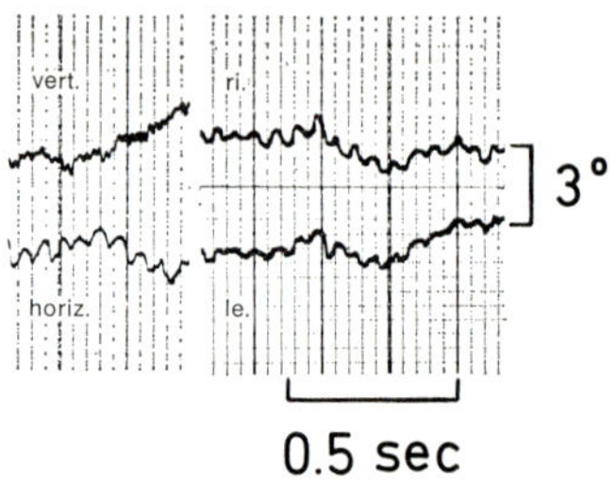

Fig. 12. Voluntary nystagmus in a normal person. Left: upper trace vertical, lower trace horizontal leads. Right: monocular recordings of horizontal movements of the right eye (upper trace) and left eye (lower trace). The frequency of the nystagmus in this case is 17 Hz (From KORNHUBER, Hals-Nasen-Ohrenheilkunde, Handbuch, Stuttgart: Thieme, 1966)

T. Dissociated Nystagmus and Internuclear Ophthalmoplegia

This syndrome is due to a lesion of the medial longitudinal fasciculus (MLF) between the pontine reticular formation and the oculomotor nucleus (BENDER and WEINSTEIN, 1944). When attempting lateral gaze, the temporally directed (abducted) eye shows more nystagmus, and when looking back and forth over an angle of about 30–40°, the adducted eye moves more slowly than the abducted one. This slowing down of the nasally directed eye during a horizontal saccade is more significant than a small amplitude difference between the two eyes in the case of gaze nystagmus. The MLF syndrome is often associated with gaze nystagmus upon looking upwards. The whole syndrome is usually caused by multiple sclerosis, rarely by a vascular lesion or syphilis. Since multiple sclerosis is one of the most common diseases of the nervous system and internuclear opthalmoplegia is a frequently occurring symptom of supraspinal involvement in this disease, the simple test of having the patient looking back and forth horizontally between the fingers of the examiner should be a standard procedure in otoneurology.

U. Seesaw Nystagmus

is actually the seesaw component of a rotatory nystagmus. If the vertical meridian of the eye shows intorsion, the eye simultaneously rises, while the other, extorting eye falls. There are two types of seesaw nystagmus, pendular and jerky. The more common pendular type is due to diencephalic lesions, mainly tumors, also causing bitemporal hemianopsia. The less common jerky seesaw nystagmus is, like other types of rotatory jerky nystagmus, due to lesions in the region of the vestibular nuclei, most often caused by syringobulbia.

V. Adversive Seizures and Epileptic Nystagmus

Deviation of the head, eyes, trunk or of all these – usually towards the contralateral side – occurs as a focal seizure or as a focal onset of a generalized seizure. Adversive seizures are indicative of an epileptogenic lesion in the frontal, parietal, temporal or occipital lobe, but not in the motor or somatosensory cortex. At the beginning and at the end of contraversive seizures with deviation of the eyes, there may be epileptic nystagmus. At the onset of the seizure it is usually towards the contralateral side, while at the end it is directed towards the ipsilateral side of the lesion (for details, see GASTAUT, 1960). The nystagmus-like clonic upward movements of both eyes and lids in the pyknoleptic petit mal epilepsy usually has a frequency of 3 per sec, the same as the spike-wave complex in the EEG.

W. Oculogyric Spasms

or crises, also called tonic eye fits, were a frequent symptom in the influenza epidemic that followed the first world war and occurred more often in post-encephalitic than genuine parkinsonism. Nowadays, such fits are sometimes due to intoxication by a neuroleptic drug. The tonic eye deviation is most often upwards but may also be to the side, downwards, central or convergent. The spasms may be treated by Biperiden injections or by L-dopa.

IV. Gaze Paralysis, Disturbance of Visually Guided Eye Movements, and Related Phenomena

A. Gaze Paralysis

Gaze paralysis should be distinguished from extraocular muscle palsies and strabismus concomitans on the one hand, and oculogyric crises on the other. But gaze paralysis is often combined with an extraocular nerve palsy, e.g. horizontal gaze palsy with a lesion of the sixth nerve, and vertical gaze palsy with lesions of the third nerve nuclei. Furthermore, extraocular muscles may be symmetrically impaired, for instance in myasthenia gravis, polyneuritis and ocular muscle dystrophy. In such cases it is important to find out whether the optokinetic nystagmus is normal over the range of free movement. In some cases there is a palsy only of voluntary gaze, or of voluntary gaze and optokinetic nystagmus, whereas the eyes can still be moved by vestibular stimuli or neck torsion.

Paralysis of conjugate gaze should be dinstinguished from hemineglect, or inattention to the side of the body contralateral to a forebrain lesion. A real gaze palsy is always connected with impairment of optokinetic nystagmus and smooth pursuit eye movement. A good test for hysterical pseudopalsy of gaze is, therefore, to move the whole visual environment by moving a large mirror in front of the patient's open eyes.

In man and in monkey both eyes are always moved simultaneously under normal viewing conditions, even in situations where it would be simpler to move only one eye. The eye movements are binocularly organized and automatically divided into two components, versions (right, left, up and down movements) and vergences (convergence and divergence). This binocular coordination occurs in a premotor neuronal apparatus of the oculomotor nuclei in the brainstem: the so-called subcortical gaze centers of the pontine and mesencephalic tegmentum and pretectal region. Consequently, there are no direct fiber connections from the cerebral cortex to the oculomotor nuclei.

Partial gaze paralysis is usually associated with gaze paretic nystagmus and with impairment of the rapid phases of optokinetic and vestibular nystagmus. In such cases vestibular nystagmus might still be present with the eyes open with Frenzel's glasses, but disappears with the eyes closed because of a deficient facilitation of the rapid phases. The velocity of the rapid phases of vestibular nystagmus and optokinetic nystagmus may be slowed down in patients with brainstem lesions.

1. Horizontal Gaze Paralysis

Since oculomotor function in the forebrain is widely distributed in the frontal, parietal, temporal and occipital lobes, cortical lesions do not usually cause gaze paralysis (PASIK and PASIK, 1964a) while subcortical lesions of the white matter in the hemisphere often result in initial gaze palsy and long-lasting impairment of optokinetic nystagmus to the contralateral side (JUNG and KORNHUBER, 1964). There are two reasons for this differential effect of cortical and subcortical lesions. First, subcortical lesions usually damage fibers coming from extensive cortical fields and running down to the brainstem. Second, while on the afferent side of the visual system up to the striate area all directions of visual motion are represented on both sides, the efferents from the occipital, temporal and parietal lobes to the brainstem — because of partial callosal crossing — consist predominantly of fibers for the optokinetic nystagmus to the contralateral side (KORNHUBER, 1966). Section of corpus callosum and optic chiasma therefore results, with monocular stimulation, in diminution of optokinetic nystagmus to the side contralateral to the unstimulated eye (PASIK and PASIK, 1964b).

Unlike lesions of the subcortical gaze centers in the tegmentum of the brainstem, forebrain lesions result only in short-lasting gaze paralysis. This fast compensation, which contrasts with the long-lasting paralysis of finger movements after forebrain lesions, is probably caused by two factors (1) compensation by subcortical mechanisms, and (2) different lateralization of the descending mechanisms for slow and fast eye movements (smooth pursuit and saccades). Following lesions in the subcortical white matter of the posterior hemisphere (which damage descending fibers to the brainstem) with defective optokinetic nystagmus to the contralateral side, both components of the optokinetic nystagmus are impaired: the fast phases (and the saccades) to the contralateral side and the slow phases (and smooth pursuit eye movements) to the ipsilateral side of the lesion. While the fibers for the smooth pursuit eye movements descend uncrossed to the pontine tegmentum, there is a functional crossing of the mechanisms for the saccadic eye movements which occurs at midbrain level (BENDER and SHANZER, 1964). Perhaps it is partially mediated by the ipsilateral pontine nuclei while crossing the midline through the cerebellum (ASCHOFF, 1974). The quick phases of nystagmus, however, are independent of the cerebellum. They are generated in the reticular nuclei fo the tegmentum (LORENTE DE NÓ, 1933; COHEN and HENN, 1972).

While this crossing awaits further analysis, it is clear, that subcortical lesions of the forebrain induce transient gaze paralysis to the contralateral side while lesions of the paramedian pontine tegmentum cause long-lasting ipsilateral gaze paralysis (BENDER and SHANZER, 1964). Lesions of the motor cortex do not impair eye movements. Lesions of the cerebellar nuclei result in long-lasting gaze nystagmus and disturbance of smooth pursuit eye movement.

2. Vertical Gaze Paralysis

occurs only in bilateral lesions of the midbrain tegmentum or pretectal region. This is because vertical eye movements are bilaterally represented in the forebrain as well as the upper brainstem. Paralysis of upward gaze occurs more often than paralysis of downward gaze. Small lesions in the posterior commissure produce paralysis of upward and/or downward gaze (PASIK et al., 1969) but perhaps the commissural symptoms are due to damage of passing fibers. According to HASSLER (1972), the center for upward gaze is the prestitial nucleus and the center for downward gaze the precommissural nucleus. In view of the results of PASIK et al. (1969), it is unlikely that the interstitial nucleus of CAJAL is the premotor apparatus for vertical gaze; this nucleus, however, probably acts as premotor apparatus for rotating eye movements (HASSLER, 1972). The optic tectum (superior colliculi) was long ago ruled out as the immediate premotor apparatus for vertical gaze (MUSKENS, 1934). However, the optic tectum plays a role as a higher center mediating visually guided eye movements, not only in the vertical, but in all directions. The neurons of the optic tectum of the monkey fire prior to saccadic eye movements of a certain size and direction, and the (usually small) receptive visual field of a given neuron is located in such a way that the saccade would bring this field into the fovea (SCHILLER, 1972). After collicular lesions monkeys are either not able to direct their eyes adequately to eccentric targets (SCHILLER, 1972) or (after small collicular lesions) they show a prolongation of the delay by 150 to 300 msec before they make accurate eye movements (WURTZ and GOLDBERG, 1972), indicating, that the indirect pathway which compensates for the defects needs more time.

Instead of a vertical gaze nystagmus, a convergence retractory nystagmus is often associated with the attempt to look upward in cases of vertical gaze paralysis. Furthermore, there is often a disturbance of the pupillary light reaction associated with vertical gaze palsy (PARINAUD's syndrome).

Unilateral hemispheric lesions do not cause vertical gaze paralysis. However, electrical stimulation of the frontal or occipital lobes may evoke vertical components of contraversive eye movements, and bilateral symmetrical stimulations evoke purely vertical eye movements.

B. Gaze Apraxia

Patients with unilateral hemispheric lesions, especially those associated with homonymous hemianopsia, may show visual inattention to the side contralateral to the lesion and be unable to move the eyes to the neglected side on command. Patients with bilateral lesions in the white matter of the posterior part of the hemispheres — even if they are not cortically blind — may have oculomotor apraxia in all directions: they cannot look at objects in the peripheral field of vision, they show disturbance of smooth pursuit eye movements, and in addition often ataxia of visually guided hand movements (Hécaen and Ajuriaguerra, 1954).

C. Disturbance of Optokinetic Nystagmus

In cases of gaze paresis optokinetic nystagmus is always impaired, but it may also be affected if a gaze disturbance is not detectable by other methods, for instance, years after a unilateral lesion of the forebrain. The diminution of optokinetic nystagmus to the contralateral side in lesions of white matter in the posterior hemispheres is often associated with homonymous hemianopsia, but it may also occur without hemianopsia. Hemianopsia per se does not cause optokinetic disturbance, e.g. complete hemianopsia due to a lesion of the optic tract does not cause any optokinetic defect. Nor does complete destruction of one striate area result in impairment of optokinetic nystagmus, even in the acute stage (Kornhuber, 1966), nor a cortical lesion of the frontal, parietal, or temporal lobe (Pasik and Pasik, 1964a). The diminution of optokinetic nystagmus to the contralateral side in subcortical hemispheric lesions, however, is as reliable as a Babinski sign to diagnose the side of the affected hemisphere.

If a large-field stimulus is used to test optokinetic nystagmus, several speeds between 40 and 140° per sec should be used since the defect is often hidden at low speeds while high speeds can give a bilateral deficient response in some patients. However, the best method for clinical testing is a small-field stimulus, like a little optokinetic drum with stripes or (for children) with figures, because a small stimulus shows the defect more clearly than a large-field stimulus. Recording and exact measurement of the slow phase speed of optokinetic nystagmus is of limited value since the intensity of the optokinetic response depends on attention and therefore varies considerably. The best method is simple bedside observation of optokinetic nystagmus by manually turning a small optokinetic drum back and forth several times at different speeds and observing the patient's eye movements together with his attention to the stimulus. Only a clear, constant unilateral diminution of optokinetic nystagmus is important. A bilateral diminution of horizontal optokinetic nystagmus is significant only in cases that show normal vertical optokinetic nystagmus, or where interspersed saccades in the direction of the slow phases indicate that the patient tries his best to follow the stimulus.

In the presence of spontaneous vestibular nystagmus of peripheral origin there is no algebraic summation of spontaneous and optokinetic nystagmus, because visual fixation to a large extent suppresses vestibular nystagmus. In severe spontaneous nystagmus of peripheral origin there might be a slight asymmetry of optokinetic nystagmus; in spontaneous nystagmus of central origin this asymmetry is often larger.

The slow phases of optokinetic nystagmus are slower than the stimulus under normal conditions of stimulation. However, in cases where one eye is immobilized and the examiner blindfolds the other, optokinetic stimulation of the immobilized eye results in an enhanced velocity of the optokinetic nystagmus of the blindfolded eye. The maximal velocity of the slow phases of normal optokinetic nystagmus in man under large field stimulus conditions is about 100° per sec, which is similar to the maximal slow-phase velocity of vestibular nystagmus.

1. Monocular Optokinetic Stimulation

In birds and rodents, which have completely crossed optic nerve fibers, optokinetic nystagmus upon monocular stimulation is stronger towards the temporal and weaker towards the nasal side. In contrast, in normal humans horizontal optokinetic nystagmus is equal in both directions with monocular stimulation. However, in persons with latent nystagmus upon monocular fixation, optokinetic nystagmus with monocular stimulation is stronger toward the side of the stimulated eye (i.e. toward the temporal side of the uncovered eye) and weaker in the opposite direction (KORNHUBER, 1960). During this test the patient should look straight ahead since gaze nystagmus may also influence the intensity of optokinetic nystagmus. Latent nystagmus upon monocular fixation can be very small, making it difficult to detect by mere closure of the other eye without an ophthalmoscope and without monocular optokinetic stimulation.

2. Inversion of the Optokinetic Nystagmus

occurs in congenital nystagmus only, not in an acquired pendular nystagmus such as miner's nystagmus or pendular nystagmus in multiple sclerosis. Inversion is often unilateral and has never, to my knowledge, been reported in a vertical direction.

D. Smooth Pursuit Eye Movements with Sinusoidal and Other Non-Unidirectional Stimuli

Eye tracking tests with sinusoidal stimuli are advantageous (as compared to unidirectional optokinetic tests) only in cases of bilateral or omnidirectional disturbance of optokinetic nystagmus, especially in intoxications. The disturbance of smooth pursuit is revealed by larger and more frequent saccades in the

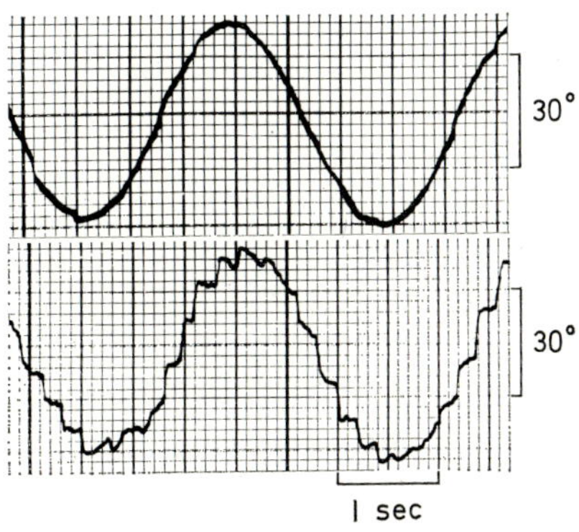

Fig. 13. Upper trace: Smooth pursuit eye movements in horizontal direction to a pendular stimulus. Lower trace: disturbance of smooth pursuit in a case of barbiturate and diphenylhydantoin intoxication; smooth pursuit is largely replaced by saccades (From KORNHUBER, Arch. Ohrenheilk. **194**, 1969)

direction of pursuit. In cases of bilateral or omnidirectional optokinetic disturbance, the disturbance of smooth pursuit is not the only symptom; there is usually gaze nystagmus and often positional nystagmus as well. If a sinusoidal horizontal movement over an angle of 30 to 40° at frequencies of about 0.3 Hz is used, the response in normal subjects is a smooth curve with only a few fine jerks at intervals of about 1 sec or more; between 0.1 and 0.3 Hz up to 10% of the total amplitude is contributed by saccades. At stimulus amplitudes of 20° pursuit eye movement is quite smooth up to 0.8 Hz, at stimulus amplitudes of 36°, up to 0.6 Hz (for further details, see Kornhuber, 1966).

The tracking characteristics, i.e. the stimulus-response relations of smooth pursuit in man, are considerably better if there is some predictable element in the motion of the stimulus. The nature of this predictive ability of the human visual system, however, has not yet been well analyzed, and it is not clear whether tests of this prediction are of clinical value.

V. Induced Vestibular Responses

A. Vestibular Nystagmus Induced by Caloric (Thermal), Galvanic and Rotatory Stimulation (Angular Acceleration)

The best method for investigating the function of a single labyrinth is, in most cases, the caloric test introduced by Robert Bárány. Galvanic stimulation is advantageous only in special cases because it still yields positive reactions even if the vestibular endorgans in the labyrinths are destroyed; galvanic nystagmus is not impaired until the peripheral neuron has degenerated (Dohlman, 1929). Electrical stimulation of the labyrinths with low-frequency square-wave alternating current (1 Hz) is useful for testing labyrinthine excitability in cases of direction-changing spontaneous nystagmus (Kirstein, 1949). The advantage of the rotatory test is not that it is more "physiological" but that it permits application of a strong stimulus (sudden stop from 90° per sec rotation after a slow, near-threshold acceleration), which reveals phenomena of vestibular release due to central lesions such as often occur in multiple sclerosis. However, most of the rotatory excitability tests are unnecessary if thorough testing is done for spontaneous, head-shaking, positional and gaze nystagmus in association with a good clinical history. A simple caloric test, on the other hand, is essential in many cases.

B. Evaluation of Caloric Responses

Nystagmography by electrical (Jung, 1953) or photoelectric methods (Torok et al., 1951) makes evaluation of the vestibular responses easier and more reliable. The parameters of the vestibular response which correspond best to the stimulus magnitude are the slow phase velocity and total amplitude of nystagmus. A simple way of evaluating these parameters is to generate the first derivation of the eye position, i.e. slow phase speed, electronically and to record it simultaneously with the original nystagmus curve at slow paper speed so that the whole caloric response can be viewed at one glance (Henriksson, 1955). With the eyes open and the gaze straight ahead with Frenzel's glasses the rate (frequency) and total number of nystagmus beats also show good correlation with slow phase velocity and total amplitude and are sensitive signs of functional impairment. Since the total number of beats is often difficult to determine without nystagmography, the rate of beats at the culmination of the caloric response (Torok, 1948, 1957) is a more convenient measure. It can be established without nystagmography using Frenzel's glasses and a stop watch: one can count the number of beats in 5-sec steps during the first 5 to 25 sec after the end of the caloric stimulus (if this consists of irrigation with water of 30° and 44° C respectively for 30 sec with the head in the optimum position for the horizontal canal, i.e. 30° forward from the supine position). The duration of nystagmus, which was previously used as a quantitative parameter, is often difficult to determine and it is less sensitive in detecting functional disturbances than slow phase speed, total amplitude, or rate of nystagmus.

If nystagmography is used, the vertical eye movements should be recorded simultaneously with the horizontal ones in order to account for lid blinks and other artifacts. There are many factors which can lead to misinterpretation of nystagmograms such as changes of the eye steady potential, galvanic skin reflex, EEG potentials, diminution of vestibular responses due to lack of alertness, deficient facilitation of the quick nystagmic phases after lid closure (especially in brainstem lesions), eye deviation toward the direction of the slow phase, and inhibition by fixation. Therefore, it is safer to carry out the caloric test with Frenzel's glasses in a dark room while continuously checking by direct observation for alertness and midposition of the eyes.

A perverted direction of caloric nystagmus occurs after lesions on the floor of the fourth ventricle, especially in the vestibular nuclei (Frenzel, 1932; Riesco-MacClure and Martinez, 1957; Fredrickson and Fernández, 1964; Uemura and Cohen, 1972). If the caloric test is applied in optimum position of the horizontal canal, a predominantly vertical or rotating nystagmus may often result.

Misinterpretations of caloric responses of the following kind are still common today.

"The caloric responses are normal; therefore, the existing spontaneous nystagmus cannot be of peripheral origin." Despite normal caloric responses a spontaneous nystagmus can still be of peripheral origin — for instance, recovery nystagmus. The patient's history must be taken into account. Only when spontaneous nystagmus has the type of form and direction found exclusively following central lesions is it possible to reach a clear decision without the history.

"The caloric responses show a directional preponderance of the nystagmus toward one side, independent of the labyrinth investigated; this is typical for a central lesion." Directional preponderance of caloric nystagmus may be of peripheral as well as central origin; moreover, directional preponderance is often found in normal persons; it is of pathologic significance only if it is connected with spontaneous nystagmus under Frenzel's glasses. The worst misinterpretation, however, is this:

"Cold caloric irrigation shows that the function of the labyrinths is normal." In the case of a totally unresponsive labyrinth, cold calorization may act as an arousal stimulus, activating spontaneous nystagmus toward the contralateral side; this can be misinterpreted if only cold irrigation is used. Therefore, if possible, both warm and cold calorization should be employed. If there is only time for one, it should be warm calorization because an existing spontaneous nystagmus due to abolished labyrinthine function has to be inhibited and reversed in order to produce an ipsilateral caloric nystagmus.

A slight hypoexcitability of one labyrinth is of no diagnostic value, unless a spontaneous nystagmus corresponds to it, or the difference exceeds 30% of nystagmus speed, amplitude or rate, or 20% of the duration (when the responses to warm and cold calorization of one labyrinth are summed and subtracted from those of the other).

In otoneurology (as in medicine and, indeed, science in general) positive findings are more significant than negative ones, because there are always many more factors which can give rise to negative results. For instance, in the case of acoustic neuroma, the caloric response is often, but not always, abolished. One should therefore not exclude the possibility of a neuroma on the basis of normal caloric responses if there are other suspicious signs.

1. Influence of Visual Fixation

If the caloric nystagmus is investigated under conditions of full visual fixation (method of FITZGERALD and HALLPIKE), the inhibition of caloric nystagmus by vision must be taken into account. This inhibition may be diminished in only one direction by subcortical lesions of the forebrain which damage corticofugal fibers to the brainstem (BADER and KORNHUBER, 1965). Therefore, in forebrain lesions the caloric nystagmus may show a slight directional preponderance to the ipsilateral side (CARMICHAEL et al., 1954), which has nothing to do with the cortical projection of the vestibular nerve. This is in contrast to caloric responses after eye closure which in forebrain lesions show a directional preponderance to the contralateral side slightly more often than to the ipsilateral side (HAKAS and KORNHUBER, 1959). In both conditions, however, the effect on the caloric nystagmus is not reliable enough for topical diagnosis, while the diminution of optokinetic nystagmus to the contralateral side is adequate to diagnose the presence and side of a subcortical forebrain lesion. Therefore, caloric tests are useless for the diagnosis of hemispheric lesions. However, a bilateral reduction of the visual inhibition of vestibular eye movements due to bilateral disseminated or brainstem lesions is of diagnostic value (LEDOUX and DEMANEZ, 1969).

2. Methods of Caloric Testing

Which kind of caloric test is the best has yet to be investigated. A modified FITZGERALD and HALLPIKE method with massive irrigation for 30 sec with water at 7° C above and below body temperature is currently popular, mainly because it does not require changes in head position (inconvenient for nystagmography) and gives stronger responses than small stimuli. However, the physical background of methods similar to the technique of VEITS is, according to the measurements of SCHMALTZ, at least as good as that of the former method, as correctly pointed out by ARSLAN. However, methods may change once the advantages of Frenzel's glasses become more widely known. A direct comparison of the FITZGERALD and HALLPIKE method with the VEITS method has been tried only by HAMERSMA, but the modification of the VEITS method he used might not be the best one.

C. Pendular Angular Acceleration and the Vestibular Frequency Response

The simple torsion swing test with its damped sine wave has the merit of requiring less expensive apparatus than a rotating chair. A still cheaper method is to observe nystagmus under Frenzel's glasses in a dark room, while turning the patient by hand back and forth on a simple office chair. The torsion swing tests used by Wüst (1956) and Greiner et al. (1961) reveal directional preponderance of vestibular nystagmus without determining whether it is of peripheral or central origin. Determination of the whole frequency response (phase and amplitude relations between stimulus and response) up to 4 Hz might be more interesting, but would need a rotating chair with much more power than those commercially available so far. From this type of device, clinically useful new information may be expected in two particular directions: Concerning impairment of the high-frequency response in bilateral peripheral lesions, and impairment of the low-frequency response in certain central lesions. In unidirectional rotatory or caloric tests the responses vary greatly, both in different persons and in the same person, depending on extravestibular factors. Therefore, it is difficult to diagnose a bilaterally symmetric incipient impairment of the labyrinths (e.g. in beginning streptomycin intoxication) by caloric or unidirectional rotatory tests. In such cases determination of the frequency response up to 4 Hz should be useful. Rotation of the head alone (Jatho, 1961) is of limited value since the gain of the cervico-ocular reflex (which is small in normal man, Meiry, 1971) increases after bilateral labyrinthectomy.

D. Unidirectional Angular Acceleration and Vestibular Release

Attempts to determine vestibular threshold by unidirectional angular acceleration (Montandon and Russbach, 1955) were claimed to be more physiological, but they are as far from being natural as other long rotation stimuli. The thresholds found by these methods tend to be the thresholds of the recording techniques rather than of the vestibular apparatus (Decher, 1962). Unfortunately, the threshold methods miss the main advantage offered by modern rotating chairs, namely to reveal signs of release after well-controlled strong stimuli. Since these signs cannot be observed by other methods, the long rotation technique with a sudden stop will be described here. The method is of greater value for neurologists than for otologists.

The patient is seated in an electronically controlled rotating chair. Eye movements are recorded. Rotational acceleration near threshold at 0.8° sec^{-2} up to a speed of 90° per sec is applied and suddenly stopped within 1 sec or less. During the slow accelerations there is usually some perrotatory nystagmus which might reveal a directional preponderance. The maximal slow phase speed of the first postrotatory nystagmus up to 120° per sec is a linear function of angular velocity prior to stop (Keser, 1950). The first postrotatory nystagmus decays with a time-constant of about 15 sec (for the horizontal semicircular canal), due to the mechanics of the cupula. However, about 27 sec after the stop (on average) the decay becomes faster than exponential (G. Stark, 1964) and the nystagmus ends about 45 sec after the stop. Several seconds later a second postrotatory nystagmus

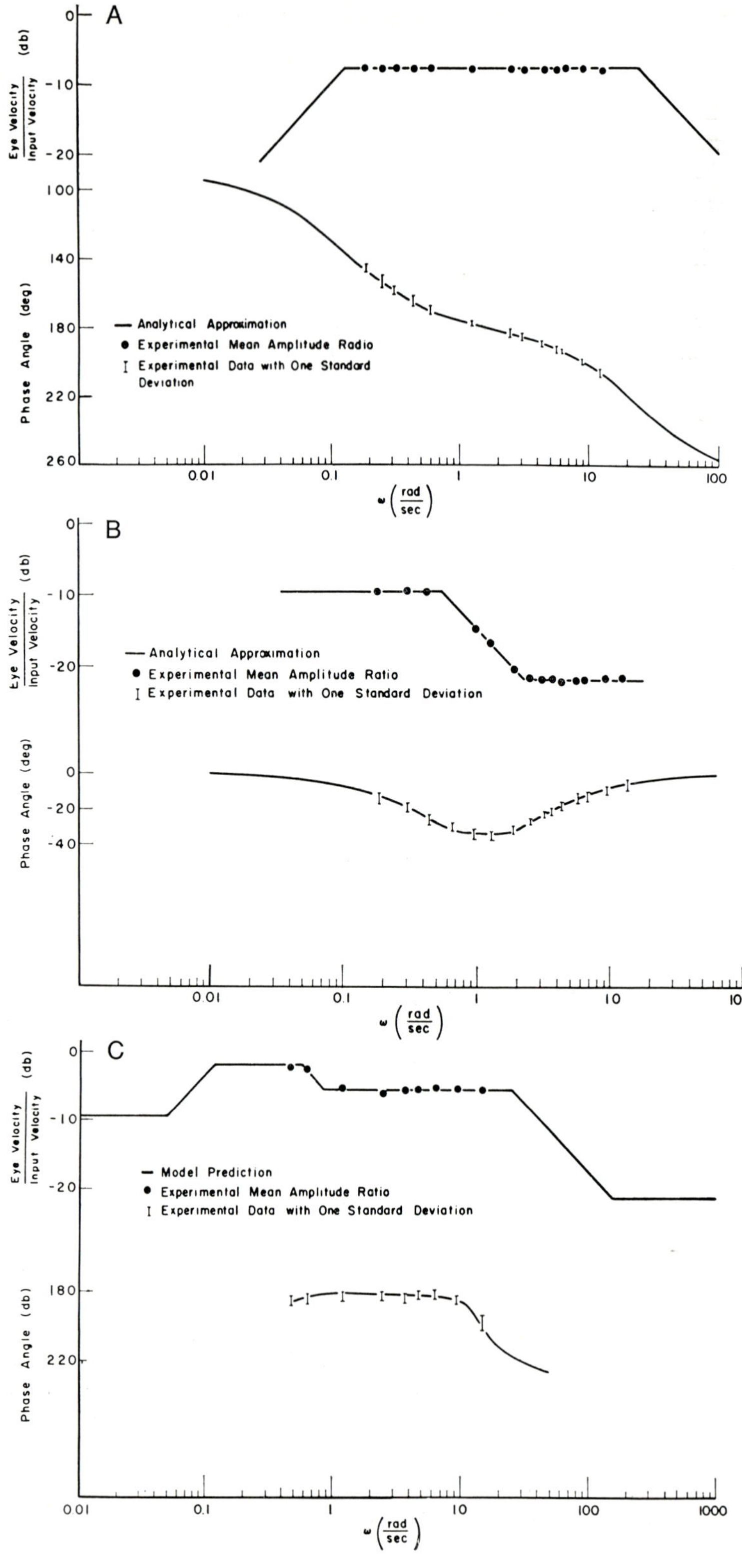
A
Eye Velocity / Input Velocity (db)
0
-10
-20
Phase Angle (deg)
100
140
180
220
260
Analytical Approximation
Experimental Mean Amplitude Radio
Experimental Data with One Standard Deviation
0.01
0.1
1
10
100
ω (rad/sec)
B
Eye Velocity / Input Velocity (db)
0
-10
-20
Analytical Approximation
Experimental Mean Amplitude Ratio
Experimental Data with One Standard Deviation
Phase Angle (deg)
0
-20
-40
0.01
0.1
1
10
100
ω (rad/sec)
C
Eye Velocity / Input Velocity (db)
0
-10
-20
Model Prediction
Experimental Mean Amplitude Ratio
Experimental Data with One Standard Deviation
Phase Angle (db)
180
220
0.01
0.1
1
10
100
1000
ω (rad/sec)

Fig. 14

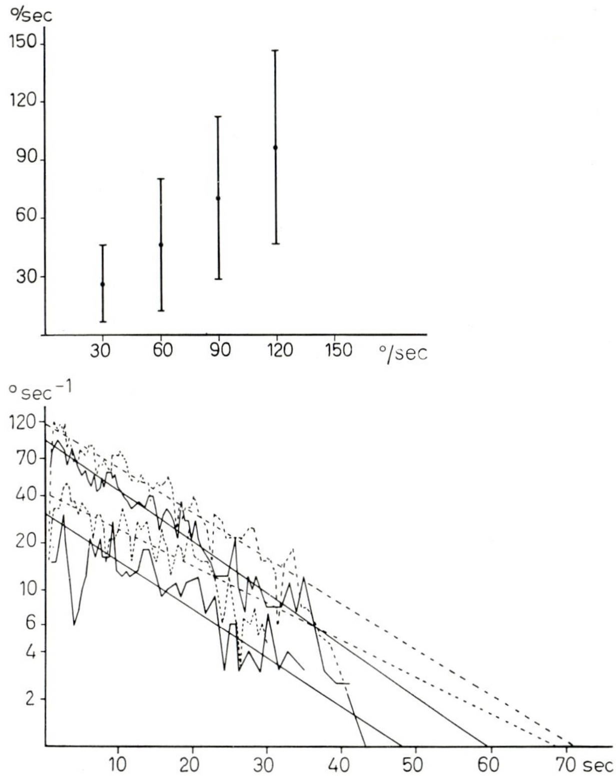

Fig. 15. Maximum speed and course of the slow phase speed of the first postrotatory nystagmus in normal man following a stop from turning speeds of 30, 60, 90 and 120° per sec. Upper figure: The maximal velocity of the slow phases of the first postrotatory nystagmus is a linear function of stimulus speed over this range. The means of 5 normal persons are plotted ± 2 SD. Lower figure: the semilogarithmic plot of the course of the slow phase speed of the first postrotatory nystagmus in one person shows exponential decay with a time constant of about 15 sec independent of the stimulus magnitude. In this person, the faster-than-exponential decay starts after 35 sec (From G. STARK, Thesis, Freiburg i. Br. 1964)

begins, beating in opposite direction; it shows a shallow intensity course and its duration is limited to about 90 to 100 sec. Such long duration, however, is reached in normal subjects on the average only after strong stimuli reaching 180° per sec prior to stop (KESER, 1950). This second postrotatory nystagmus is largely due to a central process which is projected to the labyrinths by the efferent vestibular system. A similar secondary afternystagmus may be obtained by optokinetic stimuli (KORNHUBER, 1962). The second postrotatory nystagmus shows great

Fig. 14. Frequency responses of the vestibular and neck compensatory eye movements. A: Bode plot of vestibular compensatory eye movements (slow phase). B: Compensatory eye movements by neck proprioception; the phase is plotted with respect to body rotation (instead of head rotation) hence the negative phase angles; note that neck proprioception (like vestibular mechanisms) turns the eyes to the left if the head is rotated to the right; there is phase lead around $\omega = 1$, but the amplitudes are very small above $\omega = 0.5$. C: Bode plot of compensatory eye movements by vestibular and neck proprioception (From MEIRY, Thesis, MIT 1965)

variability in normal man and should always be evaluated together with the first postrotatory nystagmus since a change in alertness may occur between the right and left rotation. An interesting point is that some lesions of the brainstem or cerebellum (especially syringobulbia, multiple sclerosis, and cerebellar atrophy) induce a third and even fourth and fifth afternystagmus of periodically alternating direction.

In other cases there may be a long-lasting second afternystagmus in the direction contrary to an existing spontaneous nystagmus, or the second afternystagmus may continue for many minutes as a spontaneous nystagmus, and this after both rotations, so that one finds spontaneous nystagmus alternately to right and left (KORNHUBER, 1966). If there are several alternating phases of postrotatory nystagmus (second, third, etc.), the total cycle time (one right and one left phase) is usually about 200 sec, as in spontaneously alternating nystagmus (KORNHUBER, 1959). This periodically alternating spontaneous nystagmus is a very strong sign of vestibular release and could also be called lack of damping or hyperresponsiveness.

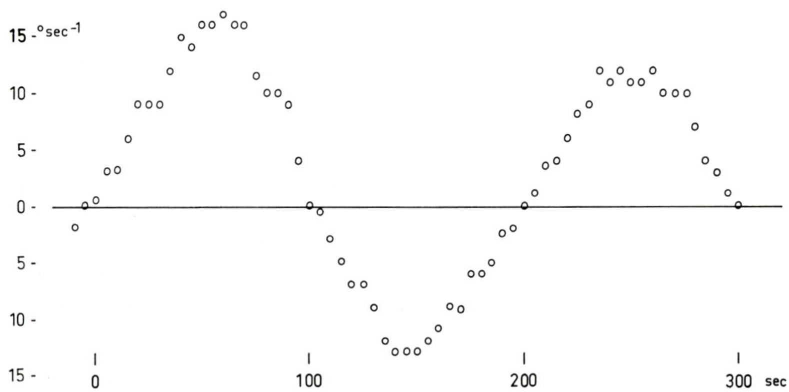

Fig. 16. Slow phase speed of a periodically alternating spontaneous nystagmus, plotted over time. The typical period of nystagmus alternans is 200 sec (From KORNHUBER, Arch. Ohrenheilk. **194**, 1969)

E. Linear Acceleration Tests

have not been found to be clinically useful and are therefore not discussed in detail. The most reliable test of otolithic function seems to be the measurement of counterrolling of the eyes after slow lateral tilt of the head and body. (For reviews, see KORNHUBER, 1966; JONGKEES, 1969; and chapters F. II. and F. IV., this volume.)

F. Vestibulo-Spinal Tests

The most useful test of spontaneous vestibulo-spinal disequilibrium is the stepping test (UNTERBERGER, 1938; see also Chapt. F. III. and F. V. this volume). A method of recording the vestibulo-spinal laterotorsion of the head during caloric tests has been devised by HENRIKSSON et al. (1962). In general, vestibulo-spinal methods are less sensitive and subject to more voluntary control by the patient than are vestibulo-ocular methods. Therefore, they are less useful in most cases. This also applies to the arm tonus reaction.

VI. Otoneurology and General Neurology

A good general neurological examination of the patient is more important than a special vestibulo-spinal test apparatus. This should include examination of the cranial nerves, cerebellar tests including finger-to-nose and heel-to-knee tests, and diadochokinesia (rapid succession of supination and pronation of the hand slapping on the patient's knee or on the doctors hand). In addition, tests should be made for paresis, spasticity, pyramidal signs, rigidity, akinesia, somatic sensation, etc. Some of the interrelations of the vestibular and the motor system in general are explained in chapter G. II. of this volume. The reader is also referred to neurological textbooks, such as BAKER, or the Handbook of Clinical Neurology.

A. Vestibulo-Oculomotor Symptoms: Peripheral or Central?

The following list summarizes some of the signs mentioned:

peripheral: unilateral caloric hypo- or unexcitability, tinnitus or hearing impairment of a cochlear or nerve type, positioning nystagmus of the peripheral type

peripheral or central: spontaneous nystagmus in the narrower sense (with the exception of long-lasting vertical or rotatory nystagmus), directional preponderance of induced nystagmus

central: positional nystagmus of the central type, intensive spontaneous nystagmus without vertigo, long-lasting vertical or rotatory spontaneous nystagmus, gaze nystagmus, gaze paresis, signs of vestibular release, periodically alternating spontaneous nystagmus, disturbances of the rapid phases of nystagmus, disturbances of optokinetic nystagmus or smooth pursuit eye movement, deficient visual inhibition of vestibular eye movements, dissociated gaze nystagmus/internuclear opthalmoplegia, dysmetria of saccadic eye movements, ocular myoclonus, perverted caloric nystagmus, fixation nystagmus including latent nystagmus upon monocular fixation, nystagmic fits, impaired consciousness, drop attacks, cerebellar dysmetria, holding tremor, dysdiadochokinesia, blurred vision, hemianopsia etc.

B. Some Key Symptoms for Topical Diagnosis

Medulla oblongata. The main vestibular sign in cases of syringobulbia is the purely rotatory nystagmus, often combined with ipsilateral diminution of the corneal reflex or pareses of the ipsilateral vocal cord. The most common vascular syndrome of the brainstem is the inferior posterior cerebellar artery syndrome with infarction of the dorsolateral medulla (Wallenberg's syndrome). Its major symptoms are vertigo, ipsi- or contralateral spontaneous nystagmus (often rotating ipsilaterally), impaired ipsilateral trigeminal sensation, hypalgesia and thermohypesthesia on the contralateral side of the body, ipsilateral Horner's syndrome and ipsilateral hemiataxia.

Cerebello-pontine angle. An acoustic neuroma usually causes early diminution of the caloric response and a slight spontaneous nystagmus to the contralateral side, especially in the head-shaking test, occurring without attacks of vertigo. In the late stage a coarse ipsilateral gaze nystagmus and facial nerve palsy appear. At this stage the patient often complains of dizziness, disequilibrium when walking and postural vertigo. Ipsilateral hemiataxia and hemiadiadochokinesia are late signs. The protein content of the cerebrospinal fluid is often high, and roentgenograms may show enlargement of the internal acoustic meatus. Eventually the cranial nerves V to X may be involved, and signs of increased intracranial pressure appear (headache, papilledema and vomiting without nausea, especially in the early morning).

Progressive bulbar palsy. This is the most frequent cause of atrophic paresis of the tongue. It also involves swallowing and causes dysarthric speech. Sooner or later lower motor neuron disease is combined with upper motor neuron disease and the masseter reflex is then enhanced.

Insufficiency of the vertebro-basilar blood supply. This can induce vertigo, especially upon rotation or hyperextension of the head, drop attacks, occipital headache, short-lasting diplopia or blurring of vision, and other transient signs of damage to the brainstem, cerebellum, thalamus and occipital lobe.

Pontine tegmentum. Ipsilateral paralysis of horizontal gaze with ipsilateral loss of optokinetic and vestibular nystagmus is accompanied by a slight contralateral spontaneous nystagmus, and often by ipsilateral paralysis of the abducens and facial nerves.

Medial longitudinal fasciculus. Internuclear opthalmoplegia (slower eye movement in the nasal direction during horizontal saccades, combined with a dissociated gaze nystagmus on attempted lateral gaze).

Mesencephalic tegmentum and pretectal region. Vertical gaze paralysis, retractory nystagmus, disturbance of pupillary light reflex (Parinaud's syndrome).

Cerebellum. Dysmetria of saccadic eye or limb movements, adiadochokinesia, cerebellar type of speech disturbance, postural (intention) tremor, pendular fixation nystagmus, gaze nystagmus; when the flocculo-nodular lobe is involved, there is positional nystagmus of the central type.

Forebrain (subcortical white matter). Diminution of optokinetic nystagmus to the contralateral side occurs without gaze nystagmus or spontaneous nystagmus. Gaze paresis is obvious only in the acute state, but gaze preference or contralateral inattention to visual and somatic stimuli may last for a long time.

C. Etiological Diagnosis

While otoneurological findings may often help in topographical diagnosis, an etiological diagnosis can be made only in the case of congenital nystagmus. In all other cases, otoneurological findings allow only diagnostic hypotheses. Rotating jerky spontaneous nystagmus occurs most often with syringobulbia or Wallenberg's syndrome. Vestibular hyperresponsiveness and periodically alternating spontaneous nystagmus occur most often in multiple sclerosis and syringobulbia.

Internuclear opthalmoplegia is most often due to multiple sclerosis. Positional nystagmus of the central type without additional spontaneous nystagmus in the upright sitting position is often due to intoxication. Gradually occurring unilateral loss of caloric reaction without vertigo should arouse suspicion of an acoustic neuroma. There are also many negative correlations, for instance, Menière's disease does not cause gaze nystagmus.

References

ALESSI, D.: Lesioni parenchimatose del cerbelleto da carcinoma uterino (Gliosi carcinotossica) Sintom atologia dissinergico-mioclonica. Riv. Pat nerv. ment. **55**, 148–174 (1940).

ARSLAN, M.: On the renewing of the methodology for the stimulation of the vestibular apparatus. Acta oto-laryng. (Stockh.) Suppl. **122** (1955).

ASCHAN, G., BERGSTEDT, M., STAHLE, J.: Nystagmography. Acta oto-laryng. (Stockh.) Suppl. **129** (1956).

ASCHOFF, J.C.: Reconsideration of the oculomotor pathway. pp. 305–310. In: F. O. SCHMITT and F.G. WORDEN, Eds. The neurosciences, Third Study Program. Cambridge: MIT press 1974.

ASCHOFF, J.C., CONRAD, B., KORNHUBER, H.H.: Acquired pendular nystagmus with oscillopsia in multiple sclerosis: a sign of cerebellar nuclei disease. J. Neurol., Neurosurg. Psychiat. **37**, 570–577 (1974).

BADER, W., KORNHUBER, H.H.: Großhirnläsionen und vestibulärer Nystagmus. Vergleichende elektronystagmographische Untersuchungen bei geschlossenen Augen und mit visueller Fixation. Acta oto-laryng. (Stockh.) **60**, 197–206 (1965).

BAKER, A.B. (Ed.): Clinical Neurology, 2nd Edition. New York: Hoeber-Harper reprinted 1965.

BÁRÁNY, R.: Physiologie und Pathologie des Bogengangsapparates. Wien: Deuticke 1907.

BARBER, H.O., WRIGHT, G.: Positional nystagmus in normals. Advanc. Oto-rhino-laryng. **19**, 276–285 (1973).

BARTELS, M.: Beobachtungen an Wirbeltieren und Menschen über unwillkürliche Augenbewegungen bei Störungen des Sehens. 2. Beobachtungen an Menschen. Klin. Mbl. Augenheilk. **80**, 145–176 (1928).

BECKER, W., KLEIN, H.M.: Accuracy of saccadic eye movements and maintenance of excentric eye positions in the dark. Vision Res. **13**, 1021–1034 (1973).

BECHINGER, D., KRIEBEL, J., SCHLAGER, M.: Das Schlafentzug-EEG, ein wichtiges diagnostisches Hilfsmittel bei cerebralen Anfällen. Z. Neurol. **205**, 193–206 (1973).

BENDER, M. B., SHANZER, S.: Oculomotor pathways defined by electrical stimulation and lesions in the brain stem of monkey. pp. 81–140. In: M. B. BENDER, Ed. The Oculomotor System. New York: Hoeber 1964.

BENDER, M.B., WEINSTEIN, E.A.: Effects of stimulation and lesion of the median longitudinal fasciculus in the monkey. Arch. Neurol. Psychiat. (Chic.) **52**, 106–113 (1944).

BRAY, P.F., ZITER, F.A., LAHEY, M.E., MYERS, G.G.: The coincidence of neuroblastoma and acute cerebellar encephalopathy. Trans. Amer. neurol. Ass. **94**, 106–109 (1969).

CARMICHAEL, E.A., DIX, M.R., HALLPIKE, C.S.: Lesions of the cerebral hemispheres and their effects upon optokinetic and caloric nystagmus. Brain **77**, 345–372 (1954).

COHEN, B.: Vestibulo-ocular relations. pp. 105–148. In: P. BACH-Y-RITA and C. C. COLLINS, Eds. The Control of Eye Movements. New York: Academic Press 1971.

COHEN, B., HENN, V.: The origin of quick phases of nystagmus in the horizontal plane. Bibl. ophthal. (Basel) **82**, 36–55 (1972).

COHEN, L.A.: Role of eye and neck proprioceptive mechanisms in body orientation and motor coordination. J. Neurophysiol. **24**, 1–11 (1961).

CHOW, K.L., RIESEN, A.H., NEWELL, F.W.: Degeneration of retinal ganglion cells in infant chimpanzees reared in darkness. J. comp. Neurol. **107**, 27–40 (1957).

DECHER, H.: Zur Bestimmung der Drehreizschwellen bei Normalfällen. Z. Laryng. Rhinol. **41**, 838–844 (1962).

DICHGANS, J., KORNHUBER, H.H.: Eine seltene Art des hereditären Nystagmus mit autosomal-dominantem Erbgang und besonderem Erscheinungsbild: vertikale Nystagmuskomponente und Störung des vertikalen und horizontalen optokinetischen Nystagmus. Acta genet. (Basel) **14**, 240–250 (1964).

DIX, M.R., HALLPIKE, C.S.: The pathology, symptomatology and diagnosis of certain common disorders of the vestibular system. Proc. roy. Soc. Med. **45**, 341–354 (1952).

DOHLMAN, G.: Experimentelle Untersuchungen über die galvanische Vestibularisreaktion. Acta oto-laryng. (Stockh.) Suppl. **8** (1929).

FERNÁNDEZ, C.: Interrelations between flocculonodular lobe and vestibular system. pp. 285–296. In: G. L. RASMUSSEN and W. F. WINDLE, Eds. Neural mechanisms of the auditory and vestibular systems. Springfiled: C. C. Thomas 1960.

FITZGERALD, G., HALLPIKE, C.S.: Studies in human vestibular function: I. Observations on the directional preponderance ("Nystagmusbereitschaft") of caloric nystagmus resulting from cerebral lesions. Brain **65**, 115–137 (1942).

FLUUR, E., ERIKSSON, L.: Nystagmographic recording of vertical eye movements. Acta oto-laryng. (Stockh.) **53**, 486–492 (1961).

FREDRICKSON, J.M., FERNÁNDEZ, C.: Vestibular disorders in fourth ventricle lesions. Arch. Otolaryng. **80**, 521 (1964).

FREDRICKSSON, J.M., SCHWARZ, D., KORNHUBER, H.H.: Convergence and interaction of vestibular and deep somatic afferents upon neurons in the vestibular nuclei of the cat. Acta oto-laryng. (Stockh.) **61**, 168–188 (1965).

FRENZEL, H.: Tumoren im Bereich des 4. Ventrikels mit regelwidriger Schlagrichtung des kalorischen Nystagmus. Klin. Wschr. 802 (1932).

FRENZEL, H.: Spontan- und Provokationsnystagmus als Krankheitssymptom. Berlin-Göttingen-Heidelberg: Springer 1955.

FRENZEL, H.: Zur Systematik, Klinik und Untersuchungsmethodik der Vestibularisstörungen. Arch. Ohr.-, Nas.-, u. Kehlk.-Heilk. **177**, 353–395 (1961).

GASTAUT, H.: Un aspect méconnu des décharges neuroniques occipitales: la crise oculoclonique ou "nystagmus épileptique". In: T. H. ALAJOUANINE, Ed. Les grandes activités du lobe occipital. Paris: Masson et Cie. 1960.

GRANT, G., ASCHAN, G., EKVALL, L.: Nystagmus produced by localized cerebellar lesions. Acta oto-laryng. (Stockh.) Suppl. **192**, 78–84 (1964).

GREINER, G.F., CONRAUX, C., PICART, P.: La stimulation vestibulaire rotatoire de forme pendulaire et ses applications cliniques. Confin. neurol. (Basel) **21**, 438–446 (1961).

GÜNTHER, W.: Das Verhalten des Nystagmus im Anfall bei der Menière'schen Krankheit. HNO-Wegweiser (Berl.) **9**, 97–101 (1961).

HAKAS, P., KORNHUBER, H.H.: Der vestibuläre Nystagmus bei Großhirnläsionen des Menschen. Arch. Psychiat. Nervenkr. **200**, 19–35 (1959).

HAMERSMA, H.: The Caloric Test. Bergen-op-Zoom: Gebr. Juten 1957.

HASSLER, R.: Supranuclear structures regulating binocular eye and head movements. Bibl. ophthal. (Basel) **82**, 207–219 (1972).

HÉCAEN, H., AJURIAGUERRA, J. DE: Balint's syndrome (psychic paralysis of visual fixation) and its minor forms. Brain **77**, 373–400 (1954).

HENRIKSSON, N.G.: An electric method for registration and analysis of the movements of the eyes in nystagmus. Acta oto-laryng. (Stockh.) **45**, 25–41 (1955).

HENRIKSSON, N.G., DOLOWITZ, D.A., FORSSMAN, B.: Studies of cristospinal reflexes (laterotorsion). I. A method for objective recording of cristospinal reflex. Acta oto-laryng. (Stockh.) **55**, 33–40 (1962).

JATHO, K.: Experimentelle Untersuchungen zum objektiven Nachweis des Dandy'schen Symptoms bei einseitigem und beiderseitigem Verlust der Vestibularisfunktion. Arch. Ohr.-, Nas.-, u. Kehlk.-Heilk. **177**, 230–254 (1961).

JONG, J.M.B.V. DE: Over cervicale nystagmus en aanverwante verschijnselen. Amsterdam: Thesis 1967.

JONG, P.T.V.M. DE: Cervical proprioceptive nystagmus; its central pathways. Amsterdam: Thesis 1973.

JONGKEES, L.B.W.: Physiologie und Pathophysiologie des Vestibularorganes. Arch. Ohr.-, Nas.-, u. Kehlk.-Heilk. **194**, 1–110 (1969).

JUNG, R.: Nystagmographie: Zur Physiologie und Pathologie des optisch-vestibulären Systems beim Menschen. In: G. v. BERGMANN et al., Eds. Handbuch der inneren Medizin, 4. Ed., Vol. V/1, p. 1325. Berlin-Göttingen-Heidelberg: Springer 1953.

JUNG, R., KORNHUBER, H.H.: Results of electronystagmography in man: the value of optokinetic, vestibular and spontaneous nystagmus for neurologic diagnosis and research. pp. 428–482. In: M. B. BENDER, Ed. The Oculomotor System. New York: Hoeber 1964.

KAMEI, T., KORNHUBER, H.H.: Spontaneous and head-shaking nystagmus in normals and in patients with central lesions. Canad. J. Oto-laryng. **3**, 372–380 (1974).

KESER, H.: Untersuchungen über die physiologischen Eigenschaften des Drehnystagmus beim Gesunden. Freiburg i. Br.: Thesis 1950.

KIRSTEIN, R.: Zur klinischen Bedeutung der Vestibularisprüfung mit niederfrequentem Wechselstrom. Arch. Ohr.-, Nas.-, u. Kehlk.-Heilk. **155**, 75–81 (1949).

KLEYN, A. DE, VERSTEEGH, C.: Über die Unabhängigkeit des Dunkelnystagmus der Hunde vom Labyrinth. Graefes Arch. Ophthal. **101**, 228 (1920).

KNAPP, E.: Kommt Spontannystagmus bei Gesunden vor? HNO-Wegweiser (Berl.) **2**, 17–19 (1950).

KORNHUBER, H.H.: Der periodisch alternierende Nystagmus (Nystagmus alternans) und die Enthemmung des vestibulären Systems. Arch. Ohr.-, Nas.-, u. Kehlk.-Heilk. **174**, 182–209 (1959)

KORNHUBER, H.H.: Über Begleitschielen und latenten Nystagmus aus neurologischer Sicht. Sitzungsber. Rhein.-Westf. Augenärzte, 102. Versammlung. Balve i. W.: Gebr. Zimmermann 1960.

KORNHUBER, H.H.: Optic and vestibular factors in motor coordination Proc. 22. Internat. Congr. Physiol. Sci. Excerpta Med. int. Congr. Ser. No. **47**, 1, 515 (1962).

KORNHUBER, H.H.: Über häufige, aber wenig beachtete Arten von Nystagmus und Schwindel: paroxysmaler Lageschwindel und latenter Fixationsnystagmus. Nervenarzt **36**, 361–362 (1965).

KORNHUBER, H.H.: Physiologie und Klinik des zentralvestibulären Systems (Blick- und Stützmotorik). In: J. BERENDES, R. LINK and F. ZÖLLNER, Eds. Hals-Nasen-Ohrenheilkunde, Handbook, Vol. III, part 3, pp. 2150–2351. Stuttgart: G. Thieme 1966.

KORNHUBER, H.H.: Physiologie und Klinik des vestibulären Systems. Arch. klin. exp. Ohr.-, Nas.-, u. Kehlk.-Heilk. **194**, 111–148 (1969).

KORNHUBER, H.H.: Das vestibuläre System, mit Exkursen über die motorischen Funktionen der Formatio reticularis, des Kleinhirns, der Stammganglien und des motorischen Cortex sowie über die Raumkonstanz der Sehdinge. pp. 173–204. In: W. D. KEIDEL and K.-H. PLATTIG, Eds. Vorträge der Erlanger Physiologentagung 1970. Berlin-Heidelberg-New York: Springer 1971.

KORNHUBER, H.H., WALDECKER, G.: Akute isolierte periphere Vestibularisstörungen. Arch. Ohr.-, Nas.-, u. Kehlk.-Heilk. **173**, 340–346 (1958).

LANGE, G., KORNHUBER, H.H.: Zur Bedeutung peripher- und zentral-vestibulärer Störungen nach Kopftraumen. Arch. Ohr.-, Nas.-, u. Kehlk.-Heilk. **179**, 366–385 (1962).

LEDOUX, A., DEMANEZ, J.P.: Nystagmographie les yeux ouverts ou fermés au cours de l'épreuve calorique. Acta oto-rhino-laryng. belg. **21**, 31–40 (1969).

LORENTE DE NÓ, R.: Vestibulo-ocular reflex arc. Arch. Neurol. (Chic.) **30**, 245–291 (1933).

MEIRY, J.L.: Vestibular and proprioceptive stabilization of eye movements. pp. 483–496. In: P. BACH-Y-RITA and C. C. COLLINS, Eds. The control of eye movements. New York: Academic Press 1971.

MIEHLKE, A.: Tierexperimentelle Untersuchungen über die Ursache und den Ort der Auslösung des peripheren Lagenystagmus. Arch. Ohr.-, Nas.-, u. Kehlk.-Heilk. **166**, 327–349 (1955).

MILOJEVIC, B.: Electronystagmographical study of vertigo. Pract. oto-rhino-laryng. (Basel) **29**, 85–94 (1967).

MONTANDON, A., RUSSBACH, A.: L'épreuve giratoire liminaire. Pract. oto-rhino-laryng. (Basel) **17**, 224–236 (1955).

MUSKENS, L.J.J.: Das supra-vestibuläre System bei den Tieren und beim Menschen, mit besonderer Berücksichtigung der Klinik der Blicklähmungen, der sog. Stirnhirnataxie, der Zwangsstellungen und der Zwangsbewegungen. Amsterdam: N.V. Noord-Hollandsche Uitgeversmaatschappij 1934.

NYLEN, C.O.: A clinical study on positional nystagmus in cases of brain tumour. Acta oto-laryng. (Stockh.) Suppl. **15** (1931).

OHM, J.: Nachlese auf dem Gebiete des Augenzitterns der Bergleute. Stuttgart: F. Enke 1954.

PASIK, P., PASIK, T.: Oculomotor functions in monkeys with lesions of the cerebrum and the superior colliculi. pp. 40–80. In: M. B. BENDER, Ed. The Oculomotor System. New York: Hoeber 1964a.

PASIK, T., PASIK, P.: Optokinetic nystagmus: an unlearned response altered by section of chiasma and corpus callosum in monkeys. Nature (Lond.) **203**, 609–611 (1964b).

PASIK, P., PASIK, T., BENDER, M.B.: The pretectal syndrome in monkeys. I. Disturbances of gaze and body posture. Brain **92**, 521–534 (1969).

RATLIFF, F., RIGGS, L.A.: Involuntary motions of the eye during monocular fixation. J. exp. Psychol. **40**, 687–701 (1950).

RIESCO-MACCLURE, J.S., MARTINEZ, A.: Nistagmus pervertido: Estudio clinico e histopatológico. Rev. Otorrinolaring. (Santiago) **17**, 1 (1957).

RIESEN, A.H.: Effects of stimulus deprivation on the development and atrophy of the visual sensory system. Amer. J. Orthopsychiat. **30**, 23–26 (1960).

SANDSTRÖM, J.: Cervical syndrome with vestibular symptoms. Acta oto-laryng. (Stockh.) **54**, 207–226 (1961).

SATTLER, C.H., BLOHMKE, A.: Zur Ätiologie des Dunkelzitterns. Z. Augenheilk. **54**, 282–286 (1925).

SCHILLER, P.H.: Some functional characteristics of the superior colliculus of the rhesus monkey. Bibl. ophthal. (Basel) **82**, 122–129 (1972).

SCHMALTZ, G.: The physical phenomena occurring in the semicircular canals during rotatory and thermic stimulation. Proc. roy. Soc. Med. **25**, 360–381 (1932).

SOLOMON, G.E., CHUTORIAN, A.M.: Opsoclonus and occult neuroblastoma. New Engl. J. Med. **279**, 475–477 (1968).

STARK, G.: Die normale vestibuläre Übergangsfunktion, eine experimentelle Untersuchung des Ablaufs des postrotatorischen Nystagmus. Freiburg i. Br.: Thesis 1964.

STENGER, H.H.: Über Lagerungsnystagmus unter besonderer Berücksichtigung des gegenläufigen transitorischen Provokationsnystagmus bei Lagewechsel in der Sagittalebene. Arch. Ohr.-, Nas.-, u. Kehl.-Heilk. **168**, 220–268 (1955).

STENGER, H.H.: Erholungsnystagmus nach einseitigem Vestibularisausfall, ein dem Bechterew-Nystagmus verwandter Vorgang. Arch. Ohr.-, Nas.-, u. Kehlk.-Heilk. **175**, 545–549 (1959).

SZENTÁGOTHAI, J.: Die zentrale Innervation der Augenbewegungen. Arch. Psychiat. Nervenkr. **116**, 721–760 (1943).

TOROK, N.: Significance of the frequency in caloric nystagmus. Acta oto-laryng. (Stockh.) **36**, 38–50 (1948).

TOROK, N.: The culmination phenomenon and frequency pattern of thermic nystagmus. Acta oto-laryng. (Stockh.) **48**, 530–535 (1957).

TOROK, N., GUILLEMEN, V., BARNOTHY, I.M.: Photoelectric nystagmography. Ann. Otol. (St. Louis) **60**, 917–926 (1951).

UEMURA, T., COHEN, B.: Vestibulo-ocular reflexes: effects of vestibular nuclear lesions. pp. 515–528. In: A. BRODAL and O. POMPEIANO, Eds. Basic Aspects of Central Vestibular Mechanisms, Progress in Brain Research, Vol. 37. Amsterdam: Elsevier 1972.

UNTERBERGER, S.: Neue objektiv registrierbare Vestibularis-Drehreaktion, erhalten durch Treten auf der Stelle. Der "Tretversuch". Arch. Ohr.-, Nas.-, u. Kehlk.-Heilk. **145**, 478–492 (1938)

VEITS, C.: Zur Technik der kalorischen Schwachreizuntersuchung. Z. Hals-, Nas.- u. Ohrenheilk. **19**, 542 (1928).

VISSER, S.L.: Some aspects of evaluating electronystagmographic examination in clinical neurology. Psychiat. Neurol. Neurochir. (Amst.) **66**, 24–44 (1963).

VLIET, A.G.M. VAN, WAARDENBURG, P.J., FORSIUS, H., ERIKSSON, A.W.: Nystagmographical studies in Åland eye disease. Acta ophthal. (Kbh.) **51**, 782–790 (1973).

WAGMAN, I.H.: Eye movements induced by electrical stimulation of cerebrum in monkeys and their relationship to bodily movements. pp. 18–39. In: M. B. BENDER, Ed. The Oculomotor System. New York: Hoeber 1964.

WÜST, H.: Untersuchungen des Vestibularapparates mit neuen Drehschwachreizmethoden. Arch. Ohr.-, Nas.-, u. Kehlk.-Heilk. **168**, 414–428 (1956).

WURTZ, R.H., GOLDBERG, M.E.: Activity of superior colliculus in behaving monkey. IV. Effects of lesions on eye movements. J. Neurophysiol. **35**, 587–598 (1972).

YOUNGERMANN, W.M.: Kommt Spontannystagmus bei Gesunden vor? Arch. Ohr.-, Nas.-, u. Kehlk.-Heilk. **136**, 314–317 (1933).

Chapter II.

Measurement of Otolith Function in Man* **

By

A. Graybiel, Pensacola, Florida (USA)

With 19 Figures

Contents

I. Introduction

Despite the great importance of defining the isolated role of the otolithic system in man, progress toward a definition has been predictably slow due to difficulties inherent in the study of its input-output relations. These difficulties include the

* First published under the title "Otolith Function and Human Performance" in Adv. Oto-Rhino-Laryng., vol. 20, pp. 485–519 (Basel: Karger, 1973).

** This research was conducted under the sponsorship of the Biomedical Research Office, Order No. T–81633, and the Space Life Sciences Office, Order L–43518, National Aeronautics and Space Administration.

need to manipulate and measure stimuli to the otolithic receptors eliciting specific quantifiable responses, at the same time taking into account the roles played by other sensory systems, notably the canalicular and visual systems and the components of the somatosensory system serving touch, pressure, and kinesthesis. The difficulties in measuring otolithic influence on behavior must also be included, and paradoxically, this applies more to enhancement than to decrement in performance. The discussion to follow is divided into two parts, the first dealing briefly with experimental variables and the second with some experimental and clinical findings with implications for the role of the otolith system in the human economy.

II. Experimental Methods

A. Manipulation of Stimulus Variables

1. Human Subjects

In our laboratory we use a battery of vestibular tests designed to provide a comprehensive assessment of all persons used as research subjects or referred with possible vestibular disorders. Speech discrimination and SISI tests are conducted in addition to audiometry; loss of hearing that cannot be explained by acoustic trauma raises the question of whether the nonacoustic labyrinth has also been affected by the same disease process because of the structural proximity and the commonality of certain features of these two divisions of the inner ear. Intra- and extraocular muscle function is tested, and is considered to be more important than tests of visual acuity because of the great vestibular influence on eye-muscle tonus. Reliance is placed on a routine neurological examination for the functional evaluation of receptor systems serving touch, pressure, and kinesthesis (TPK systems); it is evident that under some stimulus conditions, e.g., weightlessness, water immersion, and supragravity states, distinctions can and should be made among the individual roles of these systems. Functional tests of the canalicular system are usually limited to evaluation of the horizontal pair of canals, but these are now being extended to include tests of vertical canal function, especially in the presence of any vestibular defect. Normal responses to usually suprathreshold stimulation of the canals are commonly interpreted as indicating "normal function of the vestibular organs," but in some instances abnormal counterrolling test values are found in association with normal canalicular responses [38]. The generalization stems from the fact that most clinicians do not possess the necessary equipment and procedures to test otolith function properly. In our laboratory we use ocular counterrolling [36, 37] and a postural equilibrium test battery [20] routinely, and, sometimes the oculogravic illusion test [18]. Very recently, the possibility of using earth-horizontal [5, 30, 32] or off-vertical rotation has been explored [23, 24, 52]. Occasionally, compensatory eye movements evoked by changes in the direction and magnitude of inertial force generated by four-pole swing are measured [34].

In evaluating subjects with vestibular defects, it is important to take into account the age at onset and the period over which active disease or its residual effects, i.e., hypo- or hyperexcitability with its resultant imbalance, was present. It is also important to determine the subject's susceptibility to motion sickness (history) prior to disease or injury, inasmuch as this reflects the basic or innate susceptibility of the person afflicted, for comparison with the existing susceptibility level. Off-vertical rotation makes it possible to explore the stressor effect of primary if not exclusive otolithic stimulation [52].

2. Mode of Stimulation

The effective stimulus to the otolith organs is generally agreed to be gravity or other inertial forces. However, the manner in which these organs are stimulated by these forces has not been established. Three general theories as to the possible modes of action of gravity upon the otoliths have been advanced: pull or traction, pressure, or stratification. While these theories have had their supporters, none can explain all the known facts. In addition, there has been some controversy over whether one of the pairs of otolith organs (saccules) has any equilibrial function at all. Anatomical and physiological evidence, however, indicates that the saccule functions in a similar and complementary way to the utricle [14, 36]. A theory based upon the ocular counterrolling response in man has been proposed by MILLER; he postulates that the otoliths (utricles and saccules) are stimulated maximally (in accord with a cosine^2 function of lateral tilt), by a shearing force applied inwardly, i.e. toward the median sagittal plane [36]. In some respects this theory conforms with that advanced by BREUER, who specified that "the 'gliding direction' of the otolith is that of its macular planes" [36]. He assumed that these "planes" were horizontal for the utricles and vertical for the saccules in a frontal section, and claimed that the effect of gravity on the nerve endings was proportional to the sine of the angle between the gliding direction and horizontal. BREUER also proposed that the otoliths (cilia) could be stimulated in opposite directions, giving rise to "behaviors" that were the reverse of each other. Recent investigations on the cat have indicated that distinct areas of otolithic sensory cells are activated when the stereocilia deviate toward the kinocilia (13, 14).

The majority of evidence to date, including data gathered in Menière's disease and in unilaterally labyrinthectomized patients [28, 57], tends to support the general theory of inward shearing: i.e. substantially less counterrolling in response to lateral tilt when the affected ear is superior. It should be noted, however, that a small percentage of patients have manifested the opposite response and even in the typical response, counterrolling when the affected ear is superior has never been found to be completely absent. An asymmetry index

$$\left(AI = \frac{\Sigma\, CR_1}{\Sigma\, CR_2} - 1.00 \times 100\right)$$

has been introduced to measure the relative difference between eye roll response to rightward and leftward tilt [38]. Clinically, these measurements are of value since they offer the means to differentiate the relative function of the right and left otolith organs in a manner analogous to (although not as clear-cut as) independent investigation of each lateral canal by caloric irrigation.

3. Manipulating the Force Environment

Subgravity levels can be generated in parabolic flight, and supragravity levels are readily generated and manipulated on human centrifuges. Water immersion minimizes stimulation of TPK receptor systems [8, 234] without influencing the gravitational load on the otolith receptors, and centrifugation under water with

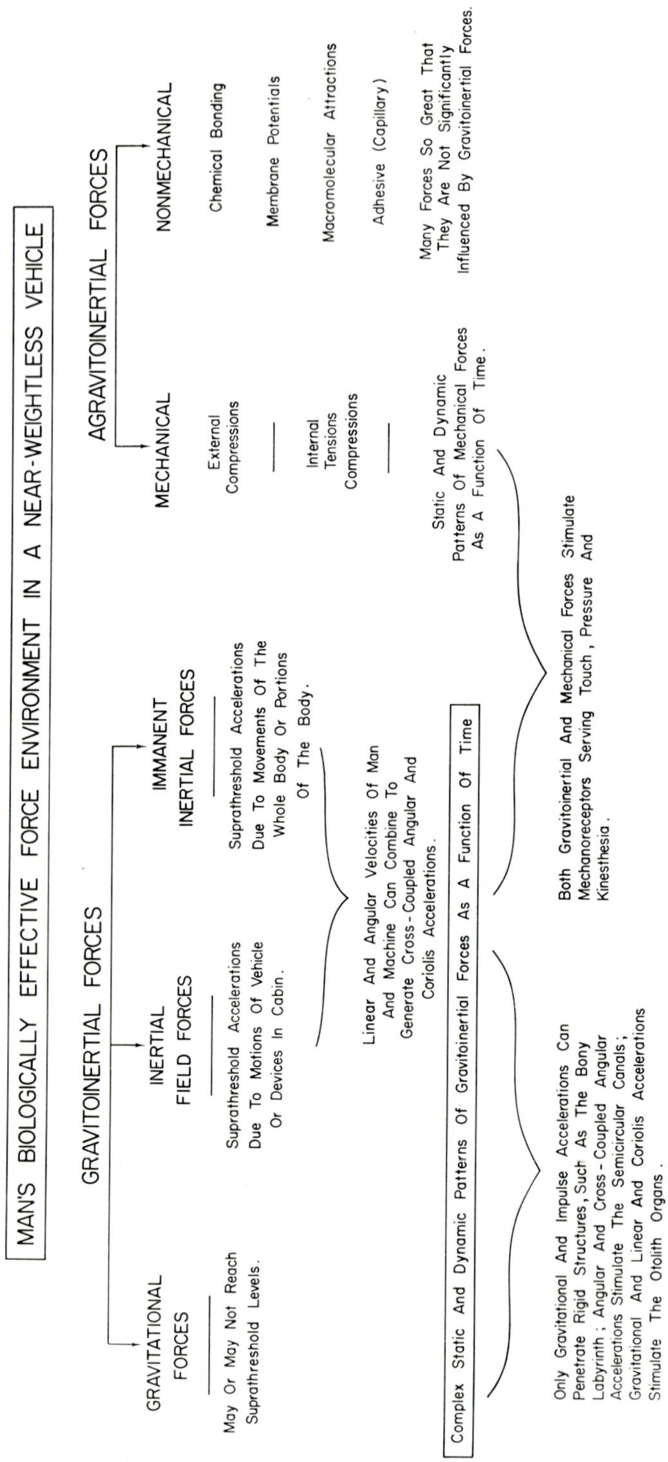

Fig. 1. Man's biologically effective force environment in a near-weightless state

proper subject support [26] can increase the gravitoinertial load on the otoliths without a comparable effect on the TPK systems.

Among the procedures for manipulating the force environment, none equals the transition into weightlessness in elegance and importance, especially in orbital flight but also in parabolic flight. The effects of this transition are highly instructive and will be briefly summarized with the aid of Fig. 1. In near-weightlessness the distinction between gravitoinertial and agravitoinertial forces represents a logical and convenient dichotomy. Gravitoinertial forces are so small in near-weightlessness that they do not contribute significantly to total body weight, a circumstance standing in sharp contrast to stimulus conditions on Earth: The gravitational potential is minute and inertial field forces likewise minute, unless generated by man. Only the accelerations generated in the course of man's work and housekeeping activities, resulting in immanent inertial forces, are of practical significance, and this is mainly because they stimulate sensory receptors and thus contribute to the flow of information to the nervous system.

The reduction of gravitoinertial forces in near-weightlessness has sharply different effects on the otolith organs and semicircular canals. In the case of the semicircular canals, these transient impulse angular accelerations are virtually identical to those generated under terrestrial conditions. By contrast, stimulation of the otolith receptors (by transient linear accelerations) is very different from that under terrestrial conditions, and stimulation of receptors serving touch, pressure, and kinesthesia (TPK) by gravitoinertial forces is also far less than under terrestrial conditions.

The preservation of man's well-being in a weightless spacecraft is heavily dependent on the second major category we distinguish, the agravitoinertial forces, which can in turn be divided into agravitoinertial forces of mechanical and non-mechanical origin (Fig. 1). With regard to the latter, further distinctions are possible, ranging between one extreme where forces are so great that absence of gravitational force is of no practical consequence, and the other extreme where its influence is felt.

The agravitoinertial mechanical forces are generated by tensions and compressions, and along with gravitoinertial forces they contribute to bodily deformations and to stimulation of TPK mechanoreceptors but not the receptors in the vestibular organs.

B. Elicitation of Meaningful Responses

Behavioral responses always challenge the investigator not only to elucidate the central nervous system mechanisms underlying them, but also to evaluate their beneficial or harmful effects. It is generally agreed that one of the useful ways in which the otolith organs serve man is in his perception of space.

Figure 2 shows a simplified analysis of the source of cues for the perception of personal and extrapersonal space based on earth reference. The direction and sense of the vector representing gravitational force indicates the upright, and the addition of mutually perpendicular lines forms the spatial frame of earth reference. Changes in position of the body relative to gravity introduce dynamic effects. The great concordance between cues from the gravitational and visual environments is

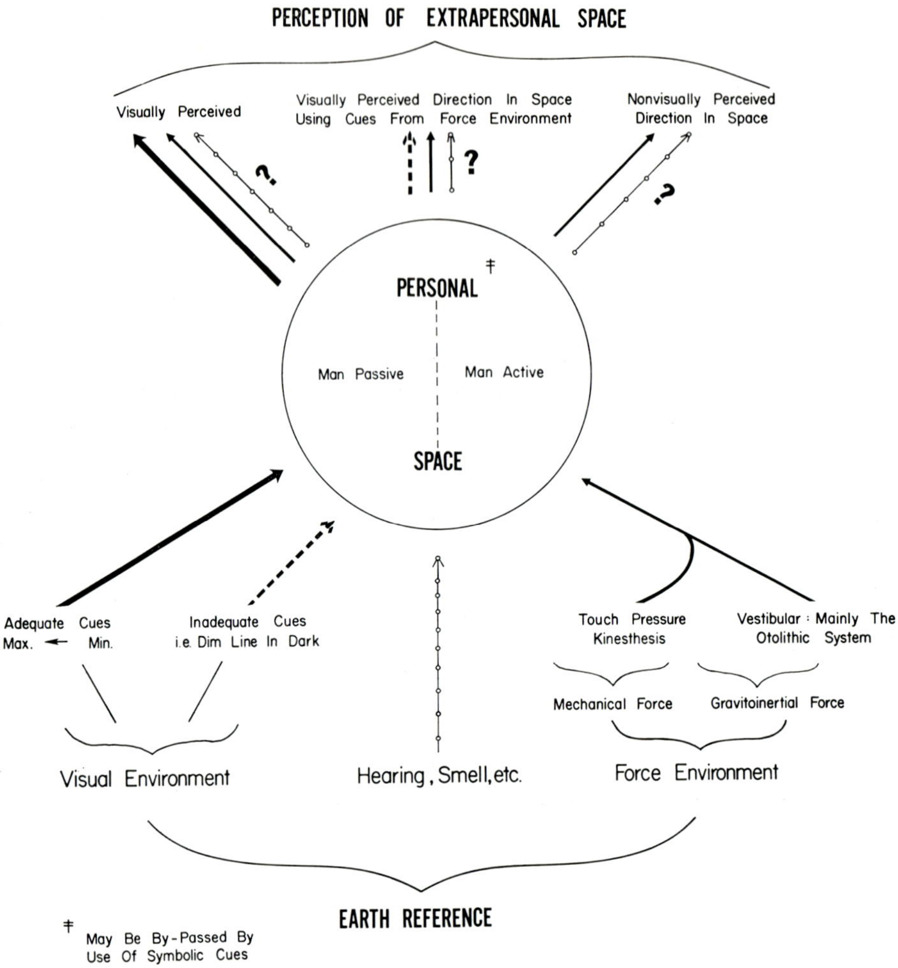

Fig. 2. Perception of extrapersonal space

obvious in natural environments and even more so in artificial ones based on the gravitational coordinate system. Both the perceived direction of personal and extrapersonal space have been investigated, with the aid of either a dim line of light in darkness or a rod or pointer to indicate the vertical. Interactions between the visual and force environments have been studied in darkness and in lighted cubicles and rooms.

The influence of otolithic cues on perception of the upright can be determined by the subject's perception of the postural vertical when a tilt device is used, and by his ability to maintain postural equilibrium under static and dynamic conditions.

Decrements in performance have been investigated by exposure of the subject to unusual gravitoinertial force environments, with particular emphasis on selective stimulation of the otolithic component of the non-acoustic labyrinth so as to elicit illusions, abnormal eye motions, postural disequilibrium, pastpointing, and motion sickness.

III. Selected Experimental Findings

A. Ocular Counterrolling

Ocular torsion can be defined as the involuntary conjugate rolling movement of the eyes around their lines of sight in the direction opposite to the leftward or rightward tilted position of the head (and body) relative to the gravitational or gravitoinertial upright. The measurements of ocular counterrolling can be made from photographs of natural iris landmarks obtained in the upright and tilt positions. The subject's participation is confined to the unilateral fixation of a dim light in the darkness just prior to recording by means of an electronic flash; hence, counterrolling qualifies as a naturally elicited reflex response. The amount of roll is measured in minutes of arc and often expressed as an index [43] defined as one half the sum of the maximum roll associated with the range of leftward and rightward tilt employed. With a tilt range of 50° the index in 95% of apparently normals subjects varies from about 120 to 500, with a mode of 320 and a mean of 344 min of arc [38]. In a group of deaf persons with bilateral labyrinthine defects (L–D subjects) the index varied from 15 to 131, with a mean of 69.

Ocular counterrolling has been measured in normal persons and L–D subjects tilted relative to the gravitational upright under terrestrial conditions [12, 43], under fractional gravitational levels in parabolic flight [44, 55], and during tilting relative to the gravitoinertial upright on a human centrifuge [48, 71]. Figure 3 compares the amount of roll as a function of G loading (0 G, 0.5 G, and 1.0 G) in

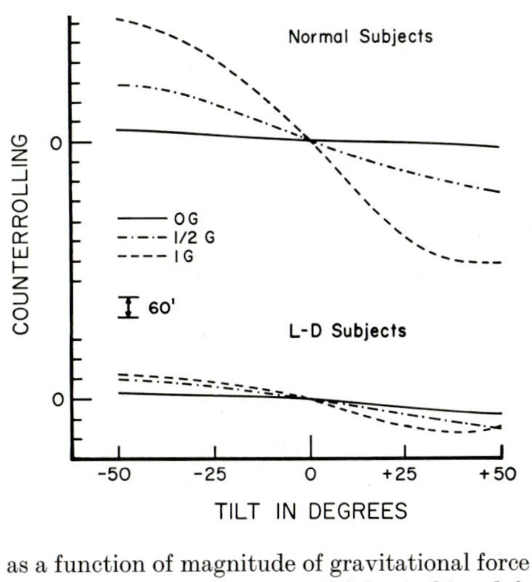

Fig. 3. Counterrolling as a function of magnitude of gravitational force and body position with respect to direction of force in normal and labyrinthine-defective subjects

seven normal and six labyrinthine-defective (L–D) subjects. (Note the lack of linearity in normal subjects and the relatively small change in L–D subjects). Figure 4 [48] compares the amount of roll during tilt as a function of G loading

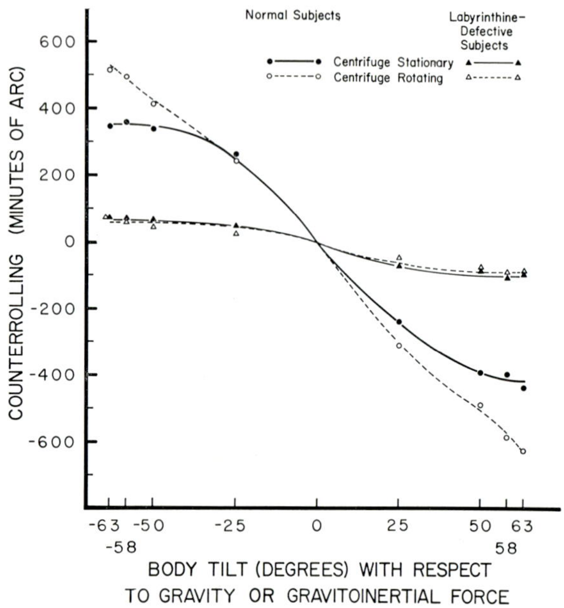

Fig. 4. Counterrolling of normal and labyrinthine-defective subject groups as a function of body tilt with respect to gravitational or gravitoinertial force

in six normal and five L–D subjects. It is interesting to note that although in normal subjects there is a meaningful relationship between the degrees of tilt and counterroll throughout the entire range of G levels, in L–D subjects there was little change in roll associated with hypergravic forces. However, the small residual amount of counterrolling manifested by the L–D subjects in 1 G could be even further reduced, in a manner qualitatively similar to that in normal subjects, by counteracting the normal gravitational effect [55].

Figure 5 shows a log plot with extensions into the supragravity range based on data from other experiments [38, 44]. At the lunar standard of gravity (under static conditions) the amount of counterroll is just detectable above the mean level of spontaneous variations; the response becomes linear, i.e. proportional to the log of the stimulus, at around 0.6 G. The upper limit to this logarithmicity has not been determined. The problem of response decline as a function of length of exposure has been the subject of another experiment. The findings clearly demonstrate that while there was considerable intrasubject variation in response, there was no significant decline in ocular counterrolling on exposure over a period of about 8 hours, implying that the behavioral effect of the stimulus of gravity was continuous [50].

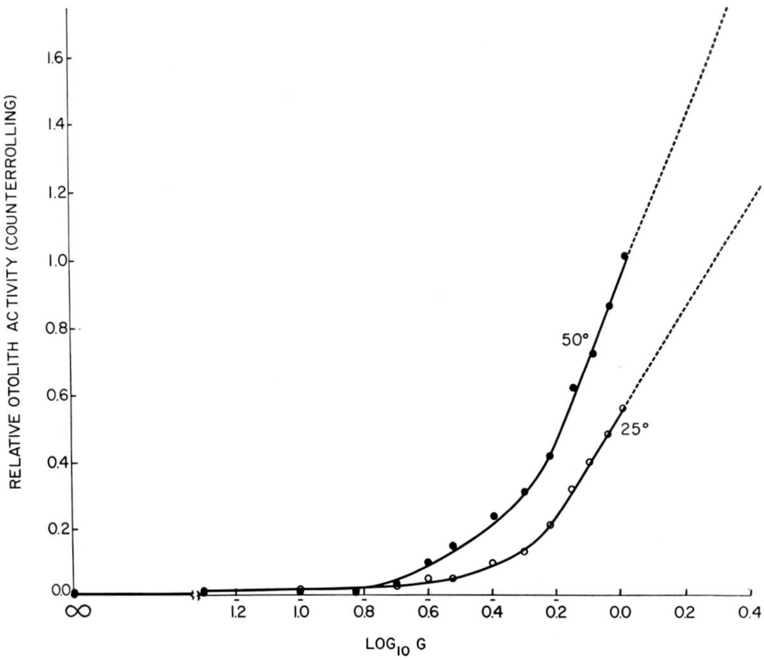

Fig. 5. Relation of otolith activity to the logarithm of the gravitational stimulus

B. The Influence of Nonvisual Cues on the Visually Perceived Direction of Space

A dim line of light in darkness does not furnish an adequate visual cue to the vertical or horizontal, but by causing it to rotate a subject has a means of indicating his estimates of the upright with reference to his body or the external world. A miniature line-target system incorporated in a goggle device has recently been developed and used in our laboratory for measuring the perceived direction of space in the pitch as well as the roll plane under static and dynamic test conditions [51].

1. E and A Phenomena

Many investigators [4, 12, 39, 40, 42, 46, 63, 68, 70] since Aubert [3] and Müller [58] have explored the effects on perception of the apparent vertical or horizontal of tilting subjects in the gravitational field. With leftward or rightward tilt in the frontal plane a bias appears as an over-compensation and later as an under-compensation, respectively termed the E and A phenomena.

Bauermeister [4] has also demonstrated the effect of body tilt on apparent verticality in normal subjects (Fig. 6). His findings clearly indicate the existence of an internal and external spatial reference system.

Figure 7 shows curves depicting typical E and A phenomena obtained on a sophisticated subject. Curves were obtained on different days. Note that the curves tend to be nearly flat at small angles of tilt from the upright.

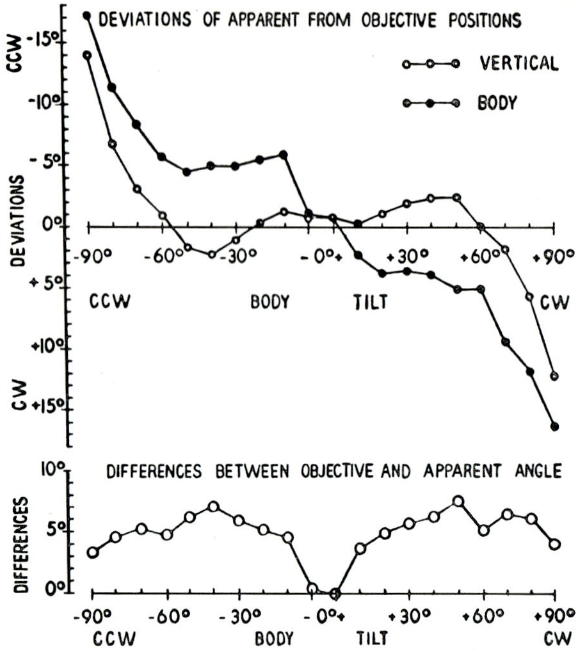

Fig. 6. Deviations of apparent from objective vertical and of apparent from objective body position under body tilt (upper part) and differences between apparent and objective angle of tilt (apparent angle always larger than objective angle) (lower part)

The change in E and A bias as a function of increasing G load was measured on the centrifuge by controlling the deviation of a freely swinging platform from the gravitoinertial upright [45]. In Fig. 8, the family of curves obtained from eight normal subjects shows the increase in E bias with increasing magnitude of force, and Fig. 9 shows the findings under similar conditions for two L–D subjects. Note that the change in the E and A phenomena occurs with smaller angles of tilt in L–D subjects than in normal subjects, and that the bias tends to be greater and the variance in the settings far greater.

When subjects fixate the luminous line while lying on their side, not only is the A phenomenon prominent, but also for some subjects, the line appears to rotate slowly clockwise and counterclockwise, a form of apparent motion (Fig. 10) [27, 42]. This rotary autokinesis and autokinesis for a point source of light was significantly greater in a group of individuals with bilateral vestibular defects, suggesting that the otolithic input tended to stabilize visual space [41]. This conclusion seems to be further supported by the disappearance of significant magnitudinal and variable differences in the judgments of visual upright by normal and L–D groups of subjects when their heads were inverted. In this position gravitational stimulation of the so-called otolithic blind spot was approached [46].

Fig. 7. Mean curves represent E and A phenomena of individual test sessions of one subject

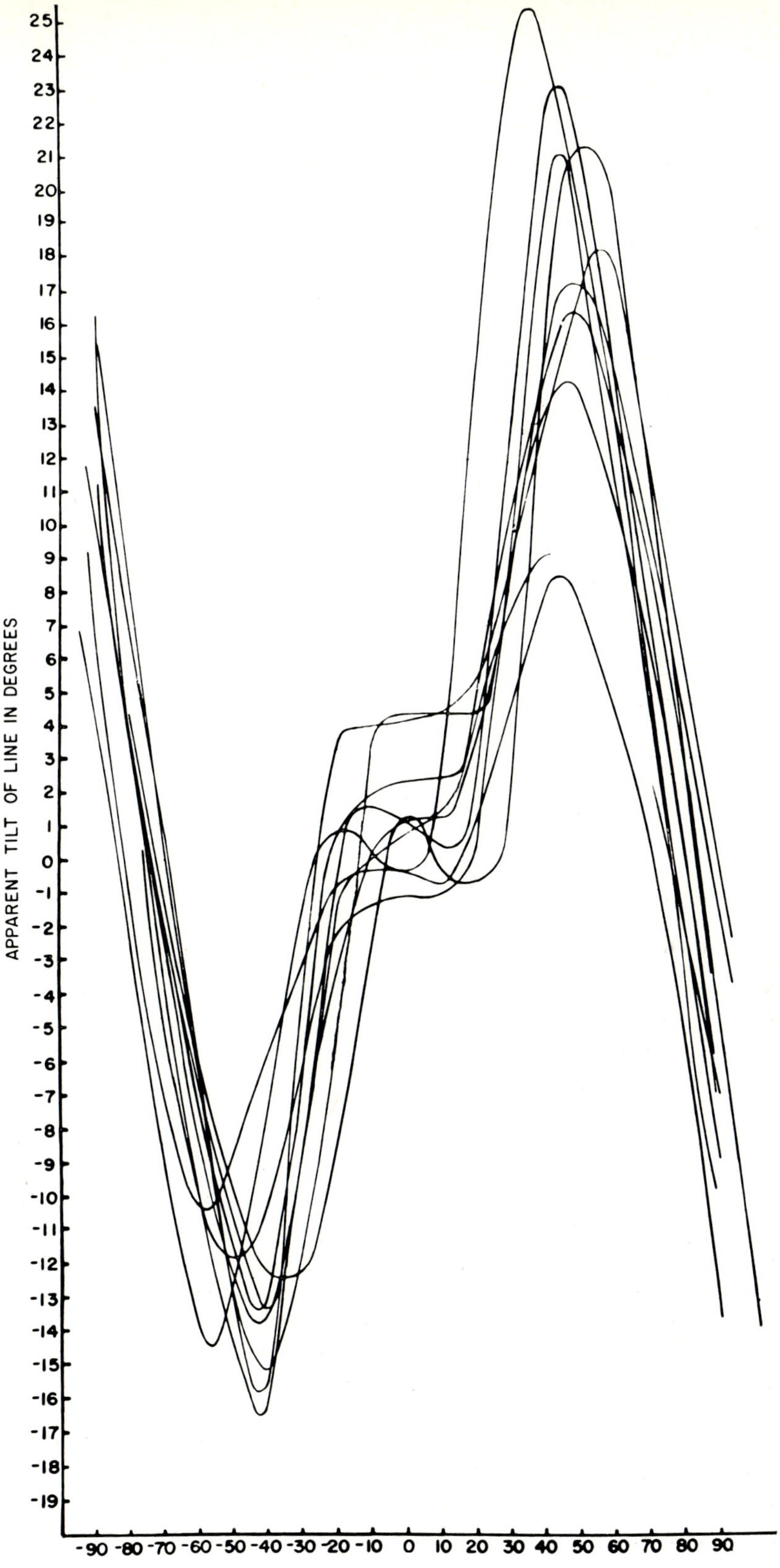
APPARENT TILT OF LINE IN DEGREES
25
24
23
22
21
20
19
18
17
16
15
14
13
12
11
10
9
8
7
6
5
4
3
2
1
0
-1
-2
-3
-4
-5
-6
-7
-8
-9
-10
-11
-12
-13
-14
-15
-16
-17
-18
-19
-90 -80 -70 -60 -50 -40 -30 -20 -10 0 10 20 30 40 50 60 70 80 90

Fig. 7

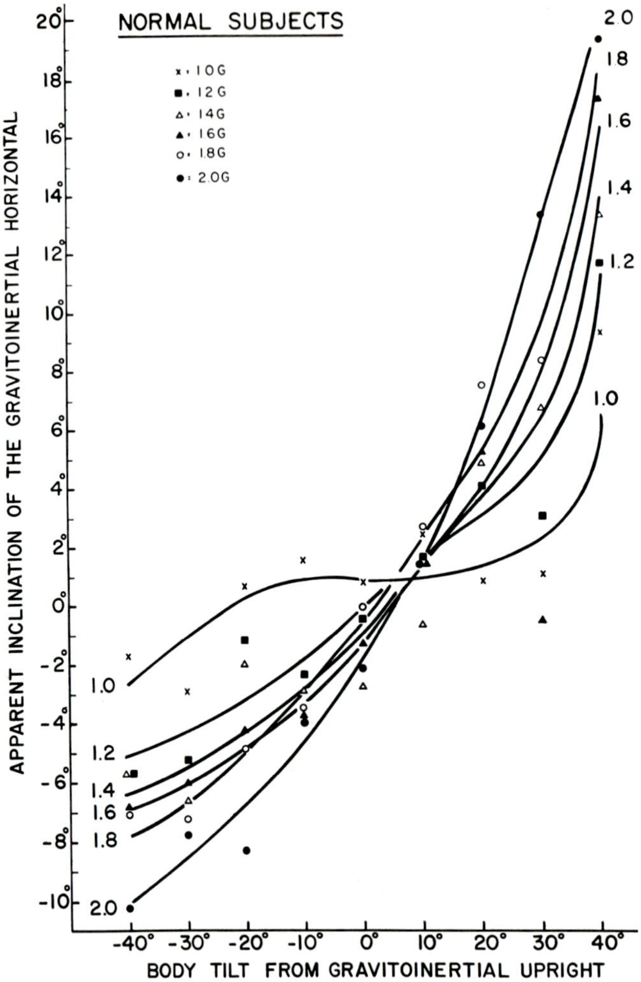

Fig. 8. Change in E phenomenon as a function of increasing G level in normal subjects

On the basis of this experience, we suggested that astronauts be given the task of setting a dim line of light in an otherwise dark field to an external horizontal reference; in weightlessness this reference was the recollection of an element of the spacecraft horizontal with respect to their seat. This was done in Gemini V and VII flights [27]. The settings of all of the astronauts during flight were similar in one important respect; namely, the variance in a single series of trials was usually smaller, but never greater, than under control conditions pre- and post-flight. The accuracy of the settings in terms of the horizontal of the spacecraft was excellent in three astronauts; one revealed a strong but constant bias. Our tentative conclusions were that three of the astronauts at least, and probably all, had adequate "sensory anchoring" to their couches but that the greatly reduced TPK sensory input had little influence on visual mechanisms.

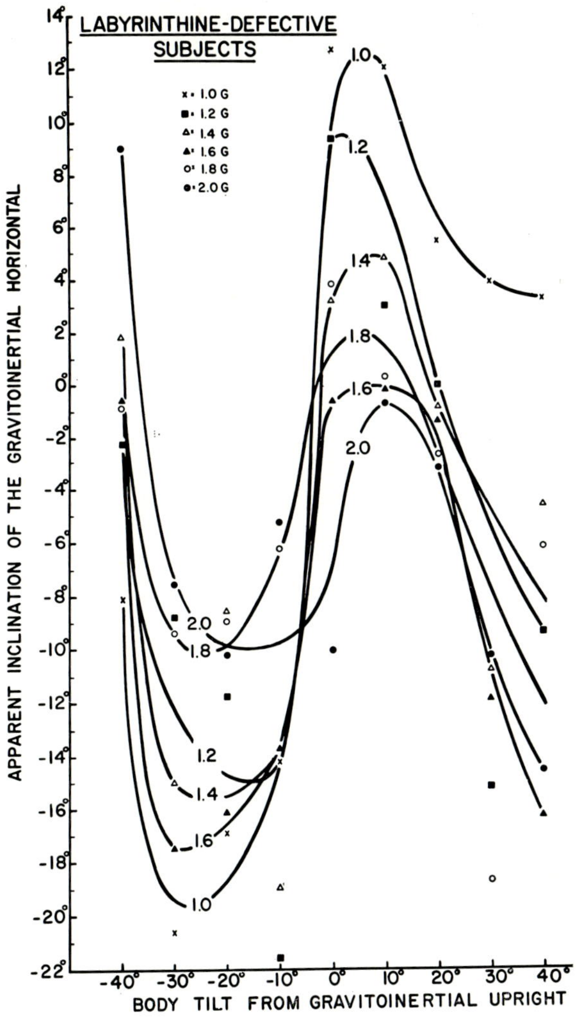

Fig. 9. Change in E and A phenomena as a function of increasing G level in labyrinthine-defective subjects

2. Oculogravic Illusion

When a person is subjected to a change in direction of the gravitoinertial vertical with reference to himself, this circumstance is rightly interpreted as body tilt away from the upright, but the perceived visual framework tends to tilt concordantly. The latter phenomenon has been termed the oculogravic illusion [18]. In apparent contrast to the E and A phenomena, the oculogravic illusion is mainly dependent on the integrity of the otolith system, although TPK systems contribute to its perception.

The threshold for perception of the oculogravic illusion by a subject seated upright with regard to the earth vertical is deflection of the gravito-inertial vertical

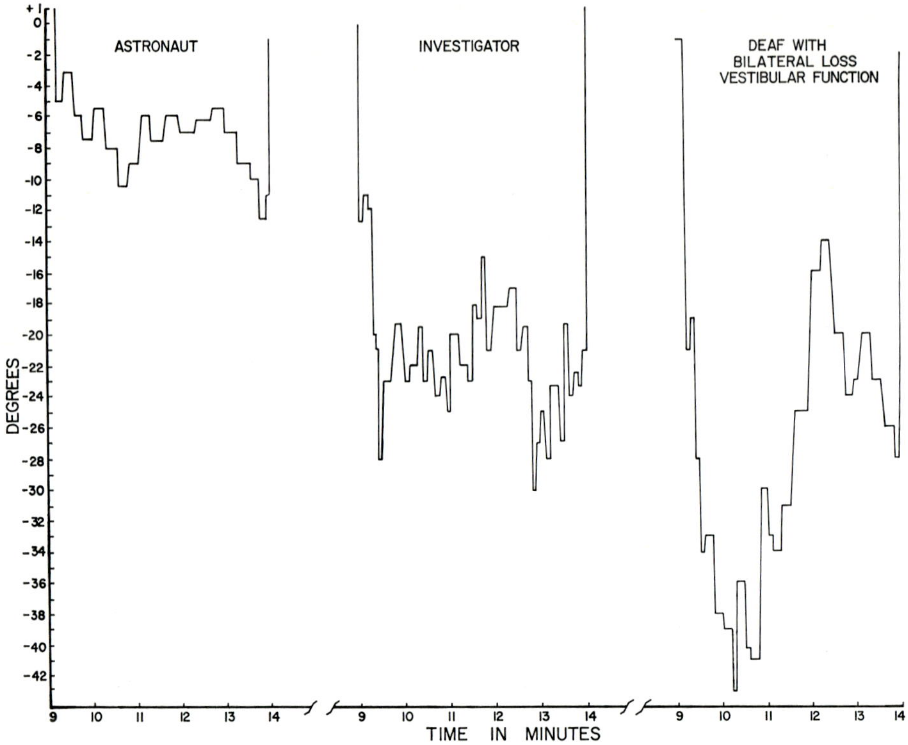

Fig. 10. Localization of a dim line of light in the dark to the horizontal by three subjects lying on their left side

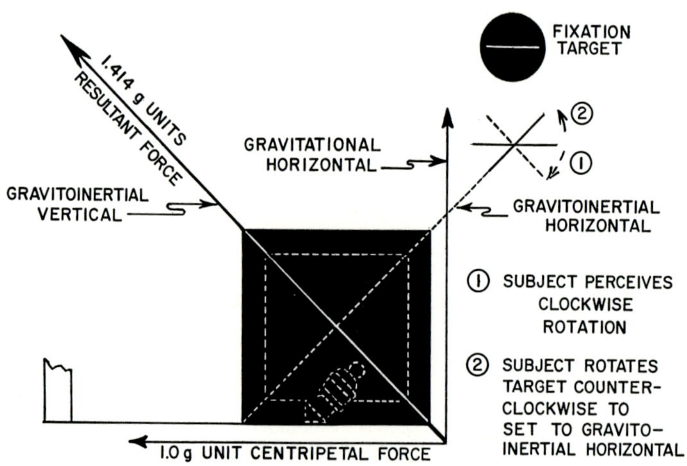

Fig. 11. Subject in the dark facing away from direction of rotation fixating a luminous line regards himself as tilted in an upright room

through an angle phi of 1.50° (1.00034 G units) from the gravitational vertical. Thresholds for subjects lying on their side were 8.9° and thresholds were unobtainable for subjects with head down [25].

In Fig. 11 a subject with eyes closed is shown seated facing the direction of rotation while exposed to a centripetal force of 1.0 G unit. He regards himself as tilted (rightward) in a room that is upright. With eyes open the fixation target will appear to have rotated to position 1. If requested to set the line to the earth horizontal, he rotates it counterclockwise from its original setting toward the gravitoinertial horizontal (position 2), usually overcompensating at this level of force.

Figure 12 shows a comparison between the settings of naive normal and L–D subjects exposed to gravitoinertial forces corresponding to deviations from the gravitational vertical (angle phi) of 20 degrees [19]. The variance was great in the case of the ten L–D subjects but not in the normal subjects. The group differences were attributed to the presence and absence of vestibular, and in particular otolith, function.

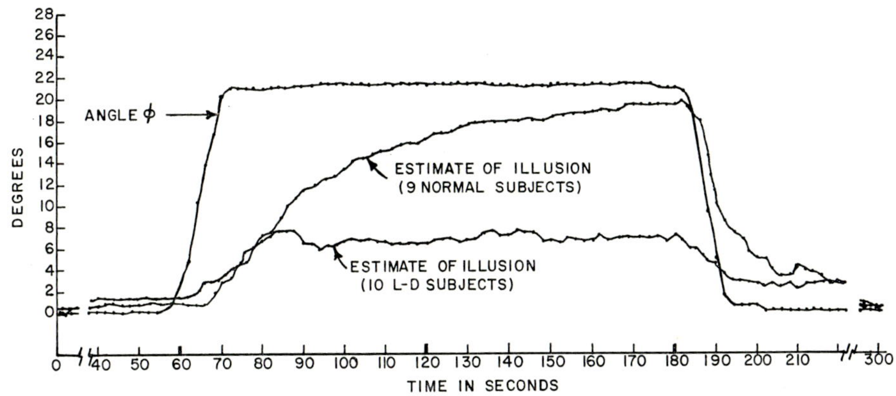

Fig. 12. Change in setting of star as a function of time compared with change in direction of resultant force of 20°. Curves depict mean values

Over a period of time the L–D subjects demonstrated "improvement" in the correspondence of their settings with the gravitoinertial horizontal. In addition to a possible practice effect (although the means of monitoring were not evident) the settings were greatly improved with prolonged exposure [9,11] and when the subjects were encased in Fiberglas molds.

Some of these factors were evident in the experimental findings upon comparison of the settings of the luminous line between normal and L–D subjects exposed to identical changes in the gravitoinertial upright, once when submerged in water to the neck, and again under dry conditions [26]. In the latter circumstance the use of Fiberglas molds tended to maximize the area of good contact with the centrifuge, while under water these contacts were minimal.

The curves in Fig. 13 summarize the findings. Three normal subjects manifested little difference in setting the line to the gravitoinertial horizontal under dry and wet conditions. On the other hand, the L–D subjects manifested a great difference: when submerged, they set the line very close to the earth horizontal, which coincid-

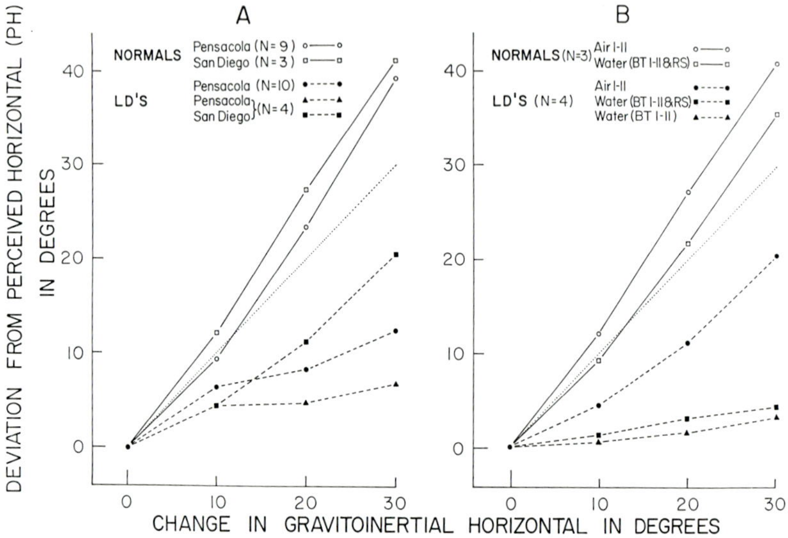

Fig. 13. Comparison between mean settings made by normal and labyrinthine-defective subject under wet and dry conditions. BT = bathing trunks, RS = rubber suit, I, II = series of trialss

ed closely with their internal horizontal coordinate; when they were dry, the settings were qualitatively similar but quantitatively about half the values indicated by the normal subjects. In other words, the loss of cues from the receptor organs responding to mechanical force had only a slight effect in the normal subject, inasmuch as the distance receptors in the otolith organs were functioning normally; the quantitatively slight decrease might be said to represent the contribution of the nonotolith receptors under dry conditions. The L–D subjects under dry and favorable conditions demonstrated that the nonotolith receptor organs provided good cues to the force environment despite the absence of distance receptors, and their settings were a measure of these cues alone. Under water the cues were greatly diminished, and in the absence of distance receptors there was shown to be little influence from gravitoinertial cues.

Schock [62] compared the ability of normal subjects to set a luminous rod in darkness to the apparent vertical (or horizontal) when in or out of water (Table 1). Except for the body-tilted-28°-left condition, in which the differences in "wet" and "dry" settings were insignificant, the mean total errors were approximately twice as great during water immersion.

Table 1. *Mean Total Errors in Setting a Luminous Rod in Darkness when Immersed and not Immersed under Water*[a]

Condition	Seated Erect	Head Tilted 45° L	Body Tilted 25° L	Body Tilted 42° L
	N=5	N=6	N=6	N=5
Dry	1.2	3.4	4.5	3.6
Wet	3.9	6.5	3.5	7.3

[a] Modified from SCHOCK [62].

C. Nonvisually Perceived Direction in Space

1. Postural Upright

In the absence of visual cues normal persons are only slightly superior to L–D subjects in their ability to restore a tilt chair to the vertical both immediately and after prolonged tilt [10]. It is interesting that the degree of improvement with practice was not significantly different in the two groups (Fig. 14) [65], implying

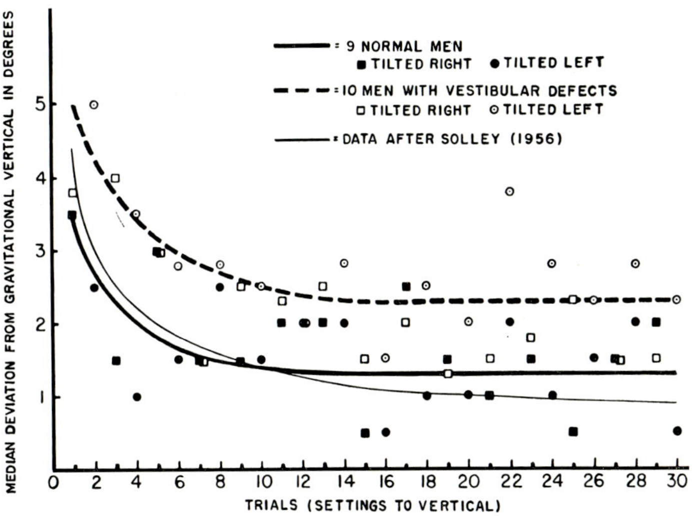

Fig. 14. Errors in setting to the postural vertical. (Solley data, ref. 62)

that a common factor, TPK systems, were operant. The data also support the notion that the tilt chair, as used in this study, is not useful in identifying subjects without otolith function.

2. Orientation to the Vertical Under Water

BROWN [8] rotated subjects in a "tucked position" on a rod under water through 3, 4, or 5 revolutions at a rate of approximately one revolution in 2 sec, ending with the subject's head up, down, forward, or backward. On cessation of rotation the subject attempted to point to the top of the tank; after approximately 5 sec, on signal, he was required to tilt his head slowly backward and forward, then "correct" his estimate of "up" if necessary. Lastly, he was required to swim slowly toward the surface. Initially, there were errors as great as 180°, greatest with the head down and back and least with the head up or forward. Nodding of the head was followed by consistent improvement. By contrast, there was little indication of difficulty in swimming toward the surface. The author regarded the initial "pointing" results as an indication that the otolithic apparatus serves to indicate the upright better when the head is in some positions than in others, and the second pointing results as an indication that the otoliths function better under dynamic than under static conditions. The possibility that canalicular influences affected the initial responses was not considered. The author pointed out that greater density of the legs compared with the trunk resulted in an automatic tendency toward vertical orientation upon release from the rod.

D. Postural Equilibrium

As we view the "scale" from primitive fish to man, the essential structure and cardinal "purpose" of the organs of equilibrium remain unchanged; namely, they are organs of equilibrium. The ordinary demands of present-day living may not challenge the vestibular system severely, but this challenge is readily provided under laboratory conditions and in the worlds of arts, entertainment, and sports.

Although a variety of behavioral tests have been proposed to demonstrate the effects of loss of vestibular function, only a few well-controlled systematic investigations have been conducted. We have used a standardized postural equilibrium test battery to aid in demonstrating the independent roles of the visual, TPK, and vestibular systems in the maintenance of equilibrium under static and dynamic conditions. The test battery, described elsewhere in detail [15] and comprising five to seven individual items, requires the patient to stand or walk in the stringent position of body erect, arms folded against chest, wearing shoes with flat heels and soles. The tests are administered in the following sequence:

Sharpened Romberg (SR): Stand on floor, eyes closed, feet in heel-to-toe position for 60 sec. Maximum score 240.

Rail Test Battery (short version):

Walk eyes open (E/O): Walk heel-to-toe, eyes open, on 3/4-inch by 8-foot rail. Maximum score 15 (steps).

Stand eyes open (E/O): Stand heel-to-toe, eyes open, on the 3/4-inch wide rail. Maximum score 180 (sec).

Stand eyes closed (E/C): Stand heel-to-toe eyes closed on $2^1/_4$ inch by 30-inch rail. Maximum score 180 (sec).

Stand on a leg eyes closed (SOLEC): First right leg (SOLEC-R), then left leg (SOLEC-L) for 30 sec. Maximum score 150 (sec).

Walk a straight 12-foot line on the floor heel-to-toe, eyes closed WALEC). Maximum score zero (inches deviation from line).

Walk on floor heel-to-toe with eyes closed (WOFEC) without side stepping. Administered simultaneously with WALEC. Maximum score 30 (steps).

A previous report [16] has described the findings in normal populations and in patients with disease, defect, or disorder involving the vestibular system. If ocular counterrolling responses are used as an index of otolithic function, persons with typically normal or low normal values but impaired function of the semicircular canals had scores similar to those of L–D subjects.

NASHNER [59] investigated postural sway under near-normal baseline conditions. On the basis of available information, he developed a general postural control model that, in turn, was used in devising a series of experiments dealing with postural sway resulting from rotation about the ankle. The experimental findings were combined with the general model to develop specific models for the sensory-motor interfaces. Three normals and one L–D individual participated. The L–D subject was 20 years of age and had compensated "to the extent possible" following bilateral transection of the VIIIth nerve 2 years prior to testing. Four types of tests were conducted:

(1) Reflex response gains. In normal subjects the average gain of the stretch reflex response induced by small rotations was about one third that necessary for postural stability. In the L–D subject with eyes open the gains were larger than in the normals but below those necessary for postural stability; with eyes closed the average gain increased markedly, and, for extensor muscles, resulted in "rigid" postural stability.

(2) Induced sway: thresholds for perception with eyes open. Threshold values in terms of response time and body angle are shown in Fig. 15 [59].

(3) Continuous recording of postural response and body angle motion. With eyes open the "control strategy" is the same for the L–D subject and normal controls, but when corrections were made for transient disturbances (higher center commands) performance was better for the normals than the L–D subject. With eyes closed the strategy remains the same for normal subjects (periods of reflex stability and transient disturbances) but changes for the L–D subject in that reflex stability gives way to continuous oscillation.

(4) Frequency spectra of body angle motions. Comparative values are shown in Fig. 16 A and B [59].

In summary, the normal subject regulates posture with a combination of high-frequency (canal and somatosensory receptors) stabilization and low-frequency (otolith and optic receptors) stabilization; with eyes closed he still has otoliths functioning. The L–D subject with eyes closed is without low-frequency stabilization, resulting in a "rigid" stability.

E. Relevant Observations and Experiments in the Exploration of Space

1. Near-Weightless State

Transition into weightlessness constitutes in effect an elegant experimental procedure for abolishing the stimulus of gravity. In the absence of gravitoinertial forces the TPK receptors can still be stimulated by agravitoinertial mechanical forces, but the bony labyrinth prevents these mechanical forces[1] from reaching

---

1 A possible exception to this is seen in minute motions such as those produced by pulsations of blood vessels.

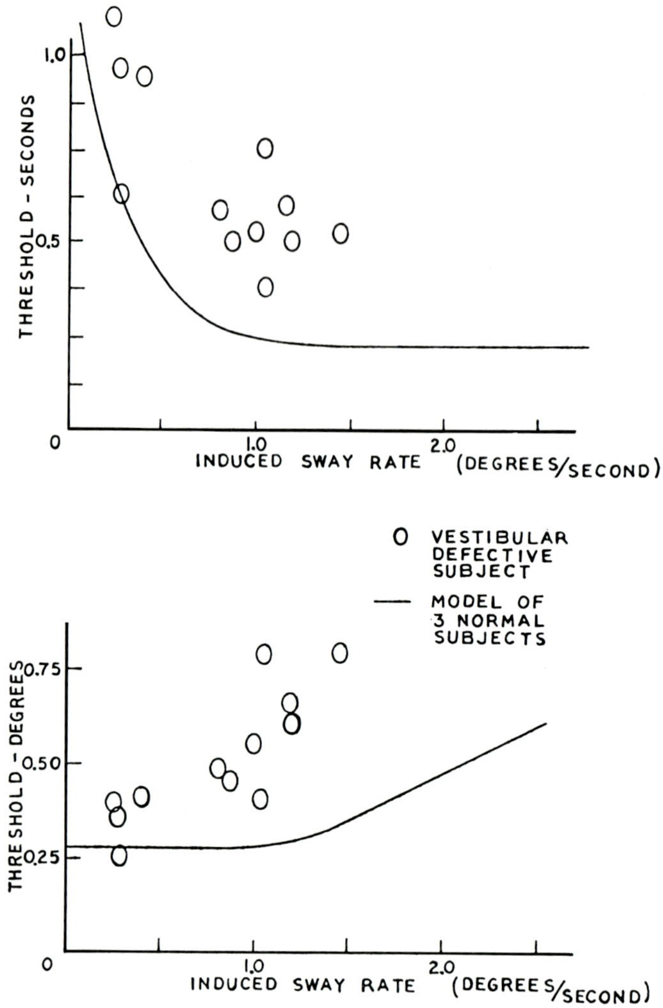

Fig. 15. Response threshold to induced sway motion of the vestibular-defective subject

macular receptors. If the abolition of ocular counterrolling in the weightless phase of parabolic flight is accepted as evidence that the tonic sensory input due to the stimulus of gravity is lost, a resting discharge (presumably of chemical origin) remains.

The dynamics of the otolith organs during the transition into weightlessness has been the object of speculation but not experimentation. In the presence of gravity, linear acceleration of about 0.03 G unit is required to change the direction of the gravitoinertial vertical by about 1.5°, the threshold for perception of the oculogravic illusion under favorable circumstances [25]. In the absence of gravity as reflected by ocular counterrolling [56] an acceleration of this magnitude would be many times above this threshold measurement for stimulation of the receptors.

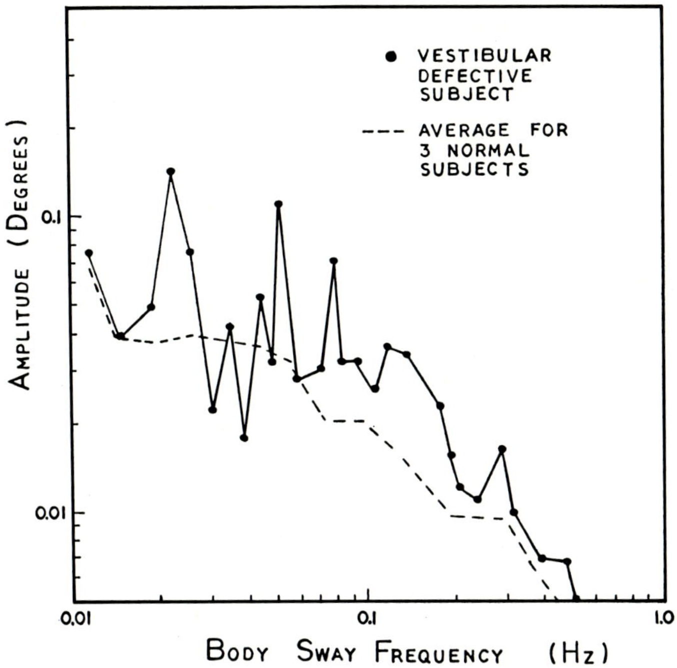

A.

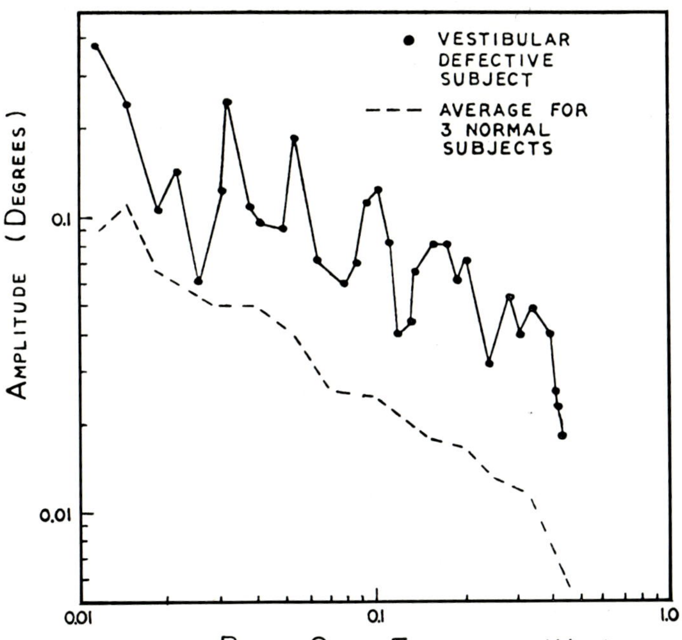

B.

Fig. 16. A. Fourier coefficients of body-sway motion for the vestibular-defective subject standing on a rigid, flat surface with eyes open. B. Fourier coefficients of body sway motion for the vestibular-defective subject standing on a rigid, flat surface with eyes closed

The stimulus situation becomes complicated in the absence of gravity that might act to restore the otoconial membrane in a manner (but not a mechanism) analogous to the behavior of the cupuloendolymph system in the semicircular canals. Even if some analogous mechanism existed, stimulation of the receptors would seem to have little behavioral significance unless or until adaptation in the processing of this information could provide the necessary "relevance" to the visual framework.

On transition into orbital flight [67] and on transition into the weightless phase of parabolic flight the inversion illusion [22] is experienced by some persons. The Russian cosmonaut Feoktistov had the curious experience of feeling upside down in a visually upright spacecraft environment, and this feeling persisted until reentry [17]. Persons with bilateral loss of labyrinthine function have not experienced the inversion illusion and have reported somewhat different experiences from normal subjects when subjected to small fractional G loadings in parabolic flight.

2. Lunar Walk

The performance of American astronauts in carrying out their tasks under the lunar standard of gravity was accomplished with remarkably little difficulty in view of the novel stimulus conditions; Armstrong was the first to walk, Aldrin the first to run, Conrad the first to fall, and Shepard the first to kneel. The force environment did not directly affect the visual and canalicular systems but had differential effects on the otolithic and TPK systems. Only the latter was affected by their back packs, which were approximately equal to body weight. With regard to the otolith organs, under static conditions the lunar standard of gravity is barely sufficient to elicit an ocular counterrolling response according to observations in parabolic flight.

The astronauts have reported that it was necessary to "jog" continuously on the lunar surface in order to maintain their equilibrium since their inner ears appeared to provide little information regarding the upright. Under dynamic conditions a linear acceleration of 0.18 G unit, sufficient to cause a change of 10 degrees in direction of the angle phi under terrestrial conditions, would only require 0.03 G unit under lunar conditions (Fig. 17). Assuming the sensory inputs from the otolith organs played a role in the lunar walk, it seems that a period of adaptation would be necessary before their contribution became beneficial, but further study of the role of the otolithic system under these conditions is necessary. In addition to observations under static and dynamic conditions, the plasticity of the central nervous system should be taken into account in serial observations over the longest feasible periods.

F. Vestibular Input-Output Relations

The schemata in Fig. 18 represent an attempt to identify important elements determining input-output relations in which the vestibular organs play either the essential role or a contributory role under different stimulus conditions. The bottom of the chart shows a brief categorization of circumstances giving rise to normal or abnormal vestibular responses. Here our attention will be focused mainly on the responses elicited in normal persons on exposure to unusual grav-

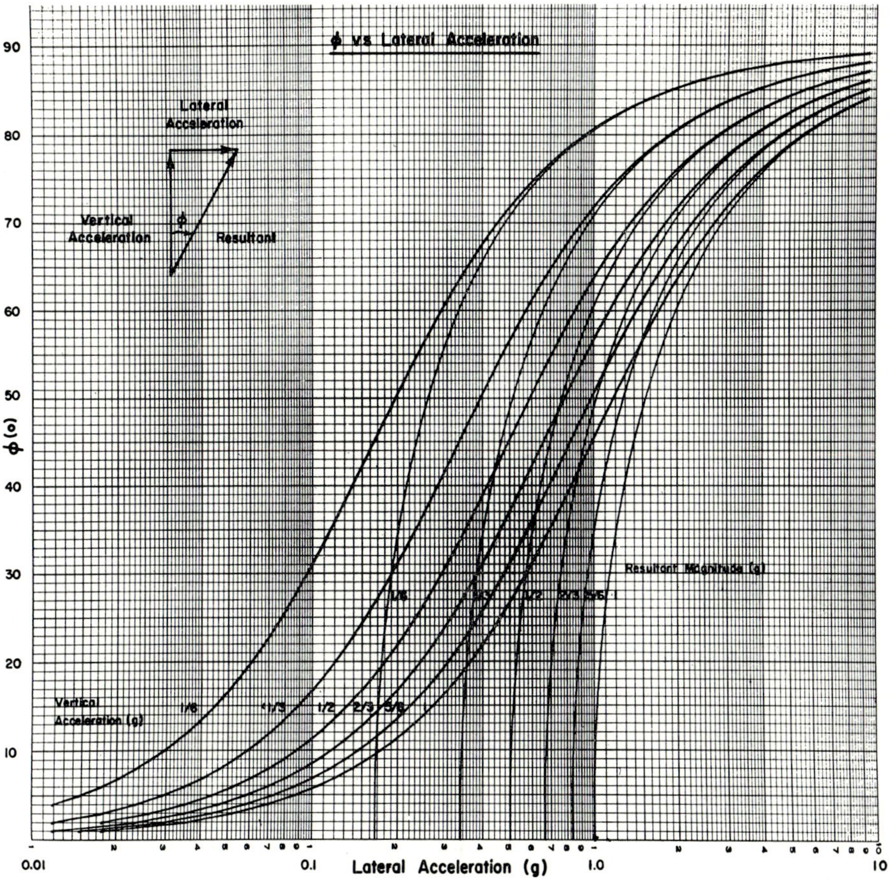

Fig. 17. Nomogram showing changes in direction of the gravitoinertial upright (angle phi) on exposure to horizontal acceleration at lunar ($^1/_6$ G) and terrestrial (1.0 G) standards of gravity and points between

itoinertial force environments (shown in Block I). The very important contribution to the stimulus patterns made by man's motions, especially those involving rotation of the head, should be emphasized. The cupuloendolymph and cilio-otolith mechanisms (Block II) involved in the conversion of mechanical to electrical energy have been described in terms of their response characteristics and models have been assembled. It is important to recall that the mechanical events interposed between cessation of the accelerative stimulus and the discharge of afferent impulses is sometimes greatly prolonged in the canal, depending on antecedent events, giving rise to "illusory" after-effects and modulating otolithic influences.

In Block III the canalicular and otolithic systems are shown as separate and interacting, although the combining term "vestibular system" is commonly used inasmuch as the central nervous system pathways of the two components have not been fully traced, and behavioral responses often represent a "combined" effect. Note the arrow indicating the efferent or return flow of impulses to the end organs, which thus closes a loop. Interactions between the canalicular and otolithic systems have been demonstrated between vestibular and nonvestibular systems (notably vision) [18, 26, 69] under abnormal stimulus conditions [5, 7, 35, 66]. When man is engaged in natural activities under terrestrial conditions, the main chain of events involves Blocks I to IV, and the loop is closed by virtue of 1) gravity, 2) man's motion generating immanent accelerations, and 3) changes in position of the otolith apparatus relative to the direction of the gravitational or gravitoinertial vertical and gravity. The vestibular influences find expression mainly through articulating motor effector systems concerned with postural stability and stabilization of the retinal image and have been termed "normal system-bound responses."

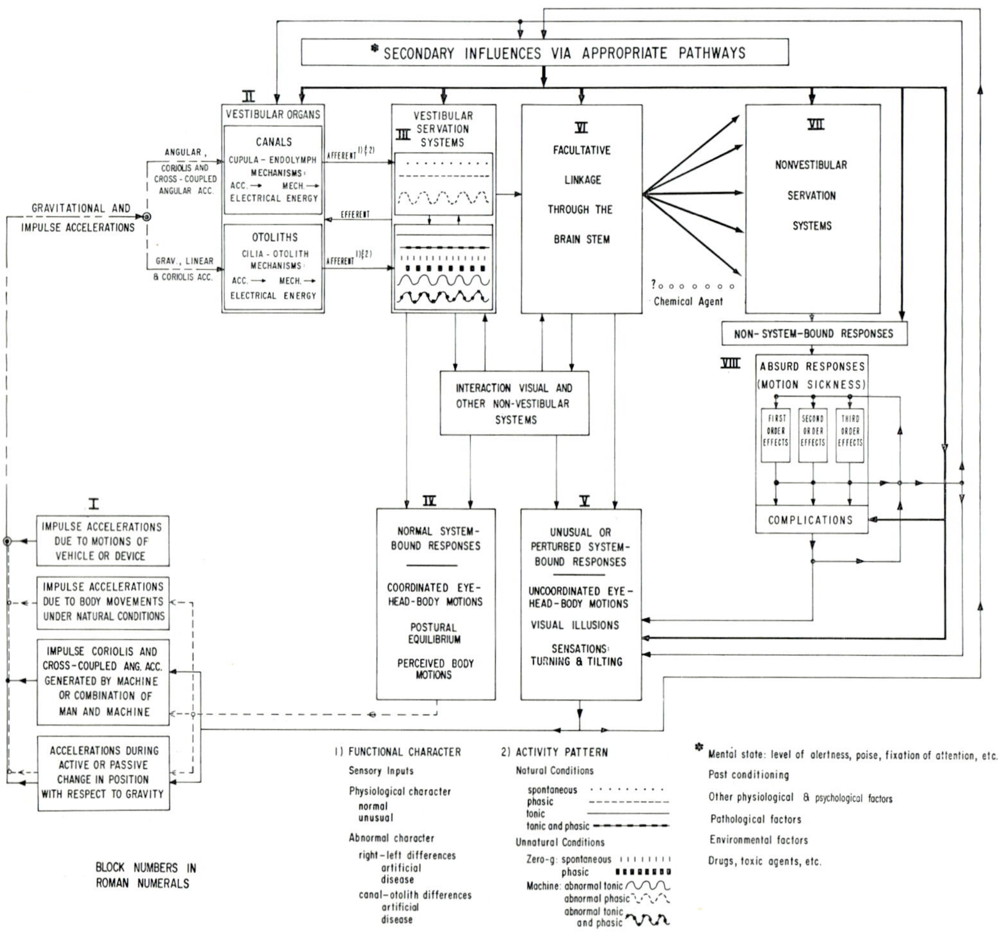

Fig. 18. Schemata showing vestibular input-output relations

In unnatural gravitoinertial force environments the canals or otolith organs or both are stimulated in an unusual manner (Fig. 18, footnote 2) eliciting "perturbed system-bound responses" (Block V), and, under certain stimulus conditions, an epiphenomenon may occur in which vestibular influences reach nonvestibular servation systems (Block VI) via a facultative linkage (Block V) and elicit "non-system-bound responses" (Block VIII) that include the well-known symptomatology of motion sickness [24, 49, 56], which can change dramatically as a function of G loading [53, 56].

Little is known about the precise nature of the facultative linkage. The fact that irradiating vestibular activity is demonstrably open to modulating influences points to the use of common pathways in the brain-stem reticular formation. This common meeting ground between somatic and visceral systems is essential not only for coordination at the reflex level but also to provide for some voluntary control over otherwise autonomic responses. What makes the vestibular linkage unusual (but not unique) is the readiness with which vestibular activity may get "out of bounds" and elicit the widespread responses that include the typical symptoms of motion sickness. The sometimes long delay between the onset of stimulation and the appearance of motion sickness suggests that a chemical linkage may also be involved [49]

Otolithic aspects of these input-output relations will be emphasized, but here it is important to point out some of the distinguishing characteristics of system-bound and non-system-bound responses and to indicate the principal ways in which they are related. In general, reflex vestibular disturbances (RVD) reflect instability of the vestibular system, and typical manifestations include nystagmus, strong oculogravic illusions (see Fig. 19), eye-head-body incoordination, and postural disequilibrium. Systematic studies reveal characteristics of the various responses that may be observed or inferred. In general, these responses are characterized by: 1) short latencies typical of reflex phenomena, 2) maximal responses to the initial stimulus, 3) modulation by secondary influences, 4) little evidence of temporal perseveration on cessation of the stimulus (with explicable exceptions), and 5) a response decline indicating the effects of adaptation.

In the case of stimulus patterns that have the potential for precipitating motion sickness (as well as RVD), the symptoms of motion sickness may nevertheless be avoided, e.g. by short exposure, making it possible to elicit reflex vestibular disturbances as "isolated" vestibular responses.

The typical overt symptoms of motion sickness are well known [31], and systematic studies reveal that they have the following characteristics: 1) delay in appearance of symptoms after the onset of the stressful stimuli, 2) gradual or rapid increase in severity of symptoms, 3) modulation by secondary influences, 4) perseveration after sudden cessation of stimuli, and 5) response decline, indicating recovery. Further abstractions reveal: 1) wide individual differences in susceptibility and in the acquisition and decay of adaptation, 2) transfer of adaptation effects, 3) learning, and 4) conditioning.

The appearance of symptoms always indicates that the adaptation capacity of the vestibular system has been exceeded. Indeed, even prior to the appearance of overt responses it can be shown that the individual's susceptibility has risen. Moreover, the order of appearance of symptoms is affected by the strength of the

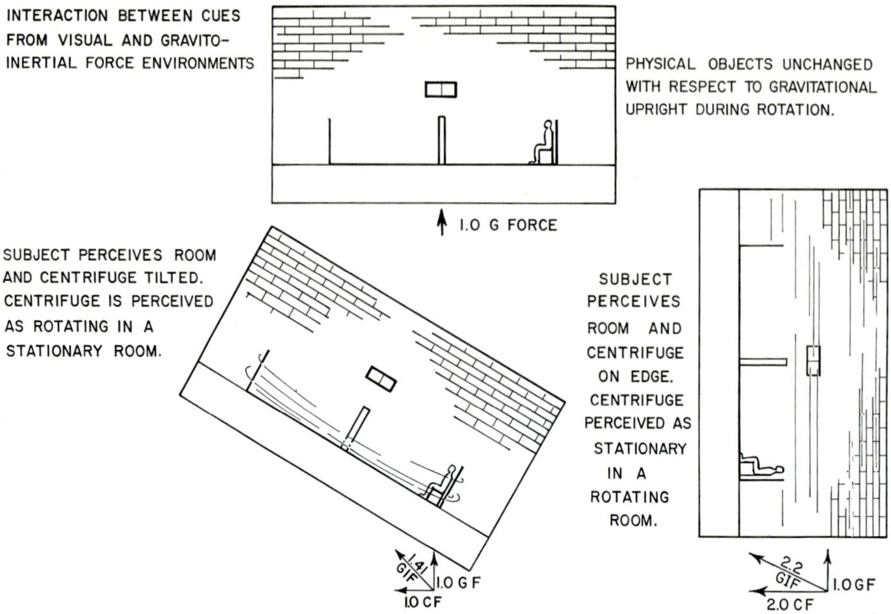

Fig. 19. Above: a normal subject rotating in a fixed position on an open centrifuge, as viewed by an outside observer. When (below) the centripetal force reaches a level of 1.0 G unit, the subject feels as if he were tilted backward and perceives the centrifuge and room tilted concordantly. At 2.0 G units (right) the subject feels as if he were stationary lying on his back and perceives the room rotating around him, analogous to experiences of aviators in certain types of spin

stressful stimuli and length of exposure. Secondary etiologic influences, categorized in Fig. 18, are always present, tending either to raise or to lower susceptibility.

G. Effect of Drugs

Otolith organ function as indicated by ocular counterrolling was completely or nearly completely resistant to the direct effect of several drugs, including those with well-known antimotion sickness properties that were administered in twice the usually recommended doses [47]. The results indicated that these drugs acted on neural centers involved in the genesis of motion sickness rather than directly on the otolithic receptor organs. Alcohol (1 ml/lb body weight), on the other hand, had a marked and progressive depressant effect on the amount of eye roll during the intoxication period, complete recovery being recorded after six hours. Alcohol releases positional nystagmus by some unknown mechanism, and judging from the evidence of this study it also suppresses otolith organ activity. JONGKEES and PHILIPSZOON [33] reported suppression of compensatory eye movement in man following oral administration of 250 mg cinnarizine.

IV. Discussion

A. Functional Tests

Reliable tests of otolithic and canalicular function are a prerequisite for the elucidation of the individual and combined roles of the two vestibular systems in man. The advantages of using a natural behavioral response rather than a provocative response dependent on "disturbing" the canalicular or otolithic system include the fact that natural mechanisms and reflex pathways are used, and serial tests do not lead either to (temporary) decrease in thresholds of response or to adaptation effects. Ocular counterrolling meets the qualifications of a natural behavioral test, but accurate measurement is difficult and interpretation of the results (in the absence of a normal baseline value) is complicated by the wide range of apparently normal values and the overlap between the abnormal and normal ranges. One possibility of overcoming these handicaps consists in exposure of the person to an increased G loading on a human centrifuge. In these circumstances the amount of roll not only increases but tends in the direction of linearity in response, as shown in Fig. 4. This modest increase in G loading does not have the disadvantage attributable to a provocative test. Admittedly, this test cannot be used as a clinical procedure, but it might help in validating a simpler test that is suitable for clinical use.

The oculogravic illusion test also escapes the provocative test category. Although clearly artificial in character, it probably depends on natural reflex mechanisms at low levels of stimulus intensity.

The results obtained on the counterrolling and oculogravic illusion tests in four L–D and three normal subjects are compared in Table 2. Although the amount of information is small, the point can be made that differences in responses between the two groups are magnified under centrifugation in the case of the counterrolling index and centrifugation during head-out water immersion in the case of the oculogravic illusion. Fortunately, JO and ZA represent the opposite extremes among the L–D group, and it is interesting that JO with the highest counterrolling index has the lowest, or nearly the lowest, settings for perception of the oculogravic illusion; this situation is nearly reversed in the case of ZA. The otolith apparatus seems to be involved in both tests, but the nonotolithic factors appear to be somewhat different. It seems desirable to make a systematic collection of more data under centrifugation, possibly using some type of foam material as a substitute for water in the oculogravic illusion test. These determinations could be validated by means of clinical and pathological studies and in turn might be used to validate a variety of simpler tests that could be used in the clinic.

B. The Constant Stimulus of Gravity

There is general agreement that if the head is rotated in the gravitational field, causing the (shearing) forces acting on the macular plates to change direction, an effective stimulus to the otolith receptors is generated in addition to whatever tangential accelerations accompany the change in direction. However, the fact that even if the head is "fixed," the otolithic reflexes measured by ocular torsion and the oculogravic illusion undergo no decay over a time period measured in

Table 2. *Comparison of Counterrolling Indices and Estimates of Gravitoinertial Horizontal of Labyrinthine-Defective and Normal Subjects under Different g Loadings*

Subjects	Ocular counterrolling (minutes of arc)				Oculogravic illusion (apparent gravitoinertial horizontal angle $\varphi = 30°$, magnitude 1.12 g units)		
	Maximum tilt 50° % earth standard of gravity			Human centrifuge angle $\varphi = 63°$ 2.2 g units	Early[c] tests	Fiberglas mold[d]	
	0%[a]	50%	100%			Dry	Head-out water immersion
Bilateral labyrinthine defects							
JO	78′	130′	126′		−3.2°	−9.1°	−3.1°
MY	32′	60′	63′	98′	2.2°[b]	−13.1°	−4.1°
PE			21′		−21.0°	−20.1°	2.5°[b]
ZA	28′	76′	14′	21′	−1.1°	−39.9°	−11.1°
Normal labyrinthine function							
CU	♯82′		267′	♯570′		−51.2°	−38.2°
DI	♯82′		241′	♯570′		−38.3°	−33.5°
HU	♯82′		336′	♯570′		−34.1°	31.9°

[a] In parabolic flight
[b] Wrong direction
[c] Each value a mean of 20 settings in 2 series
[d] Mean of 15 settings in 3 series 2 in bathing trunks 1 in rubber suit

hours demonstrates that the stimulus of gravity or of gravitoinertial force under static conditions generates a tonic sensory input, presumably in addition to a resting discharge. Whether the same receptor units generate this tonic discharge or whether continual slight (unavoidable) changes in the position of the head cause stimulation of different receptor units is a matter of speculation.

It is interesting to speculate whether the stimulus of gravity to otolith receptors is effective during sleep. If it is not effective, there will be some resemblance to the stimulus condition in weightlessness. The systematic studies of REDING and FERNÁNDEZ [61] on five sleeping children bear upon this factor. They observed that nystagmus was present, although depressed, in half the trials in which REM sleep was manifested, with the important implication that the presence of nystagmus might be associated with facilitation of impulses travelling from the pontine reticular formation to the vestibular nuclei. Moreover, this finding lends support to the conclusion of ADEY and co-workers [1] that the paradoxical phase of sleep might involve as "internalization of attention." REDING and FERNÁNDEZ [61] pointed out that the temporal relations between the appearance of nystagmus and REM during sleep might be the counterpart of "arousal nystagmus" during the waking state.

C. Contributions to Enhancement of Performance

There is evidence that the otolithic system contributes to man's perception of personal and extrapersonal space and that the best concordance between otolithic and visual cues to the gravitational vertical is provided when man is upright or nearly upright. Presumably, this match is the result of much practice with excellent monitoring possibilities. A constancy bias with regard to nonvisual cues can be demonstrated with increasing angles of tilt from the upright and with increasing G load for the same angle of tilt. In most of these circumstances the bias is greater and the variance in the settings greater in persons without than in those with normal vestibular function. A noteworthy finding, however, is the extent to which TPK receptors are able to compensate for loss of the otolith function.

The results of a recent case study suggest that the contribution of the otolithic system to postural equilibrium may be greater than has hitherto been assumed. The evidence is fragmentary, however, and the relative roles of the canalicular and otolithic systems in postural equilibrium need further study. There have been remarkable instances of complete or nearly complete loss of vestibular function in young persons with normal hearing who were unaware of any handicap [29], which illustrates the great role of vision and, to a lesser extent, the role of nonvestibular somatic sensory mechanisms. The successful lunar walks also suggest that the essential mechanisms subserving the astronauts' activities under these conditions of near-weightlessness served them well and without any overt manifestation of disturbance in the canalicular and otolithic systems.

The role of the otolith organs in stabilizing the retinal image is difficult to evaluate in man.

D. Contributions to Decrement in Performance

In man there seems to be a disparity between the great potentialities of the vestibular system he has inherited and its useful servation. This disparity disappears, however, when we come to consider reflex vestibular disturbances and motion sickness, which may create turmoil throughout the body as a result of exposure to an abnormal but otherwise physically harmless stimulus. Under these artificial stimulus conditions, to which man cannot adapt quickly, the vestibular system is disturbed, and the question arises of to whether the otolithic system alone can elicit nystagmus and motion sickness or whether the presence, at least, of the canalicular system is essential.

Loss of the stimulus of gravity resulting from transition into weightlessness may render a person susceptible to motion sickness when making normal head motions or when engaged in general activities [53, 56]. It appears that under these conditions the otolithic system is indirectly responsible.

The inversion illusion in weightlessness and the oculogravic illusion and elevator illusion [60] are almost surely mainly of otolithic origin.

The evidence collected in recent reports [29, 30] strongly suggests that exposure to earth-horizontal rotation elicited nystagmus in a young man who had apparently lost all function of the horizontal pair of semicircular canals and in whom function of the vertical canals was reduced. Motion sickness was also elicited during some of the exposures.

Normal persons exposed in a variety of devices designed to stimulate the otolith organs but to avoid stimulation of the semicircular canals become motion sick [2, 6, 21, 23, 24, 52, 64] and a few persons demonstrate differences in susceptibility when exposed to provocative tests designed to stimulate mainly the otolith organs or mainly the semicircular canals. It may be that otolith sickness and canal sickness will prove to be convenient terms. Susceptibility to off-vertical rotation and primarily otolithic stimulation [52] was found to change in direct proportion to the shear angle of the rotating linear acceleration vector and at a constant tilt angle of 10° to be maximal at rates between 15 rpm and 20 rpm. At 40 rpm and 45 rpm, subjects were not only much less susceptible, but began to lose their sensation of being tilted.

V. Summary

It is a greater undertaking to define the isolated role of the otolith than to define that of the canalicular system in man. One reason is the greater difficulty in manipulating the stimulus and eliciting specific responses, and another reason is the overlapping function of receptors serving touch, pressure, and kinesthesis (for which there is no counterpart in the case of the canals). Benefits such as contributions to perception of the upright and to the maintenance of postural equilibrium may be of significant value. Harmful effects on exposure to unusual force environments or to labyrinthine disease or irritative disorder may be severe. The abolition of the gravitational stimulus in the Skylab orbital flights has provided a unique opportunity for investigation of the otolithic system [54].

References

1. Adey, W.R., Kado, R.T., Rhodes, J.M.: Sleep: cortical and subcortical recordings in the chimpanzee. Science, **141**, 932–933 (1963).
2. Alexander, S.J., Cotzin, M., Hill, C.J., Jr., Ricciuti, E.A., Wendt, G.R.: Wesleyan University studies of motion sickness. III. The effects of various accelerations upon sickness rates. J. Psychol. (Provincetown) **20**, 3–8 (1945).
3. Aubert, H.: Eine scheinbar bedeutende Drehung von Objecten bei Neigung des Kopfes nach rechts oder links. Arch. path. Anat. Physiol. **20**, 381–393 (1861).
4. Bauermeister, M.: Effect of body tilt on apparent verticality, apparent body position, and their relation. J. exp. Psychol. **67**, 142–147 (1964).
5. Benson, A.J., Bodin, M.A.: Interaction of linear and angular accelerations on vestibular receptors in man. Aerospace Med. **37**, 144–154 (1966).
6. Benson, A.J., Whiteside, T.C.D.: The effect of linear acceleration on the response to angular acceleration in man. J. Physiol. (Lond.) **156**, 6P–7P (1961).
7. Bergstedt, M.: Studies of positional nystagmus in the human centrifuge. Acta oto-laryng. (Stockh.) Suppl. **165**, 1–144 (1961).
8. Brown, J.L.: Orientation to the vertical during water immersion. Aerospace Med. **32**, 209–216 (1961).
9. Clark, B., Graybiel, A.: Visual perception of the horizontal during prolonged exposure to radial acceleration on a centrifuge. J. exp. Psychol. **63**, 294–301 (1962).
10. Clark, B., Graybiel, A.: Perception of the postural vertical following prolonged bodily tilt in normals and subjects with labyrinthine defects. Acta oto-laryng. (Stockh.) **58**, 143–148 (1964).
11. Clark, B., Graybiel, A.: Perception of the visual horizontal in normal and labyrinthine defective observers during prolonged rotation. Amer. J. Psychol. **79**, 608–612 (1966).
12. Colenbrander, A.: Eye and otoliths. A centrifuge study on the ocular response to otolith stimulation. Thesis, Utrecht, 1964.
13. Fluur, E., Mellstrom, A.: Utricular stimulation and oculomotor reactions. Laryngoscope (St. Louis) **80**, 1701–1712 (1970).
14. Fluur, E., Mellstrom, A.: Saccular stimulation and oculomotor reactions. Laryngoscope (St. Louis) **80**, 1713–1721 (1970).
15. Fregly, A.R., Graybiel, A.: An ataxia test battery not requiring rails. Aerospace Med. **38**, 277–282 (1968).
16. Fregly, A.R., Graybiel, A.: Labyrinthine defects as shown by ataxia and caloric tests. Acta oto-laryng. (Stockh.) **69**, 216–222 (1970).
17. Gazenko, O.: Medical studies on the cosmic spacercafts "Vostok" and Voskhod". NASA TT F-9207. Washington, D.C.: National Aeronautics and Space Administration 1964.
18. Graybiel, A.: Oculogravic illusion. Arch. Ophthal. **48**, 605–615 (1952).
19. Graybiel, A., Clark, B.: The validity of the oculogravic illusion as a specific indicator of otolith function. Aerospace Med. **36**, 1173–1181 (1965).
20. Graybiel, A., Fregly, A.R.: A new quantitative ataxia test battery. Acta oto-laryng. (Stockh.) **61**, 292–312 (1966).
21. Graybiel, A., Johnson, W.H.: A comparison of the symptomatology experienced by healthy persons and subjects with loss of labyrinthine function when exposed to unusual patterns of centripetal force in a counter-rotating room. Ann. Otol. (St. Louis) **72**, 357–373 (1963).
22. Graybiel, A., Kellogg, R.S.: The inversion illusion in parabolic flight: Its probable dependence on otolith function. Aerospace Med. **38**, 1099–1103 (1967).
23. Graybiel, A., Miller, E.F. II: Off-vertical rotation: A convenient precise means of exposing the passive human subject to a rotating linear acceleration vector. Aerospace Med. **41**, 407–410 (1970).

24. Graybiel, A., Miller, E.F. II: The otolith organs as a primary etiological factor in motion sickness: with a note on "off-vertical" rotation. NASA SP-187, pp. 53–64. Washington, D.C.: U. S. Government Printing Office 1970.

25. Graybiel, A., Patterson, J.L., Jr.: Thresholds of stimulation of the otolith organs as indicated by the oculogravic illusion. J. appl. Physiol. **7**, 666–670 (1955).

26. Graybiel, A., Miller, E.F. II, Newsom, B.D., Kennedy, R.S.: The effect of water immersion on perception of the oculogravic illusion in normal and labyrinthine-defective subjects. Acta oto-laryng. (Stockh.) **65**, 599–610 (1968).

27. Graybiel, A., Miller, E.F. II, Billingham, J., Waite, R., Berry, C.A., Dietlein, L.F.: Vestibular experiments in Gemini flights V and VII. Aerospace Med. **38**, 360–370 (1967).

28. Graybiel, A., Schuknecht, H.F., Fregly, A.R., Miller, E.F. II, McLeod, M.E.: Streptomycin in Menière's disease. Long-term follow-up. Arch. Otolaryng. **85**, 156–170 (1967).

29. Graybiel, A., Smith, C.R., Guedry, F.E., Jr., Miller, E.F. II, Fregly, A.R., Cramer, D.B.: Idiopathic progressive vestibular degeneration in a young man: Loss of vestibular servation not the basis for detection. Ann. Otol. (St. Louis) **81**, 165–178 (1972).

30. Graybiel, A., Stockwell, C.W., Guedry, F.E., Jr.: Evidence for a test of dynamic otolith function considered in relation to responses from a patient with idiopathic progressive vestibular degeneration. Acta otolaryng. (Stockh.) **73**, 1–3 (1972).

31. Graybiel, A., Wood, C.D., Miller, E.F. II, Cramer, D.B.: Diagnostic criteria for grading the severity of acute motion sickness. Aerospace Med. **39**, 453–455 (1968).

32. Guedry, F.E., Jr.: Orientation of the rotation-axis relative to gravity: Its influence on nystagmus and the sensation of rotation. Acta oto-laryng. (Stockh.) **60**, 30–48 (1965).

33. Jongkees, L.B.W., Philipszoon, A.J.: Some nystagmographical methods for the investigation of the effect of drugs upon the labyrinth. Acta physiol. pharmacol. neerl. **9**, 240–275 (1960).

34. Jongkees, L.B.W., Philipszoon, A.J.: Nystagmus provoked by linear accelerations. Acta Physiol. pharmacol. neerl. **10**, 239–247 (1962).

35. Lansberg, M.P., Guedry, F.E., Jr., Graybiel, A.: The effect of changing the resultant linear acceleration relative to the subject on nystagmus generated by angular acceleration. Aerospace Med. **36**, 456–460 (1965).

36. Miller, E.F. II: Counterrolling of the human eyes produced by head tilt with respect to gravity. Acta oto-laryng. (Stockh.) **54**, 479–501 (1962).

37. Miller, E.F. II: Ocular counterrolling. In: The Vestibular System and Its Diseases, R.J. Wolfson, Ed., p. 229–241. Philadelphia, Pa.: University of Pennsylvania Press 1966.

38. Miller, E.F. II: Evaluation of otolith organ function by means of ocular counterrolling measurements. In: Vestibular Function on Earth and in Space, J. Stahle, Ed., p. 97–107. Oxford, England: Pergamon Press 1970.

39. Miller, E.F. II, Fregly, A.R., Graybiel, A.: Visual horizontal perception in relation to otolith function. Amer. J. Psychol. **81**, 488–496 (1968).

40. Miller, E.F. II, Fregly, A.R., van den Brink, G., Graybiel, A.: Visual localization of the horizontal as a function of body tilt up to $\pm 90°$ from gravitational vertical. NSAM-942. Pensacola, Fla.: U.S. Naval School of Aviation Medicine 1965.

41. Miller, E.F. II, Graybiel, A.: Comparison of autokinetic movement perceived by normal persons and deaf subjects with bilateral labyrinthine defects. Aerospace Med. **33**, 1077–1080 (1962).

42. Miller, E.F. II, Graybiel, A.: Rotary autokinesis and displacement of the visual horizontal associated with head (body) position. Aerospace Med. **32**, 915–919 (1963).

43. Miller, E.F. II, Graybiel, A.: A comparison of ocular counterrolling movements between normal persons and deaf subjects with bilateral labyrinthine defects. Ann. Otol. (St. Louis) **72**, 885–893 (1963).

44. Miller, E.F. II, Graybiel, A.: Otolith function as measured by ocular counterrolling. NASA SP-77, p. 121–130. Washington, D.C.: U.S. Government Printing Office 1965.

45. Miller, E.F. II, Graybiel, A.: Magnitude of gravitoinertial force, an independent variable in egocentric visual localization of the horizontal. J. exp. Psychol. **71**, 452–460 (1966).

46. Miller, E.F. II, Graybiel, A.: Role of the otolith organs in the perception of horizontality. Amer. J. Psychol. **79**, 24–37 (1966).

47. Miller, E.F. II, Graybiel, A.: Effect of drugs on ocular counterrolling. Clin. Pharmacol. Ther. **10**, 92–99 (1969).

48. Miller, E.F. II, Graybiel, A.: The effect of gravitoinertial force upon ocular counterrolling. J. appl. Physiol. **31**, 697–700 (1971).

49. Miller, E.F. II, Graybiel, A.: The semicircular canals as a primary etiological factor in motion sickness. Aerospace Med. **43**, 1065–1074 (1972).

50. Miller, E.F. II, Graybiel, A.: Ocular counterrolling measured during eight hours of sustained body tilt. Minerva otorinolaring. (In press).

51. Miller, E.F. II, Graybiel, A.: Goggle device for measuring the visually perceived direction of space. Minerva otorinolaring. **22**, 177–180 (1972).

52. Miller, E.F. II, Graybiel, A.: Perception of body position and susceptibility to motion sickness as functions of angle of tilt and angular velocity in off-vertical rotation. NAMRL-1182. Pensacola, Fla.: Naval Aerospace Medical Research Laboratory 1973.

53. Miller, E.F. II, Graybiel, A.: Altered susceptibility to motion sickness as a function of subgravity level. Space Life Sci. **4**, 295–306 (1973).

54. Miller, E.F. II, Graybiel, A.: Experiment M-131 — Human vestibular function. Aerospace Med. **44**, 593–608 (1973).

55. Miller, E.F. II, Graybiel, A., Kellogg, R.S.: Otolith organ activity within Earth standard, one-half standard, and zero gravity environments. Aerospace Med. **37**, 399–403 (1966).

56. Miller, E.F. II, Graybiel, A., Kellogg, R.S., O'Donnell, R.D.: Motion sickness susceptibility under weightless and hypergravity conditions generated by parabolic flight. Aerospace Med. **40**, 862–868 (1969).

57. Miller, E.F. II, Pulec, J.L., Wilcox, J.G., Graybiel, A.: Specific acute losses of vestibular function in man following unilateral section of one or all components of the eight cranial nerve. Ann. Otol. (St. Louis) (In press).

58. Müller, E.G.: Über das Aubertsche Phänomen. Z. Sinnesphysiol. **49**, Part II, 109–244 (1916).

59. Nashner, L.M.: Sensory feedback in human posture control. MVT-70-3. Cambridge, Mass.: Man Vehicle Laboratory, Massachusetts Institute of Technology 1970.

60. Niven, J.I., Whiteside, T.C.D., Graybiel, A.: The elevator illusion: Apparent motion of a visual target during vertical acceleration. Joint Report. FPRC 1213. NSAM-876. Flying Personnel Research Committee, Farnborough, England, and Naval School of Aviation Medicine, Pensacola, Fla., 1963.

61. Reding, G.R., Fernández, C.: Effects of vestibular stimulation during sleep. Electroenceph. clin. Neurophysiol. **24**, 75–79 (1968).

62. Schock, G.J.D.: Perception of the horizontal and vertical in simulated subgravity conditions. U. S. armed Forces med. J. **11**, 786–793 (1960).

63. Schöne, H.: On the role of gravity in human spatial orientation. Aerospace Med. **35**, 764–772 (1964).

64. Sjöberg, A.: Experimentelle Studien über den Auslösungmechanismus der Seekrankheit. Acta oto-laryng. (Stockh.) Suppl. **14**, 1–136 (1931).

65. Solley, C.M.: Reduction of error with practice in perception of the postural vertical. J. exp. Psychol. **52**, 329–333 (1956).

66. Stockwell, C.W., Guedry, F.E., Jr.: The effect of semicircular canal stimulation during tilting on the subsequent perception of the visual vertical. Acta oto-laryng. (Stockh.) **70**, 170–175 (1970).

67. VASIL'YEV, P.V., VOLYNKIN, YU., K.: Some results of medical investigations carried out during the flight of "Voskhod." NASA TT F-9423. Washington, D.C.: National Aeronautics and Space Administration 1965.

68. WERNER, H., WAPNER, S., CHANDLER, K.: Experiments on sensory-tonic field theory of perception. II. Effect of supported and unsupported tilt of the body on the visual perception of verticality. J. exp. Psychol. **42**, 346–350 (1951).

69. WHITESIDE, T.C.D., GRAYBIEL, A., NIVEN, J.I.: Visual illusions of movement. Brain **88**, 193–210 (1965).

70. WITKIN, H.A.: Perception of the upright when the direction of the force acting on the body is changed. J. exp. Psychol. **40**, 93–106 (1950).

71. WOELLNER, R.C., GRAYBIEL, A.: Counterrolling of the eyes and its dependence on the magnitude of gravitational or inertial force acting laterally on the body. J. appl. Physiol. **14**, 632–634 (1959).

Chapter III.

Measurement of Vestibulo-Spinal Responses in Man

By

E. Peitersen, Copenhagen

With 3 Figures

Contents

I. Definition

The vestibulospinal reflexes include all spinal reactions demonstrable by changes in position and movements caused by labyrinthine stimulation. Such reflexes are elicited in the head and neck, upper limbs, trunk, and lower limbs. The most important ones are the reflexes in the upper and lower limbs, i.e. deviations of the arms in various planes, deviations during walking and blindfold walking, inclination and rotation of the body.

II. Introduction

Purkinje, in 1827, seems to have been the first to observe the vestibulospinal reflexes in man, mentioning the sensation of bending in a given direction and a greater weight on one foot than the other after rotation in a given direction. In his opinion, the explanation was pressure upon the brain brought about by the rotation, but it is now well known that all vestibular reactions are responses elicited by stimulation of the semicircular canals and otolith organs.

From a clinical point of view, the vestibular reactions in man are divided most conveniently, according to Wodak (1953), into:

Vestibulo-ocular reflexes
Vestibulo-spinal reflexes
Vestibulo-autonomic reflexes

which are, of course, concurrent reactions from different organs.

The anatomical sections of this book have given exhaustive descriptions of the connections between the peripheral vestibular apparatus and the vestibular nuclei and the connection of the latter with other parts of the central nervous system. In this paper, therefore, it is sufficient to point out that the connection between the labyrinth and the spinal cord is through the vestibulospinal tract, the reticulospinal tract, and in the upper part also through the descending medial longitudinal fasciculus. The primary vestibular fibers do not proceed distal to the dorsal spine, which means that the upper and lower limbs have different vestibular "innervation" (Walberg et al., 1958; Brodal et al., 1962). By electromyography of a large number of muscles and simultaneous stimulation of various parts of Deiters' nucleus, Pompeiano (1960) demonstrated a physiological somatotropic projection entirely in keeping with the anatomical one (Pompeiano and Brodal, 1957). Another striking anatomical finding is that Deiters' nucleus receives fibers predominantly from the utricular macula and that it is intimately connected with the spinal cord through the vestibulospinal tract. The pathway of the vestibulospinal reflexes elicited by stimulation of the lateral semicircular canal is a different one, judging by animal experiments, perhaps the medial nucleus and the reticulospinal tract. This is interesting in view of the fact that the reactions of the semicircular canals are easiest to observe in man. Considering the named anatomical factors, the reactions elicited may be expected to be of unequal intensity and to be chronologically shifted in relation to each other. Indeed, Gernandt (1960) demonstrated a definite difference in electrical response, in leads from the anterior roots, following vestibular stimulation in the cervicodorsal part and in the lumbosacral part.

The effect of vestibular stimulation upon the spinal cord consists in an increase of extensor tonus and a decrease of flexor tonus (Gernandt and Thulin, 1955a, 1955b), i.e. facilitation of the antigravity muscles. This is a very important point, as it is the result of this action that is recorded in the tests used for measuring vestibulospinal responses in man. Conversely, the signs of functional loss are recorded in the event of labyrinthine destruction.

In general, vestibular reactions can be said to be extremely susceptible to the function of other organs, and thus are easily suppressed or altered, cf. for instance the influence of fixation upon nystagmus and of examination with the person's eyes open upon the deviation in walking. Furthermore, it is important to realize that the response recorded is in fact a response caused by vestibular stimulation, not a normal spontaneous reaction. This is of particular importance in pointing and walking experiments, where the spontaneous deviation has to be known before vestibular stimulation is applied. Lastly, other sources of error, such as motor paresis or articular disease, can affect the results of studying labyrinthine action upon the limbs.

III. Classification

Vestibulospinal reactions in: head and neck
upper limbs
trunk
lower limbs
tipping reactions.

IV. Methods of Measurement

A. Head and Neck

Characteristic movements of the head and neck following vestibular stimulation were described by BÁRÁNY in 1906. Rotation induces postrotatory nystagmus and simultaneous turning of the head in the direction of the slow phase. This was confirmed by MYGIND (1919) and by FISCHER and WODAK (1922).

BALDENWECK (1912) demonstrated that after irrigation with water above and below body temperature the head would also turn into the direction of the slow phase.

KRAGH's studies (1922) confirmed this finding and further showed that the response occurred when the lateral semicircular canal was in the optimal position, while it was not elicited if it was in the pessimal position.

More recent studies of head movements following caloric stimulation, termed "laterotorsion" from the torque-like action of the spinal muscles in twisting the body, have been performed by HENRIKSSON et al. (1962a), HENRIKSSON et al. (1962b), and DOLOWITZ et al. (1962). The principle is that the head rotation in the supine subject gives rise to changes in the mutual pressure between two pneumatic balloons on which the head rests. The response can be recorded on a mingograph, whether it occurs spontaneously or following vestibular stimulation; it is possible to combine this process with electronystagmography.

Laterotorsion outlasts nystagmus, but its maximum occurs later and it is less susceptible to light.

The laterotorsion is fairly consistent for a given individual, but shows interindividual variations. Slight movements often occur spontaneously in the laterotorsion test, but these movements are almost equally spread around zero, and there is no significant tendency to turn more into one direction than into the other. In normal individuals laterotorsion induced by caloric stimulation is always in the direction of the slow component of nystagmus and on average it is statistically higher than the spontaneous laterotorsion. This is of the utmost importance, since it indicates that it is a vestibular response that is being measured. Another suggestive factor is that patients with vestibular lesions show reduced nystagmus reaction and laterotorsion. On the other hand, it appears inexplicable why patients with Ménière's disease have normal laterotorsion but a reduced nystagmic reaction, and why patients with meningoencephalitis have normal nystagmic reaction but elevated laterotorsion values, seeing that both responses are elicited from the peripheral labyrinth.

B. Upper Limbs

Numerous pointing experiments have been reported but BÁRÁNY (1910, 1925) was the first to publish a critical analysis and objective measurements of pointing deviations following vestibular stimulation. BÁRÁNY stressed the importance of letting the subject sit down with his eyes closed, thus eliminating the uncertainty caused by standing still. He used a disk by means of which the pointing deviation could be measured in the horizontal as well as vertical plane. The subject was repeatedly made to extend his index finger and touch the disk. In this way, BÁRÁNY demonstrated that the past-pointing was into the same direction as the slow component of nystagmus following vestibular stimulation.

The "Abweichreaktion" described by BÁRÁNY (BÁRÁNY and WITTMAACK, 1911) was studied in more detail by GÜTTICH (1914). This reaction consists in lateral deviation of the forward extended arms and can be elicited by irrigation of one ear with warm or cold water. GÜTTICH demonstrated that the deviation was into the direction of the slow component of nystagmus.

THORNVAL (1917), using a disk like BÁRÁNY's, stressed the importance of performing several experiments, as there is a fairly marked variation from time to time, and also emphasized that induced tests should always be preceded by spontaneous ones. After rotation of the subject he found an overwhelming predominance of deviation into the direction of the rotation, and in half his cases he observed deviation of both arms. After irrigation with cold/warm water, the majority, but not all, showed deviation of the homolateral/contralateral arm into the direction of the slow component. In more than half the subjects, galvanic stimulation, monauricular-monopolar, elicited deviation of the homolateral arm, if the anode was placed at the ear and of the contralateral arm if the cathode was placed at the ear.

WODAK and FISCHER (1922) and FISCHER and WODAK (1924b) grouped the vestibular reactions in the upper limbs into "Armtonusreaktion" and "Abweichreaktion". The former is manifest as lowering or raising of the arm and the latter, as already mentioned (GÜTTICH, 1914), as a deviation. Irrigation with cold water induced lowering of the homolateral and raising of the contralateral arm, and the reverse phenomenon occurred on irrigation with warm water. Graphic recording was used. In galvanic stimulation anode corresponds to cold and cathode to warm water. The Abweichreaktion may also be recorded graphically by getting the subject to hold a pencil against a moving strip of paper.

TALPIS (1927) eliminated the tactile influence in pointing experiments by placing lamps on the fingers and photographing the movements. NYMAN (1945) used the same principle, but in a modified, technically more advanced form. The results revealed a wide spontaneous range in the same individual and a difference between the right and the left arm. Moreover, there was some normal outward deviation of the extended arms, mainly of the left one. The explanation may be that the right arm is used more, and therefore its movements have finer coordination, the left arm being to some extent characterized by "co-movements".

In the vertical writing test described by FUKUDA (1959a), the arm deviation can be measured when the seated subject writes letters underneath each other. Most subjects are said to write with a maximum deviation of 5°. Following calorization, there is said to be a deviation into the same direction as the slow component of nystagmus. BRUNIA and HOOPENBROUWERS (1966), however, found normal subjects wrote with a far greater deviation in the spontaneous test, and according to what has been stated above the test is of no value in assessment of the vestibulospinal reflexes in the upper limbs, let alone the tonic neck reflexes.

As is apparent from the reported pointing methods and results, no importance can be attached to a single pointing test in assessment of the vestibular influence upon the upper limbs at a given time. Several tests must be done, and tests using vestibular stimulation should always be preceded by spontaneous tests. Furthermore, extralabyrinthine factors must be eliminated from the test situation as far as at all possible. The subject must be seated and must be blindfolded. The arms must be extended horizontally forward, since the increase in extensor tonus elicited by the vestibular stimulation is most distinct in this positions, manifesting itself in an outward movement of the arm, as in the Abweichreaktion.

The finger — nose test, on the other hand, is unsuitable for investigation of past-pointing elicited by vestibular stimulation. This was shown at an early date by BÁRÁNY (BÁRÁNY and WITTMAACK, 1911) who wondered why a person subjected to calorization could put his finger to his nose every time, while showing distinct past-pointing on the pointing disk. The explanation is that the finger — nose test can be done correctly because of proprioceptive impulses.

In acute, severe vestibular actions, such as labyrinthine destruction, there will be pointing deviation into the same direction as the slow component of nystagmus. This deviation is often of only brief duration, as compensation sets in. It is also not unusual to find no demonstrable pointing deviation in patients with spontaneous nystagmus elicited from the peripheral vestibular apparatus.

C. Trunk

The vestibular reflexes which may be elicited in the trunk have to be recorded while the subject is seated as otherwise the response from the lower limbs would be manifest, and although it does not differ essentially from those of the trunk, the latter would be overshadowed. As the trunk responses are of little practical importance, not much space will be devoted to them here. BALDENWECK (1912) stated that following irrigation with cold water the trunk leans toward the irrigated ear and away from it after irrigation with warm water. KRAGH (1924) and FISCHER and WODAK (1924a), studying the response to rotation, found reflexes against the direction of rotation during rotation with postrotatory shift.

TOROK and KAHN (1960) described a method called "lateropulsion" in which sideways movements of the trunk induced by rotation could be recorded by means of an electronic amplifier, very accurately on a mingograph, simultaneously with the nystagmus. The deviations induced at the start and end of a rotation are small, equal, but into opposite directions. Initially the trunk leans away from the direction of rotation, and at the end the direction is reversed. During constant rotation there is no inclination.

This test hardly records a purely vestibular reaction, and seems rather to be a tipping reaction. The phenomenon is comparable to that of a person standing in a bus, who sways backward when the bus starts and forward when it stops. No doubt proprioceptive factors are operative.

D. Lower Limbs

The reactions elicited in the lower limbs by vestibular stimulation take the form of swaying or inclination into a given direction, a tendency to fall, or even a fall or turning of the subject on his own vertical axis, demonstrable in walking tests. Fischer and Wodak (1924a) called these movements "Körperneigungsreflexe" and "Körperdrehreflexe" respectively.

1. Walking and Stepping Tests

The turning reaction following vestibular stimulation can be assessed by direct observation, but this is an inaccurate estimate, since the angle is small. The deviation is distinct in blindfold walking, where the subject tries to walk straight forward or backward, in some cases both. In walking forward and backward the deviations are into opposite directions. In the event of a deviation, the subject may describe a stellate figure, "marche en étoile" (Babinski and Weill, 1913). A person with peripheral vestibular nystagmus, spontaneous or induced, is usually said to deviate into the direction of the slow component of nystagmus during blindfold forward walking. Wodak (1953) studied subjects who were made to walk at 4 different speeds ranging from very slow to very fast. The results showed that following cold caloric stimulation and rotatory stimulation ($10 \times 360°/20$ sec) they deviated into the direction of the slow component when walking slowly, while during fast walking they deviated now into one and now into the other direction. From this Wodak categorically concluded that walking tests were of no practical and probably not even of clinical importance. Deviations in walking following galvanic stimulation have differed according to the reports. Following bipolar-binauricular stimulation Babinski and Weill (1913) and also Hennebert (1950) found deviation into the direction of the anode in most cases. Peitersen and Zilstorff-Pedersen (1963b), on the other hand, found no definite direction of deviation after galvanic stimulation in the stepping test. No doubt the best method for assessing a subject's walking deviation is the "treading" test. Unterberger (1938) was the first to make systematic use of this test, which he called the "Tretversuch." He found that normal right-handed persons rotated slightly to the left, whereas left-handed persons rotated to the right; both groups showed some slight forward movement as well. After irrigation with 10 ml water at 27° C, Unterberger found an average deviation of 90° into the direction of the irrigated ear. After galvanic stimulation the subjects also rotated on their own axis, whereas consistent turning could not be induced by rotatory stimulation. In 1940 Hirsch published his "waltzing test" which broadly speaking is identical with Unterberger's "Tretversuch". Following caloric, galvanic, and rotatory stimulation Hirsch demonstrated rotation on the subject's longitudinal axis. After stimulation with 5 ml water at 15° C the subjects rotated through 180–360°, depending upon individual sensitivity. The rotation lasted for several minutes. If the lateral semicircular canal was in the pessimal position no rotation was elicited. FUKUDA (1959b) used the same test, but called it the "stepping test". FUKUDA studied 500 normal persons, each person only once. These persons tried to walk 50–100 steps on the same spot. Most of them succeeded, but some rotated 30–45° on their own axis and moved 0.5—, 1 m forward or—, very rarely—, backward. Following rotatory stimulation through $2 \times 360°$ the subjects turned into the direction of rotation, while after stronger stimulation, i.e. rotation through $10 \times 360°$, they turned in the opposite direction.

JORDAN (1963), reproducing the stepping test, found the subjects had turned on their own axis through 0–190° after 30 steps. Furthermore, about half of them changed their direction of rotation in the two tests performed on each. Thus, his results are in conflict with FUKUDA's.

Using both the walking and the stepping test, MILOJEVIC and WATSON (1965) found that right-handed subjects deviated predominantly to the right and left-handed persons to the left, while they found no difference in Romberg's test.

The method used by ZILSTORFF-PEDERSEN and PEITERSEN (1963) and by PEITERSEN (1965) is a modification of UNTERBERGER's and FUKUDA's test, a "stepping *in situ*" in which the blindfolded subject tries to keep in the center of two concentric circles (Fig. 1) while lifting his feet alternately as in ordinary

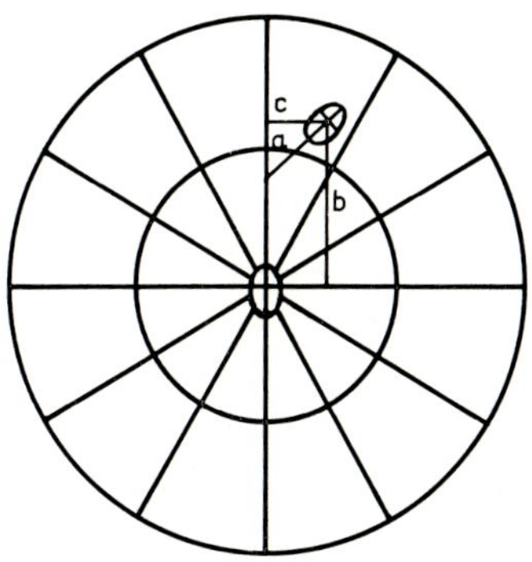

Fig. 1. Test circles: Subject's rotation on his own axis in degrees (a); movement forward in centimeters (b); and movement to the sides in centimeters (c)

walking. The tests, which were carried out in a quiet, darkened room to exclude orientation by means of acoustic and visual stimuli, lasted for one minute. The subjects walked in their own shoes, unless they were high-heeled, if they walked steadily in them. Letting the subjects walk barefoot or in their stockinged feet, as FUKUDA did, can lead to an erroneous result, as many persons can orientate by feeling the warmth of their own feet on the floor. The position of the arms is another problem. Previous investigators, such as UNTERBERGER, HIRSCH, and FUKUDA, had their subjects walk their arms extended parallel and horizontal in front of them. This is of no importance in the spontaneous test, but after vestibular stimulation there is no guarantee that deviation of the arms (BÁRÁNY, 1925; GÜTTICH, 1914; FISCHER and WODAK, 1924a) will not pull the subject around in a given direction, so that the result does not represent a reaction derived exclusively from the lower limbs. In this connection, it should be mentioned that the primary vestibular fibers supply only the upper limbs and not the lower (WALBERG et al., 1958). The present author's tests were therefore performed with the subjects' arms by their sides. The rotation on the subject's axis was recorded in degrees, and the movement forward or backward and to the sides was measured in centimeters.

In the spontaneous tests it is interesting to note that the dispersion in the rotation angle is remarkable, both from subject to subject, and in the same subject in repeated tests. This shows that a single test is of no value (ZILSTORFF-PEDERSEN and PEITERSEN, 1963; PEITERSEN, 1965; JORDAN, 1963). Among the three types of vestibular stimuli used, rotatory (PEITERSEN and ZILSTORFF-PEDERSEN, 1963a), galvanic (PEITERSEN and ZILSTORFF-PEDERSEN, 1963b), and thermal (PEITERSEN, 1963a), the thermal stimulus is definitely the best one, because it can be applied unilaterally and it is easy to vary quantitatively.

The importance of the strength of the stimulus is clearly apparent (PEITERSEN, 1963a) from Fig. 2, which shows that irrigation with water at a temperature only a few centigrade degrees different from body temperature induces the characteristic rotation in the same direction as the slow phase of nystagmus. If stronger

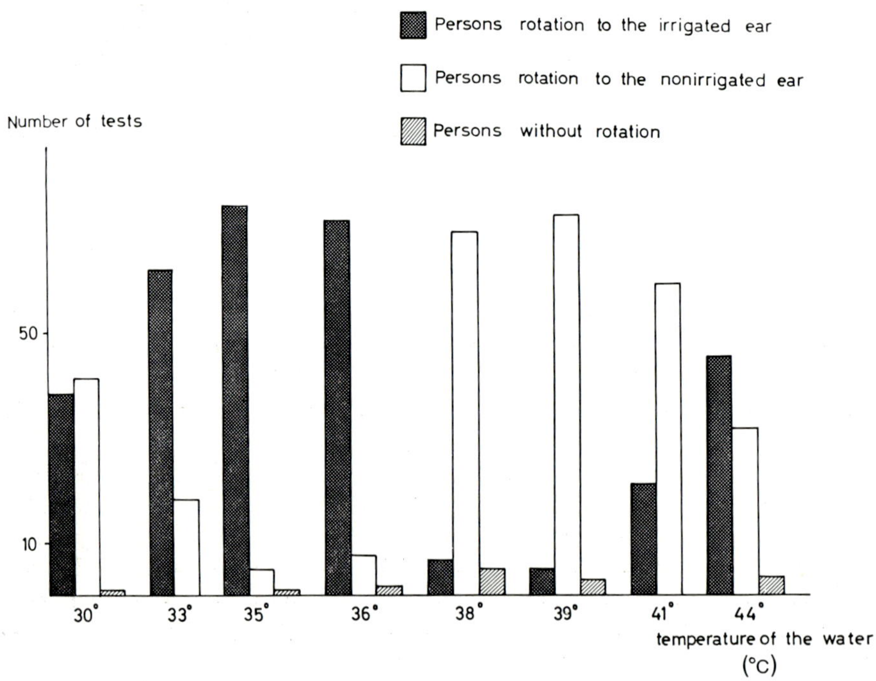

Fig. 2. Graphic representation of the direction of rotation by the subjects at different temperatures of irrigating water

thermal stimuli are used, the general unsteadiness and dizziness become so manifest that it is impossible to obtain a definite result. The outcome will be very fortuitous, and as stated by WODAK (1953): "the finer reactions, to which rotation of the body belongs, will be drowned in general dizziness". Analogous factors are manifest after surgery on the stapes for otosclerosis (PEITERSEN, 1963b). On the day after the operation, the stimulus, i.e. opening of the perilymphatic space, is more manifest than on the following days. As a result, a larger number of patients rotate toward the operated ear on the third and fourth days than on the first day after the operation (Fig. 3).

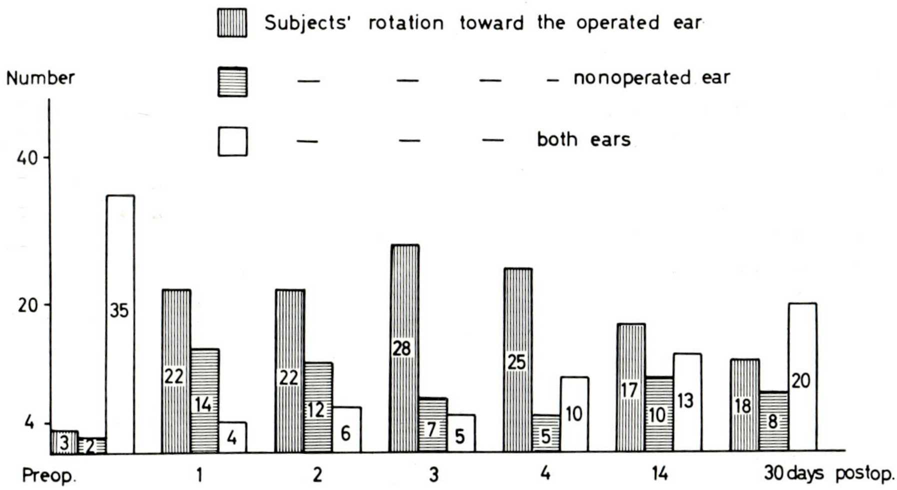

Fig. 3. Direction of the patient's rotation in the stepping tests before and after operation for otosclerosis

For similar reasons approximately the same occurs in patients with diseases of the inner ear and vestibular nerve (PEITERSEN, 1964). The three groups mentioned above are characterized by affection of the peripheral labyrinth. Patients with intracranial diseases (PEITERSEN and ZILSTORFF-PEDERSEN, 1964) and normal subjects who have ingested alcohol (PEITERSEN, 1966), in whom the action also affects the central vestibular system, show a significantly increased rotation angle in the stepping test, but not rotation into a constant direction.

It is concluded (PEITERSEN, 1965; PEITERSEN, 1967) that the stepping test, as a spontaneous routine measure, is of value, especially in patients with unilateral peripheral vestibular diseases. The most reliable results are obtained in patients who are not too unsteady or dizzy. In cases where tests for induced nystagmus are unreliable or impossible, as in external ophthalmoplegia, the stepping test is a valuable vestibular test which in these cases should be carried out after weak thermal stimulation with water at 35° and 39°C.

Of course, the stepping test should no more be used alone than other vestibular tests, but should always be supplemented by others.

2. Swaying or Inclination

Since ROMBERG (1846) reported that patients with tabes dorsalis were unable to stand with their feet together and closed eyes, this test has been widely used, and attempts have been made to assess the results objectively, first by graphic recording (e.g. by MILES, 1924), and later by photography (e.g. by GOLDBERG, 1943). HELLEBRANDT and FRANSEEN (1943) have reviewed the previously used methods.

In recent years electrical tests, in particular, have gained ground (THOMAS and WHITNEY, 1959; UCHYTIL, 1962). UCHYTIL worked out an extremely elegant and simple method in which the subject is placed in an electric field between two plate-shaped electrodes. If the position is altered, changes in the electric field occur. These changes are recorded on a mingograph. HENRIKSSON et al. (1967) use two electrical scales on which the subject stands. Alternations in the pressure of weight from the right and left feet and upon the forefoot and hindfoot are recorded by an ink writer.

On the basis of the numerous tests is has been ascertained that normal persons who stand with feet together and closed eyes sway slightly to the sides and somewhat more forward and backward. The next question is how vestibular stimuli influence the standing position. BÁRÁNY (1906) and FISCHER and WODAK (1924a) found an inclination or a tendency to fall toward the stimulated ear following stimulation with cold water, and conversely inclination toward the nonstimulated ear after irrigation with warm water. These reactions occurred when the lateral semicircular canal was stimulated. Changes in the position of the head alter the direction of the reactions or abolish them. Galvanic stimulation induced swaying toward the anode and away from the cathode (BÁRÁNY, 1906; FISCHER and WODAK, 1924a). HENNEBERT (1950) also found this to be the main rule, while some subjects swayed in the opposite direction or not at all. PEITERSEN and ZILSTOFF-PEDERSEN (1963b) found swaying in the direction of the current in monopolar-monauricular stimulation and swaying in the opposite direction to the current upon bipolar-binauricular stimulation, while following bipolar-monauricular stimulation the swaying was away from the stimulated ear. The current required to induce swaying was lowest with bipolar-binauricular stimulation, on average 0.5 mA.

Postrotatory inclination is into the direction of the rotation as demonstrated by BREUER (1874), BÁRÁNY (1910, 1922), and other authors.

UCHYTIL (1962), supplementing the spontaneous tests with tests following caloric stimulation, found swaying in the direction of the slow component of nystagmus. He also demonstrated swaying towards the ear in which vestibular function was reduced in a patient with acute labyrinthitis.

3. Deep Reflexes

As early as 1912 it was demonstrated by BECK and BIACH that the deep reflexes respond to vestibular stimuli. For instance, irrigation with cold water increases the ipsilateral patellar reflex. Reversely, the contralateral patellar reflex will become brisker after irrigation with warm water.

WIGAND and STRUPPLER (1962) carried out very elegant studies on the susceptibility of the Achilles tendon reflex to calorization with 20 ml water at 20°C.

The excursions of the reflex were recorded on an oscillograph, and electronystagmography was performed at the same time. It was found that the reflex induced mechanically by striking the tendon was increased, whereas the reflex induced by stimulation of the posterior tibialis nerve was not definitely affected. These findings were taken to mean that vestibular stimulation in man increases the irritability of the muscle spindles by way of the gamma-system, in this case making the gastrocnemius reflex brisker.

V. Tipping Reactions

Unter the heading of vestibulospinal reflexes it seems appropriate to mention also the righting and balance reactions elicited by way of the labyrinth through proprioceptive impulses when the subject is suddenly taken off his balance by tipping or tilting the couch. VON STEIN (1894) was the first to carry out systematic studies on compensatory righting reactions in man. Since then McNALLY and TAIT (1925), TAIT (1926), DE KLEYN and VERSTEEGH (1936), RÅDMARK (1944), NYMAN (1945) and others have studied the same phenomena, although the tipping tables, the speed of tipping, and the recording methods have differed. NYMAN's tipping table and recording methods are technically the most refined. The tipping reaction in normal persons is distinctly different from that in persons with destroyed labyrinths, who are unable to keep their balance without the aid of vision if the couch is suddenly tipped. If one labyrinth is functioning the person will respond normally. The tipping reaction is not now much used for diagnosis, but it is worth bearing in mind that, as demonstrated by RADEMARKER and GARCIN (1932), patients with cerebellar ataxia do not fall during this test.

In contradistinction to the above methods, in which the subjects are usually positioned on their hands and knees, KITAHARA (1965) studied head deviation with the subjects standing erect on a platform. The platform could be turned with an angular speed of 1°/sec to the right, to the left, forward, and backward. Most normal subjects then move their head in the opposite direction, whereas the majority of patients with Ménière's disease show no deviation when the platform is turned into the direction of the affected ear.

Concerning the results of this method, called "acceleration registrography," normal persons tipped in this way obviously try to maintain the position of the head in relation to the perpendicular line, and this causes the compensatory movement. However, persons who have only one functioning labyrinth will make the same movement, so that it is difficult to understand why patients with unilateral Ménière's disease cannot. Furthermore, the speed of inclination is constant, 1°/sec, so that an accelerative action upon the labyrinth is possible only at the start and end of the tipping. On the whole, it seems doubtful whether this method, as claimed, has any practical value as a clinical test of the labyrinthine righting reflexes.

VI. Concluding Remarks

As pointed out, the vestibulospinal reflexes are clearly defined reactions which are nonetheless difficult to record owing to the influence by extralabyrinthine factors. This is presumably why it was not until quite recently that clinical interest again became focused on this aspect of vestibulology, which flourished in the early part of this century.

The increasing attempts at objective recording, as in nystagmus tests, are of great importance.

It is of fundamental importance also to look upon the vestibular system as an entity, though of a widely ramified mosaic pattern with its possibilities of response. Accordingly, a single reaction should not be studied alone, but supplemented by a wide choice of tests. This opens up the possibility of assessing not only the peripheral vestibular apparatus, but also its central part, and of making a topical diagnosis in this part.

References

Babinski, J., Weill, G.A.: Désorientation et déséquilibration spontanée et provoquée. La déviation angulaire. C. R. Soc. Biol. (Paris) **74**, I, 852–855 (1913).

Baldenweck, L.: L'inclinaison et la rotation de la tête pendant l'épreuve calorique. Ann. Mal. Oreil. Larynx. **38**, 240–245 (1912).

Bárány, R.: Untersuchungen über den vom Vestibularapparat des Ohres reflektorisch ausgelösten rhythmischen Nystagmus und seine Begleiterscheinungen. Mschr. Ohrenheilk. **40**, 193–297 (1906).

Bárány, R.: Neue Untersuchungsmethoden, die Beziehungen zwischen Vestibularapparat, Kleinhirn, Grosshirn und Rückenmark betreffend. Wien. med. Wschr. **60**, 2033–2037 (1910).

Bárány, R.: Zur Zerlegung der Fallreaktion in zwei Komponenten. Acta oto-laryng. (Stockh.) **4**, 73–75 (1922).

Bárány, R.: 1. Der Zeigeversuch. 2. Die Abweichereaktion. 3. Der Einstellungsversuch, nebst Bemerkungen zur Theorie des Vestibularapparates und Kleinhirns. Acta oto-laryng. (Stockh.) **7**, 139–160 (1925).

Bárány, R., Wittmaack, K.: Funktionelle Prüfung des Vestibularapparates. Verh. dtsch. otol. Ges. **20**, 38–184 (1911).

Beck, O., Biach, P.: Labyrinth und Sehnenreflexe. Berl. klin. Wschr. **49**, 300–303 (1912).

Breuer, J.: Ueber die Function der Bogengänge des Ohrlabyrinthes. Med. Jahrb. (Wien) 1874.

Brodal, A., Pompeiano, O., Walberg, F.: The vestibular nuclei and their connections, anatomy and functional correlations, 1st ed. Edinburgh: Oliver and Boyd 1962.

Brunia, C.H.M., Hoppenbrouwers, T.: In search of tonic cervical reflexes. An evaluation of Fukuda's vertical writing test. Acta oto-laryng. (Stockh.) **61**, 547–554 (1966).

Dolowitz, D.A., Forssman, B., Henriksson, N.G.: Studies of cristospinal reflexes (laterotorsion). III. Patterns of cristoocular and cristospinal reflexes in clinical oto-neurology. Acta oto-laryng. (Stockh.) **55**, 496–504 (1962).

Fischer, M.H., Wodak, E.: Experimentelle Untersuchungen über Vestibularisreaktionen. Z. Hals-, Nas.- u. Ohrenheilk. **3**, 198–215 (1922).

Fischer, M.H., Wodak, E.: Beiträge zur Physiologie des menschlichen Vestibularapparates. I. Die vestibulären Körperreflexe und die Fallreaktion. Pflügers Arch. ges. Physiol. **202**, 523–552 (1924a).

Fischer, M.H., Wodak, E.: Beiträge zur Physiologie des menschlichen Vestibularapparates. II. Die Grundlagen und grafischen Registriermethoden der „vestibulären Körperreflexe". Pflügers Arch. ges. Physiol. **202**, 553–565 (1924b).
oto-laryng. (Stockh.) **50**, 26–36 (1959a).

Fukuda, T.: Vertical writing with eyes covered: A new test of vestibulo-spinal reaction. Acta oto-laryng. (Stockh.) **50**, 26–36 (1959a).

Fukuda, T.: The stepping test: Two phases of the labyrinthine reflex. Acta oto-laryng. (Stockh.) **50**, 95–108 (1959b).

GERNANDT, B.E.: Generation of labyrinthine impulses, descending vestibular pathways, and modulation of vestibular activity by proprioceptive, cerebellar, and reticular influences. In: G.L. RASMUSSEN and W.F. WINDLE, Eds. Neural mechanisms of auditory and vestibular systems. Springfield/Ill.: Ch.C. Thomas 1960.

GERNANDT, B.E., THULIN, C.-A.: Reciprocal effects upon spinal motoneurons from stimulation of bulbar reticular formation. J. Neurophysiol. **18**, 113–129 (1955a).

GERNANDT, B.E., THULIN, C.-A.: Effect of vestibular nerve section upon the spinal influence of the bulbar reticular formation. Acta physiol. scand. **33**, 120–131 (1955b).

GOLDBERG, L.: Quantitative studies on alcohol tolerance in man. Acta physiol. scand. **5**, Suppl. 16, 1–128 (1943).

GÜTTICH, A.: Beitrag zur Physiologie des Vestibularapparates. Beitr. Anat. ect., Ohr. **7**, 1–18 (1914).

HELLEBRANDT, F.A., FRANSEEN, E.B.: Physiological study of the vertical stance of man. Physiol. Rev. **23**, 220–255 (1943).

HENNEBERT, P.E.: L'épreuve galvanic. Acta oto-rhino-laryng. belg. **4**, 409–417 (1950).

HENRIKSSON, N.G., DOLOWITZ, D.A., FORSSMAN, B.: Studies of cristospinal reflexes (laterotorsion). I. A method for objectiv recording of cristospinal reflexes. Acta oto-laryng. (Stockh.) **55**, 33–40 (1962a).

HENRIKSSON, N.G., FORSSMAN, B., DOLOWITZ, D.A.: Studies of cristospinal reflexes (laterotorsion). II. Caloric nystagmus and laterotorsion in normal individuals. Acta oto-laryng. (Stockh.) **55**, 116–128 (1962b).

HENRIKSSON, N.G., JOHANSSON, G., OLSSON, L.G., ÖSTLUND, H.: Acta oto-laryng. (Stockh.) Suppl. **224**, 272–279 (1967).

HIRSCH, C.: A new labyrinthine reaction: "The waltzing test". Ann. Otol. (St. Louis) **49**, 232–238 (1940).

JORDAN, P.: Fukuda's stepping test: A preliminary report on reliability. Arch. Otolaryng. **77**, 243–245 (1963).

KITAHARA, M.: Acceleration registrography. A method of examinations concerned with the labyrinthine righting reflex. Ann. Otol. (St. Louis) **74**, 203–214 (1965).

DE KLEYN, A., VERSTEEGH, C.: Über labyrinthäre Gleichgewichtsreaktion bei Menschen und Tieren nach schnellem Kippen um die longitudinale Achse. Acta oto-laryng. (Stockh.) **24**, 34–52 (1936).

KRAGH, J.: La réaction vestibulaire de la tête. Acta oto-laryng. (Stockh.) **4**, 209–218 (1922).

KRAGH, J.: Sur la réaction vestibulaire du tronc humain mesurée pendant la rotation. Acta oto-laryng. (Stockh.) **6**, 178–181 (1924).

MCNALLY, W.J., TAIT, J.: Ablation experiments on the labyrinth of the frog. Amer. J. Physiol. **75**, 155–179 (1925).

MILES, W.R.: Alcohol and human efficiency. Publ. No. 333. Washington D.C.: Carnegie Institution 1924.

MILOJEVIC, B., WATSON, J.L.: Vestibular asymmetries in right- and left-handed people. Acta oto-laryng. (Stockh.) **60**, 322–330 (1965).

MYGIND, S.H.: Hovednystagmus hos mennesket. Bibl. Laeger **111**, 254–261 (1919).

NYMAN, H.: A grafic registration of tipping and pointing reaction. Acta oto-laryng. (Stockh.) Suppl. **60**, 1–131 (1945).

PEITERSEN, E.: Vestibulospinal reflexes. IV. Alterations in stepping test after thermal stimulation in normal subjects. Arch. Otolaryng. **78**, 59–67 (1963a).

PEITERSEN, E.: Vestibulospinal reflexes. V. Acute disturbances of vestibular function after operations on the stapes, especially as evaluated by stepping test. Arch. Otolaryng. **78**, 642–648 (1963b).

PEITERSEN, E.: Vestibulospinal reflexes. VII. Alterations in stepping test in various disorders of the inner ear and vestibular nerve. Arch. Otolaryng. **79**, 481–486 (1964).

PEITERSEN, E.: Vestibulo-spinale reflexer: Kliniske og eksperimentelle undersøgelser ved hjælp af steppingtesten. Copenhagen: Munksgaard 1965.

PEITERSEN, E.: Vestibulospinal reflexes. IX. Alterations in stepping test during alcohol intoxication. Arch. Otolaryng. **83**, 332–334 (1966).

PEITERSEN, E.: Vestibulospinal reflexes. X. Theoretical and clinical aspects of the stepping test. Arch. Otolaryng. **85**, 192–198 (1967).

Peitersen, E., Zilstorff-Pedersen, K.: Vestibulospinal reflexes. II. Alterations in stepping test after rotatory stimulation in normal subjects. Arch. Otolaryng. **77**, 353–358 (1963a).

Peitersen, E., Zilstorff-Pedersen, K.: Vestibulospinal reflexes. III. Alterations in stepping test following galvanic stimulation. Arch. Otolaryng. **77**, 586–591 (1963b).

Peitersen, E., Zilstorff-Pedersen, K.: Vestibulospinal reflexes. VIII. Alterations in stepping test in various intracranial diseases. Arch. Otolaryng. **79**, 600–605 (1964).

Pompeiano, O.: Organizzazione sommatotopica delle riposte posturali alla stimolazione elettrica del nucleo di Deiters nel gatte decerebrato. Arch. Sci. biol. (Bologna) **44**, 497–511 (1960).

Pompeiano, O., Brodal, A.: The origin of vestibulospinal fibres in the cat. An experimental-anatomical study, with comments on the descending medial longitudinal fasciculus. Arch. ital. Biol. **95**, 166–195 (1957).

Purkinje, J.E.: Über die physiologische Bedeutung des Schwindels und die Beziehung desselben zu den neuesten Versuchen über die Hirnfunctionen. Rufts Magazin ges. Heilk. **23**, 284–310 (1827).

Rademaker, G.G.J., Garcin, R.: Note sur quelques réactions labyrintiques des extrémites chez l'animal et chez l'homme. Étude physiologique et clinique. Rev. neurol. **39**, 637–653 (1932).

Rådmark, K.: Tipping reaction in cases of vertigo after head injury. Acta oto-laryng. (Stockh.) Suppl. **52**, 1–133 (1944).

Romberg, M.H.: Lehrbuch der Nervenkrankheiten des Menschen. Berlin: A. Duncker 1846.

von Stein, S.: Die Lehren von den Funktionen der einzelnen Theile des Ohrlabyrinthes. Jena: Fischer 1894.

Tait, J.: Ablation experiments on the labyrinth of frogs. Arch. Otolaryng. **4**, 281–295 (1926).

Talpis, L.: Zur Methode der grafischen Registrierung des Zeige- und Einstellungsversuches, der Armtonus und Abweichreaktion. Arch. Ohr.-, Nas.-, u. Kehlk.-Heilk. **116**, 255–265 (1927).

Thomas, D.P., Whitney, R.J.: Postural movements during normal standing in man. J. Anat. (Lond.) **93**, 524–539 (1959).

Thornval, A.: Funktionsundersøgelser af Vestibularorganet og Cerebellum. Copenhagen: Busk 1917.

Torok, N., Kahn, A.: Vestibular lateropulsion. Ann. Otol. (St. Louis) **69**, 61–72 (1960).

Uchytil, B.: Methode der objectiven Aufzeichnung vestibulospinaler Reflexe. Mschr. Ohrenheilk. **96**, 554–558 (1962).

Unterberger, S.: Neue objectiv registrierbare Vestibularis-Körperdrehreaktion, erhalten durch Treten auf der Stelle: „Der Tretversuch". Arch. Ohr.-, Nas.-, u. Kehlk.-Heilk. **145**, 478–492 (1938).

Walberg, F., Bowsher, D., Brodal, A.: The termination of primary vestibular fibers in the vestibular nuclei in the cat. An experimental study with silver methods. J. comp. Neurol. **110**, 391–419 (1958).

Wigand, M.E., Struppler, A.: Elektrophysiologische Untersuchungen über die Eigenreflex-Erregbarkeit des Menschen bei Vestibularisreizung. Arch. Ohr.-, Nas.-, u. Kehlk.-Heilk. **179**, 273–282 (1962).

Wodak, E.: Physio-pathologische Probleme des menschlichen Vestibularapparates. Fortschr. Hals-Nas.-Ohrenheilk. **1**, 166–263 (1953).

Wodak, E., Fischer, M.H.: Eine neue Vestibularisreaktion. Münch. med. Wschr. **69**, 193–194 (1922).

Zilstorff-Pedersen, K., Peitersen, E.: Vestibulospinal reflexes. I. Spontaneous alterations in the position of normal persons doing the stepping test. Arch. Otolaryng. **77**, 237–245 (1963).

Chapter IV.

Modification of the Response to Angular Accelerations by Linear Accelerations

By

A. J. Benson, Farnborough, Hampshire (England)

With 14 Figures

Contents

I. Introduction

The specialized receptors of the vestibular apparatus provide the animal with information about its motion and its orientation with respect to the gravitational vertical. By evolutionary processes the dynamic responses of this end-organ subserving equilibratory function have been optimized for the environment in which the animal lives (Mayne, 1965). But man has developed mechanical aids to locomotion which expose him to linear and angular accelerations differing in magnitude and time course from those for which the end-organ and its central integrative mechanisms are functionally adapted. Thus, when he is exposed to such unnatural force environments the vestibular apparatus may generate signals which are no longer appropriate to the motion of the vehicle; illusory sensations and inappropriate vestibular reflexes serve to disorientate the operator and degrade his control.

In the study of spatial disorientation in flight, as in the more fundamental studies of vestibular function which the applied problems have engendered the anatomical and functional differentiation of the vestibular apparatus has led to a dichotomous approach. The precision with which the separate responses to angular and linear acceleration can now be described (YOUNG, 1968) has not been matched by an adequate description of the responses to the motions in a terrestrial environment in which angular and linear accelerations are concomitant. Certain simple interactions are well substantiated and will be described in the following pages, but our knowledge about the underlying mechanisms is rudimentary. This situation has arisen because most of the experimental work in this area has been carried out on the intact animal or human subject. Although the physical stimulus can be defined, there is uncertainty about which end-organs are stimulated and only speculation about the way in which the afferent signals are processed and integrated with the central nervous system.

II. Receptors Stimulated by Linear and Angular Acceleration

It is now firmly established that the ampullar receptors of the semicircular canals are exquisitely sensitive to angular accelerations and the receptors of the utricular and saccular maculae, to linear accelerations (LOWENSTEIN, Chap. B.II.). However, it is not axiomatic that responses elicited by angular accelerations of the whole animal are initiated solely by canal receptors or that the effect of a linear acceleration is mediated solely by the otolith organs.

Linear accelerations can stimulate, by virtue of inertial forces, not only the sensory epithelium of the otolithic maculae but also other mechanoreceptors. These are the touch and pressure receptors in the skin and deeper supporting tissues, and receptors in the capsules of joints which signal the position and rate of change of position of the articulation. In addition to these end-organs, which engender sensations, there are also the specialized sensory endings in the somatic musculature which respond to changes in muscle length brought about by alteration of the force environment. Thus in the majority of experimental studies the response evoked by variation in the direction or magnitude of the linear acceleration vector cannot be regarded as a specific manifestation of stimulation of the otolithic maculae, rather it represents the stimulation of the specialized gravireceptors of the otolith organs and the activity of the more generally distributed gravireceptors. Proof of the role of vestibular receptors in a response engendered by linear accelerations is in some experiments provided by repetition of the test procedure on animals or human subjects in whom the vestibular receptors have been rendered non-functional either by disease, operative procedures, or congenital defect. However, there are many more observations in which the relative importance of vestibular and non-vestibular gravireceptors cannot be proved.

With angular motion about an earth vertical axis there is usually less ambiguity about which sensory end-organs are stimulated, for the sensitivity of the ampullar receptors of the semicircular canals to angular accelerations is well documented. However, there are occasions when the linear accelerations associated with angular motion, namely the centripetal and tangential accelerations, may be an adequate stimulus to vestibular and somatesthetic gravireceptors. Because the threshold stimulus to the otolithic maculae is of the order of 0.01 g (g = 9.81

msec^{-2}) (MEIRY, 1966) and these are situated approximately 45 mm (IGARASHI, 1966) from the longitudinal axis (*foramen magnum*) of the body, then rotation about this axis at angular velocities greater than about 1.5 rad sec^{-1} would be an adequate stimulus. Similarly, effective tangential accelerations would require an angular acceleration of the order of 2.2 rad sec^{-2}. The linear accelerations experienced by other receptors is a function of their distance from their axis of rotation and their instantaneous angular velocity and acceleration. Thus the subject without vestibular function, or a normal man who is accelerated at a subthreshold rate, can detect rotation about an earth vertical axis more readily when the axis of rotation coincides with the anteroposterior (x) or transverse (y) body axes than with the longitudinal (head-foot or z) axis. However, when the ampullar receptors are stimulated by adequate angular accelerations, the thresholds for the detection of angular motion are similar about the three orthogonal body axes (MELVILL JONES et al., 1964).

When angular motion occurs about an axis which is not aligned with the gravitational vertical, then the body experiences a linear acceleration vector of changing orientation for as long as rotation continues. The magnitude of the component of the linear acceleration vector normal to the axis of rotation is proportional to the sine of the angle by which the rotation axis deviates from the vertical. Accordingly, at angles greater than 0.6° adequate stimulation of macular receptors should occur (assuming a threshold value of 0.01 g); at an angle of 90°, i.e., when the axis of rotation is horizontal, the changing vector has a magnitude of 1 g and is a powerful stimulus to both vestibular and somatesthetic gravireceptors.

It is important to recognize that in the course of everyday life motions to which the animal is exposed are complex. Rarely does it experience a simple linear acceleration or a simple angular acceleration; even a pure rotational movement of the head in one plane engenders angular acceleration and deceleration with a concomitant reorientation to gravity, if the plane of rotation is other than horizontal. Translational or angular motion occurring in the presence of rotation in another plane induces Coriolis accelerations which may be an additional stimulus to the vestibular apparatus. The coexistent modulation of the spontaneous discharge of both ampullar and macular receptors is thus the normal neural input to the central nervous system, the isolated stimulation of one group of receptors is an artifact of the laboratory or clinic.

III. Are the Ampullar Receptors Stimulated by Linear Accelerations?

The preceding discussion of the receptors stimulated by linear and angular motions is based on simple physical principles and the established Mach-Breuer-Brown theory of the functional differentiation of the vestibular apparatus (CAMIS, 1930). The electrophysiological studies of the afferent activity in the primary neurons from the sensory epithelium of the cristae and maculae have substantiated the general propriety of the theory (ROSS, 1936; LOWENSTEIN and SAND, 1940a; b; LEDOUX, 1949; LOWENSTEIN and ROBERTS, 1950; GROEN et al., 1952). However, several workers have, on the basis of observations made on intact man or on experimental animals, adduced that the cristae were adequately stimulated by linear accelerations (DE KLEIJN and MAGNUS, 1921; LORENTE DE NÓ, 1931; TER BRAAK, 1937; GERNANDT, 1950; TIMM 1953). This largely indirect evidence will be discussed in detail in the following pages, but before the variety of the observed interactions of linear and angular accelerations are presented, it is germane to consider the less ambiguous information provided by studies of isolated primary afferent neurons.

A. Evidence from Primary Afferent Neurons

Recording from dissected branches of the vestibular nerve within the cranial cavity of the frog, ROSS (1936) reported that the activity of fibers from the cristae of lateral and vertical canals were "substantially independent of gravity". This finding was not supported by LEDOUX (1949), who found that the spontaneous activity of canal afferents was influenced by the orientation of the head to gravity. The resting discharge was decreased when the plane of the canal was vertical and the ampulla superior, and increased when the ampulla was inferior. The alteration of activity which occurred on moving from one position to the other was not immediate but took several seconds to reach a maximum and was maintained for 1 min or longer before the discharge frequency began to return to its initial level. LOWENSTEIN had observed comparable positional responses in canal afferents during his detailed studies of the behavior of the vestibular receptors in elasmobranchs (LOWENSTEIN and SAND, 1940a, b) but considered it to be a sign of functional deterioration of the isolated preparation. LEDOUX on the other hand found that the responses to gravity disappeared as the preparation aged and took place before degradation of its response to angular accelerations was apparent. Yet in a preliminary account of recent experiments in which positional tests were carried out 15 min after decapitation of the fish, LOWENSTEIN (1968) reported a distinct response to gravity in fibers from the cristae of the majority of vertical canals and in about 50% of the fibers from the lateral canals. As in the frog, the discharge frequency was greatest when the ampulla was in an inferior, and least when in a superior, position.

Both LEDOUX and LOWENSTEIN employed an experimental technique which required that an opening be made into the perilymphatic space, whereas ROSS preserved the integrity of the labyrinthine capsule. It may thus be argued that the positional response of the ampullar receptors is an artifact consequent to the loss of perilymph and to the support which it offers to the endolymph-containing membranous system. Traction by the unsupported utriculus and sacculus at the base of the cristae, when the ampulla is in a superior position, could cause relative displacement of the sensory cells of the cristae with respect to the cupula and so alter the excitability of the sensory epithelium.

Alternatively the cupula itself may be deflected by the linear acceleration. This view has been put forward by TIMM (1953) and TER BRAAK (1937) who calculated that a difference in specific gravity of 0.0001 between cupula and endolymph is required if an acceleration of 1 g is to produce the same cupula deflection as an angular acceleration of 0.0009 rad sec^{-2} (0.05° sec^{-2}), i.e., a threshold stimulus.

Measurements of the specific gravity of the cupula carried out by MONEY (personal communication) in a density gradient column capable of measuring specific gravity to an accuracy of 0.0004 (MONEY et al., 1966) revealed that the density of the cupula was indistinguishable from that of endolymph. The force attributable to gravity which may deflect the cupula is therefore small and unlikely to account for the substantial alteration in discharge frequency reported by LEDOUX and LOWENSTEIN.

This suggestion is supported by the apparent lack of a positional effect on the time constant of decay in activity of canal afferents following an angular impulse, such as a sudden stop from rotation at constant velocity (LOWENSTEIN, 1968). If a significant difference in density between endolymph and cupula did exist, then the couple which restores the cupula from the deflected to the neutral position would be either assisted or opposed by a force proportional to the product of linear acceleration and the difference in density between endolymph and cupula. The absence of an alteration in the time constant of restoration (the π/Δ of VAN EGMOND et al., 1949) or the long time constant T_1 (YOUNG, 1968) of the cupula as indicated by the behavior of the isolated ray labyrinth or the postrotational nystagmus response (*vide infra*) favors the conclusion that the cupula *per se* is not normally deflected by a linear acceleration vector of constant magnitude which maintains a constant orientation to the vestibular apparatus.

B. Evidence from Neurons Relaying Canal Afferents

The problems and uncertainties which accompany the interpretation of the experiments on the primary afferents are compounded when the activity of neurons of the vestibular nuclei of the brain stem is examined. For one can no longer be certain that the cell body whose activity is recorded by an adjacent microelectrode is innervated only by primary afferents from the sensory epithelium of the cristae or maculae of the ipsilateral vestibular apparatus. Though the behavior of such second-order neurons, particularly in the medial and superior vestibular nuclei (ADRIAN, 1943; GERNANDT, 1949; ECKEL, 1954; MELVILL JONES, 1967; MELVILL JONES and MILSUM, 1970), can reflect with apparent precision the specific activity of the ampullar receptors of one canal, alterations in excitability of the cell by other neuronal systems cannot be positively excluded. In addition the response of the peripheral receptors may be modified by the activity of the efferent vestibular system (SCHMIDT, 1962; SALA, 1965).

Recording from cell bodies in the vestibular nerve of the decerebrate cat, GERNANDT (1950) showed a difference in the response of neurons innervated by the lateral canal, according to the position of the animal on the turntable. When the head of the animal was close (0.1 m) to the axis of rotation, all the cells studied behaved in an "Ewaldian" manner, that is, their resting discharge was increased during angular acceleration in an ipsilateral direction (e.g. clockwise rotation if recording on the right side) and decreased when the angular acceleration was in the contralateral direction. However, when the head of the animal was 0.4 m from the axis of rotation, and presumably pointing outwards along the radius, rotation in the contralateral direction was found not to inhibit activity but to increase it above the resting level. GERNANDT argued that this phenomenon was a manifestation of the effect of the centripetal acceleration on the cupula with ipsilateral rotation the centrifugal force assisted the cupular deflection produced by the ampullopetal flow of endolymph; with contralateral rotation, the centrifugal force opposed and overcame the utriculofugal movement of the cupula engendered by the angular acceleration. Unfortunately, it was not made clear whether the augmentation of the resting discharge was sustained during rotation at constant speed or was time dependent and hence a function of angular acceleration or the changing magnitude of the tangential and centripetal linear accelerations.

Gernandt's observations were not substantiated by Crampton (1966). He examined unitary activity of "Ewaldian" cells in the vestibular nuclei of cats under deep pentobarbital anesthesia. The evoked activity produced by an angular acceleration of 0.07 rad sec^{-2} ($4°sec^{-2}$) to a constant velocity of 2.1 rad sec^{-1} ($120°sec^{-1}$) did not differ in any consistent way when the head of the animal was placed at the center of rotation and when it was exposed to a centripetal acceleration of 0.24 *g*. The animal was aligned at right angles at the radius, in order to optimize the couple which might deflect the cupulae of the lateral canals. Although

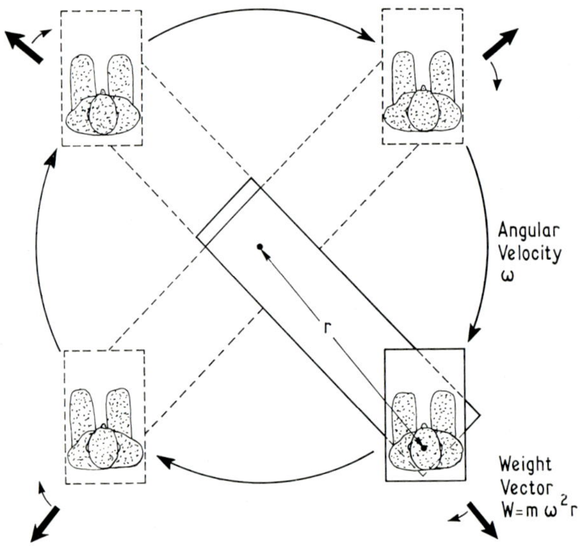

Fig. 1. Counterrotation. Diagram to illustrate the manner in which the subject, or experimental animal, may be exposed to a rotating linear acceleration vector without angular acceleration. The seat at the end of the centrifuge arm (radius r) rotates with respect to the arm at an equal but opposite angular velocity (ω) to that of the arm. The subject thus maintains the same geographical orientation while moving in a circular path, and experiences a linear acceleration (magnitude ω^2r) which rotates in the horizontal (xy) plane in the same direction as the centrifuge arm

facilitation and inhibition of unitary activity were observed in some cells, not one showed an alteration of activity, according to head position and direction of rotation, which was in accord with the hypothesis that the cupula is deflected by a constant linear acceleration.

The contradictory findings of GERNANDT and CRAMPTON can probably be explained by differences in the recording sites and excitability of the preparation. Pentobarbital depresses transmission within the central nervous system, and only those neurons with many synaptic boutons from lateral canal afferents would respond to angular stimuli and hence be selected for study. In addition, alteration in excitability of these cells consequent to changes in otolithic and other gravireceptor stimulation (DUENSING and SCHAEFER, 1959; DUMONT, 1960; FREDRICKSON et al., 1966; FREDRICKSON and SCHWARZ, 1968) would be reduced, as would the activity in the efferent vestibular pathway. Thus, in the study of CRAMPTON the unitary activity of cells in the vestibular nuclei probably reflected more closely the physical behavior of the cupula than did the units examined by GERNANDT. The inference, albeit circumstantial, is that the cupula is not deflected by a constant linear acceleration of 0.25 g.

So far consideration has been given only to the effect of linear accelerations, of constant magnitude and direction, on the activity in first- and second-order neurons of the ampullar receptors.

The response to more complex dynamic stimuli in which there are changes in the magnitude and direction of the acceleration vector is perhaps of greater physiological significance, for such changes in the force environment are the normal concomitants of head and body movement of the animal; sustained linear accelerations, other than the gravitational acceleration, are primarily confined to assisted locomotion in mechanical vehicles.

Preliminary studies by LOWENSTEIN (1968, 1970), who placed his isolated elasmobranch preparation on a counterrotating platform (Fig. 1) with a radius of 0.3 m from the principal axis of rotation, failed to show any significant alteration in activity of primary canal afferents at speeds of rotation of up to 3.1 rad sec^{-1} (180° sec^{-1}) giving, a centripetal acceleration of 0.3 g. This lack of effect of a rotating vector, with angular frequency of 0.5 Hz, on units which showed a well-defined positional response is in accord with the relatively slow development of the response to gravity noted by LEDOUX (1949). Presumably, at rotational frequencies within the dynamic range of the canal response to linear acceleration, the radius was too short to allow a centripetal acceleration of sufficient magnitude to be developed. In the cat, however, a comparable stimulus (a centripetal acceleration of 0.4 g, with a rotational frequency of 0.5 Hz) was found to cause a consistent alteration of the activity of lateral canal units in the region of the medial vestibular nuclei (BENSON et al., 1970). These observations were made on decerebrate cats with intact cerebellum, the study being confined to those units which responded only to angular accelerations in the horizontal plane in which the lateral canals lay. Units which exhibited convergence (DUENSING and SCHAEFER, 1959) of canal and gravireceptor inputs, that is, those cells which responded to both angular and translational motion during initial testing on a six degree of freedom motion platform, were discarded.

All the lateral canal dependent cells examined showed a differential alteration in activity during exposure to the rotating linear acceleration vector. Irrespective of whether the cells reflected the activity of the ipsilateral or contralateral cristae, rotation of the linear acceleration vector in the opposite direction to the excitatory angular acceleration always evoked a higher discharge frequency of the cell than

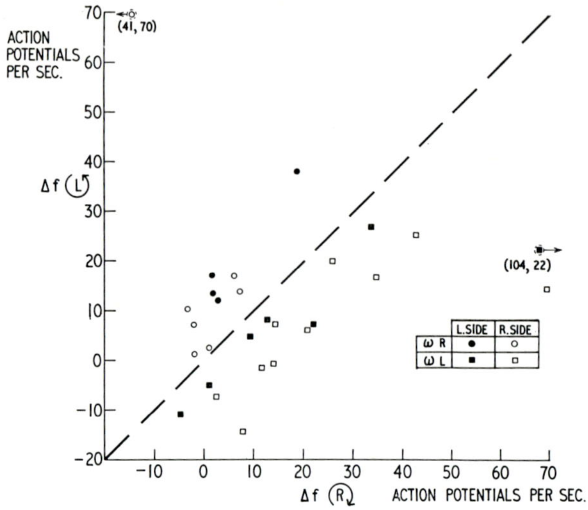

Fig. 2. Alteration in frequency of discharge of 'lateral canal' units according to the direction of rotation of the linear acceleration vector. Each point compares the increment or decrement in activity (Δf) with respect to resting activity, when the cat was exposed to a linear acceleration which rotated to the left (ordinate) and to the right (abscissa). Data from 8 decerebrate unanesthetized cats which were exposed to a linear acceleration of 0.4 g which rotated at 0.5 Hz in the horizontal plane. Note that all units which responded during initial testing to angular acceleration to the right by an increase in activity (indicated by ○ and ●) lie above the line of parity; these units stimulated by angular acceleration to the left (□ and ■) lie below the line. From BENSON et al. (1970)

when the vector rotated in the opposite direction (Fig. 2). The "Ewaldian" cells (whose activity corresponded to the ipsilateral canal) showed, on the average, facilitation and inhibition of the resting activity according to the direction of rotation of the vector. The "non-Ewaldian" cells (whose activity corresponded to the contralateral canal) were facilitated in both directions of rotation of the vector, though the differential alteration of activity was clearly defined as was a cyclical modulation of the discharge frequency (Fig. 3).

Prima facie, these findings support the hypothesis advanced by BENSON and BODIN (1966a) to explain the sustained unidirectional nystagmus observed in man during rotation at constant velocity about a horizontal, head-foot (z) body axis. They suggested that because of the density difference between perilymph and endolymph with its containing membranous duct (MONEY et al., 1966), a linear acceleration vector which rotates in the plane of the canal would cause a continuous redistribution of the endolymph within the membranous duct. Such a "roller pump" type model has been analyzed mathematically by STEER (1967), who concluded that an alteration in cross-sectional area of the duct of only 3% would be required to produce a cupular deflection appropriate to the nystagmic response. Lack of information about the mechanical properties of the membranous duct and the trabeculae which support it within the bony canal did not allow the relevance of this analysis to be extended to the living vestibular system.

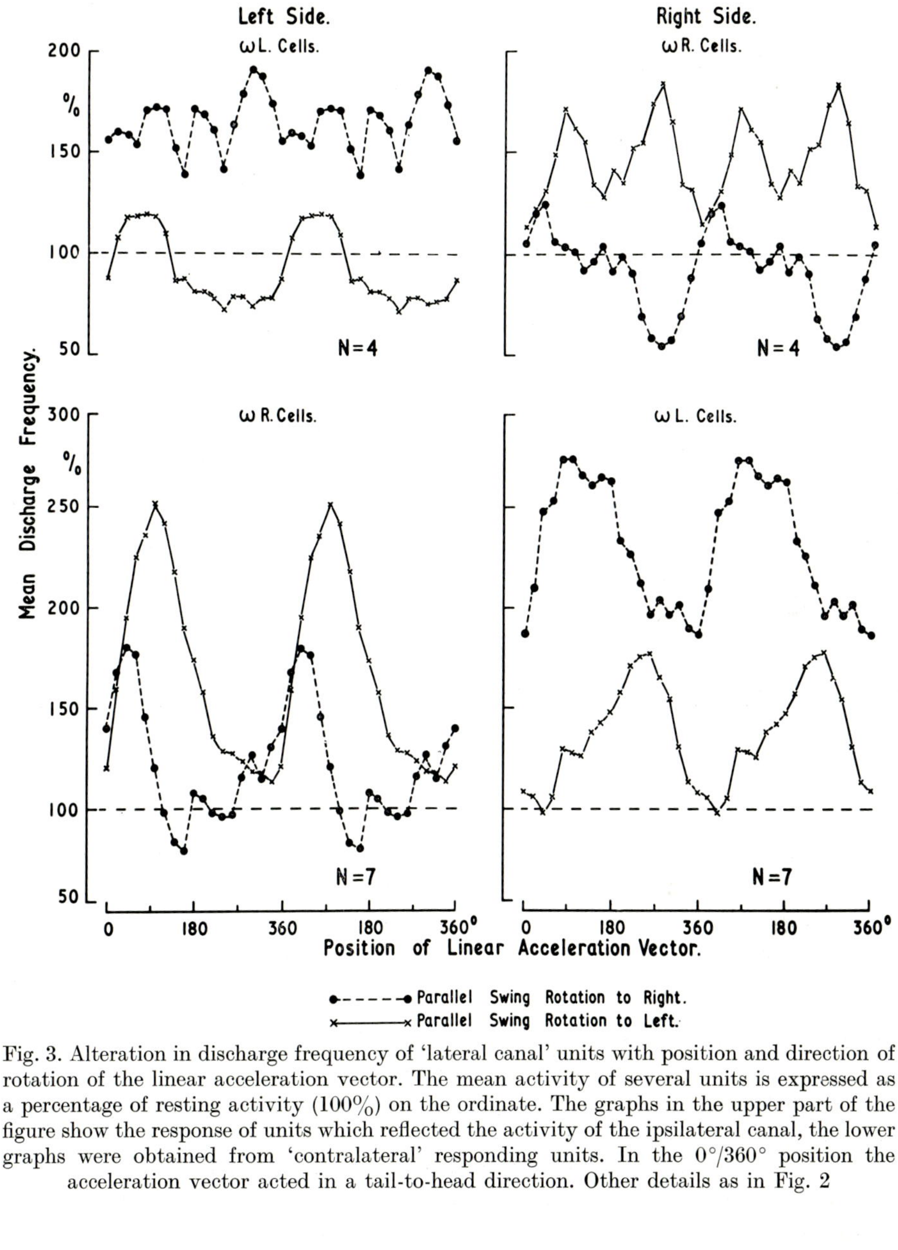

Fig. 3. Alteration in discharge frequency of 'lateral canal' units with position and direction of rotation of the linear acceleration vector. The mean activity of several units is expressed as a percentage of resting activity (100%) on the ordinate. The graphs in the upper part of the figure show the response of units which reflected the activity of the ipsilateral canal, the lower graphs were obtained from 'contralateral' responding units. In the 0°/360° position the acceleration vector acted in a tail-to-head direction. Other details as in Fig. 2

A similar problem confronted the author when he constructed a physical model of a canal with "endolymphatic" and "perilymphatic" systems. Dimensional analysis allows (SPELLS, 1961) a model to be built with a rigid "membranous duct" which has a dynamic behavior close to that exhibited by man, but the scaling of perilymph viscosity and simulation of the properties of the membranous duct were quite empirical. With a thin rubber latex tube as the "membranous duct" cemented to the larger radius wall of the "bony canal", and a density difference of 3% between "endolymph" and "perilymph", there was no sustained deflection of the model "cupula" during rotation of the canal in a vertical plane at constant velocity. The absence of a response to a rotating linear acceleration in such a model does not disprove the hypothesis that adequate stimulation of ampullar receptors can be caused by rotation of the acceleration vector, though it does little to strenghten it.

An alternative explanation of the findings of Benson et al. (1970) is that the differential alteration of lateral canal unit activity was a manifestation, not of the behavior of the ampullar receptors, but of the activity in gravireceptor and other afferents which converged on the neurons of the medial vestibular nuclei or upon internuncials in the commissural pathways (Shimazu and Precht, 1966). Although the resting activity of the neurons studied by Benson et al. (1970) was not apparently changed by sinusoidal linear oscillations during initial test procedures, the rotating vector was a more potent and sustained stimulus to the maculae and other mechanoreceptors and hence more likely to produce changes in excitability of 'canal' units than was the translational motion used when such units were selected.

It is not difficult to understand how the direct modulation of lateral canal neurons by macular afferents could account for the cyclical alteration in excitability observed when the animal was exposed to a rotating linear acceleration vector, for with such a stimulus, macular receptors show a sinusoidal alteration in activity (Lowenstein and Roberts, 1950; Milsum and Melvill Jones, 1967) as the magnitude of the specific force in the direction which accords with the 'directional sensitivity' of the sensory cell (Spoendlin, 1965; Lindeman, 1969) changes in a sinusoidal manner. However, this simple concept does not account for the differential alteration in the mean activity of canal units according to the direction of rotation of the vector.

A recent theoretical analysis (Benson and Barnes, 1973; Barnes, 1971) of the motion of the statoconial mass under the influence of a linear acceleration vector rotating in the plane of the macula, has suggested that this mechanical stimulus could produce torsion of the statoconial mass relative to the base of the macula as well as the expected translational motion in the plane of the macula. Consideration of the morphological polarization of receptors and the possible neural organization of macular afferents led to the hypothesis that torsion of the statoconial plaque was responsible for the bias in the neural signals from the maculae which impinged upon 'lateral canal' neurons in the vestibular nuclei. This hypothesis, whilst accounting for the quantitative differences in the oculomotor responses found in several experimental situations where there was rotation of the linear acceleration vector, awaits validation from neurophysiological studies of the dynamic behavior of macular receptors.

There remains the possibility that the bias or directional asymmetry in the response of canal-dependent units to a rotating vector is a manifestation neither of cupular deflection nor of torsion of the statoconial plaque but of the activity of other neural centers which resolve, presumably by the integration of the sequential response of gravireceptors, the direction of rotation of the vector. Certainly man, with normal vestibular function, is able to perceive the direction of rotation of a linear acceleration vector, at least at rotational frequencies of up to 0.3 Hz (Guedry, 1965a; Correia and Guedry, 1966). Bias was observed in vestibular units of decerebrate cats, so the locus of such a postulated neural mechanism must lie either in the brain stem or cerebellum.

C. Evidence from Nystagmus and Sensations of Turning

For over a 100 years (Purkinje, 1820; Flourens, 1824) eye movements have been used to assess in either a qualitative or quantitative manner the response of the vestibular apparatus to adequate stimulation. The equilibratory function of the vestibulo-ocular reflex arc is now well understood (Chap. F. I.). As a generality, angular accelerations produce nystagmus appropriate to the plane and direction of the stimulus, linear accelerations, a sustained compensatory eye movement and no nystagmus. Direct mechanical stimulation of the cupula gives rise to nystagmus (Ewald, 1892) and direct stimulation of the maculae (Maxwell, 1923; Ulrich, 1934; Szentágothai, 1952), to an angular displacement of the eye. Accordingly, nystagmus has come to be regarded as a manifestation of deflection of the cupulae, and eye deviation as an indicant of otolith organ activity. The inadequacy of this concept has been made apparent by many experiments in which the oculomotor response to changing linear accelerations has been studied, but it will serve as a premise for a discussion of the way linear acceleration vectors of constant magnitude and direction modify the responses to angular accelerations.

If the cupula is deflected, or the sensory epithelium of the crista stimulated in some other way, by a linear acceleration of 1 g, then nystagmus which alters direction according to the orientation of the canals to gravity should occur; there should be a positional nystagmus. The frequency with which this occurs in healthy subjects without disease of the vestibular apparatus or of the central nervous system is variable and depends *inter alia* upon the care taken to prevent visual fixation and upon the sensitivity of the observational technique. For example, in normal aircrews, positional nystagmus has a reported incidence of from 2% (Kiorboe, 1959) to 25% (King, 1960, personal communication). Stahle (1958) and Jongkees (1960), however, using electro-oculography, claimed that positional nystagmus does not occur in the normal subject, while Bergstedt (1961a) found that 27% of his clinically normal subjects had positional nystagmus. Analysis of his figures showed that in the right lateral position the mean nystagmus slow-phase velocity was 0.5° sec^{-1} beating with slow phase to the right, and in the left lateral position, 1.2° sec^{-1} to the right. There was no significant difference between the nystagmus velocities in the right and left lateral positions. It must therefore be concluded that in the normal subject the acceleration of gravity is not an adequate stimulus to the ampullar receptors. In individuals with disease of the vestibular apparatus the sensory epithelium of the cristae may be stimulated by gravity (Jongkees, 1960; Schuknecht, 1962; Hallpike, 1967), and the characteristics of the positional nystagmus can be of pathogonomic significance; however, a discussion of the theories which attempt to explain this clinical sign is outside the scope of this section.

IV. Effect of the Acceleration of Gravity on Responses to Rotation

Although a linear acceleration of 1 g applied in a fixed direction is unable to evoke nystagmus in a normal subject or experimental animal, it can modify the nystagmus engendered by stimulation of the semicircular canals.

According to Markaryan (1967) it was Khilov (1929, 1936) who first demonstrated that the duration of nystagmus following a stopping stimulus was dependent upon the orientation of the head to gravity in the postrotational period. Subsequently Koella (1947) found that when a rabbit was rotated about an axis inclined at 45° to the vertical, the postrotational nystagmic response was 40% shorter and the mean frequency 30% less than when the axis of rotation was vertical. Similarly, Correia and Guedry (1964) and Benson and Bodin (1966a) showed that in subjects who were rotated about their longitudinal (head-foot or z) axis the postrotational nystagmus was less when the axis of rotation was horizontal than when vertical. This difference was demonstrated by Benson and Bodin (1966c) to be caused, principally, by a more rapid decay of nystagmus slow-phase velocity when the gravitational acceleration was approximately coplanar with the lateral canals, than when the head was in the normal upright position and the acceleration vector approximately normal to the plane of the lateral canals (Fig.4).

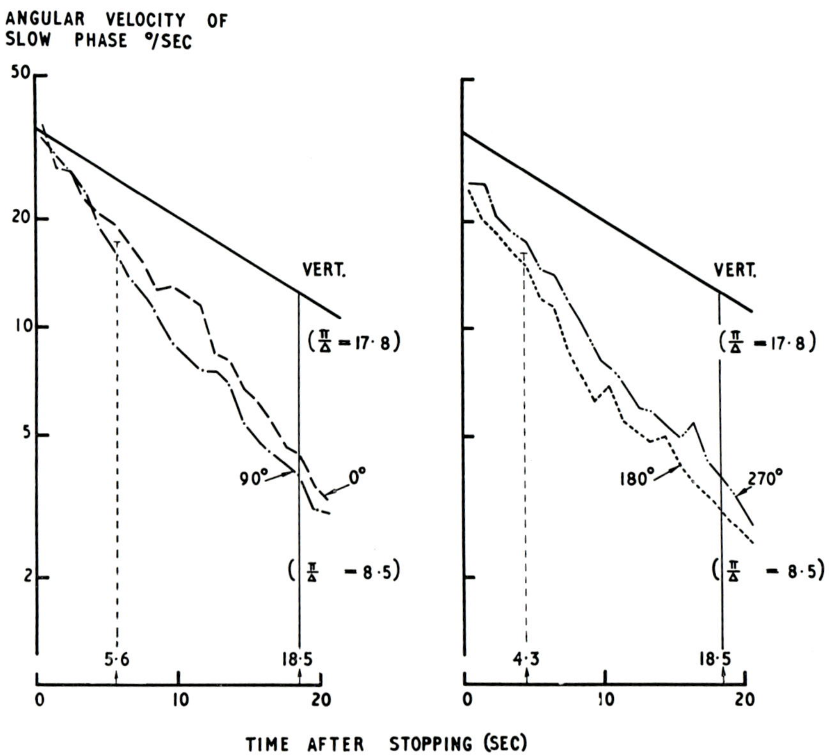

Fig. 4. Comparison of decay of nystagmus following rotation about a head-foot (z) axis, when the axis of rotation was vertical and when horizontal. Mean values from 14 subjects, each of whom experienced an impulsive deceleration from 60°/sec at t = 0 sec. Angular velocity of slow phase is plotted on a logarithmic scale. Time constants of decay (π/Δ) were consistently shorter ($p = 0.001$) when the axis of rotation was horizontal than when vertical. There was no significant effect attributable to the position in which the stretcher was stopped: 0° = supine, 180° = prone, 90° and 270° = right- and left-side-down, respectively. From Benson and Bodin (1966c)

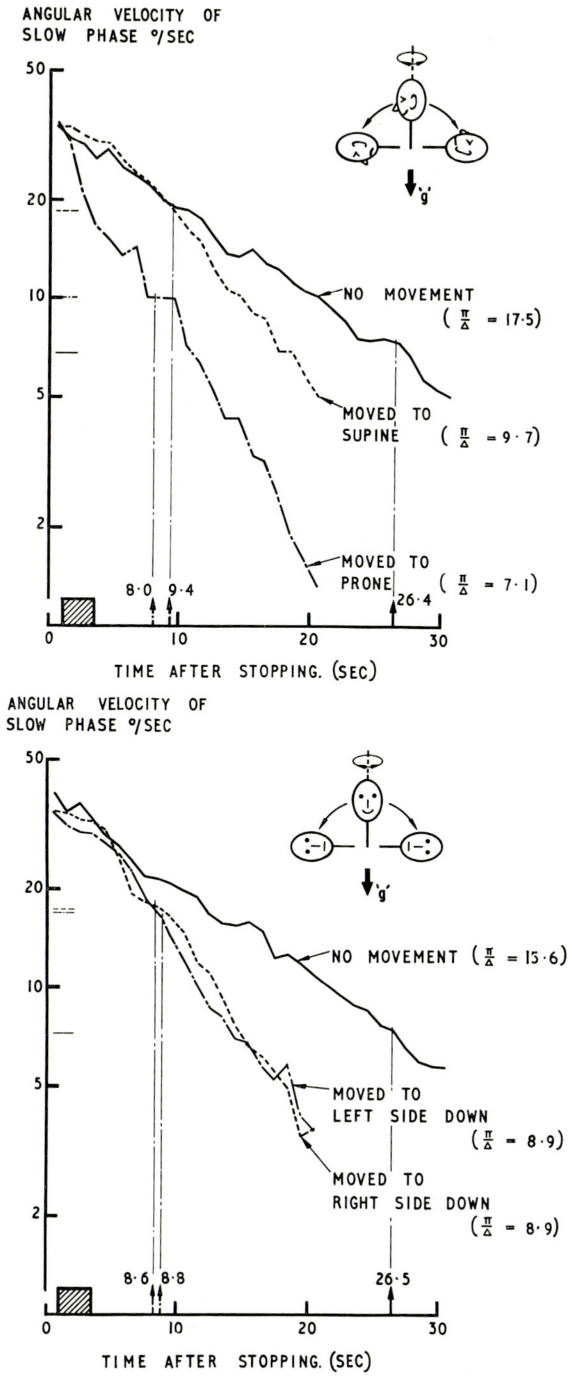

Fig. 5. Effect of orientation to gravity on decay of nystagmus following rotation at 60°/sec. The shaded block on the abscissa indicates the period in which the subject was moved from the vertical to a horizontal position. Figures on abscissa indicate the mean durations of the after-sensation in seconds. π/Δ = mean time constant of decay in seconds. Mean values from 8 subjects. From Benson and Bodin (1966b)

A comparable reduction in the time constant of decay was observed (Fig. 5) when the subject was rotated about a vertical axis and shortly after stopping was moved through 90° to one of the four orthogonal horizontal positions employed in the previous experiment (Benson and Bodin, 1966b). In all these experiments the time constant of decay of the lateral nystagmus was approximately halved when cupular restoration occurred with the subject in the horizontal position.

If the cupulae of the lateral canals were deflected by gravity, the decay of nystagmus following rotation to the right should have been prolonged when the subject was in the right-side-down position, and reduced in the left-side-down position; but there was no significant difference in the rates of decay in the right or left lateral positions. There was, however, a small yet significantly higher rate of decay in the prone than in the supine position (Fig. 5). This difference was more apparent in the rabbit (Janeke, 1968), since the postrotational nystagmus was all but absent in the prone position (duration 2 sec) yet quite intense when the animal was stopped in the supine position (duration 14 sec) following rotation at 2.5 rad sec^{-1} about a horizontal axis. Similarly in subjects who were rotated about a horizontal axis which was aligned with the x (roll) axis of the skull, Udo de Haes and Schöne (1970) demonstrated a greater suppression of postrotational nystagmus when the subject was stopped with his body in the prone position than when supine.

If slow-phase eye velocity bears a constant, linear relationship to cupular deflection, these experiments might imply that the orientation of the stimulated canal to gravity can influence the dynamics of the canal-cupula-endolymph system since restoration of the cupula is more rapid when the linear acceleration is coplanar with the lateral canals than when it is normal to the plane of the canal. Alternatively if, as suggested by Groen (1957, 1962) and Stahle (1957), the "coupling" between the signal from the ampullar receptors and eye velocity is capable of modification by other neural inputs, these findings are but a manifestation of the central suppression or adaptation of the signal from the lateral canals. This hypothesis was favored by Guedry (1965a, b), who pointed out that when the subject is in the horizontal position, otolithic and other gravireceptor information contradicts the inappropriate signal from the lateral canals, while in the vertical position there is no competing gravireceptor signal. Support for this latter mechanism was afforded by the results of an experiment in which subjects, following rotation at constant velocity in the head vertical position, were moved in the saggittal (x, z) plane either 30° forwards or 30° backwards (Benson, 1966). If the magnitude of the linear acceleration in the plane of the canals was of importance then the time constant of decay should have been increased in the 30° forward position and decreased in the 30° back position. It was found that nystagmus decayed at a significantly higher rate in both the 30° forward and the 30° back positions.

The magnitude of the suppression is related to the intensity of the competing gravireceptor signal (Udo de Haes and Schöne, 1970). Thus in an experiment in which subjects were rotated about a vertical axis with the head in the 30° forward position, and on stopping were moved backwards (in the sagittal plane) through an angle ranging from 30° to 180°, the greatest reduction in the time constant of decay occurred when they had been moved through 90° (Benson, 1966). With larger angles of tilt the time constant again increased, but following movement to the 180° position, which brought the plane of the stimulated canal and also the illusory sensation of turning once again to the horizontal, where there should have been no competing gravireceptor signal, the time constant was still significantly lower than when cupula restoration occurred in the 30° forward position. KOELLA (1947) reported a comparable decrease in the duration of postrotational nystagmus in the rabbit, as the inclination of the axis of rotation to the vertical was increased from 0° to 45°.

The sensation of turning evoked by the stopping stimulus showed greater suppression than the nystagmic response. On the average, the duration of the after-sensation was reduced by about 60% when cupular restoration (lateral canals) occurred in the horizontal as opposed to vertical position. Indeed, some subjects had no illusory sensation of turning about their longitudinal (z) body axis following rotation about an earth horizontal axis at 1.1 rad sec^{-1} (GUEDRY, 1965a; BENSON and BODIN, 1966a). As is shown in Fig. 5, where the mean time at which the after-sensation was reported to have disappeared is marked on the nystagmus decay curve, the reduction in the duration of the sensation could not be equated with the more rapid decay of nystagmus, when the subject was horizontal. There was a dissociation of the sensation of turning and the nystagmic response engendered by the same vestibular signal, the sensory response being the more susceptible to the influence of antagonistic gravireceptor information than the nystagmus. This finding was in agreement with a number of other studies in which subjective and objective indicants of canal function were compared (BENSON, 1967).

When the vertical canals are stimulated by angular accelerations in the coronal (yz) or sagittal (xz) planes of the head, the postrotational nystagmus and sensation are apparently less readily modified by the concomitant linear acceleration than are the responses of the lateral canals. Subjects who were rotated in the right or left lateral positions about an earth vertical axis and reorientated immediately after stopping to the head vertical position, showed only a small reduction in the time constant of decay of the vertical nystagmus (7.5 sec to 5.9 sec) and in the duration of the after-sensation (12.1 sec to 9.5 sec) (BENSON and BODIN, 1966b). Likewise there was no significant difference in the nystagmic response following rotation in the sagittal plane about a horizontal axis with that which occurred when the rotation axis was vertical (time constants 12.3 sec and 10.2 sec, respectively) (BODIN, personal communication).

The differing susceptibilities of vertical and lateral canal responses to gravireceptor stimulation may be a manifestation of the differing organizations of the compensatory vestibular responses to angular motion about the yaw (z) axis compared to those in the pitch (y) and roll (x) axes. For man, with his upright posture, motion in yaw can commonly occur without changes in the direction of the gravity vector, whereas with rotation in the other two orthogonal axes there is usually concordant information from vertical canals and gravireceptors. Stimulation of the vertical canals by rotation about a vertical axis is an unnatural stimulus because of the lack of synergistic information from gravireceptors. Accordingly in such test situations the decay of nystagmus will be enhanced over that which occurs when the canal and gravireceptor signals are in accord. This opinion was supported by the finding (BODIN, 1968) of a longer time constant of decay (12.6 sec) of the per-rotational nystagmus when the axis of rotation was earth horizontal than when it was vertical (time constant = 9.2 sec), and is in accord with the more rapid decay of postrotational responses observed by MELVILL JONES et al. (1964), in the pitch and roll axes than in the yaw axis, with angular stimuli about an earth vertical axis.

V. The Mechanism of Suppression

The notable feature of the suppression of the postrotational nystagmic response by gravireceptor signals is that it is manifest as an alteration in the time constant of decay. The inhibitory process cannot be described as a simple subtractive or proportional function, for these would both produce a change in eye velocity when the subject was reorientated to the gravity vector and should not influence the time constant of decay. Likewise it is not due to a change in the bitemporal component of the corneoretinal potential, or to the small alteration in the plane of the nystagmus relative to the skull noted by KOELLA (1947), for these would cause a sudden alteration in the apparent eye velocity. Unless these factors varied as a non-linear function of time they should not bring about a reduction in the time constant of decay of the recorded nystagmus.

It is known from a number of studies (GROEN, 1957, 1962; STAHLE, 1957; BENSON, 1967) that the responses evoked in different effector systems on stimulation of the semicircular canal receptors do not have the same dynamic behavior. For example, the time constant of decay of the sensation of turning following an angular stimulus is commonly half that of the nystagmus decay which in turn is shorter than the time constant of decay of end-organ activity. Thus the neural coupling between end-organ and response cannot be considered as an immutable link, but must contain elements which modify the transmission of the neural signal as a function of time and hence behave in an adaptive manner.

Recently mathematical models of the adaptive coupling between semicircular canal and response have been developed by YOUNG and OMAN (1969) and MALCOLM and MELVILL JONES (1970) which, when used in conjunction with the established second-order canal equation, have allowed the responses to step and ramp angular velocity inputs to be calculated with considerable accuracy. The adaptive term, expressed as a transfer function, has the form:

$$\frac{R(s)}{\theta(s)} = \frac{K.s}{s + \frac{1}{T_a}}$$

Where R is the response

θ is the neural signal from the ampulla or cupula deflection

T_a is the adaptation time constant

K is a constant of proportionality.

It would appear that the adaptative time constant for nystagmus normally has a value of 80–120 sec; the sensation of turning exhibits greater adaptation and accordingly has a shorter time constant, i.e., about 30 sec.

It would thus seem most likely that the supression of canal response by antagonistic gravireceptor signals is brought about by an alteration of the adaptive mechanism which relays afferent signals from ampullar receptors. The reduction of the time constant of decay of postrotational responses can be expressed as a shortening of the adaptation time constant (T_a), the magnitude of the reduction in T_a being a function of the disparity between canal and gravireceptor information.

Changes in the adaptive coupling occur rapidly and are reversible, as was demonstrated in an experiment in which subjects were moved from the vertical to the right or left lateral position immediately after rotation about a vertical

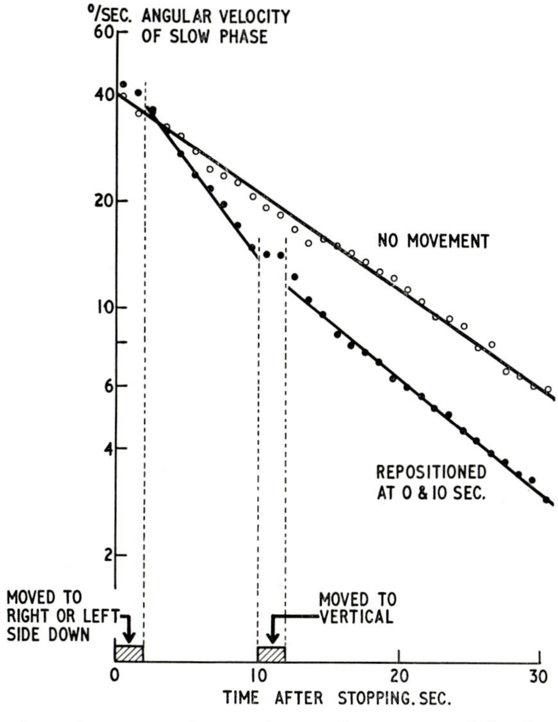

Fig. 6. Effect of orientation to gravity on decay of nystagmus following rotation about a vertical, head-foot (z) axis at 60°/sec. Shortly after stopping the subject was moved from the vertical to the right-or left-side-down position and 10 sec later was returned to the vertical position. Mean values from 12 subjects. From Benson (1968)

axis (Fig. 6). When moved to the lateral position the rate of decay of the postrotational nystagmus was approximately twice as fast as when the subject remained in the vertical position. Yet, on returning to the vertical position, the rate of nystagmus decay returned to a value close to that which was observed when the subject was not repositioned in the postrotational period.

Although the concept of an adaptive coupling and its expression as a simple transfer function allow the experimentally observed responses to be modelled with a fair degree of accuracy, the neural organization of such a mechanism remains obscure.

VI. The Effect of Sustained Accelerations other than 1g on Responses to Rotation

A. Weightlessness

From the foregoing discussion it would perhaps be expected that when the body is deprived of information from gravireceptors, as occurs during weightlessness, the response to angular acceleration would be modified. During the prolonged weightlessness of orbital flight there have been no reports of alteration of vestibular function which can be unambiguously equated to an alteration of canal responses. The obnormal vestibular sensations reported by the Russian astronauts (Billingham, 1966) are more likely to have been caused by Coriolis accelerations acting on the canals or abnormal stimulation of the macular receptors of individuals who were not well habituated to complex motion stimuli.

Controlled observations of canal responses have only been made during the brief periods (up to 55 sec) of zero gravity obtained by flying an aircraft in a Keplerian trajectory. Roman et al. (1963) used a rolling manoeuvre of the aircraft (angular acceleration in the x body axis) as the test stimulus, and measured the duration of per- and postrotatory sensations, whereas Jackson and Sears (1965) examined eye movements evoked by rotation of their subjects about a head-foot (z) axis. In neither study were significant differences detected between the per- or postrotational responses elicited during zero gravity and those produced by the same angular stimuli administered during level flight, i.e., in a 1 g environment. Similarly Oosterveld and van der Laarse (1969), using rabbits, found no change in the nystagmus evoked by torsional (z axis) oscillation during 9 sec periods of weightlessness achieved by parabolic flight.

In contrast, Yuganov (1965) claimed that weightlessness brought about a reduction in the excitability of the semicircular canal mechanism. He found that in ten subjects the duration of postrotational nystagmus during zero gravity had a mean value of 13.3 sec whereas the apparently comparable measure obtained on the ground (i.e. at 1 g) was 23.1 sec. A significant reduction in the duration of postrotational sensations was also observed, the mean values being 6.1 sec in zero gravity and 11.9 sec at 1 g. It is inferred that these experiments were carried out in aircraft, but unfortunately no details were given of the nature of the angular stimulus or of the temporal relationship of the stimulus to the flight path of the aircraft, so it is not possible to determine whether Yuganov's findings contradict those of Roman et al. (1963) and Jackson and Sears (1965) or represent the behavior of the vestibular system in a different experimental situation.

It is clearly difficult to generate precise angular stimuli in parabolic flight, and the relatively brief period of weightlessness must of necessity be preceded by an increase in aircraft normal acceleration, which may of itself modify the vestibular response evoked during zero gravity. Results of more detailed and better controlled studies of vestibular function during prolonged weightlessness, such as is provided by an orbiting laboratory, are awaited with interest.

B. Linear Accelerations Greater than 1g

Eccentric rotation has been widely employed in the study of linear and angular accelerations, indeed it is the only way in which sustained linear accelerations can be produced in the confines of the laboratory.

Irrespective of whether the sensation of turning evoked by the initial acceleration (JONGKEES, 1956; BENSON and WHITESIDE, 1961) or the oculogyral illusion (GRAYBIEL et al., 1956; GRAY and CROSBIE, 1958) was used as an indicant of semicircular canal activity, centripetal acceleration failed to produce a significant alteration in the duration of the subjective response. This, in part, was attributable to the difficulty experienced by subjects, when seated at the end of a centrifuge arm, in discriminating a sensation of turning from the more potent and unusual sensations of increased weight and apparent tilt associated with a change in the magnitude and direction of the linear acceleration vector. In some subjects these competing sensory stimuli reduced the duration of the rotatory sensation, but in others it was prolonged so that the variance of the measure was increased and a probable reduction in the subjective response obscured.

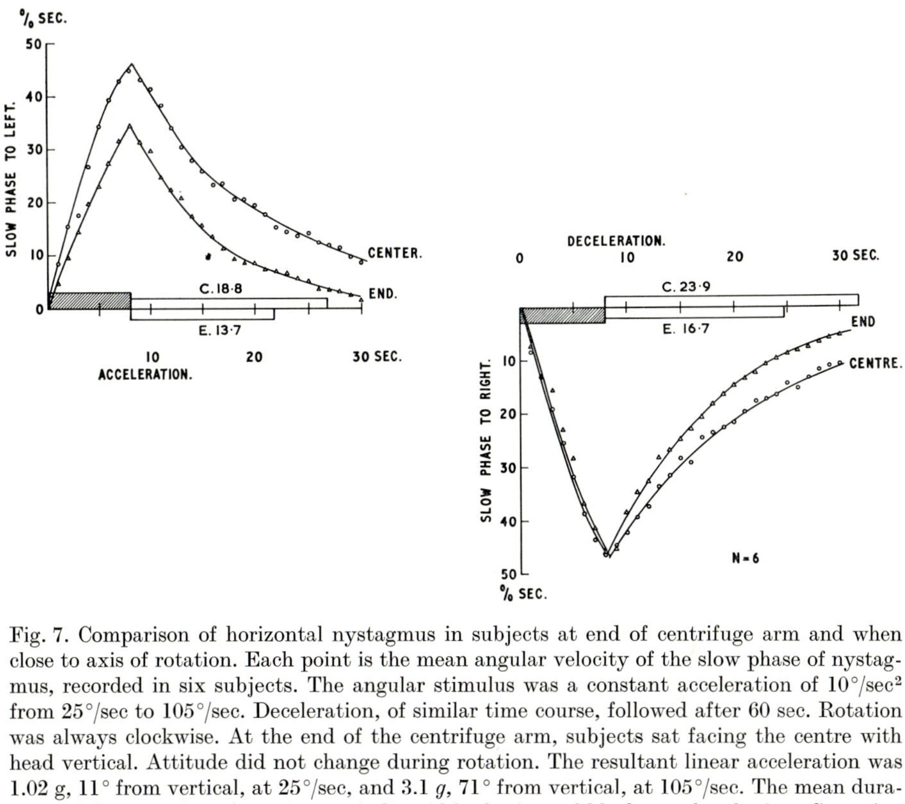

Fig. 7. Comparison of horizontal nystagmus in subjects at end of centrifuge arm and when close to axis of rotation. Each point is the mean angular velocity of the slow phase of nystagmus, recorded in six subjects. The angular stimulus was a constant acceleration of 10°/sec² from 25°/sec to 105°/sec. Deceleration, of similar time course, followed after 60 sec. Rotation was always clockwise. At the end of the centrifuge arm, subjects sat facing the centre with head vertical. Attitude did not change during rotation. The resultant linear acceleration was 1.02 g, 11° from vertical, at 25°/sec, and 3.1 *g*, 71° from vertical, at 105°/sec. The mean durations of the sensation of turning are indicated by horizontal blocks on the abscissa. Sensation times did not differ significantly from one another between conditions. From BENSON (1966)

In contrast to the subjective measures, the nystagmus evoked by an angular acceleration has been found to be modified by linear accelerations greater than 1 *g*. Popov (1939) and Bakhvalova (1950) showed that the duration of the nystagmus induced by an angular acceleration was less when the subject was exposed to a linear acceleration greater than 1 *g* than when the same angular stimulus was administered in a 1 *g* environment. With the advent of electro-oculography and more precise qualifications of the nystagmus response it was found that the reduction in the duration of nystagmus was caused both by a fall in peak slow-phase eye velocity and by an increase in the rate of decay of the nystagmic response (Benson and Whiteside, 1961; Benson, 1966). Figure 7 contains the results of an experiment in which lateral nystagmus was recorded in subjects who were either close to the axis of rotation or were at the end of a centrifuge arm and facing the center of rotation. In these experiments the resultant of the radial acceleration due to rotation of the centrifuge and to the acceleration of gravity lay in the sagittal (xz) plane of the subject's head, but in later experiments it was found that the rate of decay of rotation-induced nystagmus could be either increased or decreased according to the orientation of the subject to the resultant (Benson, 1962; Lansberg et al., 1964; Crampton, 1966).

When the subject faced the direction of rotation so that the centripetal acceleration lay in his coronal (yz) plane, Crampton (1966), in a well-controlled experiment, demonstrated that the nystagmus with slow-phase velocity directed towards the subject's left was enhanced when the centripetal acceleration was directed from the subject's left to right, and conversely decreased when the acceleration acted in the opposite direction. Likewise, when the initial acceleration produced a nystagmus with slow phase to the right, this response was facilitated when the acceleration vector was directed from right to left. These systematic effects were observed with a resultant acceleration of only 1.06 *g* (centripetal y axis component = 0.35 *g*) which, apparently, was insufficient to cause the sustained right or left beating nystagmus reported by Lansberg et al. (1964) with a resultant of about 1.6 *g* in the coronal plane (centripetal y axis component = 1.3 *g*), and by Benson (1962) in subjects who faced 40° away from the radius and were exposed to a resultant of 3.1 *g* (centripetal y axis component = 1.9 *g*).

The sustained nystagmus which varied in direction according to the orientation of the subject to the linear acceleration persisted for at least 40 sec and had the characteristics of a *positional* nystagmus. Unfortunately detailed positional tests (in a 1 *g* environment) were not carried out by either Lansberg et al. or Benson, so it is not known whether the nystagmus recorded under increased accelerations was a potentiated positional response or not. However, Bergstedt (1961a) claimed that clinically healthy subjects without positional or spontaneous nystagmus did not have nystagmus when exposed to transverse (y axis) accelerations ranging from 1.25 to 2.6 *g* when the centrifuge was accelerated at less than 0.016 rad sec^{-2} (0,9° sec^{-2}); furthermore the nystagmus evoked by higher angular accelerations of 0.02 to 0.05 rad sec^{-2} (1.1–3.0° sec^{-2}) soon died away once a constant speed of rotation was achieved. Those subjects who had nystagmus during ordinary positional tests showed a change in intensity of the response when exposed to increased transverse accelerations. Because Lansberg et al. and Benson employed initial angular accelerations of the order of 0.17 rad sec^{-2} (10° sec^{-2})

for some 8 sec, one could argue that the sustained nystagmus is only evoked when there is a substantial stimulus to the cristae of the lateral canals in addition to the linear acceleration greater than 1 g acting in the transverse (y) axis on the head.

It had previously been suggested (BENSON, 1962) that the sustained nystagmus was a manifestation of deflection of the cupula by the linear acceleration, but this view is no longer tenable. When the decay of nystagmus to its basal level (4° sec^{-1})

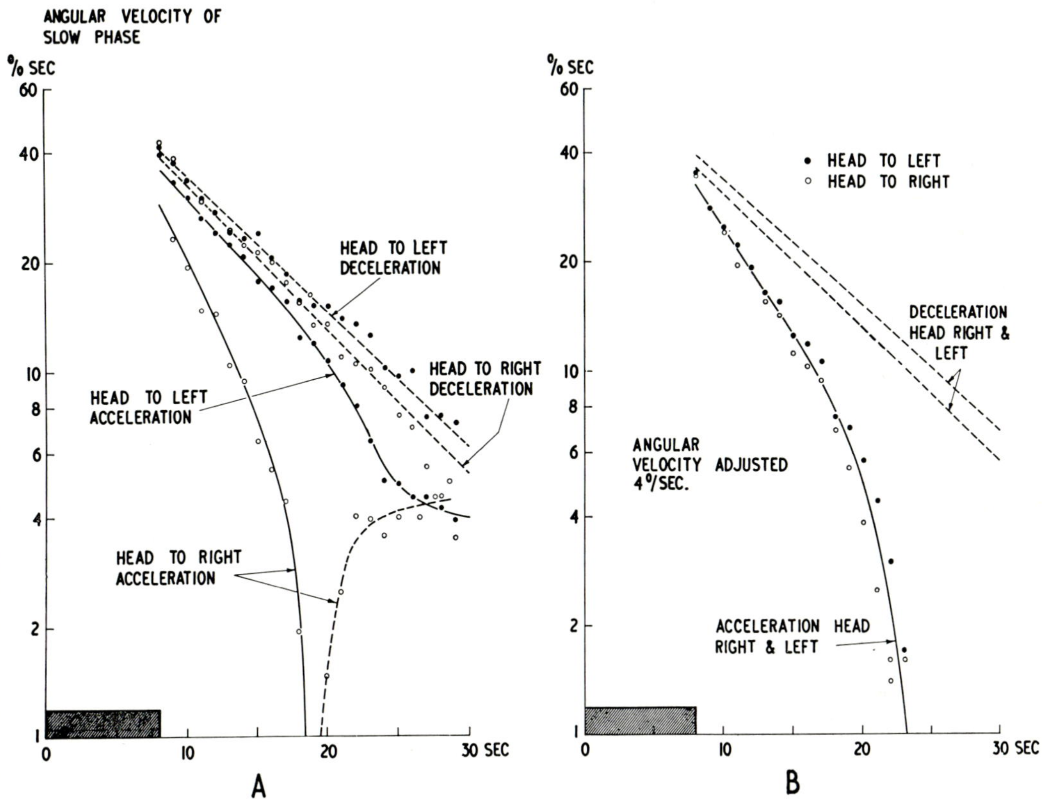

Fig. 8. Modification of horizontal nystagmus by the direction of a linear acceleration of 3.1 g. The subject sat at the end of the centrifuge arm, with head vertical, and faced 40° to the right or left of the radius. Angular motion was the same as in Fig. 7. Each point is the mean slow-phase velocity obtained in eight runs from four subjects and is plotted on a logarithmic ordinate scale. Reversal of nystagmus in head right position following acceleration is indicated by a broken line. When nystagmus recorded at 3.1 g was adjusted by +4°/sec and –4°/sec in head right and left positions, respectively, the decay followed a similar time course which was not a simple exponential function. From BENSON (1966)

rather than zero was plotted (Fig. 8), it was found that the decay curves for the head-to-left and head-to-right positions were identical. If there were a force acting on the cupula of the lateral canals, it should have increased the time constant of decay in the head-to-left position and decreased it in the head-to-right position, following angular acceleration to the right. The finding of a more rapid decay, irrespective of whether the linear acceleration vector lay in the sagittal plane or had components in both coronal and sagittal planes, must be regarded as another example of the suppression of the ampullar responses when the organism is provided with gravireceptor information that is not in accord with information from the semicircular canals.

In view of the appreciable suppression of postrotational nystagmus brought about by a linear acceleration of only 1 g, a more profound inhibition might have been expected with the more potent stimuli provided by a centrifuge. However, under the conditions of the experiment, the conflict between canal and gravireceptor information was more subtle and unfamiliar. Angular motion about a vertical axis would be correctly sensed by the canals, but this would be incompatible, at least on the basis of a habitual association between canal and gravireceptor signals occurring in every day life, with the powerful signals from the maculae and other gravireceptors which would indicate a maintained reorientation of the body to the gravitational vertical (i.e., backwards or sideways tilt).

The departure of the decay of the nystagmus slow-phase velocity from the normal exponential (Fig. 8) may have been caused by an alteration in the plane of the nystagmus, as a compensatory deviation (a counterrolling response) developed appropriate to the direction of the resultant linear acceleration. Lansberg et al. (1964), who recorded both vertical and horizontal components of the corneoretinal potential, reported that the nystagmus was in a vertical direction when the initial horizontal nystagmus, initially beating with slow phase to the right, changed to a predominantly leftwards directed response. The absence of a comparable alteration in the plane of the nystagmic eye movement when the subject faced in the opposite direction, suggests that these results may be more an artifact of the electro-oculographic technique than a veridical measure of the plane of the nystagmus.

Most of the studies carried out have been made on the lateral nystagmus induced by angular stimulus about the longitudinal (z) body axis. However, the nystagmus evoked by angular acceleration in both the roll (x) and pitch (y) axes was reported by Markaryan (1967) to be influenced by the magnitude and direction of the centripetal acceleration in the z body axis. This author claimed that a positive (G_2) acceleration increased the intensity of the nystagmic response, as measured by the amplitude, duration and number of beats, and conversely that a negative (G_2) acceleration decreased the response. These conclusions are questionable, because the recording technique employed was insensitive to roll axis nystagmus and the experimental measures, though carried out on nine subjects, were not apparently analyzed statistically.

Studies of the modification of canal nystagmus by constant linear acceleration vectors in experimental animals have, like the experiments carried out on man, produced somewhat conflicting results. In the rabbit the direction-changing nystagmus evoked by angular acceleration about a z (yaw) axis was found to be suppressed by the initial increase of linear acceleration in the z axis of the head (Oosterveld and van der Laarse, 1969; Janeke and Oosterveld, 1969). Yet some 12 sec after the acceleration was applied the amplitude of the nystagmic response was essentially the same as that obtained under control (1 g) conditions. The intensity of the transitory suppression was linearly related to the magnitude of the G_2 acceleration and was complete at 4.8 *g*. In contrast, KURASHVILI and BABIYAK (1970), who also worked with rabbits, found that the amplitude and slow-phase velocity of nystagmus was increased during the time the linear acceleration was increasing, but once the acceleration had stabilized the nystagmic response diminished. These authors do not give information about orientation of the animal in the centrifuge so it is not possible to correlate their observations with those of other workers.

VII. Modification of the Thermal Response by Linear Accelerations

The nystagmus induced by the irrigation of the external meatus with water above or below body temperature is widely used in clinical practice as a test of the functional integrity of the vestibular end-organ and its afferent projections. Most authors agree with the hypothesis (BÁRÁNY, 1906) that nystagmus is caused by a

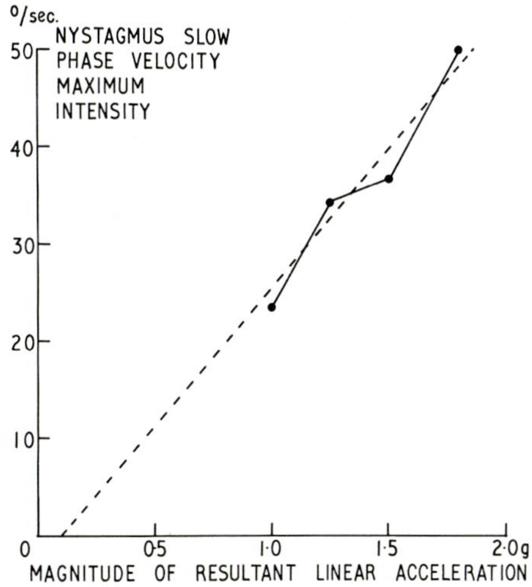

Fig. 9. Relationship between intensity of caloric nystagmus and magnitude of the linear acceleration. Mean values from 4 subjects. Peak slow-phase velocity of lateral nystagmus in response to irrigation with water at 20°C was determined during exposure to increased linear acceleration in a centrifuge. The subject was orientated so that the resultant acceleration was always in the anteroposterior (x) axis of the skull. The extrapolated line through the points intercepts the abscissa at 0.1 *g* and indicates that a caloric response should not be elicited during weightlessness. From BERGSTEDT (1961a)

local alteration in the specific gravity of the endolymph, principally of the lateral canal. If the canal is other than in a plane normal to the linear acceleration (commonly gravity), a pressure differential will be developed across the cupula which will be deflected and the ampullar receptors stimulated. Thus, this admittedly unphysiological method of stimulating the cristae is dependent upon the presence of a linear acceleration.

The physical model predicts, *inter alia*, that the intensity of the response is a function of the direction and magnitude of the acceleration vector. With regard to the magnitude of the acceleration, the findings of BERGSTEDT (1961b) were unambiguous, for on performing the caloric tests on subjects exposed to sustained accelerations of 1.0 to 1.8 g in a centrifuge, he was able to demonstrate a linear relationship between the maximum intensity of the nystagmic response and the magnitude of the resultant acceleration vector (Fig. 9). Extrapolation indicated that there would be no response at accelerations of less than 0.1 g, or when the subject was weightless. Experiments by KELLOGG and GRAYBIEL (1967) and OOSTERVELD and VAN DER LAARSE (1969) carried out during parabolic flight in an aircraft, have sustained this view; however, their finding that the nystagmic response disappeared as soon as the subject was exposed to zero gravity is not entirely compatible with the physical model, for this would predict that on entering the weightless state the nystagmus should decay at a rate determined by the dynamics of the canal-cupula-endolymph system.

Consideration of the effect of the direction of the acceleration vector reveals further limitations of the physical model. In a number of experiments (VON BEHRMAN, 1940, 1942; JONGKEES, 1949; MCLEOD and CORREIA, 1964; MILOJEVIC and VOOTS, 1965; COATS and SMITH, 1967) in which the caloric test was performed with the head in various angular positions in the sagittal (xz) plane, differences in the duration and the intensity of the nystagmic response were observed, which were not in accord with the prediction that they should be related to the cosine of the angle (θ) between the plane of the canal and the gravitational vertical. Certainly, when θ was close to 90°, as occurs in man when his head is tipped forward 30° from the vertical, the caloric reaction was negligible, but over large arcs the *duration* of the response did not differ appreciably. For example, in the experiment of JONGKEES (1949) the duration of caloric nystagmus was 135 sec when the subject was in the supine position, 130 sec when the head was vertical, and 125 sec in the two intermediate positions. He also reported that the response was shorter when the test was performed with the subject in the prone than in the supine position, an observation which was supported by MCLEOD and CORREIA (1964) who showed that the nystagmus slow-phase velocity was, on the average, reduced by a factor of 0.43 when the subject was prone as opposed to supine. Similarly, in the cat (MILOJEVIC and VOOTS, 1965) the nystagmus was of significantly longer duration, though not of greater amplitude, when the caloric test was performed with the fronto-occipital axis of the cat's head (corresponding to the plane of the lateral canal) pointed 45° backwards from the vertical (i.e., towards the supine position) than when the head was tilted forwards through 45°.

The detailed study (COATS and SMITH, 1967) of the effect of position in the sagittal plane on the nystagmus velocity achieved during the caloric test confirmed these earlier observations. The relationship between the intensity of the response, as indicated by peak slow-phase velocity, and position was shown to be of sinusoidal form (Fig. 10), with peaks at the 30° and 210° positions, but it was not symmetrical, larger responses to both warm and cold irrigations occurring when the subject was close to the supine position (30°) than when nearly prone (210°).

There is thus a parallel between these differences in thermal responses with position and the more rapid decay of the postrotational horizontal nystagmus in

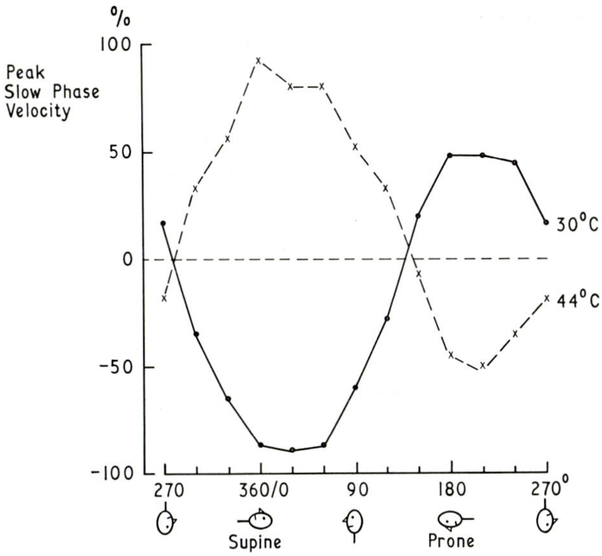

Fig. 10. Relationship between intensity of caloric nystagmus and orientation of subject to gravity. The peak slow-phase velocity of the lateral nystagmus obtained in each position was expressed as a percentage of the peak response in the optimum position, usually 30°. Mean values from 5 subjects who each had warm and cold irrigations in twelve positions in the sagittal (xz) plane. From COATS and SMITH (1967)

the prone than in the supine position, as described earlier. From the arguments already adduced it would seem most likely that the smaller caloric response in the prone position is the manifestation of more intense, or less familiar, gravireceptor stimulation which causes a greater suppression of inappropriate signals from the stimulated cristae in the prone than in the supine position. Likewise, the evocation of a caloric response in the head vertical position comparable in duration to that which was elicited by a theoretically more potent stimulus when the subject was supine (JONGKEES, 1949), can be explained by the absence of competing gravireceptor signals when the longitudinal axis of the body was aligned with gravity.

The nature of the inhibitory mechanism remains obscure. The isolated observation of JONGKEES (1960) that the nystagmus induced by a caloric stimulus administered in the normal supine position was replaced by a nystagmus of opposite sign when the subject was moved to the vertical position some 200 sec after the initial stimulus, suggests that the suppression is due to the development within the central nervous system of a signal in opposition to that from the ampullar receptors. When the thermal stimulus to the canal is reduced, as occurs when the head is vertical, the nystagmus evoked by the opposing signal is seen in isolation.

However neither of these ‘adaptive’ mechanisms readily account for the fact that the ‘neutral points’ (i.e. the positions where thermal stimulation gave no nystagmus) were not equiangular from the positions where peak responses were obtained. Accordingly, COATS and SMITH (1967) suggested that the asymmetry was caused by the direct effect of the thermal stimulus on the sensory cells of the crista: warm irrigation would increase the discharge frequency and produce a nystagmus with fast phase towards the stimulated side, a cold irrigation would have the opposite effect. Irrespective of whether the change in temperature of the crista is enough to engender the considerable difference in eye velocity occurring in the prone and supine positions, this hypothesis does not account for the change in direction of the nystagmus reported by JONGKEES (1960). It would appear that both central adaptive mechanisms and direct thermal stimulation of the ampullar receptors have to be invoked in order to explain the departure of the observed thermal responses from those which theory predicts.

The presence of adaptive mechanisms, though clearly recognized in the analysis of responses to angular stimuli (YOUNG and OMAN, 1969; MALCOLM and MELVILL JONES, 1970), has not been extended to the caloric response. Yet the comparatively long time scale over which thermal stimuli act, implies that the relationship between ampullar signal and nystagmic response is likely to be considerably modified by adaptive mechanisms. Irrespective of whether adaptation is achieved by the development of opposing signal within the central nervous system or a shift in the zero eye velocity 'reference' level, as proposed by YOUNG and OMAN (1969), the nystagmic response will tend to decay more rapidly than the afferent signal from the ampullar receptors exposed to the thermal stimulus. Thus the duration and to a lesser extent the peak slow-phase velocity of caloric nystagmus will, in part, be determined by intensity of the adaptive process, which itself is dependent upon the time integral of the response (YOUNG and OMAN, 1969) and, as suggested in this review, upon the disparity between canal and gravireceptor information.

Evidence for adaptation in the caloric response was demonstrated by an experiment carried out by YUGANOV (1965). He found that the duration of caloric response in ten subjects had a mean value of 95.5 sec when the z axis acceleration was 1 g, and that the duration of the response was increased to 118.6 sec when the test was carried out at 2 g. However when the z axis acceleration was increased gradually from 1 g to 2 g during the period of the caloric reaction, the nystagmus lasted some 139 sec and was significantly longer than when a 2 g acceleration was held constant. Yet when the linear acceleration declined from 2 g to 1 g during the test procedure, the nystagmus had a mean duration of only 80.4 sec, a value which was significantly less than the duration at 1.0 g.

The results of experiments carried out in flight by OOSTERVELD and VAN DER LAARSE (1969) also point to the modification of the caloric response by adaptive processes. They found that a +2.5 g z axis acceleration applied for 30 sec could evoke nystagmus for up to 16–20 min after an irrigation which gave nystagmus for only 2 min in a constant 1 g environment.

These findings imply that a caloric stimulus produces changes in the vestibular apparatus which take a considerably longer time to return to normal than is manifest by the oculomotor response, provided the force environment is constant. Following irrigation the afferent signal from vestibular receptors changes relatively slowly and adaptive processes, appropriate to the specific neural input, attenuate the nystagmic response. Thus nystagmus ceases long before the activity of ampullar receptors has returned to the resting level. But with a change in the force environment there is an alteration of the vestibular signal from the adapted level, and nystagmus will again become manifest. Obviously, the stimulus causes an alteration in the macular signal, yet it is also likely that the ampullar signal will be modified because of residual density differences within the canal-cupula-endolymph system.

VIII. Positional Alcohol Nystagmus

Nystagmus as a symptom of intoxication with ethyl alcohol was observed by FLOURENS (1824), but despite the continued investigation of the phenomenon, in particular the positional alcohol nystagmus (PAN), it is still not known for certain whether alcohol acts on the end-organ or through more central mechanisms (ASCHAN et al., 1964). There is no doubt, however, that the functional integrity of the vestibular receptors is a prerequisite for the evocation of PAN, and that the plane and direction of the nystagmus are intimately related to the orientation of the head to the gravitational vertical (DE KLEIJN and VERSTEEGH, 1930; ASCHAN et al., 1956).

When the subject is placed in the right lateral position (gravity vector in the y axis) shortly after taking alcohol, the lateral nystagmus beats with fast phase to the right, and conversely, fast phase to the left when the subject is in the left lateral position. In man, this initial response (PAN I) commonly disappears some 2.5 to 3 hr after taking alcohol and is replaced after 4 to 5 hr by a positional nystagmus (PAN II) in which the relationship between the direction of the nystagmus and orientation to gravity is opposite to that of PAN I.

In a systematic study of positional alcohol nystagmus, BERGSTEDT (1961a) found that the nystagmus in both phase I and phase II was augmented when the magnitude of the resultant linear acceleration was increased. There was not, however, a linear relationship between the nystagmic response and the magnitude of the acceleration comparable to that exhibited by the caloric response (BERGSTEDT, 1961b), for the degree of facilitation was found to depend upon both the angular acceleration of the centrifuge and the level of the sustained acceleration. Furthermore, following the initial facilitation of the nystagmus, it tended to decrease in an irregular manner during the period in which the linear acceleration was kept constant.

The effect of alteration of the force environment on positional alcohol nystagmus in man and rabbit has also been studied by OOSTERVELD (1970), who confirmed BERGSTEDT's observations of the potentiation of PAN I and II by increased y axis acceleration. He demonstrated that during the period when PAN could no longer be produced by a 1 g stimulus (i.e. 6 hrs after taking 30 ml of alcohol), the application of a 2.5 g acceleration elicited the typical nystagmic response at times of up to 48 hr after the administration of alcohol. Brief periods of weightlessness were found to abolish both PAN I and II in much the same way as caloric nystagmus. But whereas caloric nystagmus returned with the restoration of normal gravity, PAN remained suppressed for several minutes; nystagmus did not return for about 240 sec after exposure to zero gravity for 45 sec.

BERGSTEDT (1961b) concluded, as did ASCHAN et al. (1964), that alcohol induces a positional nystagmus by disordering the central integration of vestibular signals, and that an alteration in signals from the maculae was the principal input which "released" the nystagmic response. This view was challenged by NITO et al. (1963) and MONEY et al. (1965), who argued that the nystagmus was initiated by signals from the cristae, since PAN I was abolished in cats when all six semicircular canals were blocked (MONEY and SCOTT, 1962). If, as they postulated, alcohol allowed the cristae to be stimulated by gravity, either by a change in the relative density of cupula and endolymph or by some other mechanism, it is difficult to explain why the intensity of PAN I was not closely linked to the magnitude of the linear acceleration, and why PAN I disappeared in rabbits when they were rotated about at earth horizontal axis at 1 rad sec^{-1} (JANEKE, 1968). Likewise the prolonged suppression of PAN following a brief period of weightlessness is an enigma.

For the present, it must be concluded that the mode of action of ethyl alcohol on the peripheral and central components of the vestibular system has yet to be resolved.

IX. Effect of Time-Varying Linear Accelerations

A. Linear Oscillation

Whereas in the normal subject, sustained linear accelerations do not provoke nystagmic eye movements but only a compensatory deviation of the eye, it is now well established that a time-varying linear acceleration vector, in the absence of angular accelerations, can evoke nystagmus. When placed on a platform which oscillates sinusoidally in a horizontal path, a lateral nystagmus may be recorded when the transverse (y) axis of the subject's head is aligned with the motion. Thus NIVEN et al. (1966) found a direction-changing lateral nystagmus in four subjects who experienced sinusoidal linear oscillations with peak accelerations of $\pm$ 0.58 g at 0.2, 0.4 and 0.8 Hz. In contrast, when subjects were positioned so that the sinusoidal linear acceleration acted in the head-foot (z) axis of the body, a comparable vertical nystagmus did not occur. With the lower accelerations provided by a parallel swing, JONGKEES and PHILIPZOON (1962, 1963) and GUEDRY and HARRIS (1963) had earlier demonstrated a lateral nystagmus in rabbit and man, but this was not readily defined unless the nystagmic response was potentiated by an alteration of gaze in the direction of the quick phase (Alexander's Law). The nystagmus velocity and direction were coupled closely to the sinusoidal motion, peak slow-phase velocity to the right occurring shortly after the peak acceleration was directed from right to left. That is eye velocity showed a phase lag with respect to acceleration of 9° at 0.2 Hz and 16° at 0.8 Hz. Because peak eye velocity did not differ at the three test frequencies, it was concluded that the magnitude of the linear acceleration in the y axis was the principal determinant of nystagmus slow-phase velocity (NIVEN et al., 1966).

Changes in the magnitude of the linear acceleration without rotation of the vector also cause a nystagmic response. Thus, using a vertical oscillator with a peak acceleration of $\pm$ 0.6 g (resultant +1.6 g to –0.4 g) in the head-foot (z) axis, MCCABE (1964) observed a vertical nystagmus in the chinchilla, cat and man. This was usually unidirectional with a peak slow-phase velocity at the lowest position of each vertical oscillation, i.e. when the acceleration was at a maximum. The persistence of the nystagmic response in animals whose semicircular canal mechanisms were impaired by streptomycin or intense noise, and the disappearance of the response following labyrinthectomy were regarded as evidence that the nystagmus resulted from stimulation of the saccular or utricular maculae, rather than of the cristae or non-vestibular gravireceptors.

B. Continuous Rotation of the Linear Acceleration Vector

With continuous rotation of the linear acceleration vector with respect to the subject, such as occurs when the axis of rotation is inclined to the vertical (MACH, 1875; LORENTE DE NÓ, 1931, 1932; KOELLA, 1948), or during counterrotation about an eccentric axis (GRAYBIEL and JOHNSON, 1963) (Fig. 1), nystagmus of labyrinthine origin may be elicited.

During rotation about an earth horizontal axis at speeds of less than about 2 rad sec^{-1}, the nystagmus was unidirectional and sustained for as long as the animal continued to be reorientated to gravity. The slow component of the

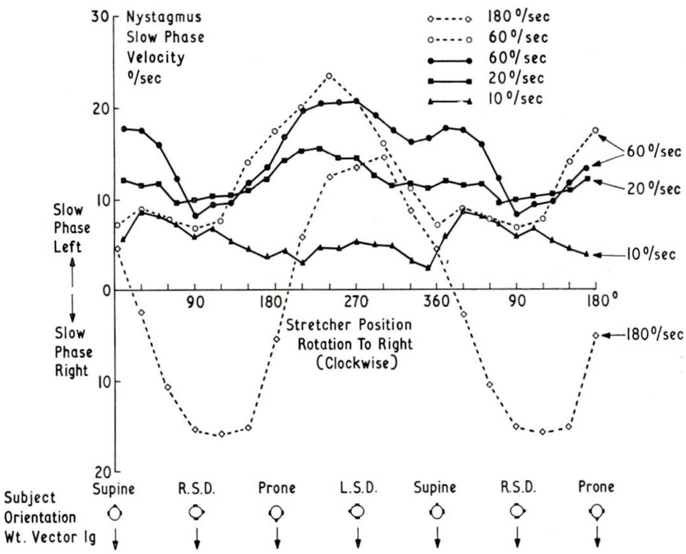

Fig. 11. Alteration of nystagmus slow-phase velocity according to orientation of subject to gravity during rotation about a horizontal, head-foot (z) axis at constant speed. Data from BENSON and BODIN (1966a) shown by a solid line, and from CORREIA and GUEDRY (1966) by a broken line. Note: The unidirectional nature of the nystagmus at speeds of rotation up to 60°/sec (1.1 rad sec^{-1}), and the appearance of maxima and minima in the left-side-down (L.S.D.) and right-side-down (R.S.D.) positions, respectively

nystagmus was in a compensatory direction. Thus in man, when the axis of rotation was coincident with the longitudinal (z) axis of the body, the eye movements were in a vertical plane (corresponding to a lateral nystagmus) with a slow phase in the opposite direction to that of the rotation (GUEDRY, 1965a; BENSON and

BODIN, 1966a); in rabbit the nystagmus had vertical and horizontal components, although the former predominated (JANEKE, 1968). Similarly, when the axis of rotation passed through the transverse (y) body axis, so that the subjects rotated 'head-over-heels', there was a vertical compensatory nystagmus (BODIN, 1968).

During horizontal axis rotation at constant speed, the slow-phase eye velocity varies in a cyclical manner (KOELLA, 1948). Figure 11, which summarizes the findings of GUEDRY (1965a), BENSON and BODIN (1966a) and CORREIA and GUEDRY (1966), shows that maxima and minima occurred when the acceleration vector lay close to the transverse (y) axis of the skull, as also noted by SAITO et al. (1968). When the rotation was to the right, peak slow-phase velocity to the left occurred as the subject passed through the left-side-down position, and was at a minimum in the right-side-down position. With rotation in the opposite direction, the positions in which the maxima and minima occurred were reversed. As the speed of rotation was increased the mean nystagmus velocity also increased, as did the amplitude of the modulation, but at rotational speeds in excess of about 2 rad sec^{-1} the mean eye velocity fell due to the appearance of a direction-changing nystagmus. At 3 rad sec^{-1} the nystagmus was symmetrical with essentially equal right and left beating components (CORREIA and GUEDRY, 1966). In the rabbit, the unidirectional nystagmus gave way to a direction-changing nystagmus at speeds of rotation in excess of 6 rad sec^{-1} (JANEKE, 1968).

The nystagmus evoked by a rotating linear acceleration vector of less than 1 g, achieved by counterrotation of a subject about a vertical (z) body axis at the end of a centrifuge arm, had 'bias' and 'sinusoidal' components comparable to the eye movements obtained during horizontal axis rotation (MONEY, 1966; NIVEN et al., 1966; STEER, 1967; BENSON, 1968). The relative magnitude of the asymmetry (bias) and cyclical oscillation of eye velocity have been found to depend upon the magnitude of the acceleration vector in the transverse (xy) plane of the skull and upon the rotational frequency. Figure 12 contains a summary of the data from the several experiments carried out on man.

There is thus a close similarity between the lateral nystagmus produced by the continued reorientation of the subject to the linear acceleration vector and that caused by a sinusoidal linear oscillation (GUEDRY, 1966). For with either method of stimulation, the lateral nystagmus is maximal when the changing component of the acceleration vector lies in, or close to, the bitemporal (y) axis of the skull, and the intensity of the response is a function of the magnitude of this component. Furthermore, when the acceleration vector is directed from right to left, nystagmus with slow phase to the right is evoked or augmented, or nystagmus in the opposite direction diminished. The converse applies when the acceleration is directed from left to right.

There is no doubt that the nystagmus produced by a rotating vector is caused by adequate stimulation of the vestibular apparatus, for it was absent in subjects without labyrinthine function (GUEDRY, 1965a). But the relative roles of the otoliths and canals in the genesis of the nystagmus have until recently been conjectural. Experiments on rabbits in which the utricular nerve was sectioned and the saccule destroyed bilaterally (JANEKE, 1968) revealed that in seven out of fifty animals, which postoperatively had unimpaired canal function (indicated by a normal response to torsional stimuli and no spontaneous nystagmus), parallel

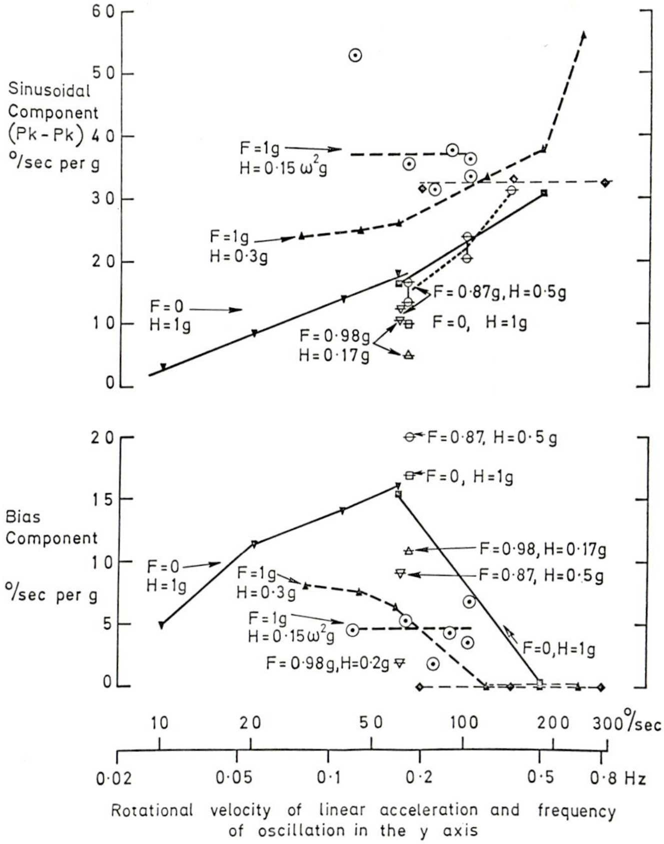

Fig. 12. Summary of normalized data on the nystagmus evoked in man by a linear acceleration vector (H) which rotated in the transverse plane (xy) of the head. The peak-to-peak amplitude of the slow-phase velocity wave form (as in Fig. 11), normalized for a 1 g rotating vector, is shown in the upper part of the figure, and the mean eye velocity, normalized for a 1 g stimulus, in the lower part. The solid lines connect mean values from experiments in which the magnitude in the vector was 1 g, and the interrupted lines, for data where the resultant acceleration was of excess of 1 g. F is the magnitude of the constant linear acceleration in the z axis.

▽ = Benson and Bodin (1966a) Horizontal z axis rotation, 8 subjects

□ = Correia and Guedry (1966) Horizontal z axis rotation, 7 subjects

⊖ = Stockwell et al. (1971) Rotation about z axis inclined to gravitational vertical, 8 subjects

$\overline{\nabla}$ = Benson (unpublished) Rotation about z axis inclined to gravitational vertical, 6 subjects

△ = Steer (1967) Rotation about z axis at end of centrifuge arm, radial acceleration (in xy plane) = 0.3 g, 6 subjects

⊙ = Benson (1968) Counterrotation, magnitude of the xy acceleration dependent on speed of rotation (ω), 6 subjects

◊ = Niven et al. (1966) Linear oscillation on horizontal track, peak acceleration in y axis = ± 0.58 g, 4 subjects. (Shown for comparison) From Benson and Barnes (1970)

swing oscillation and rotation about a horizontal axis failed to evoke nystagmus or the cyclical alteration of eye position seen in the normal animal. Conversely, CORREIA and MONEY (1970) found that on preventing endolymph flow by blocking all six endolymphatic ducts, a rotating linear acceleration vector still produced a sustained unidirectional nystagmus, although angular acceleration had no effect.

It must therefore be concluded that the nystagmic eye movements evoked by a cyclical alteration in the direction or magnitude of the linear acceleration vector are the manifestation of adequate stimulation of the macular receptors. The ampullar receptors, if stimulated at all by the linear acceleration, do not appear to make a significant contribution to the response. A theoretical analysis of the motion of the statoconial plaque under the influence of a rotating vector was made by BARNES (BENSON and BARNES, 1973), who suggested that the sinusoidal and bias components of the oculomotor response were, respectively, the manifestation of translational and torsional movement of the statoconial plaque relative to the sensory epithelium of the maculae. Solution of equations of motion for normal and shear accelerations appropriate to the different experimental conditions (e.g. horizontal axis rotation, counterrotation, etc.) yielded curves which were in qualitative agreement with the results depicted in Fig. 12. However, agreement between model predictions and experimental results does not necessarily imply that the physiological mechanism is the same as the theoretical model.

X. Interaction of Time-Varying Linear Accelerations and Angular Accelerations

When a subject is rotated about an earth horizontal axis, the initial angular acceleration from rest to constant velocity is combined with rotation of the gravity vector. These two stimuli are synergistic, so the nystagmus velocity immediately after an angular impulse should be higher than that elicited by the same angular impulse about an earth vertical axis. Experiments carried out on subjects rotated about a horizontal axis coincident with a longitudinal (z) or bitemporal (y) body axis, lend support to this opinion, for the mean initial nystagmus velocity was higher when the axis of rotation was horizontal than when vertical. However, because of the small number of observations, the effect did not reach statistical significance (BODIN, personal communication). Examination of the data also suggested that the separate contributions of the angular acceleration and the rotating vector to the response did not summate algebraically or facilitate one another, rather they exhibited occlusion. The subsequent decay of the per-rotational nystagmus was slightly prolonged when the axis of rotation was horizontal.

A more detailed study of the interaction of synergistic signals from ampullar and macular receptors was carried out by BENSON and STERNFELD (BENSON, 1968). They examined the lateral eye movements produced by a sinusoidal angular oscillation in the yaw (z) axis in two experimental configurations. In one, the oscillation axis was vertical, so the otoliths provided no information about rotation; but in the other, the axis of rotation was horizontal, so macular receptors were stimulated by the changing direction of the gravity vector in the transverse (xy) plane of the skull. Determination of the gain (expressed as the ratio between peak eye velocity and peak stimulus velocity) and of the phase relationship

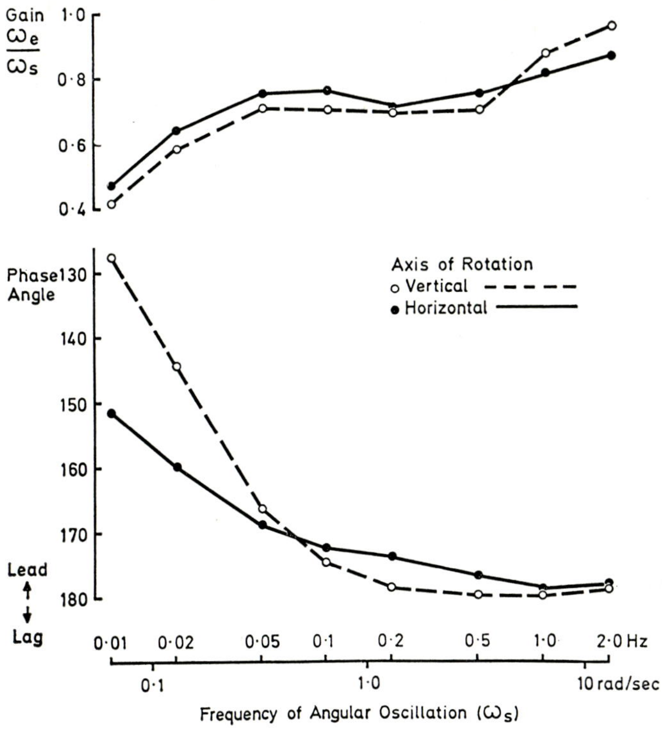

Fig. 13. Gain and phase plots of lateral eye movements produced by sinusoidal angular oscillation in yaw (rotation in longitudinal or z body axis) about vertical and horizontal axes. The peak angular velocity of the stimulus was (ω_s) $\pm$ 0.52 rad sec (30°/sec) at all frequencies. The ratio of peak eye velocity (ω_e) to ω_s was used to calculate the gain of the vestibulo-ocular system. Phase angle was determined from positions of zero eye and stimulus velocity; a phase angle of π rad (180°) represents zero phase error of the *compensatory* eye movement, which at low frequencies was phase advanced with respect to stimulus. See also Fig. 14. From Benson (1969)

between stimulus and response over the frequency range 0.01 to 2.0 Hz yielded the Bode plot shown in Fig. 13. At low frequencies (0.01 to 0.05 Hz), the presence of a changing otolithic stimulus produced a significant reduction in the phase advance of the compensatory eye movement attributable to the time constant (T_1 or π/Δ) of the canals and the adaptive time constant (T_a), but at 0.2 and 0.5 Hz the phase error was increased by about 5°. On the average the peak velocity of the slow phase of nystagmus was slightly higher when the axis of oscillation was horizontal than when it was vertical, but this effect was not sufficiently consistent to be statistically significant.

At low frequencies, rotation of the linear acceleration vector not only reduced the phase error but also produced a modulation of eye velocity which was temporarily related to the orientation of the head to gravity (Fig. 14). Maxima and minima of the modulating wave form occurred when the subject was close to the left- or right-side-down position (i.e. when the acceleration of gravity acted in the y axis of the skull) and hence was comparable to the oculomotor response which

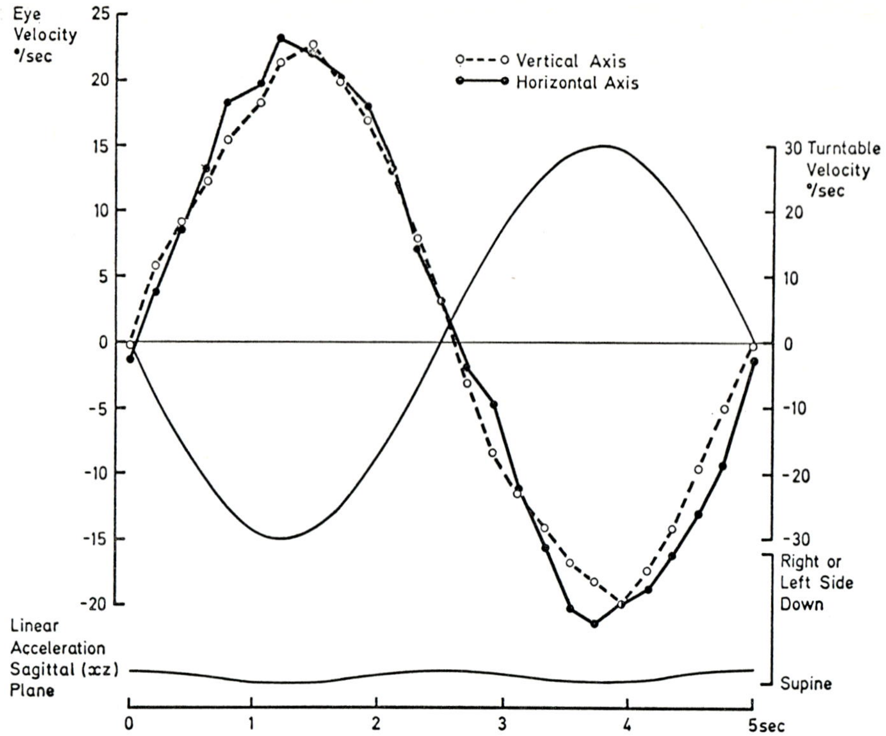

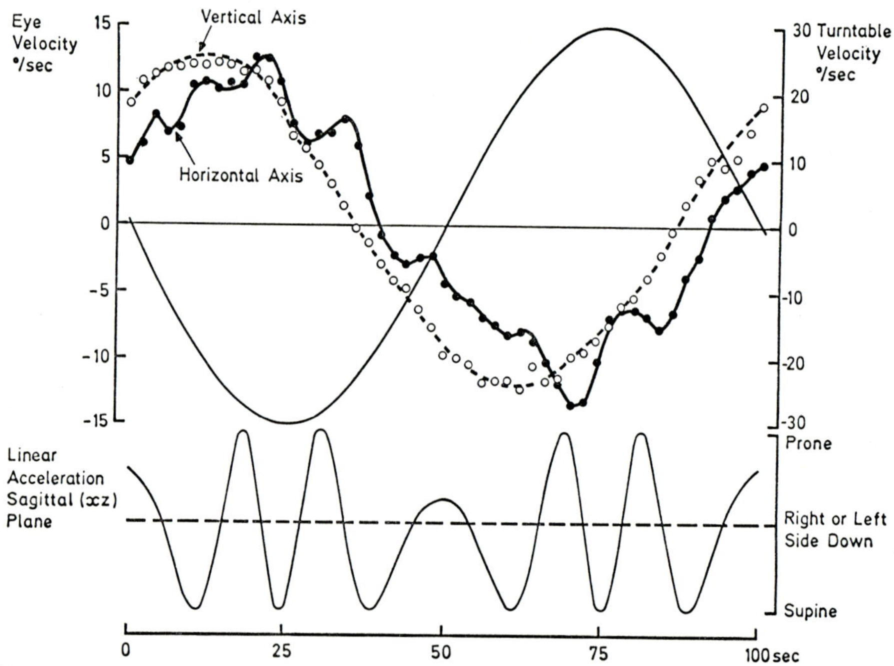

Fig. 14. Comparison of slow-phase eye velocities during oscillation about vertical and horizontal axes at 0.2 Hz (A) and 0.01 Hz (B). Each point is the mean eye velocity of three subjects during 5 stimulus cycles in A and 2 cycles in B. The continuous lines show turntable velocity and the orientation of the subjects to gravity during horizontal axis oscillation. From BENSON (1969)

occurs with continuous rotation of a linear acceleration vector in the xy plane. At higher frequencies the magnitude of the y axis linear acceleration was comparatively small, so the otolithic contribution to the eye velocity wave form was insignificant.

The form of the oculomotor response observed during horizontal axis oscillation can be accounted for by the simple summation of semicircular canal and otolithic components (BARNES, 1971), though lack of quantitative information about the dynamic behavior of the macular receptors prevents the accurate modelling of the phase relationship between stimulus and response. The reduction in phase error at low frequencies may also be accounted for by an increase in the adaptative time constant (i.e. less adaptation). It was argued earlier that when signals from the maculae and canals are antagonistic, the adaptive time constant is decreased; conversely when information from these two end-organs is in accord, is synergistic, then it is likely that the adaptive time constant will increase.

The combination of angular motion about a vertical axis with concomitant rotation about a horizontal axis presents a complex stimulus to the cristae and the maculae because of the development of Coriolis accelerations. However, by employing a slow (0.02 Hz) sinusoidal oscillation about a vertical axis and continuous rotation about the orthogonal horizontal axis, JANEKE (1968) was able to discriminate between the cyclical eye deviation and nystagmus evoked by the rotating vector, and the nystagmus attributable to canal stimulation by the angular Coriolis accelerations. When the speed of rotation about the horizontal axis was 0.7 rad sec^{-1}, the observed eye movement corresponded to the separate contributions of the rotating vector and the canal stimulus, though at a higher speed (2.5 rad sec^{-1}) there was apparently a selective depression of the response attributed to the rotating linear acceleration. These findings await confirmation and qualification, but they do suggest that in certain circumstances the response engendered by gravireceptor stimulation may be modified by signals from the semicircular canals.

References

ADRIAN, E.D.: Discharges from vestibular receptors in the cat. J. Physiol. (Lond.) **101**, 389–407 (1943).

ASCHAN, G.M., BERGSTEDT, M., GOLDBERG, L., LAURELL, L.: Positional nystagmus in man during and after acute alcohol intoxication. Quart. J. Stud. Alcohol **17**, 381–405 (1956).

ASCHAN, G., BERGSTEDT, M., GOLDBERG, L.: Positional alcohol nystagmus in patients with unilateral and bilateral labyrinthine destruction. Confin. neurol. (Basel) **24**, 80–102 (1964).

BAKHVALOVA, T.D.: O funkchional'noii svyazi otolitovogo apparata i polukruzhn'ikh kanalov. (On the functional state of the otolith apparatus and semicircular canals). Vestn. Otorino-laring. **4**, 35–37 (1950).

BÁRÁNY, R.: Untersuchungen über den vom Vestibularapparat des Ohres reflektorisch ausgelösten rythmischen Nystagmus und seine Begleiterscheinungen. Mschr. Ohrenheilk. **40**, 193–297 (1906).

BARNES, G.R.: Theoretical model of the utricular otolith and its response to angular motion with respect to an acceleration in shear. Report No. 506. Farnborough, Hants: R.A.F. Inst. Av. Med. 1971.

VON BEHRMAN, W.: Über Indifferenzlagen und Nystagmusgebiete, I. Acta oto-laryng. (Stockh.) Suppl. **40** (1940).

VON BEHRMAN, W.: Über Indifferenzlagen und Nystagmusgebiete, II. Acta oto-laryng. (Stockh.) **30**, 298–310 (1942).

Benson, A.J.: Effect of linear acceleration on labyrinthine nystagmus in man. Proc. 22nd Int. Cong. Physiol. Sci., Com. 1016, 1962.

Benson, A.J.: Modification of the per- and post-rotational responses by the concomitant linear acceleration. In: 2nd Symposium on the Role of the Vestibular Organs in Space Exploration. Washington, D.C.: NASA SP–**115**, 199–213 (1966).

Benson, A.J.: Post-rotational sensation and nystagmus as indicants of semicircular canal function. In: 3rd Symposium on the Role of the Vestibular Organs in Space Exploration. Washington, D.C.: NASA SP–**152**, 421–432 (1967).

Benson, A.J.: Lateral eye movements produced by a rotating linear acceleration vector. J. Physiol. (Lond.) **197**, 85–86P (1968).

Benson, A.J.: Interactions between semi-circular canals and gravireceptors. In: Recent Advances in Aerospace Medicine, D.E. Busby, Ed. Dordrecht: D. Reidel, p. 249–261, 1970.

Benson, A.J., Barnes, G.R.: Responses to rotating linear acceleration vectors considered in relation to a model of the otolith organs. In: 5th Symposium on the Role of the Vestibular Organs in Space Exploration. Washington, D.C.: NASA SP–**314**, 221–236 (1973).

Benson, A.J., Bodin, M.A.: Interaction of linear and angular accelerations on vestibular receptors in man. Aerospace Med. **37**, 144–154 (1966a).

Benson, A.J., Bodin, M.A.: Comparison of the effect of the direction of the gravitational acceleration on post-rotational responses in yaw, pitch and roll. Aerospace Med. **37**, 889–897 (1966b).

Benson, A.J., Bodin, M.A.: Effect of orientation to the gravitational vertical on nystagmus following rotation about a horizontal axis. Acta oto-laryng. (Stockh.) **61**, 517–526 (1966c).

Benson, A.J., Guedry, F.E., Melvill Jones, G.: Response of semi-circular canal dependent units in vestibular nuclei to rotation of a linear acceleration vector without angular acceleration. J. Physiol. (Lond.) **210**, 475–494 (1970).

Benson, A.J., Whiteside, T.C.D.: The effect of linear acceleration on the response to angular acceleration in man. J. Physiol. (Lond.) **156**, 6–7P (1961).

Bergstedt, M.: Studies of positional nystagmus in the human centrifuge. Acta oto-laryng. (Stockh.) Suppl. **165** (1961a).

Bergstedt, M.: The effect of gravitational force on the vestibular caloric test. Acta oto-laryng. (Stockh.) **53**, 551–562 (1961b).

Billingham, J.: Russian experience of problems in vestibular physiology related to the space environment. In: 2nd Symposium on the Role of the Vestibular Organs in Space Exploration. Washington, D.C.: NASA SP–**155**, 5–14 (1966).

Bodin, M.A.: The effect of gravity on human vestibular responses during rotation in pitch. J. Physiol. (Lond.) **196**, 74–75P (1968).

Bos, J.H., Jongkees, L.B.W., Philipszoon, A.J.: On the action of linear accelerations upon the otoliths. Acta oto-laryng. (Stockh.) **56**, 477–489 (1963).

Camis, M.: The physiology of the vestibular apparatus. Tr. Creed, R.S., Oxford: University Press 1930.

Coats, A.C., Smith, S.Y.: Body position and the intensity of caloric nystagmus. Acta oto-laryng. (Stockh.) **63**, 515–532 (1967).

Collins, W.E.: Special effects of brief periods of visual fixation on nystagmus and sensations of turning. Aerospace Med. **39**, 257–266 (1968).

Correia, M.J., Guedry, F.E.: Influence of labyrinth orientation relative to gravity on responses elicited by stimulation of the horizontal semi-circular canals. Report No. 905. Pensacola, Fla.: Nav. Sch. Aviat. Med. 1964.

Correia, M.J., Guedry, F.E.: Modification of vestibular responses as a function of rate of rotation about an earth-horizontal axis. Report No. 957. Pensacola, Fla.: Nav. Aerospace Med. Inst. 1966.

Correia, M.J., Money, K.E.: The effect of blockage of all six semi-circular canal ducts on nystagmus produced by dynamic linear acceleration in the cat. Acta oto-laryng. (Stockh.) **69**, 7–16 (1970).

Crampton, G.H.: Does linear acceleration modify cupular deflection? In: 2nd Symposium on the Role of the Vestibular Organs in Space Exploration. Washington, D.C.: NASA SP–**115**, 169–184 (1966).

DUENSING, F., SCHAEFER, K.P.: Über die Konvergenz verschiedener labyrintharer Afferenzen auf einzelne Neurone des Vestibulariskerngebietes. Arch. Psychiat. Nervenkr. **199**, 345–371 (1959).

DUMONT, S.: Effects extralabyrinthique sur l'activité des cellules des noyaux vestibulaire. J. Physiol. (Paris) **52**, 87–98 (1960).

ECKEL, W.: Elektrophysiologische und histologische Untersuchungen im Vestibulariskerngebiet bei Drehreizen. Arch. Ohr.-, Nas.-, u. Kehlk.-Heilk. **164**, 487–513 (1954).

VAN EGMOND, A.A.J., GROEN, J.J., JONGKEES, L.B.W.: The mechanics of the semi-circular canal. J. Physiol. (Lond.) **110**, 1–17 (1949).

EWALD, J.R.: Physiologische Untersuchungen über das Endorgan des Nervus octavus. Wiesbaden: Bergmann 1892.

FLOURENS, J.P.M.: Recherches expérimentales sur les propriétés du système nerveux dans les animaux vertébrés, 2nd ed. Paris: Crevot 1842.

FREDRICKSON, J.M., SCHWARZ, D.: Multisensory influence upon single units in the vestibular nucleus. In: 4th Symposium on the Role of the Vestibular Organs in Space Exploration. Washington, D.C.: NASA SP–**187**, 203–208 (1968).

FREDRICKSON, J.M., SCHWARZ, D., KORNHUBER, H.H.: Convergence and interaction of vestibular and deep somatic afferents upon neurons in the vestibular nuclei of cat. Acta oto-laryng. (Stockh.) **61**, 168–188 (1966).

GERNANDT, B.E.: Response of mammalian vestibular neurons to horizontal rotation and caloric stimulation. J. Neurophysiol. **12**, 173–184 (1949).

GERNANDT, B.E.: The effect of the centrifugal force upon the nerve discharge from the horizontal canal. Acta physiol. scand. **21**, 61–72 (1950).

GRAY, R.F., CROSBIE, R.J.: Variation in duration of oculogyral illusions as a function of the radius of turn. Report NADC-MA-5806. Johnsville, Pa.: Nav. Air. Develop. Ctr. 1958.

GRAYBIEL, A., JOHNSON, W.H.: A comparison of the symptomatology experienced by healthy persons and subjects with loss of labyrinthine function when exposed to unusual patterns of centripetal force in the counter-rotating room. Ann. Otol. (St. Louis) **72**, 1–17 (1963).

GRAYBIEL, A., NIVEN, J.I., MACCORQUODALE, K.: The effect of linear acceleration on the oculogyral illusion. Report NSAM-443. Pensacola, Fla.: Nav. Sch. Aviat. Med. 1956.

GROEN, J.J.: Adaptation. Pract. oto-rhino-laryng. (Basel) **19**, 524–530 (1957).

GROEN, J.J.: Inhibitory mechanism of the vestibular system in man in comparison with hearing. J. acoust. Soc. Amer. **14**, 1497–1503 (1962).

GROEN, J.J., LOWENSTEIN, O., VENDRICK, A.J.H.: The mechanical analysis of the responses from the end-organs of the horizontal semi-circular canal in the isolated elasmobranch labyrinth. J. Physiol. (Lond.) **117**, 329–346 (1952).

GUEDRY, F.E.: Orientation of the rotation-axis relative to gravity; its influence on nystagmus and the sensation of rotation. Acta oto-laryng. (Stockh.) **60**, 30–49 (1965a).

GUEDRY, F.E.: Psychophysiological studies of vestibular function. In: Contributions to Sensory Physiology. W.D. NEFF, Ed. New York: Academic Press 1965b.

GUEDRY, F.E.: Influence of linear and angular accelerations on nystagmus. In: 2nd Symposium on the Role of the Vestibular Organs in Space Exploration. Washington, D.C.: NASA SP–**115**, 185–198 (1966).

GUEDRY, F.E., HARRIS, C.S.: Labyrinthine function related to experiments on the parallel swing. Report, NSAM-86. Pensacola, Fla.: Nav. Sch. Aviat. Med. 1963.

HALLPIKE, C.S.: Some types of ocular nystagmus and their neurological mechanisms. Proc. roy. Soc. Med. **60**, 1043–1054 (1967).

IGARASHI, M.: Dimensional study of the vestibular end-organ apparatus. In: 2nd Symposium on the Role of the Vestibular Organs in Space Exploration. Washington, D.C.: NASA SP–**115**, 47–54 (1966).

JACKSON, M.M., SEARS, C.W.: The effect of weightlessness upon the normal nystagmic reaction. Proc. 36th Meeting Aerospace Med. Assoc., 138–139, 1965.

JANEKE, J.B.: On nystagmus and otoliths. A vestibular study of responses as provoked by a cephalo-caudal horizontal axial rotation. Dissertation: University of Amsterdam 1968.

JANEKE, J.B., OOSTERVELD, W.J.: The effect of gravity on central and vestibular eye movements. Med. Proc. **15**, 449–453 (1969).

JONGKEES, L.B.W.: Which is the preferable method of performing the caloric test? Arch. Otolaryng. **49**, 594–608 (1949).

JONGKEES, L.B.W.: On centric and eccentric rotatory examination. Svensk Otolaryng. Förenings Förhandlingar, 98–105, 1956.

JONGKEES, L.B.W.: On positional nystagmus. Acta oto-laryng. (Stockh.) Suppl. **159**, 78–83 (1960).

JONGKEES, L.B.W., PHILIPSZOON, A.J.: Nystagmus provoked by linear accelerations. Acta physiol. pharmacol. neerl. **10**, 239–247 (1962).

JONGKEES, L.B.W., PHILIPSZOON, A.J.: The influence of position upon the eye-movements provoked by linear accelerations. Acta oto-laryng. (Stockh.) **56**, 414–420 (1963).

KELLOGG, R.S., GRAYBIEL, A.: Lack of response to thermal stimulation of the semi-circular canals in the weightless phase of parabolic flight. Aerospace Med. **38**, 487–490 (1967).

KHILOV, K.L.: Zh. ushn. nos. gorlov Bolezn. **6**, 289–299 (1929).

KHILOV, K.L.: In: Sb. trudov tsentral'noy nauchnoy psikhofiziologicheskoy laboratorii po izucheniyu letnogo truda grazhdanskogo vozdushnogo flota SSSR. (Collection of papers by the Central Psychophysiological Laboratory on the study of the activities of the civil air-force of the USSR). **1**, 5–72 (1936).

KISLYAKOV, V.A., ORLOV, I.V.: The physiology of the vestibular analyzer of centrifugal force on caloric nystagmus. In: Fiziologiya Vestibulyarnago Analizatora. V.V. PARIN and M.D. YEMEL'YANOV, Moscow: 'Nauka' Press, 86–89, 1968. English translation: Physiology of the Vestibular Analyzer. Washington, D.C.: NASA TT, F–**616**, 81–84 (1970).

KIØRBOE, F.: The significance of nystagmus observed in routine otological examination of flight personnel. In: Medical Aspects or Flight Safety. E. EVRARD, P. BERGERET and P.M. VAN WULFTEN PALTHE, Eds. London: Pergamon, 290–295, 1959.

KURASHVILI, A. YE., BABIYAK, V.P.: On the functional relationship between the semi-circular canals and the otolithic apparatus. In: Fiziologiya Vestibulyarnago Analizatora. V.V. PARIN and M.D. YEMEL'YANOV, Eds. Moscow: 'Nauka' Press, 119–122, 1968. English translation: Physiology of the Vestibular Analyzer. Washington, D.C.: NASA TT, F–**616**, 115–119 (1970).

DE KLEIJN, A., MAGNUS, R.: Labyrinthreflexe auf Progressivbewegungen. Pflügers Arch. ges. Physiol. **186**, 39–60 (1921).

DE KLEIJN, A., VERSTEEGH, C.: Experimentelle Untersuchungen über den sogenannten Lagenystagmus während akuter Alkoholvergiftung beim Kaninchen. Acta oto-laryng. (Stockh.) **14**, 356–377 (1930).

KOELLA, W.: Experimentell-physiologischer Beitrag zum Nystagmusproblem. Helv. physiol. pharmacol. Acta **5**, 154–168 (1947).

KOELLA, W.: Das Verhalten des perrotatorischen Augennystagmus beim Kaninchen bei Drehung um nicht lotrechte Achsen. Helv. physiol. pharmacol. Acta **6**, 280–291 (1948).

LANSBERG, M.P., GUEDRY, F.E., GRAYBIEL, A.: Effect of changing resultant linear acceleration relative to the subject on nystagmus generated by angular acceleration. Aeromed. Acta (Soesterberg) **9**, 97–122 (1964). Also Aerospace Med. **36**, 456–460 (1965).

LEDOUX, A.: Activité électrique des nerfs des canaux semi-circulaires, du saccule et de l'utricule chez la grenouille. Acta oto-rhino-laryng. belg. **3**, 335–349 (1949).

LINDEMAN, H.H.: Studies on the morphology of the sensory regions of the vestibular apparatus. Ergebn. Anat. Entwickl.-Gesch. **42**, 1–113 (1969).

LORENTE DE NÓ, R.: Ausgewählte Kapitel aus der vergleichenden Physiologie des Labyrinthes. Die Augenmuskelreflexe beim Kaninchen und ihre Grundlagen. Ergebn. Physiol. **32**, 73–242 (1931).

LORENTE DE NÓ, R.: The regulation of eye positions and movements induced by the labyrinth. Laryngoscope (St. Louis) **42**, 233–330 (1932).

LOWENSTEIN, O.E.: Electrophysiological experiments on the isolated surviving labyrinth of elasmobranch fish to analyse the responses to linear accelerations. In: 4th Symposium on the Role of the Vestibular Organs in Space Exploration. Washington, D.C.: NASA SP–**187**, 161–166 (1968).

LOWENSTEIN, O.E.: Electrophysiological experiments on the isolated surviving labyrinth of elasmobranch fish to analyse the responses to linear acceleration. In: Vestibular Function on Earth and in Space. J. STAHLE, Ed. Oxford and New York: Perganmo, 35–41, 1970.

Lowenstein, O., Roberts, T.D.M.: The equilibrium function of the otolith organs of the Thornback Ray *Raja clavata*. J. Physiol. (Lond.) **110**, 392–415 (1950).

Lowenstein, O., Sand, A.: The mechanism of the semi-circular canal. A study of the responses of single-fibre preparations to angular accelerations and to rotation at constant speed. Proc. roy. Soc. B **129**, 256–275 (1940a).

Lowenstein, O., Sand, A.: The individual and integrated activity of the semi-circular canals of the elasmobranch labyrinth. J. Physiol. (Lond.) **99**, 89–101 (1940b).

Mach, E.: Grundlinien der Lehre von den Bewegungsempfindungen, Leipzig: Engelmann 1875.

Malcolm, R., Melvill Jones, G.: A quantitative study of vestibular adaptation in humans. Acta oto-laryng. (Stockh.) **70**, 126–135 (1970).

Markaryan, S.S.: The problem of the interrelationship between the function of the semicircular canals and that of the otolith apparatus. In: Problemy kosmicheskoy biologii, 4th. N.M. Sisakyan, Ed. Moscow: "Nauka" Press, 176–181, 1967. English Translation, Problems of Space Biology, 4. Washington, D.C.: NASA TT–**528**, 185–190 (1969).

Maxwell, S.S.: Labyrinth and equilibrium. Philadelphia and London: Lippincott 1923.

Mayne, R.: The "match" of the semi-circular canals to the dynamic requirements of the various species. In: First Symposium on The Role of the Vestibular Organs in the Exploration of Space. Washington, D.C.: NASA SP–**77**, 57–67 (1965).

McCabe, B.F.: Nystagmus response of the otolith organs. Laryngoscope (St. Louis) **74**, 372–381 (1964).

McLeod, M.E., Correia, M.J.: Use of caloric test in evaluating the effects of gravity on cupula displacement. Report, NSAM-94. Pensacola, Fla.: Nav. Sch. Aciat. Med. 1964.

Meiry, J.L.: The vestibular system and human dynamic space orientation. Washington, D.C.: NASA Contractor Report No. 628, 1966. Also Sc. D. Thesis Massachusetts Institute of Technology.

Melvill Jones, G.: Neural reflection of vestibular mechanics. In: 3rd Symposium on the Role of the Vestibular Organs in the Exploration of Space. Washington, D.C.: NASA SP–**152**, 169–180 (1967).

Melvill Jones, G., Barry, W., Kowalsky, N.: Dynamics of the semi-circular canals compared in yaw, pitch and roll. Aerospace Med. **35**, 984–989 (1964).

Melvill Jones, G., Milsum, J.H.: Further relations between neural and mechanical responses of the semi-circular canal. Proc. 37th Aerospace Med. Assoc. Meeting, 252–253, 1967.

Melvill Jones, G., Milsum, J.H.: Characteristics of neural transmission from the semi-circular canal to the vestibular nuclei of cats. J. Physiol. (Lond.) **209**, 295–316 (1970).

Milojevic, B., Voots, R.J.: Simultaneous stimulation of the otolith organs and semi-circular canals. Acta oto-laryng. (Stockh.) **61**, 92–100 (1965).

Milsum, J.H., Melvill Jones, G.: Trigonometric resolution of neural responses from the vestibular otolith organ. Digest 7th Int. Conf. Med. Biol. Eng., Stock., 203, 1967.

Money, K.E.: Discussion of F.E. Guedry. In: 2nd Symposium on the Role of the Vestibular Organs in Space Exploration. Washington, D.C.: NASA SP–**115**, 196–197 (1966).

Money, K.E., Johnson, W.H., Corlett, B.M.A.: Role of semi-circular canals in positional alcohol nystagmus. Amer. J. Physiol. **208**, 1065–1070 (1965).

Money, K.E., Scott, J.W.: Functions of separate sensory receptors of nonauditory labyrinth of the cat. Amer. J. Physiol. **202**, 1211–1220 (1962).

Money, K.E., Sokoloff, M., Weaver, R.S.: Specific gravity and viscocity of endolymph and perilymph. In: 2nd Symposium on the Role of the Vestibular Organs in Space Exploration. Washington, D.C.: NASA SP–**115**, 91–98 (1966).

Morimoto, M.: Otoneurological study on the brain tumour. Acta med. biol. (Niigata) **3**, 243–262 (1955).

Nito, Y., Johnson, W.H., Money, K.E., Ireland, P.E.: The non-auditory labyrinth and positional alcohol nystagmus. Acta oto-laryng. (Stockh.) **58**, 65–67 (1963).

Niven, J.I., Hixson, W.C., Correia, M.J.: Elicitation of horizontal nystagmus by periodic linear acceleration. Acta oto-laryng. (Stockh.) **62**, 429–441 (1966).

Oosterveld, W.J.: Effect of gravity on positional alcohol nystagmus (PAN). Aerospace Med. **41**, 557—560 (1970).

Oosterveld, W.J., van der Laarse, W.D.: Effect of gravity on vestibular nystagmus. Aerospace Med. **40**, 382–385 (1969).

OWADA, K., OKUBU, K.: The otolith reactions on nystagmus by caloric stimulations. Acta oto-laryng. (Stockh.) Suppl. **179**, 1–6 (1963).

OWADA, K., SHIIZU, S., KIMURA, K.: The influence of the utricle on nystagmus. Acta oto-laryng. (Stockh.) **52**, 215–220 (1960).

POPOV, A.P.: Voprosy meditsinskogo obespecheniye aviatsii. **1**, 99 (1939) (Problems of medical supervision in aviation). Quoted by MARKARYAN 1967.

PURKINJE, J.E.: Beiträge zur näheren Kenntnis des Schwindels. Jahrbücher d. öster. Staates **6**, 79 (1820). Quoted by M. CAMIS 1930.

ROMAN, A.J., WARREN, B.H., GRAYBIEL, A.: The sensitivity to stimulation of the semi-circular canals during weightlessness. Report NSAM-84. Pensacola: Fla. Nav. Sch. Aciat. Med. 1963.

ROSS, D.A.: Electrical studies on the frog's labyrinth. J. Physiol. (Lond.) **86**, 117–146 (1936).

SAITO, I., WADA, H., YAGURA, S., KATO, N.: On the influences of gravitational acceleration to nystagmus. Jap. J. Aerospace Med. Psy. **6**, 6–12 (1968).

SALA, O.: The efferent vestibular system. Acta oto-laryng. (Stockh.) Suppl. **197** (1965).

SCHMIDT, R.S.: Frog labyrinthine efferent impulses. Acta oto-laryng. (Stockh.) **56**, 51–64 (1962).

SCHUKNECHT, H.F.: Positional vertigo: clinical and experimental observations. Trans. Amer. Acad. Ophthal. Otolaryng. **66**, 319–332 (1962).

SHIMAZU, H., PRECHT, W.: Inhibition of central vestibular neurons from the contralateral labyrinth and its mediating pathway. J. Neurophysiol. **29**, 467–492 (1966).

SPELLS, K.E.: Calculations for the design of large-scale working models of the semi-circular canal. Report No. S. 34. Farnborough, Hants.: RAF Inst. Aviat. Med. 1961.

SPOENDLIN, H.H.: Ultrastructural studies of the labyrinth in squirrel monkeys. In: First Symposium on the Role of the Vestibular Organs in the Exploration of Space. Washington, D.C.: NASA SP–**77**, 7–22 (1965).

STAHLE, J.: Electronystagmography in the rotary test. A study in a series of normal individuals. Acta Soc. Med. upsalien. **62**, 77–103 (1957).

STAHLE, J.: Electro-nystagmography in the caloric and rotatory tests. Acta oto-laryng. (Stockh.) Suppl. **137**, (1958).

STEER, R.W., JR.: The influence of angular and linear acceleration and thermal stimulation on the human semi-circular canal. Sc.D. Thesis. Massachusetts Institute of Technology 1967.

STOCKWELL, C.W., TURNIPSEED, G.T., GUEDRY, F.E.: Nystagmus responses during rotation about a tilted axis. Army-Navy Joint Report No. NAMRL–1129. Pensacola, Fla.: Nav. Aerospace Med. Res. Lab. 1971.

SZENTÁGOTHAI, J.: Die Rolle der einzelnen Labyrinthrezeptoren bei der Orientation von Augen und Kopf in Raume. Budapest: Akademai Kiado 1952.

TER BRAAK, J.W.G.: Kann der Bogengangsapparat durch geradlinige Beschleunigung gereizt werden? Pflügers Arch. ges. Physiol. **238**, 327–332 (1937).

TIMM, C.: Physikalische Vorgänge bei der Labyrinthreizung. Z. Laryng. Rhinol. **32**, 237–251 (1953).

UDO DE HAES, H.A., SCHÖNE, H.: Interaction between statolith organs and semi-circular canals on apparent vertical and nystagmus. Acta oto-laryng. (Stock.) **69**, 25–31 (1970).

ULRICH, H.: Die Funktion der Otolithen, geprüft durch direkte mechanische Beeinflussung des Utriculusotolithen am lebenden Hecht. Pflügers Arch. ges. Physiol. **235**, 545–553 (1934).

YOUNG, L.R.: A control model of the vestibular system. Symposium on technical and biological problems in cybernetics. Yerivan, Armenia, USSR 1968.

YOUNG, L.R., OMAN, C.M.: Model for vestibular adaptation to horizontal rotation. Aerospace Med. **40**, 1076–1080 (1969).

YUGANOV, YE. M.: The problem of the functional characteristics and interaction of the otolith and cupular portions of the vestibular apparatus under conditions of altered gravity. In: Problemy kosmicheskoy biologii, 4. N.M. SISAKYAN, Ed. Moscow: ‚Nauka' Press, 54–69, 1965. English translation. Problems of Space Biology 4. Washington, D.C.: NASA TT F–**368**, 48–63 (1966).

Chapter V.

Vestibular Ataxia and its Measurement in Man*

By

A. R. FREGLY, **Pensacola, Florida (USA)

With 11 Figures

Contents

I. Introduction

The designation of vestibular ataxia as a distinct phenomenon[1] hinges upon reliable evidence of a person's limited ability to coordinate voluntary muscular movements while walking or standing due to the absence, disturbance or loss of function of the vestibular apparatus *per se*. One probably distinct and well-known qualitative characteristic of such an ataxia is the difficulty experienced by individuals with extensive loss of labyrinthine functions in walking at night or in darkness. This particular form of vestibular ataxia can be recognized readily in the laboratory or clinic when such individuals attempt to walk tandemly (heel-to-toe) with eyes closed.

Recent applications of a new, standardized, multifaceted quantitative ataxia test battery (GRAYBIEL and FREGLY, 1966; FREGLY and GRAYBIEL, 1968a) to highly selected groups of individuals with various degrees of loss of labyrinthine function have afforded the opportunity to describe this and the other aspects of spontaneous vestibular ataxia in quantitative terms, as well as the many mani-

* From the Naval Aerospace Medical Laboratory, U.S. Naval Aerospace Medical Institute, Pensacola, Florida. Opinions and conclusions contained herein are those of the author and do not necessarily reflect the views or the endorsement of the Navy Department. The research summarized herein was conducted under the sponsorship of the Office of Advanced Research and Technology, National Aeronautics and Space Administration, Order Nos. R-37 and R-93.

** Present address: Chief of Naval Education and Training Support, Pensacola, Florida 32509, USA.

1 A comprehensive review of this phenomenon appears elsewhere (IGARASHI et al., 1974. In Press).

festations of induced vestibular ataxia. But it should be emphasized that the impossibility of delineating the vestibular contributions *per se* to ataxia test responses of man with technical accuracy means present definitions of vestibular ataxia are only tentative at best. In addition, definitive accounts of ataxia test responses are at least hampered by the following overlapping factors: (1) there are methodological problems in sampling ataxia test performances; (2) the factorial nature of ataxia test performance skills has not yet been studied adequately; (3) there are unsettled statistical problems of defining abnormal ataxia test behavior.[2] In this presentation spontaneous vestibular ataxia is defined in terms of some characteristic differences between "vestibular normal" and "vestibular defective" individuals in their performance skills on a particular battery of ataxia tests.

II. The Ataxia Test Battery

The following considerations of methodology appear to be important when the sole purpose of vestibular ataxia testing is to establish reliable quantitative differences between individuals in relation to one or more indicators of vestibular functioning, e.g. in relation to calorically-induced or rotation-induced nystagmus, so that the normal can be separated from the pathological: (1) high sensitivity to individual differences in performance within a wide range of age and ability such as can be determined by means of walking and standing platforms of various widths (rails and the floor) coupled with a stringent body position of feet tandemly aligned in strict heel-to-toe position, arms folded against the chest, and the body erect or nearly erect; (2) multidimensional sampling of vestibular-dependent stimulus-response relationships, for example, by means of stance and gait tests performed with and without the use of vision; (3) simplicity and economy of apparatus to insure wide and frequent use; (4) brevity and ease of test administration; (5) objectivity of scoring, e.g. by timing the duration of standing and counting the number of steps walked; (6) task novelty, to minimize the measurement of over-practiced skills; (7) high test-retest reliability; (8) high task interest to insure ego involvement, or motivation; (9) face and construct validity.

An ataxia test battery taking all such matters into account was devised to test large numbers of individuals for the purpose of establishing normal standards of performance (GRAYBIEL and FREGLY, 1966; FREGLY and GRAYBIEL, 1968a)[3]. The test administration and scoring procedures are redescribed here in sufficient detail to greatly facilitate the understanding of the presentation of the data which follow. The ataxia test items, in the order they were administered, consisted of:

1. Sharpened Romberg (SR): standing on the floor while eyes were closed and with arms folded against chest, feet aligned in strict tandem heel-to-toe position, and body very nearly, if not completely, erect for a period of 60 sec. A maximum of four trials was administered.

---

2 For the convenience of investigators particularly interested in these and numerous other problems related to vestibular research, a bibliography containing selected references to a variety of methods and results of posture, postural equilibrium and ataxia testing is appended to the chapter.

3 New normative standards have been reported recently (FREGLY et al., 1972; FREGLY et al., 1973).

Testing was discontinued when the criterion score of 60 sec standing time was met on any trial. A score of 60 sec on the first trial was weighted 4, and a perfect test score of 240 (60 sec $\times$ 4 trials) was assigned; a perfect score on the second trial was weighted 3, and 180 (60×3) plus the score obtained on the first trial became the assigned test score, etc. Subjects were always credited with perfect scores on the remaining (nonadministered) trials.

2. Walk Eyes Open (Walk E/O[4]) (short version)[5]: walking heel-to-toe with feet in a strictly tandem position on a rail 3/4 $\times$ 96 inch. with arms folded against chest while in a body-erect position. The number of heel-to-toe steps taken (maximum 5 per trial) during the best three out of the five trials administered constituted the test score. Maximum score obtainable was 15 steps.

3. Stand Eyes Open (Stand E/O) (short version): standing heel-to-toe with feet in a strictly tandem position and arms folded against the chest while in a body-erect position on the 3/4-inch-wide rail for 60 sec. The best three trials out of the five administered were totalled and became the test score. Maximum score equalled 180 sec.

4. Stand Eyes Closed (Stand E/C) (short version): standing, as for the Stand E/O test, on a 30 $\times$ 2–1/4 inch. rail 60 sec. Scoring was identical to the Stand E/O test.

5. Stand One Leg Eyes Closed (SOLEC-R and SOLEC-L): standing on each leg for 30 sec while arms were folded against chest and body was in erect, or nearly erect, position. Moving the standing foot from the start position was not permitted. A maximum of five trials was administered, and testing on each leg was discontinued when the criterion score of 30 sec was obtained on any trial. A score of 30 on the first trial was weighted 5, and the maximum test score of 150 (30 sec $\times$ 5 trials) was assigned; i.e. full credit for the remaining nonadministered trials was given, as for the SR test. Thus, a 30-sec score on the second, third, fourth, or fifth trial was weighted 4, 3, 2, or 1, respectively.

6. Walk A Line Eyes Closed (WALEC): walking a 12-foot long line on the floor as straightly as possible at a speed typical to the subject, with arms folded against chest and feet tandem, heel-to-toe. Trials during which the foot position was violated either by nontandem alignment of feet or by toe not touching heel were scored as mistrials. A maximum of five mistrials was permitted. Each quantitatively scorable trial required that the subject walk the entire 12-foot distance. On completed trials the number of inches of deviation from the line, measured to the nearest inch from the center of the foot, constituted a trial score, and the total of the two best trials out of three (best equalled least deviant from the line) constituted the test score. Maximum score equalled 0 inches. Subjects not meeting the criteria for scorable trials were scored as unable to perform (UTP).

7. Walk On Floor Eyes Closed (WOFEC): Because the WALEC appeared to be as much a test of spatial orientation as a test of ataxia if not more, and because the performances of notably ataxic individuals were qualitatively often more deviant from normal than was indicated quantitatively by the scoring procedure, the WOFEC was subsequently added to the test battery (Fregly and Graybiel, 1968a). In the stringent body and foot position assumed for the WALEC, ten tandem, heel-to-toe steps beyond the first two starting steps without side-stepping were scored as a perfect trial. The scores obtained on the best three out of the five trials administered constituted the test score. The best test score that could be obtained was 30 (10 steps $\times$ 3 trials).

8. Supplementary ataxia tests: Individuals with unusually poor eyes-closed-test performance scores also were given the Classical Romberg (CR) test with eyes closed, followed by the eyes-open versions of any or all the standardized test battery items, viz. SR E/O, SOLEO-R and/or SOLEO-L, WALEO, WOFEO, and CR E/O.

All male subjects wore military or military-type dress shoes, whereas all female subjects wore flats. Soft-soled footwear, such as tennis or basketball shoes, was not permitted during testing.

---

4 Often designated the Walk H/T (heel-to-toe) test in previous publications.

5 In the long version (Graybiel and Fregly, 1966) six 8-foot long, wooden or metal rails of different widths (in inches) were used as follows: 2–3/4, 2–1/4, 1–3/4, 1–1/4, 3/4, and 1/2, and the Stand E/O and Stand E/C tests were also included. Maximum scores obtainable were 60 steps on Walk E/O, and 720 seconds on Stand E/O and Stand E/C in the best two out of three trials.

The test battery was standardized through testing both large and small samples of normal individuals varying in age and occupation who were in good to excellent physical health as attested to by recent medical evaluations. In addition to an otological history, audiograms were recorded at the time of ataxia testing. A large number of subjects were also given a threshold caloric test (McLEOD and MEEK, 1962; FREGLY and GRAYBIEL, 1970), and in many instances ocular counterrolling determinations (MILLER, 1961) were also made. The normal examinees included military officers and enlisted male and female personnel; student aviators; "Project Astronaut Candidates"; several of the Mercury, Gemini, and Apollo astronauts; test pilots, and test pilot candidates; the longitudinally studied (since 1940) "Thousand Aviators" (FREGLY et al., 1968); and male and female civilians. Other normals included two groups who had experienced occupational stresses and who were tested to determine their vestibular status, i.e. Navy deep sea divers and individuals who had been exposed to high-G forces on centrifuges.

The clinical populations sampled included individuals with total, or near total, bilateral loss of labyrinthine functions due to meningitis or mastoiditis in early life (bilateral labyrinthine-defectives, or BL-Ds), individuals treated with streptomycin sulfate for Ménière's syndrome, individuals treated surgically for acoustic neuroma (unilateral labyrinthine-defectives, or UL-Ds) patients in whom vertigo was a major symptom or complaint and who had been referred by otologists or neurologists, and a young man with normal hearing but with no evidence of vestibular function (GRAYBIEL, 1964, 1965, 1966, 1968; GRAYBIEL et al., 1967, 1971). The general health and physical fitness of all individuals comprising the clinical groups were adequate, or better, for ataxia testing.

A discussion of the ataxia test findings obtained on normal subjects and on the various clinical groups under both natural and unusual conditions comprises the remaining portion of the chapter.

III. Ataxia Test Findings in Normals

Age and sex influences on the performance of normal individuals on several items of the ataxia test battery are summarized in Fig. 1. In all age groups and on all tests (WALEC[6] excepted) the performance scores of the male subjects exceeded those of the female subjects. The factors contributing to these systematic sex differences are, as yet, unknown. But these and related findings (FREGLY et al., 1968) have made it clear that both age influences and sex differences must be taken into account if results on clinical subjects are to be related to the normative standards of performance (GRAYBIEL and FREGLY, 1966; FREGLY and GRAYBIEL, 1968a).

IV. Spontaneous Vestibular Ataxia

Persons classified as having spontaneous vestibular ataxia include those with absent or reduced vestibular functions. The ataxia which appears to be characteristic of individuals with complete, or nearly complete, bilateral loss of labyrinthine functions is reflected in the data shown in Table 1. Upon initial testing,

6 Age and sex influences on this test were not apparent (FREGLY and GRAYBIEL, 1968a).

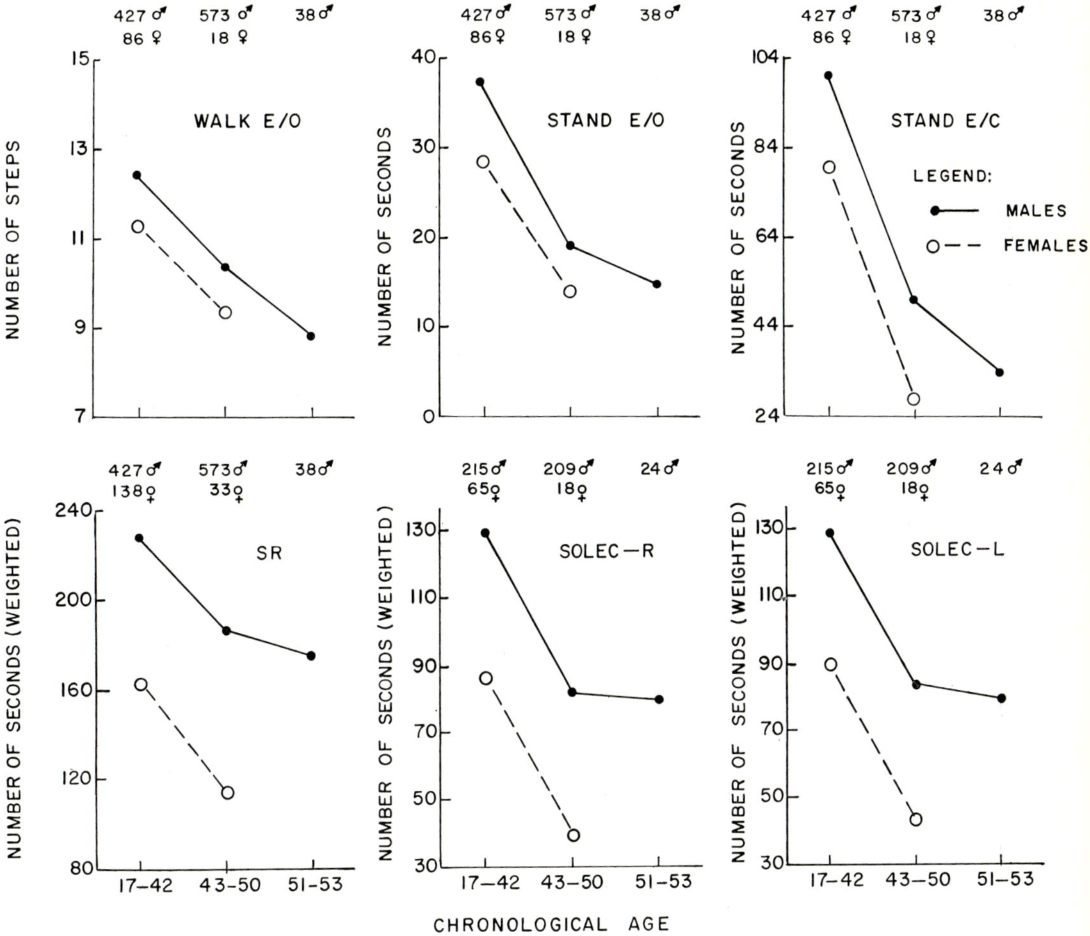

Fig. 1. Chronological age and sex influences on rail (short version) and floor ataxia test battery performance skills

all ten subjects of this elite, comprehensively studied group (for example, Clark and Graybiel, 1966, 1967; Graybiel, 1964, 1965, 1966, 1968; Graybiel and Clark, 1965; Graybiel and Johnson, 1963; Guedry, 1965; Miller et al., 1966) scored at or below the 1st percentile in relation to normative standards on all standing tests (except for ZA on SOLEC-R), including the test performed with eyes open (Stand E/O). On the remaining test, walking with eyes open (Walk E/O), all subjects except ZA produced equally poor performance scores. Eight of these subjects[7] were retested on three of the tests (those performed on rails) on nine occasions at intervals of one to several days. Results of these retests, which are summarized in Table 2, indicated that performance changes on each distinct test

7 The two oldest subjects, DO and GR, were excluded because of their higher age classification and, accordingly because of the different percentile equivalents of their performance scores in relation to the normative standards.

Table 1. *Clinical and Ataxia Test Findings in a Comprehensively Studied Group of Ten Men with Bilateral Loss of Labyrinthine Function*

Subjects	Age	Etiology	Age at onset (yrs.)	Hearing (db) R	Hearing (db) L	Threshold Caloric test responses in degrees centigrade R	Threshold Caloric test responses in degrees centigrade L	CRI[a]	SR Score	SR %-tile equiv.	Walk E/O Score	Walk E/O %-tile equiv.	Stand E/O Score	Stand E/O %-tile equiv.	Stand E/C Score	Stand E/C %-tile equiv.	SOLEC-R Score	SOLEC-R %-tile equiv.	SOLEC-L Score	SOLEC-L %-tile equiv.	WALEC Score	WALEC %-tile equiv.
DO	43	Meningitis	13	Nil	Nil	Neg. at 10.0	Neg. at 10.0	74	17	1st	9	<1st	33	<1st	29	<1st	9	1st	13	1st	UTP[b]	<1st
GR	47	Mastoiditis	12	Nil	160	No Response	No Response	60	20	1st	24	<1st	71	<1st	19	<1st	11	1st	10	1st	UTP	<1st
GU	21	Meningitis	$4\frac{1}{2}$	145	145	10.0	10.0	89	17	1st	17	<1st	34	<1st	22	<1st	17	1st	12	1st	UTP	<1st
HA	29	Meningitis	13	Nil	Nil	Neg. at 2.8	Neg. at 2.8	48	6	1st	24	<1st	44	<1st	25	<1st	14	1st	10	1st	UTP	<1st
JO	34	Meningitis	$7\frac{1}{2}$	Nil	Nil	Neg. at 3.0	Neg. at 3.0	171	20	1st	27	<1st	30	<1st	30	<1st	17	1st	14	1st	UTP	<1st
MY	25	Meningitis	8	Nil	Nil	Neg. at 2.8	7.9	99	13	1st	28	<1st	93	<1st	23	<1st	14	1st	11	1st	UTP	<1st
PE	33	Meningitis	12	Nil	Nil	Neg. at 2.6	Neg. at 2.6	77	12	1st	40	<1st	58	<1st	19	<1st	17	1st	18	1st	UTP	<1st
PI	22	Meningitis	3	Nil	Nil	9.8	Nil	116	14	1st	29	<1st	111	<1st	21	<1st	10	1st	10	1st	UTP	<1st
ST	20	Meningitis	$12\frac{1}{2}$	130	135	10.0	11.0	47	20	1st	38	<1st	122	<1st	24	<1st	12	1st	12	1st	UTP	<1st
ZA	20	Meningitis	$3\frac{1}{2}$	135	130	2.8	2.8	85	28	1st	52	30th	222	<1st	35	<1st	34	2nd	18	1st	UTP	<1st

Rail (long version) and floor ataxia test batteries: SR, Walk E/O, Stand E/O, Stand E/C, SOLEC-R, SOLEC-L, WALEC.

[a] Counterrolling index, calculated as one-half the sum of the eye roll measured in minutes of arc at the 50° rightward and leftward tilt positions.
[b] Unable to perform (could not meet criteria for scorable trials).

Table 2. *Effects of Extended Practice on the Rail Ataxia Test Battery (Long Version) Performances of a Group of Eight Males, Ages 20 to 34 Years, with Bilateral Loss of Labyrinthine Function Due to Meningitis in Early Life*

Test days	Walk E/O Test Range of Scores	Walk E/O Test Mean Score	%-tile equiv.	Percent Change[a]	Stand E/O Test Range of Scores	Stand E/O Test Mean Score	%-tile equiv.	Percent Change	Stand E/C Test Range of Scores	Stand E/C Test Mean Score	%-tile equiv.	Percent Change
1	17–40	31.9	<1st	—	30–227	89.9	<1st	—	19–35	24.9	<1st	—
2	25–58	38.6	<1st	21	33–239	83.0	<1st	–8	15–29	22.8	<1st	–9
3	27–57	42.1	1st	32	37–270	121.0	<1st	35	19–31	25.6	<1st	3
4	33–57	44.4	3rd	39	42–213	117.1	<1st	30	21–33	26.3	<1st	6
5	29–60	48.0	10th	51	43–218	113.5	<1st	26	21–34	27.5	<1st	10
6	36–57	49.1	15th	54	39–307	134.4	<1st	50	21–34	28.3	<1st	14
7	34–59	50.8	25th	59	38–244	138.3	<1st	54	17–32	25.9	<1st	4
8	29–58	48.1	10th	51	42–274	131.9	<1st	47	21–35	28.5	<1st	15
9	27–60	49.4	15th	55	48–249	126.4	<1st	41	21–40	26.5	<1st	6
10	42–58	52.0	30th	63	43–236	119.1	<1st	33	20–36	27.6	<1st	11

[a] Relative to Day 1 Scores.

were differentially influenced by the repeated exposure. Initially ataxic visual rail-walking performances became progressively and markedly improved, and by the tenth test day the average scores approached the normal range. Hence the improved Walk E/O test performance of such individuals was regarded as reflecting a partially compensated vestibular ataxia (FREGLY and GRAYBIEL, 1970). The compensation demonstrated by this group, however, was generally "hard-won" and somewhat less indicative of the skills tested than the quantitatively improved performance scores suggest. For example, these subjects readily discovered and exhaustively exploited such "gimmicks" as rapid staccato walking patterns, both to improve their timing (rhythm) and to increase their momentum, and they persistently exercised extraordinarily careful starting positions on the rail. With the exception of one outstanding subject (ZA) who initially scored at the 30th percentile level, little of the ease, poise, and grace of smooth, continuous, or well-coordinated movements at average walking speeds so characteristic of vestibular-intact individuals during unpracticed rail-walking was present in the improved, practiced performances of these BL-D subjects.

The ataxic visual rail-standing performances of this group were only minimally compensated if at all (despite the changes indicated by the noteworthy, generally progressive improvements in scores — as much as 54%), as shown by the fact that when initial performance levels were below the 1st percentile they remained at that level throughout the retest periods.

The markedly ataxic nonvisual rail-standing performances noted upon initial testing of this BL-D group failed to improve with extended practice and were thus considered to be totally uncompensated (FREGLY and GRAYBIEL, 1970).

In a control group of twelve male medical students who were free of vestibular defects and who were subjected to the same tests and retests, the changes in performance scores were as follows: Walk E/O: from 52.4 (mean) and 40–60 (range) initially to 58.5 and 53–60 on Day 9; Stand E/O: from 470.0 and 388–528 initially to 527.8 and 500–569 on Day 9; Stand E/C: from 209.2 and 67–316 initially to 309.9 and 114–404 on Day 10. The percentile equivalents of these scores changed, initially to maximally, from 32nd, 35th, and 52nd to 88th, 89th, and 84th on the Walk E/O, Stand E/O, and Stand E/C tests, respectively. In comparison with the limited improvements in performance shown by the BL-D group, the improvements shown by the normal group were not only considerably greater but also remarkably consistent from one test to another in terms of the changes in the percentile ranks.

In this same group of ten BL-D subjects, width-of-platform influences upon the initial scores obtained on more simplified tests of visual rail-walking and floor-walking and of visual and nonvisual rail-standing and floor-standing are summarized in Table 3. Generally, the magnitude of the scores was found to be positively related to the widths of the walking and standing platforms. But of equal interest was the finding of systematic differences (on all three tests) between the scores obtained on the 4-inch wide and 3-inch wide paper strips (masking tape) on the floor, the latter being slightly inferior. This apparently psychological effect (not solely a visual effect because the eyes closed test performances were influenced also) persisted throughout a five-day test-retest period in most subjects (Table 4).

Table 3. *Effects of Width of Platform on the Ataxia Test Performance Scores (Initial) of Ten Men with Bilateral Loss of Labyrinthine Function*

Ataxia tests	Masking tape[a] on floor 4[b]	3	Rails[a] 4	3	2–3/4	2–1/4	1–3/4	1–1/4	3/4	1/2
Walk E/O	10.0[c]	9.8	8.4	8.5	6.1	6.2	5.3	4.5	3.2	3.5
Stand E/O	106.6[d]	90.7	70.8	66.5	33.6	21.0	15.6	6.3	4.8	4.0
Stand E/C	8.8[d]	7.9	7.4	5.9	5.7	5.3	4.3	3.4	3.7	2.3

[a] Eight feet long.
[b] Width in inches.
[c] Mean total heel-to-toe steps on best two of three trials.
[d] Mean total time in seconds on best two of three trials.

Table 4. *Persistence of Width and Type of Platform Influences in Addition to Psychological Effects on Ataxia Test Performances of a Group of Ten Males with Bilateral Loss of Labyrinthine Function*

Test days	Walking eyes open (perfect score = 10)[a] Mean scores: Floor strips 4 inches wide	Floor strips 3 inches wide	Rails 4 inches wide	Rails 3 inches wide	Standing eyes open (perfect score = 120)[a] Mean scores: Floor strips 4 inches wide	Floor strips 3 inches wide	Rails 4 inches wide	Rails 3 inches wide	Standing eyes closed (perfect score = 120)[a] Mean scores: Floor strips 4 inches wide	Floor strips 3 inches wide	Rails 4 inches wide	Rails 3 inches wide
1	10.0	9.8	8.4	8.5	106.6	90.7	70.8	66.5	8.8	7.9	7.4	5.9
2	9.7	9.4	9.1	9.6	102.9	94.3	93.8	74.6	10.3	11.3	10.5	5.6
3	9.8	9.7	9.6	9.7	104.7	102.8	94.8	68.9	10.3	9.8	6.3	5.6
4	10.0[b]	10.0[b]	9.5	9.5	97.4[b]	110.4[b]	97.2	71.5	14.6[b]	10.4[b]	7.9	7.7
5	10.0[b]	10.0[b]	10.0	9.7	91.3[b]	92.4[b]	103.3	79.4	12.0[b]	9.1[b]	8.8	5.8
6	—	—	9.8	9.7	—	—	102.3	85.5	—	—	10.3	8.9
7	—	—	10.0[c]	9.9[c]	—	—	82.0[c]	91.2[c]	—	—	9.1[c]	7.0[c]

[a] Scoring procedure identical with rail ataxia test battery (long version) procedures.
[b] N = 7.
[c] N = 9.

It is apparent also from the data in Table 4 that (1) performances on the "floor tests" were superior to performances on the "rail tests" throughout; (2) as opposed to Walk E/O performances, neither rail nor floor performance scores on the Stand E/O or Stand E/C test became perfect (maximum score = 120), although all scores with eyes open were vastly superior to those with eyes closed; and (3) extremely minimal improvements were shown on the Stand E/C tests, but these improvements were not always maintained. Comparable data on normal individuals are not available, but it would be expected from results reported above for normals on more difficult tasks that intergroup differences would be considerably less than those observed with the standardized rail ataxia test battery (long version).

In a second group of men (N = 16) with total, or nearly total, bilateral loss of labyrinthine functions due to meningitis in early life (Fregly and Graybiel, 1970), performance scores on the rail (short version) and floor ataxia test batteries (Table 5) were nearly identical to those obtained by the BL-D group tested earlier. None of these subjects scored above the 1st percentile on any of the standing tests undertaken with eyes closed, and none scored above the 7th percentile on the Stand E/O tests (performed on the 3/4-inch wide rail). Moreover, as in the previously cited group of BL-Ds, there was considerable variability in performance skills on the Walk E/O test (3/4-inch wide rail), with percentile equivalents to the scores ranging from <1st to 40th. Interestingly, one subject scored beyond the 1st percentile on the WALEC test, although his performance was grossly inferior (4th percentile level) in relation to normal standards. That this individual alone among his peers was able to tandem walk for a distance of 12 feet without sidestepping was considered to be an outstanding accomplishment which seemed attributable either to some degree of residual otolithic function and/or outstanding nonvestibular proprioception.

Recently a 25-year-old, athletic soldier was referred for extensive vestibular evaluation (Smith, 1967; Graybiel et al., 1971). His only complaint was episodic dizziness (approximately once a month), each attack lasting only a few seconds. Audiological findings in all routine and advanced tests showed consistently normal hearing bilaterally. All neurological findings were negative. Spontaneous nystagmus was observed during the neurological, otological, and vestibular evaluations. Complete bilateral absence of horizontal semicircular canal sensitivity was indicated by negative responses to sustained caloric irrigation with 2.4°C water (for as long as three minutes) on several occasions. However, the possibility of some residual vertical canal functioning was indicated by his responses to rotation tests. His counterrolling index of 103 implied abnormal functioning of the otolithic apparatus (Miller and Graybiel, 1963). All evidence pointed to near, if not complete, bilateral absence of vestibular function. Results of initial and repeated ataxia tests (Table 6) strongly supported this conclusion. While his WALEC and/or WOFEC scores were average or near average on occasion, his performances on eyes-closed tests generally were of the caliber of the two groups of BL-Ds discussed above, even after long practice periods. That his Walk E/O scores improved most and his Stand E/O scores second-most is consistent with the previous findings in BL-Ds in terms of indicating partially compensated (Walk E/O) and minimally compensated (Stand E/O) vestibular ataxia. More extensive evaluation of this unusual

Table 5. *Threshold Caloric and Ataxia Test Findings in a Group of Sixteen Men with Bilateral Loss of Labyrinthine Function*[a] *Due to Meningitis in Early Life*

				Rail (short version) and floor ataxia test batteries													
		Threshold Caloric Test Responses		SR		Walk E/O		Stand E/O		Stand E/C		SOLEC-R		SOLEC-L		WALEC	
Subjects	Age	R	L	Score	%-tile equiv.	Score	%-tile equiv.	Score	%-tile equiv.	Score	%-tile equiv.	Score	%-tile equiv.	Score	%-tile equiv.	Score	%-tile equiv.
AD	23	Neg. at 10.0°C	Neg. at. 10.2°C	15	1st	6	5th	8	1st	14	3rd	18	1st	10	1st	UTP[b]	<1st
AI	21	24.4°C	14.0°C	10	1st	3	<1st	6	<1st	5	<1st	15	1st	14	1st	UTP	<1st
BA	24	Neg. at 9.6°C	Neg. at 9.6°C	13	1st	5	4th	8	1st	10	<1st	14	1st	12	1st	UTP	<1st
BE	42	Neg. at. 9.6°C	Neg. at 9.8°C	8	1st	4	2nd	7	<1st	6	<1st	6	1st	5	1st	UTP	<1st
BI	22	10.0°C	Neg. at 9.6°C	17	1st	6	5th	6	<1st	7	<1st	13	1st	12	1st	UTP	<1st
BU	35	Neg. at 9.6°C	Neg. at 9.8°C	13	1st	9	15th	9	3rd	16	6th	19	1st	18	1st	UTP	<1st
CR	23	Neg. at 9.8°C	10.2°C	14	1st	8	9th	7	<1st	8	<1st	12	1st	13	1st	UTP	<1st
FA	23	Neg. at 9.8°C	Neg. at 9.8°C	27	1st	12	40th	12	7th	14	3rd	19	1st	15	1st	UTP	<1st
IN	20	Neg. at 9.8°C	Neg. at 10.0°C	14	1st	10	23rd	6	<1st	6	<1st	12	1st	12	1st	UTP	<1st
KA	24	Neg. at 10.0°C	Neg. at 10.0°C	13	1st	5	4th	8	1st	8	<1st	10	1st	11	1st	UTP	<1st
JO	22	Neg. at 9.8°C	Neg. at 10.2°C	13	1st	5	4th	11	5th	7	<1st	14	1st	12	1st	UTP	<1st
LA	26	10.0°C	? No Response	8	1st	6	5th	8	1st	10	<1st	13	1st	13	1st	UTP	<1st
MO	32	Neg. at 9.6°C	Neg. at 10.0°C	22	1st	7	7th	7	<1st	4	<1st	9	1st	7	1st	UTP	<1st
OL	23	Neg. at 10.2°C	Neg. at 10.8°C	14	1st	7	7th	8	1st	6	<1st	11	1st	9	1st	UTP	<1st
OR	32	Neg. at 9.6°C	Neg. at 10.2°C	9	1st	6	5th	3	<1st	3	<1st	9	1st	13	1st	21	4th
ZE	24	Neg. at 10.8°C	Neg. at 9.8°C	9	1st	5	4th	11	5th	11	<1st	18	1st	19	1st	UTP	<1st

[a] Including total, or near total, loss of hearing.

[b] Unable to perform.

Table 6. *Ataxia Test Findings in a Young Man with Normal Hearing and Bilateral Loss of Vestibular Function*

Test sessions	SR		Walk E/O[a]		Stand E/O[a]		Stand E/C[a]		SOLEC-R		SOLEC-L		WALEC		WOFEC	
	Score	%-tile equiv.	Score	%-tile equiv.	Score	%-tile equiv.	Score	%-tile equiv.	Score	%-tile equiv.	Score	%-tile equiv.	Score	%-tile eqiuv.	Score	Range
1	16	1st	5	2nd	10	5th	9	1st	12	1st	18	1st	13	27th	23	<AV.[d]
2	12	1st	7	6th	9	3rd	7	1st	14	1st	18	1st	UTP[b]	<1st	18	<AV.
3	20	1st	7	6th	9	3rd	10	1st	27	1st	18	1st	UTP	<1st	21	<AV.
4	43	1st	13	56th	14	15th	9	1st	19	1st	20	1st	N.T.[c]	—	N.T.	—
5	19	1st	13	56th	11	7th	7	1st	25	1st	27	2nd	UTP	<1st	19	<AV.
6	20	1st	13	56th	12	9th	12	1st	28	1st	12	1st	UTP	<1st	7	<AV.
7	19	1st	10	23rd	11	7th	9	1st	18	1st	22	1st	UTP	<1st	21	<AV.
8	19	1st	11	30th	13	12th	7	1st	17	1st	14	1st	UTP	<1st	19	<AV.
9	24	1st	12	42nd	9	3rd	8	1st	17	1st	22	1st	UTP	<1st	25	<AV.
10	19	1st	14	68th	10	5th	13	1st	19	1st	20	1st	20	8th	30	AV.
11	13	1st	11	30th	10	5th	9	1st	16	1st	24	1st	15	22nd	30	AV.
12	24	1st	12	42nd	8	2nd	16	4th	28	1st	14	1st	UTP	<1st	25	<AV.
13	26	1st	12	42nd	10	5th	14	2nd	20	1st	18	1st	14	25th	30	AV.

[a] Short version of the Rail Ataxia Test Battery.
[b] Unable to perform.
[c] Not tested.
[d] Below average.

individual, is necessary before any conclusive decisions regarding the site and nature of his vestibular lesion(s) are possible (GRAYBIEL et al., 1972).

Four patients who had received streptomycin sulfate in the treatment of Ménière's syndrome were used as experimental subjects to determine the long-range effects of the therapy (GRAYBIEL et al., 1967). None had experienced any recurrence of symptoms over the entire follow-up period, which ranged from 11 to 13 years. They showed residual tinnitus, deafness ascribable to the syndrome, and ataxia ascribable to toxic effects of the drug as well as to the syndrome. In the three subjects who had one normal ear each, the streptomycin did not affect the hearing in that ear but it did suppress semicircular canal function considerably. This function recovered only partially. In all five diseased ears there was a slight but significant improvement in hearing (later lost in one), but great suppression of semicircular canal function with little recovery. Otolith function, as measured by ocular counterrolling (MILLER, 1961), was within the normal range in two subjects and greatly suppressed in two. None was susceptible to motion (canal) sickness when exposed to bizarre stimulation of the vestibular apparatus in the Pensacola Slow Rotation Room (SRR). Some of these findings, together with the quantitative findings on the rail and floor ataxia test batteris, are summarized in Table 7. In comparison with results in the BL-D groups, the tested and retested ataxia test performances of this group were identical with respect to tandem walking with eyes closed (WALEC test), highly similar but somewhat less disturbed with respect to the standing tests performed with eyes closed (SR, Stand E/C, and SOLEC-R and L), and considerably less disturbed on both tests undertaken with the assistance of vision (Walk E/O and Stand E/O on the 3/4-inch wide rail). Such results gave further substantiation to the difference in compensation of vestibular ataxia. Inasmuch as their greatly differing degrees of otolith function, as defined by the counterrolling index, bore no systematic relation to these results in the patients with Ménière's syndrome, they were considered ascribable mainly (but probably not solely) to loss of semicircular canal function. The relative roles of otoliths and canals during performance on the ataxia test battery have not been elucidated (FREGLY et al., 1972).

The importance of bilateral functioning of the vestibular mechanism for normal maintenance of postural equilibrium was made clear upon application of the rail and floor ataxia test batteries to a group of persons who had become unilaterally labyrinthine-defective as a result of surgical treatment for acoustic neuroma (HOUSE, 1964; FREGLY and GRAYBIEL, 1968a, 1970; NELSON, 1968). The ataxia test findings and the threshold caloric test responses are shown in Table 8. Except for subject LY, whose response was borderline, the caloric responses in the non-operated ears were within the normal range (FREGLY and GRAYBIEL, 1970). Hearing was also well preserved in the nonoperated ears. On the ataxia test batteries, impaired performance was consistently shown in the tests undertaken with eyes closed. Among these, the WALEC test, which is a measure of nonvisual, including vestibular-influenced, locomotor disturbance, was the most sensitive indicator of the vestibular ataxia of these individuals. Judged from the results of the WALEC test their gross impairments were identical to those observed in the BL-D subjects. Their impaired performances on the remaining ataxia tests were highly variable, but were generally not so severe as were observed in the BL-Ds.

Table 7. *Clinical and Ataxia Test Findings in a Group of Four Individuals Treated with Streptomycin for Ménière's Syndrome*

Subject	Age	Clinical findings				Rail (short version) and floor ataxia test batteries																									
		Years since streptomycin treatment	Threshold caloric test responses (degrees centigrade)		Counterrolling index	SR				Walk E/O				Stand E/O				Stand E/C				SOLEC-R				SOLEC-L				WALEC	
			Dis.	Nor.		Initial score	%-tile equiv.	Improved score[c]	%-tile equiv.	Initial score	%-tile equiv.	Improved score	%-tile equiv.	Initial score	%-tile equiv.	Improved score	%-tile equiv.	Initial score	%-tile equiv.	Improved score	%-tile equiv.	Initial score	%-tile-equiv.	Improved score	%-tile equiv.	Initial score	%-tile equiv.	Improved score	%-tile equiv.	Initial score	%-tile equiv.
OC	50	11	31.3	8.5	305	11	1st	26	3rd	12	70th	13	87th	7	5th	12	30th	8	1st	11	1st	10	1st	15	4th	11	1st	19	7th	UTP[e]	<1st
CA[a]	49	10	Neg. at 12.0	25.0	127	6	1st	16	7th	13	90th	13	90th	8	10th	13	35th	11	10th	12	15th	12	1st	12	1st	N.T.[d]	—	N.T.	—	N.T.	—
AN	56	9	8.2	32.6	235	9	1st	14	1st	3	18th	7	26th	6	7th	13	65th	6	<1st	8	<1st	13	4th	17	6th	11	1st	21	10th	UTP	<1st
KI	42	10	16.5	17.0[f]	114	14	1st	17	1st	4	2nd	13	82nd[b]	8	1st	14	43rd[b]	10	<1st	13	8th[b]	11	1st	14	4th[b]	12	2nd	16	3rd[b]	UTP	<1st

[a] Female.

[b] In relation to normative standards of the succeeding age group to which this subject advanced since initial testing.

[c] Maximum score obtained some time between the second and seventh retest periods.

[d] Not tested.

[e] Unable to perform.

[f] Diseased bilaterally.

Table 8. *Threshold Caloric and Ataxia Test Findings in a Group of Eleven Individuals with Unilateral Loss of Labyrinthine Function*[a] *Due to Surgical Treatment for Acoustic Neuroma*

Patients	Age	Time (months) since operation	Operated ear	Threshold caloric responses (degrees centigrade)		Rail (short version) and floor ataxia test batteries																			
						SR		Walk E/O		Stand E/O		Stand E/C		SOLEC-R		SOLEC-L		WALEC		SR E/O		SOLEO-R		SOLEO-L	
				Operated Ear	Good Ear	Score	%-tile equiv.	Score	%-tile equiv.	Score	%-tile equiv.	Score	%-tile equiv.	Score	%-tile equiv.	Score	%-tile equiv.	Score	%-tile equiv.	Score	Range	Score	Range	Score	Range
DA[b]	33	19	R	Neg. at 10.0	36.2	11	2nd	6	15th	8	12th	12	15th	12	1st	11	1st	UTP	<1st	118	≪AV.	135	<AV.	150	AV.
LY	36	29	L	Neg. at 9.6	34.0	27	1st	6	4th	9	3rd	20	7th	24	1st	24	1st	UTP	<1st	240	AV.	150	AV.	122	<AV.
BI[b]	40	48	R	Neg. at 10.0	36.0	14	3rd	7	25th	7	8th	9	2nd	12	1st	11	1st	UTP	<1st	221	<AV.	150	AV.	150	AV.
FI[b]	42	33	R	Neg. at 10.0	36.2	11	2nd	2	1st	8	12th	10	4th	12	1st	13	5th	UTP	<1st	240	AV.	150	AV.	150	AV.
UE	43	29	L	Neg. at 10.0	35.8	26	3rd	12	70th	9	13th	14	11th	17	5th	18	5th	UTP	<1st	240	AV.	150	AV.	150	AV.
MA	43	16	L	Neg. at 9.8	36.6	12	1st	5	7th	7	5th	14	11th	22	10th	11	1st	UTP	<1st	240	AV.	150	AV.	150	AV.
CO	47	15	R	Neg. at 9.6	36.0	63	11th	9	38th	10	19th	21	29th	33	22nd	46	34th	UTP	<1st	240	AV.	150	AV.	150	AV.
RA	49	23	L	Neg. at 9.6	36.0	36	5th	9	38th	12	32nd	13	9th	29	19th	36	24th	UTP	<1st	240	AV.	150	AV.	150	AV.
MK[b]	52	41	L	Neg. at 10.4	35.4	17	17th	4	15th	7	23rd	9	23rd	14	9th	10	1st	UTP	NSL	65	≪AV.	123	NSL	120	NSL
MR[b]	54	10	L	Neg. at 9.6	35.2	11	8th	10	69th	6	9th	9	23rd	18	27th	13	9th	UTP	NSL	240	AV.	109	NSL	145	NSL
RI[b]	58	12	R	Neg. at 10.0	35.4	13	12th	6	38th	7	23rd	10	23rd	13	9th	14	9th	UTP	NSL	162	<AV.	131	NSL	123	NSL

[a] Including complete unilateral loss of hearing.
[b] Female

Legend: UTP = Unable to perform. NSL = Normative standards lacking. <AV. = Below average. ≪AV. = Far below average.

Nevertheless, the impairments were considerable in relation to normative standards of performance. The discriminative (or diagnostic) power of each remaining standardized item of the ataxia test battery in relation to six cut-off levels on the normative curves (lowest one hundredth (1st percentile), one twentieth (5th percentile), one tenth (10th percentile), one sixth (17th percentile), one fourth (25 th percentile), and one third (33rd percentile) was hierarchically (from most to least discriminative) as follows: SOLEC-R and SOLEC-L tests: 36–45%, 45–63%, 72–81%, 90%, and 100% of the scores fell at the 1st, 5th, 10th, 25th, and 33rd percentiles, respectively; SR test: 18%, 63%, 72%, and 100% of the scores fell at the 1st, 5th, 10th, and 17th percentile levels, respectively; Stand E/C and Stand E/O tests: 0%, 18%, 27–36%, 63%, 90%, and 100% of the scores fell at the 1st, 5th, 10th, 17th, 25th, and 33rd percentile levels, respectively. Thus none of this group had scores higher than those of the lowest one third of the normal groups on any of the standardized tests, including the tests undertaken with the assistance of vision. For the most part, the performance scores obtained on the tyes-open version of the SOLEC and SR tests (SOLEO-R and L; SR E/O) were typical of those from normal individuals. Perfect scores were obtained on the Classical Romberg test, which was performed with eyes closed and with a wider base of support, which again indicated the insensitivity of this test to gross vestibular dysfunction (Fregly and Graybiel, 1968a).

Over the years we have examined 94 individuals in the age range of 19 to 70 years referred by otologists or neurologists; all these patients had intermittent vertigo as a major symptom or complaint and their medical status presented unusually difficult problems of diagnosis (Fregly and Graybiel, 1968a). Generally, the referral diagnosis was either tentative or incomplete. When tentative or final diagnoses became available, they included typical and atypical vestibular neuronitis, Ménière's syndrome, postural vertigo, positional nystagmus, labyrinthine artery occlusion, post-traumatic pseudobulbar palsy, acoustic trauma, long-standing deafness, orthostatic light-headedness, cerebral vascular insufficiency, and psychogenic disorder. The health and physical fitness of these patients were adequate or more than adequate for ataxia testing. The findings on three items of the floor ataxia test battery in the various age groups are summarized in Table 9. Without exception, the ataxia test performances of these male and female patients in each of the several age groups represented were inferior in relation to the skills of symptom-free normal individuals. In most instances (all groups with insufficient N's excepted) the group mean differences were statistically significant. Threshold caloric test findings in the majority of these patients were within or near statistically normal limits and bore no systematic relations to the ataxia test findings, whereas the great majority with below-normal caloric responses also had below-normal ataxia test performance scores (Fregly and Graybiel, 1970). As found in the BL-D, UL-D, and Ménière's groups, these patients experienced no difficulty in performing the Classical Romberg test.

In summary, spontaneous vestibular ataxia, as measured by the quantitative rail and/or floor ataxia test batteries, is readily demonstrable in individuals with clinical evidence of labyrinthine dysfunction, and its severity appears to correlate with the severity of the dysfunction: taxis was found to be less impaired in UL-Ds than in BL-Ds, and in patients with vertigo as a major symptom or complaint,

Table 9. *Floor Ataxia Test Performance Skills of Otoneurological Patients with a History of Vertigo Compared with the Skills of Symptom-Free Normal Individuals*

Subject Classification	Age Range	N	SR Test Mean	S.D.	N	SOLEC-R Test Mean	S.D.	N	SOLEC-L Test Mean	S.D.
Males										
Normal	17–42	427	228.4	32.67	215	129.2	33.29	215	129.3	32.15
Vertiginous	19–41	36	144.7[b]	88.52	36	81.0[b]	48.51	36	80.3[b]	52.84
Normal	43–50	573	185.7	71.27	209	82.1	48.96	209	83.6	49.86
Vertiginous	45–50	6	53.7[b]	27.19	6	46.3	35.79	6	46.5	15.24
Normal	51–53	38	175.9	82.06	24	78.9	48.52	24	71.3	49.95
Vertiginous	51–52	3	170.0	73.17	3	60.7	22.81	3	60.3	30.68
Normal	50–71	76	165.6	81.28	50	72.3	47.28	50	70.2	48.02
Vertiginous	56–69	7	58.6[b]	54.86	7	32.0[a]	16.72	7	25.1[a]	11.95
Females										
Normal	18–29	83	187.8	67.19	41	100.8	41.98	41	102.0	41.80
Vertiginous	20–29	8	40.8[b]	66.71	8	24.6[b]	14.69	8	25.5[b]	17.92
Normal	30–49	87	128.4	84.59	40	53.2	36.79	40	58.5	37.63
Vertiginous	32–49	20	62.6[b]	62.17	20	32.8[a]	21.53	20	37.4[a]	29.69
Normal	50–71	24	106.6	88.40	11	47.1	42.65	11	47.5	43.94
Vertiginous	50–70	14	27.7[b]	14.08	14	17.9[a]	7.58	14	16.5[a]	7.89

[a] Significantly different from the age-matched normals at $\leq .05$ level of confidence (t test).

[b] Significantly different from the age-matched normals at $\leq .01$ level of confidence (t test).

impairment was slighter than in UL-D subjects. Findings to date indicate that the floor ataxia tests alone are sufficient for making these distinctions and that of the floor ataxia tests, the tandem walking with eyes closed tests (WALEC and WOFEC) appear to be affected most by vestibular-influenced losses of postural equilibrium functioning (FREGLY et al., 1972; FREGLY et al., 1973).

V. Induced Vestibular Ataxia

In its simplest form, vestibular ataxia can readily be induced by self-rotation about one's own body axis for several revolutions while in an upright position, as evidenced by the impairment of postural equilibrium which ensues immediately upon cessation of the rotation. If, during the rotation, the head is moved out of the plane of the body's rotation, the effects of such bizarre stimulation of the vestibular apparatus will exaggerate the vestibular ataxia observable when rotation stops. Certain angular or linear motions of the visual or physical surroundings while the body remains static, such as during optokinetic stimulation, can induce similar disturbances of postural equilibrium. When the body revolves, vestibular ataxia is induced via direct (peripheral) stimulation of the vestibular organs, whereas during optokinetic and other such stimulation the vestibular ataxia is induced indirectly by processes reflecting a conflict between visual inputs and vestibular and nonvestibular proprioceptive inputs. In a more complex situation in which postural equilibrium is disturbed during attempts to stand or walk on a rotating platform, the interactions between vestibular and non-vestibular processes are even more intricate, due to influences of a complex array of accelerations (gravity, centripetal, Coriolis) on the delicately balanced peripheral and central nervous mechanisms. Another example is the induced vestibular ataxia observable on craft at sea during attempts to stand or walk. That such interactions have pronounced and long-lasting residual effects upon stringent maintenance of postural equilibrium (persisting long after return to the normal force environment) is apparent from the results of several experiments on vestibular normal individuals (Figs. 2–5, 7, 8), vestibular normals, and bilaterally labyrinthine-defective individuals (Figs. 6 and 9).

Figure 2 shows the mean rail ataxia test battery (short version) performance scores of four student aviators 72 hours after exposure to constant rotation at a speed of 10 rpm for 12 days in the Pensacola Slow Rotation Room I (SRR I) (GRAYBIEL et al., 1965). The group showed improvements over baseline scores on the two visually assisted tests (Walk E/O and Stand E/O), while there was a marked deterioration in Stand E/C test performances, which suggested that recovery from the effects of exposure in the SRR was not yet complete. It is also of interest to note that the initial performance scores of all four subjects on Walk E/O and Stand E/O were at the lower ends of the normal distributions (11th to 36th percentile levels), and that the initial Stand E/C scores of two of them also fell below the normal mean. Moreover, the subjects who consistently produced the lowest scores before rotation (11th, 3rd, and 6th percentile equivalents on the Walk E/O, Stand E/O and Stand E/C tests, respectively) showed the least change in scores on all three tests 72 hours after rotation stopped. It is noteworthy also that all qualitative indications of unsteadiness or ataxia observed by subject or experimenter had disappeared within a few hours of cessation of rotation.

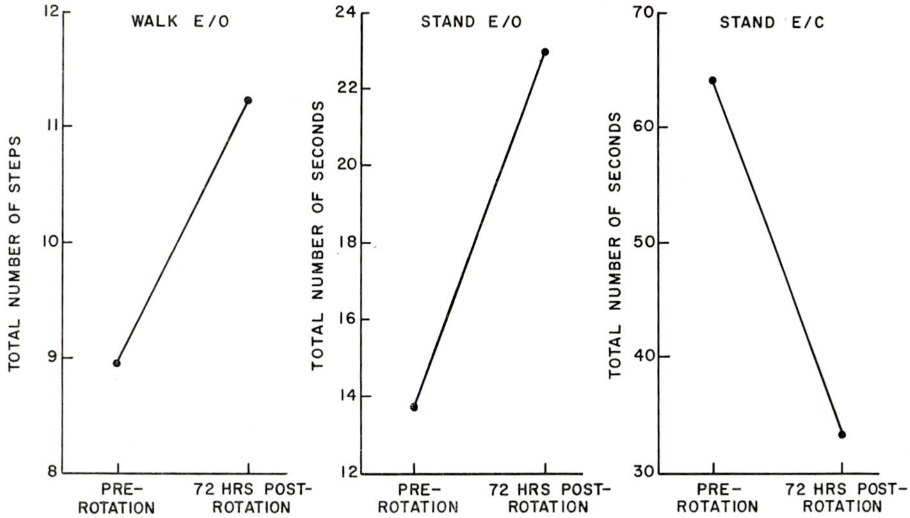

Fig. 2. Rail (short version) ataxia test battery performance scores of four aviators 72 hours after rotating at 10 rpm in the Pensacola Slow Rotation Room I for a period of 12 days

The differential effects of three different stepwise increases in rates of rotation from 0 to 10 rpm for a period of five to six days in the Pensacola SRR I (Bergstedt, 1965) on the rail (short version) and floor ataxia test battery performances of three groups of four normal subjects (student aviators) immediately upon cessation of rotation, along with the three different rotation profiles, are shown in Fig. 3. In Experiment I (rotation profile I) the differences in rpm between each step were 6.4, 2.1, and 1.5 increasing and 3.6, 2.8, and 3.6 decreasing; in Experiment II the differences were 3.3, 3.3, and 3.4 upward and 3.4, 3.3, and 3.3 downward; in Experiment III the difference in rpm between each step over a 40-hour period both increasing and decreasing was 0.25 per hour. In contrast to previous experiments in which subjects were suddenly exposed to 10 rpm and then suddenly returned to 0 rpm, thereby causing considerable disturbances in their ability to adapt, the stepwise procedures of these three experiments were designed to enhance adaptation to rotation at 10 rpm by allowing subjects to adapt to one rpm level before proceeding to the next rpm level, etc. The results of oculogyral illusion and Coriolis nystagmus tests, obtained while the subjects were in an on-board chair that could be rotated clockwise or counterclockwise, were used to estimate the adaptability of the subjects. Prerotation tests indicated that the 12 subjects differed in susceptibility to motion (canal) sickness; for example, the subjects in Experiment II were more susceptible than those in Experiment I. It was concluded on the basis of symptomatology experienced that the adaptability problems were least in Experiment II. As Fig. 3 shows, the differential changes in the performance scores on all six ataxia tests from prerotation to postrotation in the three groups of subjects were positively correlated with the differential stepwise increases in rotation. The subjects of Experiment I, where the largest initial step increase in rotation was used, showed the greatest performance decrements after rotation, whereas the subjects of Experiment III, in which the step increase in rotation was smallest, showed least impairment of their test performances after rotation. The Group II subjects, whose rotation profile was similar to that of the Group I subjects, were very similar to the Group I subjects in their postrotation ataxia test performance decrements. The intergroup differences in the performance decrements observed were smallest on the eyes-closed tests and largest on the two eyes-open tests. Interestingly, the Walk E/O performances of Group III were not affected at all by the rotation, a finding reminiscent of the hierarchically defined compensability for spontaneous vestibular ataxia discussed above.

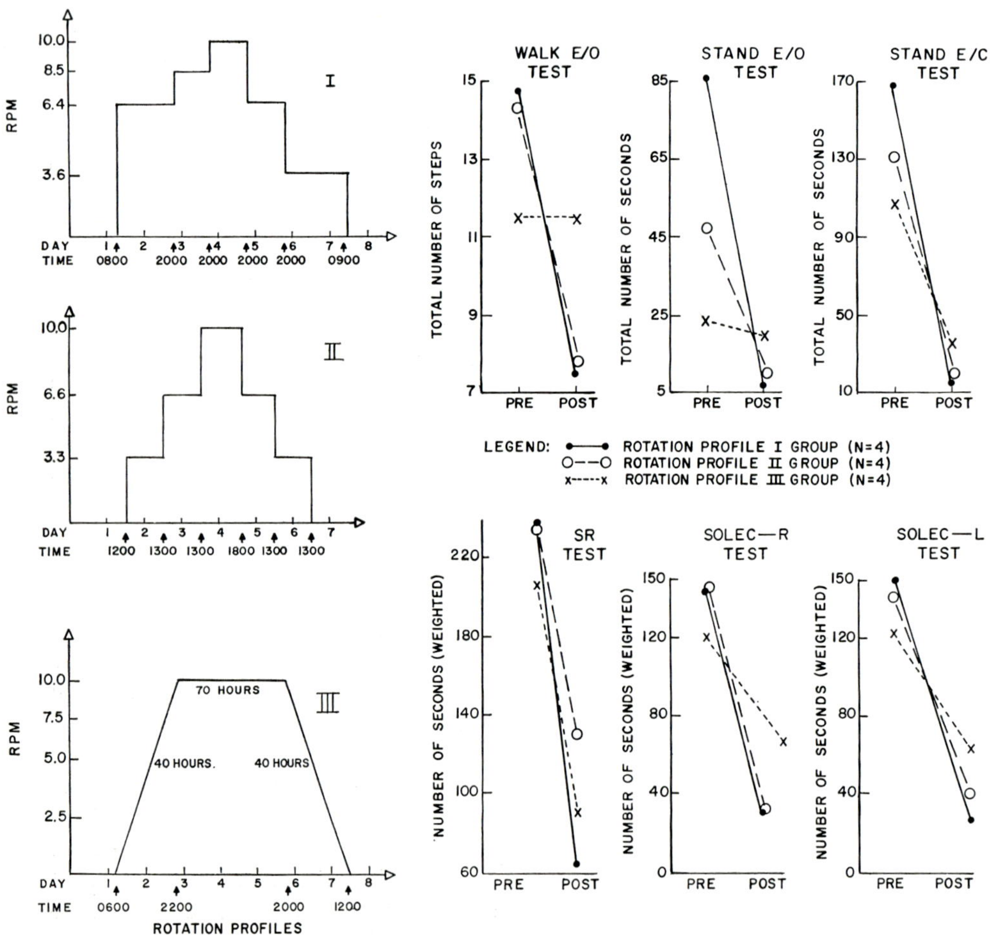

Fig. 3. Differential effects of three different stepwise increases in rates of rotation from 0 to 10 rpm for a period of 5 to 6 days in the Pensacola Slow Rotation Room I on the rail (short version) and floor ataxia test battery performances of three groups of male subjects immediately upon cessation of rotation

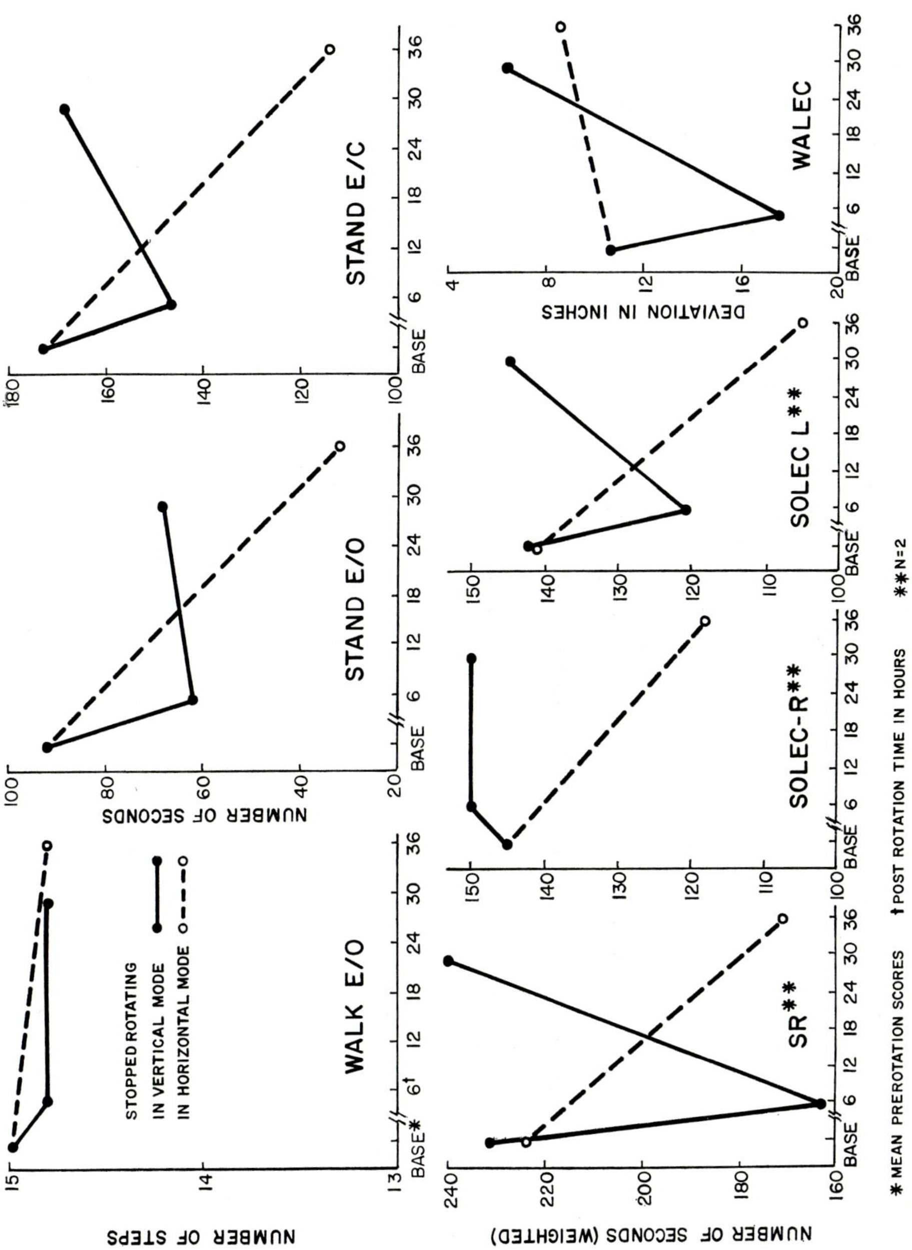

Fig. 4. Differential postrotation effects of horizontal vs. vertical body orientation assumed 2 days before cessation of rotation at 4 rpm in the Pensacola Slow Rotation Room II upon the rail (short version) and floor ataxia test battery performance scores of four normal male subjects (originally published in Aerospace Med. **39**, 960, 1968 as Fig. 13)

More recently, four Navy enlisted men in two pairs participated in an experiment involving habituation to the artificial environment in the Pensacola SRR II while rotating at 4 rpm (Graybiel et al., 1968). One pair initially in the horizontal mode (supported on air bearings) was changed to the vertical mode in the middle (days 2–3) of the perrotation period; in the second phase, 35 or more days later, they began rotating while in the vertical mode. The order was reversed for the second pair. The differences in the postrotatory perseveration of postural habituation to the rotating environment in relation to the differences in the orientation of the body 2 days prior to rotation and as long as 36 hours after cessation of rotation are shown in Fig. 4. Upon cessation of rotation the subjects moved as little as possible until the ataxia tests were administered. In the "finish-vertical" mode they were tested 5.5 hours and again 29.5 hours later. In the "finish-horizontal" mode the subjects remained in their molds as if rotation had not been discontinued, i.e. they were upright for only a few minutes before being tested on a single occasion 36 hours after rotation stopped. Rail (short version) and floor ataxia test battery performances were impaired during all postrotation test periods, but considerably more so after the finish-horizontal mode of rotation. Consistent with the findings in other rotating room experiments, walking test performances were less affected (hardly at all) by rotation than standing test performances. The process of walking undoubtedly afforded more opportunity for readaptation to the static environment, whereas in the standing tests the return to normal was severely hampered by the finer motor adjustments needed for the maintenance of postural equilibrium. On the narrow rail, particularly, errors in corrective head and body motions were poorly tolerated, even with the eyes open. Characteristically, the subjects felt that their body balance had returned to normal long before the objective, stringent ataxia test procedures demonstrated a return to normal. Postural hypotension was ruled out as a factor influencing these results. There were no systematic order effects, i.e. results of initial exposure to rotation in the vertical mode did not differ essentially from results of initial exposure to rotation in the horizontal mode. The experiment demonstrated that postural homeostasis to the rotating environment was preserved for at least 36 hours after rotation ceased. These results were corroborated in a subsequent experiment (in preparation), which involved rotation in the Pensacola SRR II at 6 rpm (Fig. 5). As in the 4 rpm experiment, postrotation impairments of ataxia test battery performances were consistently (WALEC excepted) of lesser magnitude and of shorter duration in the finish-vertical mode than in the finish-horizontal mode. The more rapid recovery of baseline levels (within 32 hours) than observed hitherto was most probably attributable to more frequently repeated testing. Walking test performances were again least affected by the rotation. The constancy or improvement in the WALEC test performance scores in this and in the previous experiment is more apparent than real. Qualitatively, WALEC and WOFEC test performances were strikingly impaired. During testing, the feet swung and landed opposite to the intended direction on each step, nearly causing the subjects to side-step, although it was apparent within a matter of seconds (on the second and third trials) that the subjects had learned appropriate corrective maneuvers. Walk E/O test performances were similarly compensable, although considerably less so in the finish-horizontal mode of rotation.

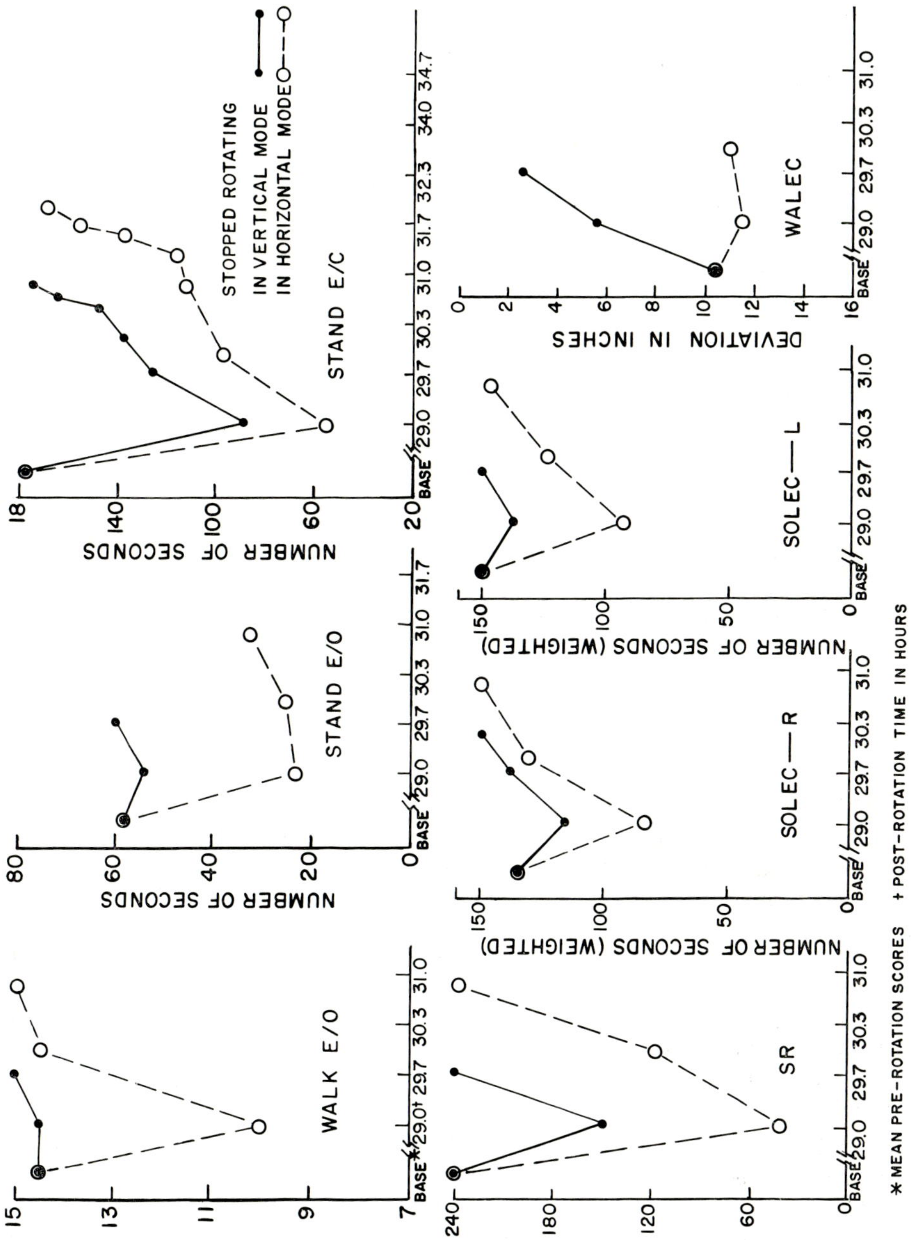

Fig. 5. Differential postrotation effects of horizontal vs. vertical body orientation assumed 2 days before cessation of rotation at 6 rpm in the Pensacola Slow Rotation Room II upon the rail (short version) and floor ataxia test battery performance scores of two normal male subjects

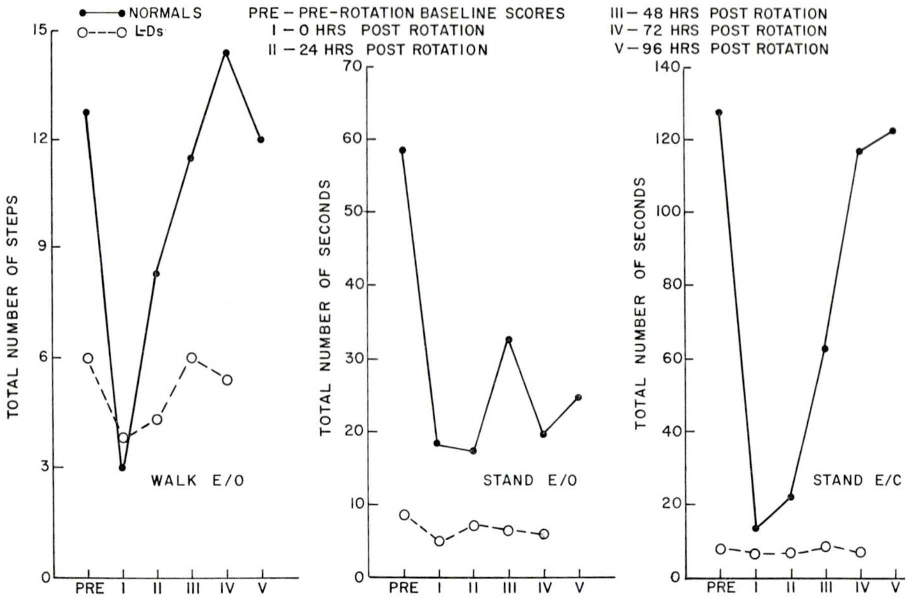

Fig. 6. Comparison of rail (short version) ataxia test battery scores of four normal males and four males with bilateral loss of labyrinthine functions (L-Ds) before and after rotation in the Pensacola Slow Rotation Room II at 10 rpm for a period of 12 days

It is apparent from the results shown in Fig. 6 that BL-D subjects were not completely "immune" to the ataxia induced by prolonged rotation (Fregly and Kennedy, 1965) because the vestibular apparatus was not solely implicated in such ataxia. The postrotation Walk E/O test performance changes in the BL-Ds, although of considerably lesser magnitude, were remarkably similar to the changes shown for the normal group. Although the magnitude differences are a reflection of the BL-D group's characteristic vestibular ataxia, thus accounting for their lower baseline scores, the nearly identical profiles of recovery in these two groups of subjects implicate the common workings of nonvestibular proprioceptive mechanisms. The fact that there were no changes in postrotation standing test performance in the BL-D group strongly suggests the likelihood that a severe rotation-induced ataxia, as was found with the normals, was of less severity than their characteristic vestibular ataxia. In other words, superimposition of rotation-induced ataxia in BL-Ds was masked by their characteristic noncompensated poor performance skills in the two standing tests.

Two indications of the magnitude and duration of ataxia induced in normal individuals while exposed to a relatively mild rotating environment (3 rpm) (Guedry et al., 1964) are shown in Figs. 7 and 8. Similar results were obtained at a higher (10) rpm in the group of four BL-D subjects discussed in the preceding paragraph (Fregly and Kennedy, 1965). Such findings provided dramatic testimony to the marked contribution of nonvestibular processes to rotation-induced vestibular ataxia.

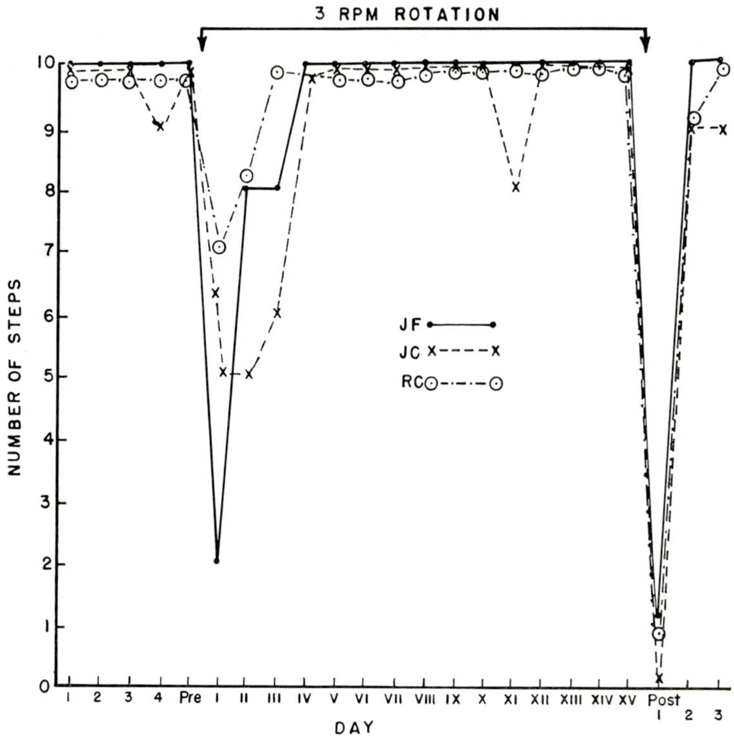

Fig. 7. Performances of three normal males on a rail-walking test (heel-to-toe, 1–1/4-inch-wide rail, eyes open) during 2 weeks of rotating at 3 rpm (originally published in Aerospace Med. **35**, 1074, 1964 as Fig. 5)

In another comparative study designed to determine differential effects of bizarre stimulation on susceptibility to motion sickness (Kennedy et al., 1965) and on postural equilibrium functions in normals vs. BL-Ds (Fregly and Graybiel, 1965), the ataxia test findings were reminiscent of those in the rotating room studies. The bizarre stimulation of the vestibular apparatus was amply provided by highly stressful storm condition of eight hours' duration at sea. Twenty hours after the storm the ship carrying the subjects was docked, and ataxia testing was undertaken within minutes. Ataxia retesting continued periodically for 36 hours. Results on the rail ataxia test battery (long version in the BL-D group) are summarized in Fig. 9. In both groups of subjects Walk E/O performances had improved over baseline levels and Stand E/O performances were impaired, although not significantly (statistically) in the BL-D group. In the Stand E/O tests (and also in the SOLEC tests, not included in the Figure), however, residual ataxia was evident for as long as 21 hours in the group of normals, whereas no such ataxia was observed in the group of BL-Ds. As after rotation, the WALEC test performances (only normals were tested) remained quantitatively unimpaired. When the scores of the normal group were divided into the top-scoring half and bottom-scoring half on each ataxia test, those in the bottom-scoring half were very similar

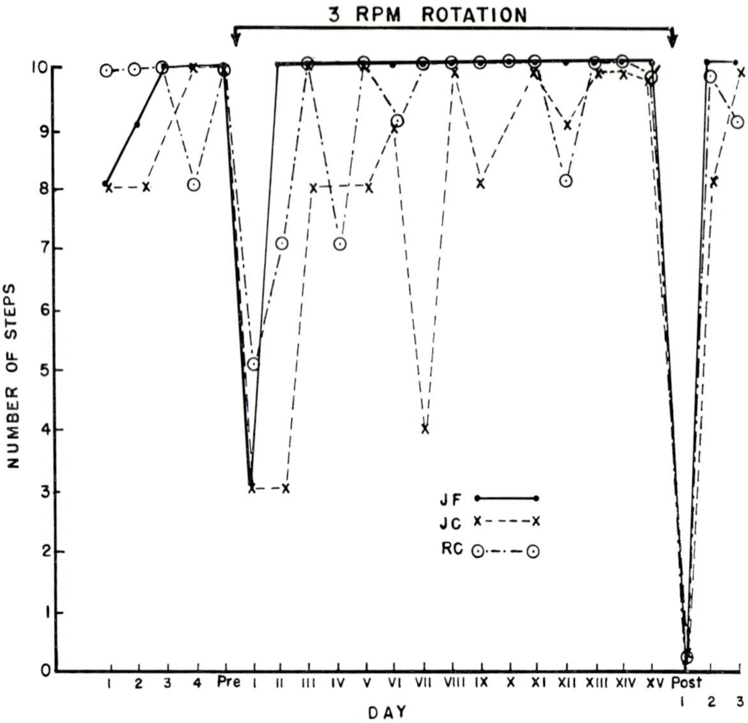

Fig. 8. Performances of three normal males on a rail-standing test (heel-to-toe, 3/4-inch-wide rail, eyes open) during 2 weeks of rotating at 3 rpm (originally published in Aerospace Med. **35**, 1075, 1964 as Fig. 5a)

to those observed in the BL-Ds (Fregly and Graybiel, 1965). Because all the normals were far from being vestibular ataxic in terms of their initial, pre-experimental performance scores, and because all presented other pre-experimental indications of normal vestibular function (e.g. normal caloric and counterrolling responses) the differential results observed in the normal group, although statistically significant, remain difficult to interpret. Cross-validation on a more comprehensively studied normal group is needed to rule out possible artifacts. Elucidation of the contributing influences in normal persons would have both practical and theoretical implications. The possibility of an otolithic explanation of these findings has not been ruled out.

VI. Alcohol-Induced Ataxia in Relation to Labyrinth Function

For the purpose of further elucidating the functional role of the vestibular organs in man, the effects of alcohol on the postural equilibrium of four BL-D subjects (DO, GR, HA, and MY; members of the group indicated in Table 1), were investigated (Fregly and Graybiel, 1968b) and compared with results on

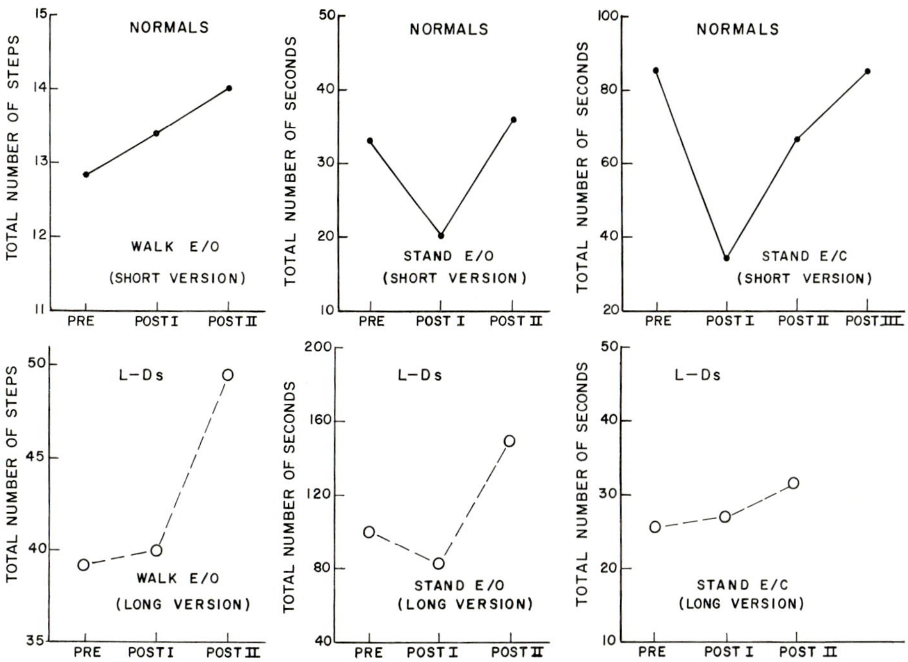

Fig. 9. A comparison of the residual effects of bizarre stimulation of the vestibular apparatus during a severe storm at sea upon rail ataxia test battery performance skills of a group of 20 normal males and a group of 9 males with bilateral loss of labyrinthine functions (L-Ds)

a previously studied group of normal individuals (Fregly et al., 1967). The differential effects in the two groups are summarized in Fig. 10. Among the standardized items of the rail and floor ataxia test batteries, visual rail-walking (Walk E/O) was the only test in which the BL-Ds demonstrated performance decrements following alcohol administration (Fig. 10B). This finding stands in marked contrast to the consistent decrements observed in the normals. During one test session two hours after ingestion of 80-proof vodka and during another three hours after ingestion of 100-proof vodka the BL-D group's baseline Walk E/O performance level was surpassed. This finding is also in contrast to the greater duration of the impairments observed in the normals. In both the 80-proof and 100-proof experiments the BL-Ds were slightly less affected (mean loss of about 2 steps) than the normals (mean loss of 3 to 4 steps). That only Walk E/O performance scores showed a decrement is consistent with the compensable nature of the skills underlying the task. Because of the provocative finding of less magnitude and shorter duration of performance decrement in BL-D subjects than was found in normals, an additional study was undertaken in an attempt to substantiate and expand on this result.

For better quantitative (numerical) intergroup comparison of magnitude effects on alcohol-influenced ataxia test behavior, three different members (JO, PE, and ZA) of the elite group of BL-Ds (see Table 1) were studied with the follow-

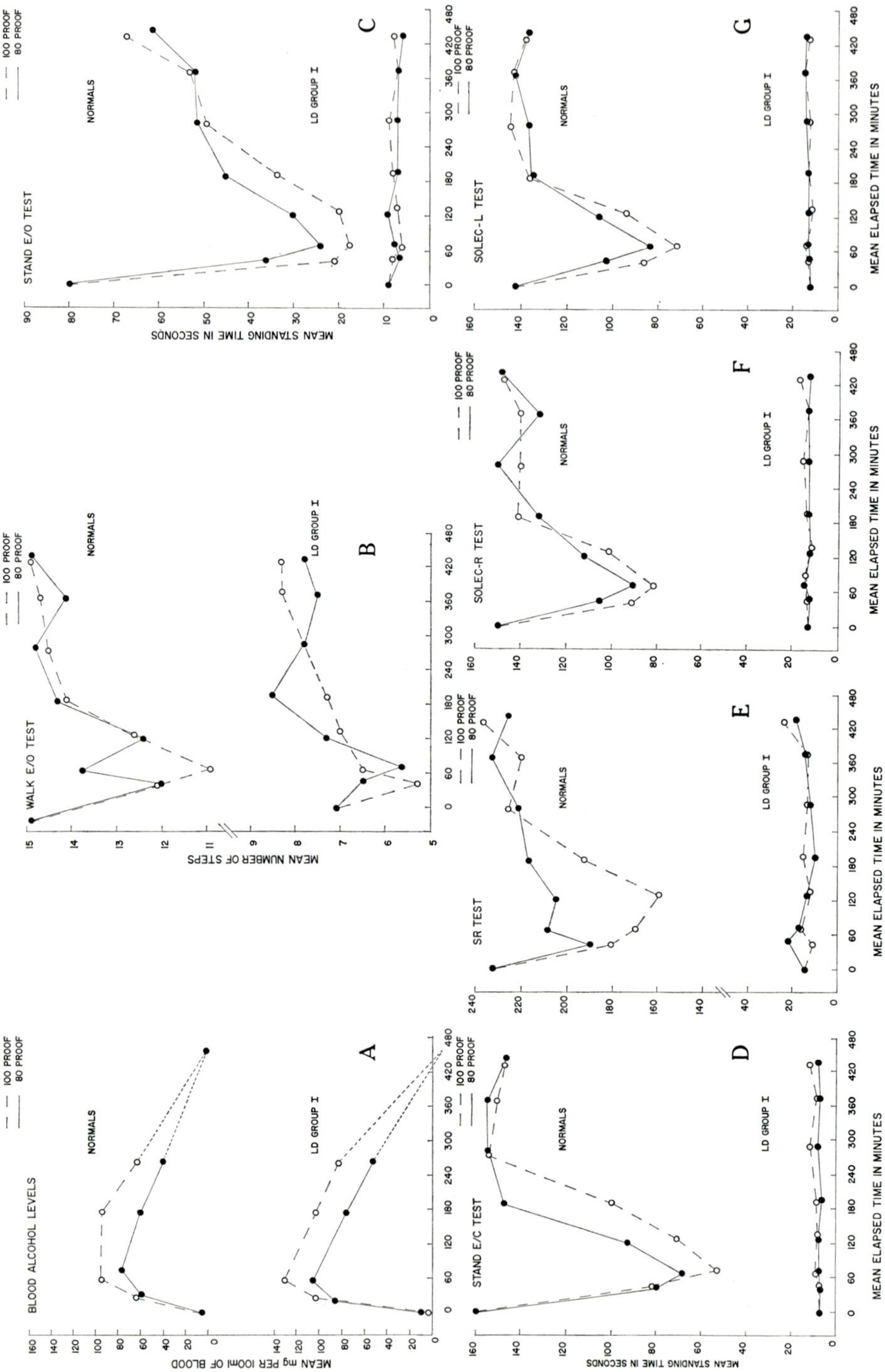

BLOOD ALCOHOL LEVELS
NORMALS
LD GROUP I
100 PROOF
80 PROOF
MEAN mg PER 100ml OF BLOOD
A
WALK E/O TEST
MEAN NUMBER OF STEPS
B
STAND E/O TEST
MEAN STANDING TIME IN SECONDS
C
STAND E/C TEST
D
SR TEST
E
SOLEC-R TEST
F
SOLEC-L TEST
G
MEAN ELAPSED TIME IN MINUTES

Fig. 10

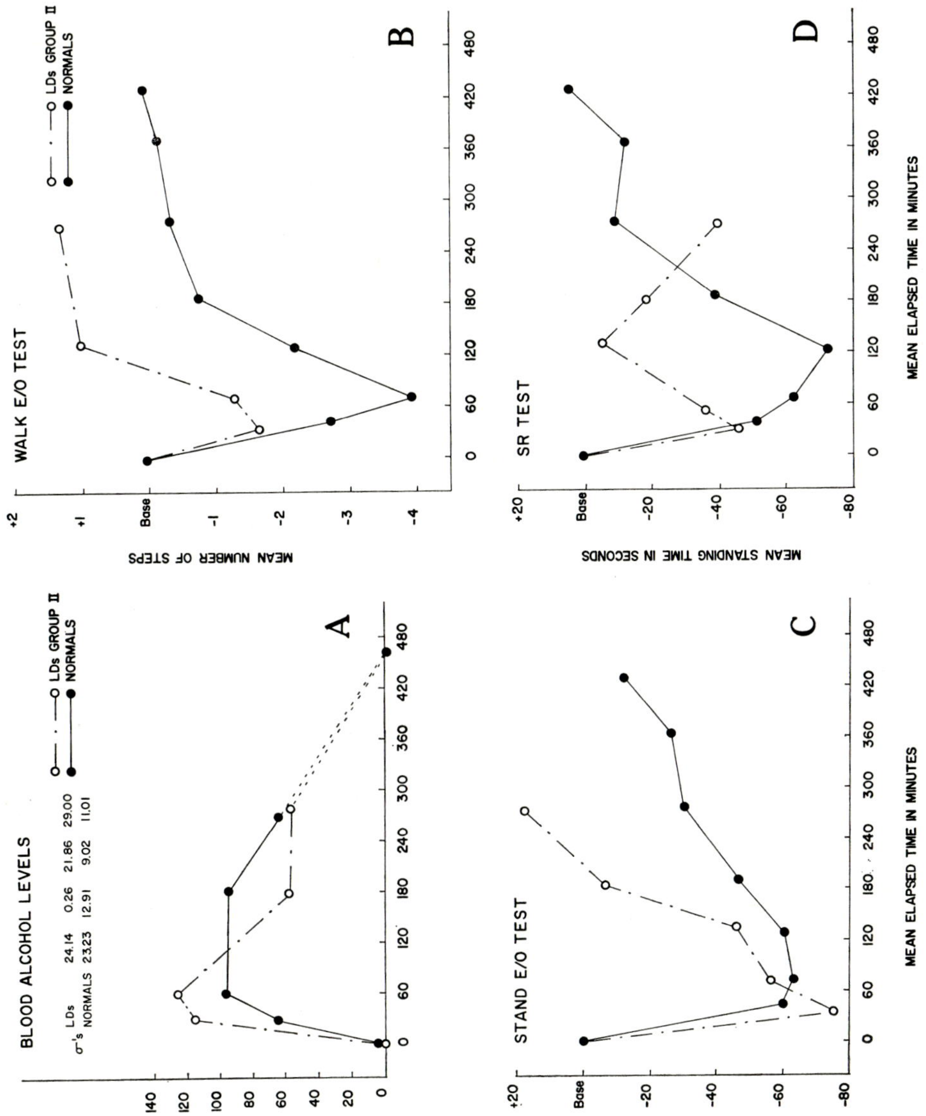

Fig. 11. Comparison of effects of 100-proof vodka in a group of 3 bilaterally labyrinthine-defective subjects (JO, PE, and ZA) with a group of 13 normal subjects: A: blood alcohol levels, B: rail-walking with eyes open, C: rail-standing with eyes open, and D: standing on floor with eyes closed (originally published in Acta oto-laryng. (Stockh.) **65**, 471, 1968 as Fig. 2)

Fig. 10. Comparisons of 80-proof and 100-proof vodka effects in a group of 4 bilaterally labyrinthine-defective subjects (DO, GR, HA, MY) with a group of 13 vestibular normal subjects: A: blood alcohol levels, B: walking with eyes open on a 3/4-inch-wide rail, C: standing with eyes open on the 3/4-inch rail, D: standing with eyes closed on a 2–1/4-inch-wide rail, E: standing on floor with eyes closed, F–G: standing on one leg (on floor) with eyes closed (originally published in Acta oto-laryng. (Stockh.) **65**, 470, 1968 as Fig. 1)

ing changes in experimental conditions: (1) visual rail-walking and visual rail-standing tasks were made easier by the use of wider rails, thereby equating their baseline scores with those of the normals (but not equating vestibular-dependent baseline abilities), and (2) one of the standardized nonvisual floor ataxia tests (SR) was repeated. "Optimum" widths of rails were selected from the long version of the rail battery (GRAYBIEL and FREGLY, 1966). Several successively narrow rails were added to each individually determined optimum rail to provide a "top" to each "tailor-made" rail battery. The BL-D group was subjected to extended practice for several days prior to the ingestion of alcohol.

Generally, the findings (Fig. 11) supported the previous results. Visual rail-walking decrements were again observed. The magnitude of the decrement and the onset and recovery periods were nearly identical to those observed previously, despite the reduced level of difficulty of the task. The results differed from those obtained in the previous BL-D group, however, in that visual rail-standing decrements also were observed; on this test recovery also occurred sooner than it did in the normal group. Surprisingly, the SR findings were also similar to those obtained with normals, although they were attributable in large part to the outstanding success of one subject (ZA) in improving his initially poor score via nonvestibular compensating processes (FREGLY and GRAYBIEL, 1968b). Results of the two investigations permitted the conclusions that (1) the intactness of the vestibular apparatus can be regarded as a factor contributing to "acute alcohol ataxia" in terms of both the magnitude and the duration of the ataxia, and (2) "acute alcohol ataxia" is apparently superimposable on pronounced vestibular ataxia only to the extent that such ataxia can be compensated via nonvestibular processes.

In a separate study (GRAYBIEL et al., 1971) in which the standardized rail (short version) and floor ataxia test batteries were used, the 100-proof vodka experiment was also conducted on the young man discussed earlier, who had normal hearing with little evidence of vestibular function. The findings were nearly identical to those observed in the group of four BL-D subjects tested initially.

VII. Summary

Spontaneous and induced vestibular ataxia in man are defined in terms of characteristic findings obtained by a quantitative ataxia test battery administered to groups of individuals with widely varying integrity of labyrinthine functions, as confirmed by results of other vestibular functional tests both under normal conditions and during and after bizarre stimulation of the vestibular apparatus. Some problems of definition and measurement of vestibular ataxia are discussed briefly. The importance of critical studies of vestibular-influenced postural equilibrium functions is implicit from an elaborate presentation of data. An extensive, but not exhaustive, bibliography of postural and postural equilibrium studies in man, which have been reported in a widely scattered literature representing many disciplines, is included as an appendix for the convenience of investigators particularly interested in this area of vestibular research.

Acknowledgement. The author is deeply indebted to Ashton Graybiel, M.D. for his close collaboration and generous support through the years in all phases of the research reported in this communication.

References

Bergstedt, M.: Stepwise adaptation to a velocity of 10 rpm in the Pensacola slow rotation room. In: The role of the vestibular organs in the exploration of space. NASA SP-77. Washington, D.C.: U.S. Government Printing Office 1965.

Clark, B., Graybiel, A.: Perception of the visual horizontal in normal and labyrinthine defective subjects during prolonged rotation. Amer. J. Psychol. **79**, 608–612 (1966).

Clark, B., Graybiel, A.: The egocentric localization of the visual horizontal in normal and labyrinthine-defective observers as a function of head and body tilt. Percept. Psychophys. **2**, 609–611 (1967).

Fregly, A.R., Bergstedt, M., Graybiel, A.: Relationships between blood alcohol, positional alcohol nystagmus and postural equilibrium. Quart. J. Stud. Alcohol **28**, 11–21 (1967).

Fregly, A.R., Graybiel, A.: Residual effects of storm conditions at sea upon the postural equilibrium functioning of vestibular normal and vestibular defective human subjects. NSAM-935. NASA Order R-93. Pensacola, Fla.: Naval School of Aviation Medicine 1965.

Fregly, A.R., Graybiel, A.: Acute alcohol ataxia in relation to vestibular function. NAMI-973. NASA Order R-93. Pensacola, Fla.: Naval Aerospace Medical Institute 1966.

Fregly, A.R., Graybiel, A.: An ataxia test battery not requiring rails. Aerospace Med. **39**, 277–282 (1968a).

Fregly, A.R., Graybiel, A.: Acute alcohol ataxia in persons with loss of labyrinthine function. Acta oto-laryng. (Stockh.) **65**, 468–478 (1968b).

Fregly, A.R., Graybiel, A.: Labyrinthine defects as shown by ataxia and caloric tests. Acta oto-laryng. (Stockh.) **69**, 216–222 (1970).

Fregly, A.R., Graybiel, A., Smith, M.J.: Walk on floor eyes closed (WOFEC): A new addition to an ataxia test battery. Aerospace Med. **43**, 395–399 (1972)

Fregly, A.R., Kennedy, R.S.: Comparative effects of prolonged rotation at 10 rpm on postural equilibrium in vestibular normal and vestibular defective human subjects. Aerospace Med. **36**, 1160–1167 (1965).

Fregly, A.R., Oberman, A., Graybiel, A., Mitchell, R.E.: Thousand aviator study: nonvestibular contributions to postural equilibrium functions. Aerospace Med. **39**, 33–37 (1968).

Fregly, A.R., Smith, M.J., Graybiel, A.: Revised normative standards of performance of men on a quantitative ataxia test battery. Acta oto-laryng. (Stockh.) **75**, 10–16 (1973).

Fregly, A.R., Smith, M.J., Wood, C.D., Cramer, D.B.: Effects of some antimotion sickness drugs and secobarbital on postural equilibrium functions at sea level and at 12,000 feet (simulated). Aerospace Med. **44**, 140–145 (1973).

Graybiel, A.: Vestibular sickness and some of its implications for space flight. In: W.S. Fields and B.R. Alford, Eds. Neurological aspects of auditory and vestibular disorders. Springfield, Ill.: C.C. Thomas 1964.

Graybiel, A.: Functional disturbances of vestibular origin of significance in space flight. In: Second International Symposium on war in Space, Paris 1965. Proceedings, pp. 8–32. Wien and New York: Springer 1967.

Graybiel, A.: Orientation in aerospace flight. Special Rpt. 66-6. NASA Order R-93. Pensacola, Fla.: Naval Aerospace Medical Institute 1966.

Graybiel, A.: Vestibular mechanisms in human behavior. Ann. Otol. (St. Louis) **77**, 772–786 (1968).

Graybiel, A., Clark, B.: Validity of the oculogravic illusion as a specific indicator of otolith function. Aerospace Med. **36**, 1173–1181 (1965).

Graybiel, A., Fregly, A.R.: A new quantitative ataxia test battery. Acta oto-laryng. (Stockh.) **61**, 292–312 (1966).

Graybiel, A., Johnson, W.H.: A comparison of the symptomatology experienced by healthy persons and subjects with loss of labyrinthine function when exposed to unusual patterns of centripetal force in a counter-rotating room. Ann. Otol. (St. Louis) **72**, 357–373 (1963).

Graybiel, A., Kennedy, R.S., Knoblock, E.C., Guedry, F.E., Jr., Mertz, W., McLeod, M.E., Colehour, J.K., Miller II, E.F., Fregly, A.R.: The effects of exposure to a rotating environment (10 rpm) on four aviators for a period of twelve days. Aerospace Med. **36**, 733–754 (1965).

Graybiel, A., Schuknecht, H.F., Fregly, A.R., Miller II, E. F., McLeod, M.E.: Streptomycin in Ménière's disease: long-term follow-up. Arch. Otolaryng. **85**, 156–170 (1967).

Graybiel, A., Smith, C.R., Guedry, F.E., Jr., Miller II, E.F., Fregly, A.R., Cramer, D.B.: Idiopathic progressive vestibular degeneration in a young man: Loss of vestibular sensation not the basis for detection. Ann. Otol. (St. Louis) **81**, 165–178 (1972).

Graybiel, A., Smith, C.R., Guedry, F.E., Jr., Miller II, E.F., Fregly, A.R., Cramer, D.B.: Idiopathic progressive vestibular degeneration. Ann. Otol. (St. Louis) **81**, 165–178 (1972).

Graybiel, A., Thompson, A.B., Deane, F.R., Fregly, A.R., Colehour, J.K., Ricks, E.L.: Transfer of habituation of motion sickness on change in body position between vertical and horizontal in a rotating environment. Aerospace Med. **39**, 950–962 (1968).

Guedry, F.E., Jr.: Orientation of the rotation-axis relative to gravity: Its influence on nystagmus and the sensation of rotation. Acta oto-laryng. (Stockh.) **60**, 30–48 (1965).

Guedry, F.E., Jr., Kennedy, R.S., Harris, C.S., Graybiel, A.: Human performance during two weeks in a room rotating at three rpm. Aerospace Med. **35**, 1071–1082 (1964).

House, W.F. (Ed.): Transtemporal bone microsurgical removal of acoustic neuroma. Monograph. Arch. Otolaryng. **80**, 597–756 (1964).

Igarashi, M., Fregly, A.R., Tokita, T.: Basic and clinical aspects of vestibular ataxia. Springfield, Ill.: C.C. Thomas, 1974 (in press).

Kennedy, R.S., Graybiel, A., McDonough, R.C., Beckwith, F.D.: Symptomatology under storm conditions in the North Atlantic in control subjects and in persons with bilateral labyrinthine defects. NSAM-928. NASA Order R-93. Pensacola, Fla.: Naval School of Aviation Medicine 1965.

McLeod, M.E., Meek, J.C.: A threshold caloric test: results in normal subjects. NSAM-834. NASA Order R-37. Pensacola, Fla.: Naval School of Aviation Medicine 1962.

Miller, II, E.F.: Counterrolling of the human eyes produced by head tilt with respect to gravity. Acta oto-laryng. (Stockh.) **54**, 479–501 (1961).

Miller, II, E.F., Fregly, A.R., Graybiel, A.: Visual horizontal perception in relation to otolith function. NAMI-989. NASA Order R-93. Pensacola, Fla.: Naval Aerospace Medical Institute 1966.

Miller, II, E.F., Graybiel, A.: A comparison of ocular counterrolling movements between normal persons and deaf subjects with bilateral labyrinthine defects. Ann. Otol. (St. Louis) **72**, 885–893 (1963).

Nelson, J.R.: Long-term effects of acoustic neuroma surgery. Arch. Otolaryng. **88**, 675–686 (1968).

Smith, C.R.: The balance mechanisms in man. Maico Audiological Library Series. **6**, Rpt. **4**, 1–3 (1967).

Appendix. A Selected Bibliography of Posture, Postural Equilibrium, and Ataxia Test Methods

The study of human standing and walking posture and postural equilibrium and of their normal variations and pathological deviations has commanded the attention of numerous investigators from such disciplines as anatomy, audiology, biophysics, engineering, gerontology, ophthalmology, neurology, neurophysiology, neurosurgery, orthopedics, otology, pharmacology, physical education, physiology, physiotherapy and physiatry, psychology and "vestibulology," among others. The bibliography is presented both as a brief historical, academic, and clinical account of the highly varied nature and scope of the literature reported by such investigators and to make available conveniently in one place a sampling of references to studies which have either definite, probable, or possible implications for vestibular research. The references are listed in seven sections and are classified, at times arbitrarily, in terms of the apparatus and/or techniques employed.

1. Non-Instrumented Floor-Standing and/or Floor-Walking Tests, such as the Classical Romberg, "Unipodic" Romberg, Mann Test, Tandem Walking, and "Star Walking"

ARLASCHENKO, N.I., BOKHOV, B.B., BUSYGIN, V.YE., VOLOKHOVA, N.A., GRIGORYEV, YU.G., POLYAKOV, B.I., FARBER, YU.V.: On tractions of the organism during prolonged action of Coriolis accelerations. FTD-TT-63-1013/1-2. Wright-Patterson Air Force Base, Ohio: Foreign Tech. Div. Translation from Byull. Eksper. Biol. Med. **6**, 28–37 (1963).

BÁRÁNY, R.: Physiologie und Pathologie des Bogengangsapparates beim Menschen. Klin. Studien. Vienna: Deuticke, 1–76, 1907.

BARBEY, E.: A propos du signe de Romberg et de ses variantes comme tests de l'équilibration statique. Confin. neurol. (Basel) **6**, 162–168 (1944).

BARON, J.: Prismatic lenses for vertigo and some experimental background for the role of the extrinsic ocular muscles in disequilibrium. Trans. Amer. Acad. Ophthal. Otolaryng. Nov.–Dec., 915–926, 1962.

BASS, R.I.: An analysis of the components of tests of semicircular canal function and of static and dynamic balance. Res. Quart. **10**, 33–52 (1939).

BIRREN, J.E.: Static equilibrium and vestibular function. J. exp. Psychol. **35**, 127–133 (1945).

BÜRGI, S.: Die Ataxien in ihrem funktionellen Aspekt. Confin. neurol. (Basel) **9**, 273–344 (1949).

CLARK, B., GRAYBIEL, A.: Human performance during adaptation to stress in the Pensacola Slow Rotation Room. Aerospace Med. **32**, 93–106 (1961).

COLLINS, V.D., HOWE, E.C.: The measurement of organic and neuromuscular fitness. Amer. Phys. Ed. Rev. **29**, 64–71 (1924).

DANDY, W.E.: The surgical treatment of Ménière's disease. Surg. Gynec. Obstet. **72**, 421–425 (1941).

DE JONG, R.N.: The neurological examination. New York: Hoeber 1967.

DE WIT, G.: Seasickness (Motion sickness). Acta oto-laryng. (Stockh.) Suppl. **108**, 1–56 (1953).

DOCKERAY, F.C., ISAACS, S.: Psychological research in aviation in Italy, France, England, and the American expeditionary forces. J. comp. Psychol. **1**, 115–147 (1921).

FARMER, T.W., MUSTIAN, V.M.: Vestibulocerebellar ataxia. A newly defined hereditary syndrome with periodic manifestations. Arch. Neurol. (Chic.) **8**, 471–480 (1963).

FISCHER, J.J.: The labyrinth. Physiology and functional tests. New York: Grune and Stratton 1956.

FISKE, D.: The ataxis. Arch. intern. Med. **83**, 593–607 (1949).

FORD, F.R., WALSH, F.B.: Clinical observations upon the importance of the vestibular reflexes in ocular movements. Bull. Johns Hopk. Hosp. **58**, 80–88 (1936).

FUKUDA, T., TOKITA, T.: A new arrangement of the vestibular examination. Acta oto-laryng. (Stockh.) Suppl. **179**, 122–137 (1963).

GLORIG, A., FOWLER, E.P., JR.: Tests for labyrinth function following streptomycin therapy. Ann. Otol. (St. Louis) **56**, 379–394 (1947).

GRAYBIEL, A., CLARK, B., ZARRIELLO, J.J.: Observations on human subjects living in a "slow rotation room" for periods of two days. A.M.A. Arch. Neurol. **3**, 55–73 (1960).

GREEN, R.E., DOUGLASS, C.C.: Intracranial division of the eighth nerve for Ménière's disease. A follow-up study of patients operated on by Dr. Walter E. Dandy. Ann. Otol. (St. Louis) **60**, 610–621 (1951).

HALLGREN, B.: Retinitis pigmentosa combined with congenital deafness, with vestibulo-cerebellar ataxia an mental abnormality in a proportion of cases. A clinical and genetico-statistical study. Acta psychiat. scand. Suppl. **136–141**, 6–101 (1959–1960).

HANCOCK, J.A.: A preliminary study of motor ability. Pedagog. Sem. **3**, 9–29 (1894).

HEAD, H.: The sense of stability and balance in the air. In: The medical problems of flying. Med. Res. Council, Spec. Rpt. Series, No. **53**, 214–256 (1920).

HENMON, V.A.C.: Air service tests of aptitude for flying. J. appl. Psychol. **3**, 103–109 (1919).

JOHNER, C.H., PERLMAN, H.B.: Hypnosis and vestibular function. Ann. Otol. (St. Louis) **77**, 126–138 (1968).

JONKEES, L.B.W.: The examination of the vestibular organ. In: Y. ZOTTERMAN, Ed. Progress in brain research. Vol. 23. Sensory Mechanisms. Amsterdam-New York: Elsevier 1967.

JONES, I.H.: Equilibrium and vertigo. Philadelphia: Lippincott 1918.

Kennedy, R.S., Graybiel, A.: Symptomatology during prolonged exposure in a constantly rotating environment at a velocity of one revolution per minute. Aerospace Med. **33**, 817–825 (1962).

Levin, P.M.: The syndrome of vestibular paralysis in man. J. nerv. ment. Dis. **89**, 335–342 (1939).

Mann, C.W.: The effects of auditory-vestibular nerve pathology on space perception. NSAM-481. Pensacola, Fla.: Naval School of Aviation Medicine 1951.

Mann, L.: Über Schwindel und Gleichgewichtsstörungen nach Commotio Cerebri und ihren Nachweis durch galvanische Reaktion. Med. Klin. **3**, 567–571, 606–609 (1907).

Milojevic, B., Watson, J.L.: Vestibular asymmetries in right- and left-handed people. Acta oto-laryng. (Stockh.) **60**, 322–330 (1965).

Monrad-Krohn, G.H.: The clinical examination of the central nervous system. New York: Harper 1938.

Newsom, B.D., Brady, J.F., Goble, G.J.: Equilibrium and walking changes observed at 7 1/2, 10 and 12 RPM in the revolving space station simulator. Aerospace Med. **36**, 322–326 (1965).

Newsom, B.D., Brady, J.F., Shafer, W.A., French, R.S.: Adaptation to prolonged exposures in the revolving space station simulator. Aerospace Med. **37**, 778–783 (1966).

Niven, J.I., Graybiel, A.: Postural equilibrium in man following unilateral labyrinthectomy. NSAM-435. Pensacola, Fla.: Naval School of Aviation Medicine 1953.

Rademaker, G.: Reactions labyrinthiques et équilibre. L'ataxie labyrinthique. Paris: Masson 1935.

Romberg, M.H.: Manual of the nervous diseases of man. London: Syndeham Trans. Vol. 2, 1853.

Seashore, H.G., Koch, G.: Postural steadiness under conditions of muscular tension and fatigue. Psychol. Rec. **2**, 317–332 (1938).

Takebayshi, H., Kuriyama, T., Imamura, H., Kurihara, M., Kishi, M.: Stereotaxic operation of superior colliculus (str. profundum) as treatment of vestibular (or vestibulo-cerebellar) ataxia. Wakayama med. Rep. **9**, 47–59 (1964).

Vaglini, F.: La prova del camino a stella in soggetti normali. Boll. Mal. Orecch. **79**, 360–366 (1961).

Vazuka, F.A.: Essentials of the neurological examination. Philadelphia: Smith, Kline and French Laboratories 1962.

Watanabe, I.: Latent vestibular ataxia. Otolaryng. (Tokyo) **37**, 315–319 (1965).

Wirth, G.: Untersuchungen über die statischen Funktionen bei Taubstummen mit und ohne Vestibularausfall. Mschr. Ohrenheilk. **97**, 501–505 (1963).

Worchel, P., Dallenbach, K.M.: The vestibular sensitivity of deaf-blind subjects. Amer. J. Psychol. **61**, 94–99 (1948).

Worchel, P., Dallenbach, K.M.: Vestibular sensitivity in the deaf. Amer. J. Psychol. **63**, 161–175 (1950).

2. *"Waltzing" and Stepping Tests*

Fukuda, T.: The stepping test: two phases of the labyrinthine reflex. Acta oto-laryng. (Stockh.) **50**, 95–108 (1959).

Fukuda, T., Tokita, T.: A new arrangement of the vestibular examination. Acta oto-laryng. (Stockh.) Suppl. **179**, 122–137 (1963).

Hinoki, M.: A new devised arrangement of vestibular examination and its results before and during treatment of Ménière's disease with ganglion stellatum blockade. Jap. J. Otol. Tokyo **63**, 2589–2608, 2625–2628 (1959).

Hirsch, C.: A new labyrinthine reaction: "The waltzing test." Ann. Otol. (St. Louis) **49**, 232–238 (1940).

Jordan, P.: Fukuda's stepping test. A preliminary report on reliability. Arch. Otolaryng. **77**, 243–245 (1963).

Peitersen, E.: Vestibulospinal reflexes. IV. Alterations in the stepping test after thermal stimulation in normal subjects. Arch. Otolaryng. **78**, 59–67 (1963a).

PEITERSEN, E.: Vestibulospinal reflexes. V. Acute disturbances of vestibular function after operations on the stapes, especially as evaluated by the stepping test. Arch. Otolaryng. **78**, 642–648 (1963b).

PEITERSEN, E.: Vestibulospinal reflexes. VII. Alterations in the stepping test in various disorders of the inner ear and vestibular nerve. Arch. Otolaryng. **79**, 481–486 (1964).

PEITERSEN, E.: Vestibulospinal reflexes. IX. Alterations in the stepping test during alcohol intoxication. Arch. Otolaryng. **83**, 332–334 (1966).

PEITERSEN, E., ZILSTORFF-PEDERSEN, K.: Vestibulo-spinal reflexes. II. Alterations in the stepping test after rotatory stimulation in normal subjects. Arch. Otolaryng. **77**, 353–358 (1963a).

PEITERSEN, E., ZILSTORFF-PEDERSEN, K.: Vestibulo-spinal reflexes. III. Alterations in the stepping test following galvanic stimulation. Arch. Otolaryng. **77**, 586–591 (1963b).

TOKITA, T.: Studies on diagnosis and treatment of Ménière's syndrome with special reference to its etiologic factors. Presented at 65th general meeting of the Japanese Otorinolaryngological Society, Tokushima City, Japan 1964.

TOKITA, T., AOKI, S., YONEKURA, E., SHIRAKI, T., KURODA, W., TAKEUCHI, T., NAKAYAMA, S., FUJIMOTO, T., AOKI, M., GOTO, T., MIZUTANI, T., SUGANUMA, Y.: Dissociation of vestibulospinal reactions. Jap. J. Otol. Tokyo **66**, 24–34 (1963).

UNTERBERGER, S.: Neue objectiv registrierbare Vestibularis-Körperdrehreaktion, erhalten durch Treten auf Stelle: Der "Tretversuch." Arch. Ohr.-, Nas.-, u. Kehlk.-Heilk. **145**, 478–492 (1938).

ZILSTORFF-PEDERSEN, K., PEITERSEN, E.: Vestibulo-spinal reflexes. I. Spontaneous alterations in the position of normal persons doing the stepping test. Arch. Otolaryng. **77**, 237–242 (1963).

3. Ataxiagraphic and Ataxiametric Methods

COLLINS, V.D., HOWE, E.C.: The measurement of organic and neuromuscular fittness. Amer. Phys. Ed. Rev. **29**, 64–71 (1924).

EDWARDS, A.S.: Effects of the loss of one hundred hours of sleep. Amer. J. Psychol. **54**, 80–91 (1941a).

EDWARDS, A.S.: Static ataxiameter for head and hips. Amer. J. Psychol. **54**, 576–577 (1941b).

EDWARDS, A.S.: The measurement of static ataxia. Amer. J. Psychol. **55**, 171–188 (1942).

EDWARDS, A.S.: Factors tending to decrease the steadiness of the body at rest. Amer. J. Psychol. **56**, 599–602 (1943).

EDWARDS, A.S.: Body sway and vision. J. exp. Psychol. **36**, 526–535 (1946).

EDWARDS, A.S.: Body sway and non-visual factors. J. Psychol. (Provincetown) **23**, 241–254 (1947).

EDWARDS, A.S.: The effect of bodily rotation upon involuntary sway and finger tremor. Amer. J. Psychol. **62**, 590–591 (1949).

EDWARDS, A.S.: A quantitative study of voluntary vs. involuntary movement. J. gen. Psychol. **46**, 93–98 (1952).

FEARING, F.S.: The factors influencing static equilibrium. An experimental study of the influence of height, weight, position of the feet on amount of sway, together with an analysis of the variability in the records of one reagent over a long period of time. J. comp. Psychol. **4**, 91–185 (1924a).

FEARING, F.S.: The factors influencing static equilibrium. An experimental study of the effects of practice upon amount and direction of sway. J. comp. Psychol. **4**, 163–183 (1924b).

FEARING, F.S.: The experimental study of the Romberg sign. J. nerv. ment. Dis. **61**, 449–465 (1925a).

FEARING, F.S.: Factors influencing static equilibrium. An experimental study of the effects of controlled and uncontrolled attention upon sway. J. comp. Psychol. **5**, 1–24 (1925b).

FISHER, M.B., BIRREN, J.E., LEGGETT, A.L.: Standardization of two tests of equilibrium: the railwalking test and the ataxiagraph. J. exp. Psychol. **35**, 321–329 (1945).

GOLDBERG, L.: Quantitative studies on alcohol tolerance in man. Acta physiol. scand. **5**, Suppl. 16, 1–128 (1943).

GRANT, W.T.: Romberg test: graphic method of recording disturbances of equilibrium. Bull. Los Angeles neurol. Soc. **8**, 25–30 (1943).

Hinsdale, G.: The station of man, considered physiologically and clinically. Amer. J. med. Sci. **93**, 478–485 (1887).

Hinsdale, G.: Observation on station with reference to respiration. N.Y. med. J. **51**, 292–294 (1890).

Husband, R.W.: The effect of musical rhythms and pure rhythms on bodily sway. J. gen. Psychol. **11**, 328–335 (1934).

McFarland, R.A., Franzen, R.: The Pensacola study of naval aviators. Final summary report. Report No. 38. Washington, D.C.: Civil Aeronautics Admin. 1944.

Miles, W.R.: Static equilibrium as a useful test of motor control. J. industr. Hyg. **3**, 316–331 (1922).

Miles, W.R.: Alcohol and human efficiency. Publ. No. 333. Washington, D.C.: Carnegie Institution of Washington 1924.

Orma, E.J.: The effects of cooling the feet and closing the eyes on standing equilibrium. Different patterns of standing equilibrium in young adult men and women. Acta physiol. scand. **38**, 288–297 (1956).

Seashore, H.G.: Some relationships of fine and gross motor abilities. Res. Quart. **13**, 259–274 (1942).

Seashore, R.H.: Individual differences in motor skills. J. gen. Psychol. **3**, 38–66 (1930).

Seashore, R.H., Buxton, C.E., McCollom, I.N.: Multiple factorial analysis of fine motor skills. Amer. J. Psychol. **53**, 251–259 (1940).

Skogland, J.E.: A quantitative study of normal and pathological station in human subjects. Med. Rec. **155**, 15–22 (1942).

Tokita, T.: Studies on diagnosis and treatment of Ménière's syndrome with special reference to its etiologic factors. Presented at 65th General Meeting of the Japanese Otorinolaryngological Society, Tokushima City, Japan, 1964.

Travis, R.C.: An experimental analysis of dynamic and static equilibrium. J. exp. Psychol. **35**, 216–234 (1945).

Uchytil, B.: Zhodnoceni fvsiologickych uchylek, vznikajicich v Rombergove postoii a pri Hautanove testu, na zaklade objektivni registrace. Čs. Otolaryng. **14**, 70–77 (1965).

Witkin, H.A., Wapner, S.: Visual factors in the maintenance of upright posture. Amer. J. Psychol. **63**, 31–50 (1950).

4. Stabilimeter (Stabilometer), Statokinesimeter, and "Dynabalometer"

Baron, J.B.: Présentation d'un appareil pour mettre en évidence les déplacements du centre de gravité du corps dans le polygone de sustentation. Arch. Mal. prof. **25**, 41–49 (1964).

Langova, J.: Statokinetische Abnormitäten bei Kindern mit verzögerter Sprachentwicklung. De therapia vocis et loquelae Vol. Societatis Internationalis Phoniatrae XVII Congressus Vindobonae, 1955.

Nayrac, P., Milbled, G., Parquet, Ph.J.: Le statokinésimètre. Etude en clinique neurologique. Lille méd. **11**, 476–480 (1966).

Penman, K.A.: A new dynamic balance testing device: The "dynabalometer." Percept. Mot. Skills **23**, 232–234 (1966).

Soulairac, A., Baron, J.B.: Étude statokinésimètrique de la régulation posturale chez l'homme. (Variations normales et pathologiques). Sem. Hôp. Paris **53**, 3365–3370 (1967).

Thiébaut, F., Isch, F., Collard, M., Conraux, C.: La statokinésimètrie (technique et résultats). Rev. neurol. **114**, 123–134 (1966).

Travis, R.C.: A new stabilometer for measuring dynamic equilibrium in the standing position. J. exp. Psychol. **34**, 418–424 (1944).

Travis, R.C.: An experimental analysis of dynamic and static equilibrium. J. exp. Psychol. **35**, 216–234 (1945).

Wapner, S., Witkin, H.A.: The role of visual factors in the maintenance of body-balance. Amer. J. Psychol. **63**, 385–408 (1950).

Witkin, H.A., Wapner, S.: Visual factors in the maintenance of upright posture. Amer. J. Psychol. **63**, 31–50 (1950).

Tilting Platforms and Other Unstable Devices, Including Goniometers, Wabble Meter, and Wabble Board

BÁRÁNY, R.: Physiologie und Pathologie des Bogengangsapparates beim Menschen. Klin. Studien. Vienna: Deuticke, 1–76, 1907.

BEGBIE, G.H.: The effects of alcohol and of varying amounts of visual information on a balancing test. Ergonomics **9**, 325–333 (1966).

BEGBIE, G.H.: Some problems of postural sway. In: A.V.S. DE REUCK and K. KNIGHT, Eds. Myotatic, kinesthetic and vestibular mechanisms. Ciba Foundation Symposium London: Churchill 1967.

CANTRELL, R.P.: Body balance activity and perception. Percept. Mot. Skills **17**, 431–437 (1963).

DE HAAN, P.: The significance of optic stimuli in maintaining the equilibrium. Acta oto-laryng. (Stockh.) **50**, 109–115 (1959).

DUSEK, E.R.: Standardization of tests of gross motor performance. Tech. Rpt. EP-81. Natick, Mass.: U.S. army Hdqtrs. Rsch. Engineer. Command 1958.

FUKUDA, T., TOKITA, T.: A new arrangement of the vestibular examination. Acta oto-laryng. (Stockh.) Suppl. **179**, 122–137 (1963).

GOTO, K.: Vestibular reflex for 200 days after unilateral labyrinthotomy in Ménière's disease. J. Oto-Rhino-Laryng. Soc. Jap. **67**, 835–842 (1964).

HONJO, S., FURUKAWA, R.: The goniometer test. Ann. Otol. (St. Louis) **66**, 440–458 (1957).

KITAHARA, M., SATO, T.: Study on the accelerations in human subjects standing on the tilting plank. J. Jibirin. **57**, 57–63 (1964).

MORSH, J.R.: Motor performance of the deaf. Comp. Psychol. Monogr. **13**, 1–51 (1936).

MORSH, J.E.: A comparative study of deaf and hearing students. Amer. Ann. Deaf. **82**, 223–233 (1937).

MOSS, F.S.: New riding-comfort research instruments and wabble meter applications. S.A.E. J. **30**, 182–184 (1932).

OMWAKE, K.T.: Effect of varying periods of sleep on nervous activity. J. appl. Psychol. **16**, 623–632 (1932).

REYNOLDS, B.: Correlation between two psychomotor tasks as a function of practice on the first. J. exp. Psychol. **43**, 341–348 (1952).

RICALDONI, M.A.: Plate-forme mobile pour l'observation et l'enregistrement graphique du phenomena de Romberg et d'autres troubles de la statique. Bull. Mem. Soc. Hôp. Paris **52**, 1138–1145 (1928).

SEASHORE, H.G.: Some relationships of fine and gross motor abilities. Res. Quart. **13**, 259–274 (1942).

SLATER-HAMMEL, A.T.: Performance of selected groups of male college students on the Reynolds' balance test. Res. Quart. **27**, 347–351 (1956).

STEIN, S.: Appareil servant à determiner les déviations des fonctions du labyrinthe de l'orielle et sa demonstration. Congres. Internat. de Zool. **2**, 208–214 (1893).

6. "Rail Method," Consisting of Standing and/or Walking on Rails, Beams, or Sticks with Eyes Open or with Eyes Closed

ALDEN, F.D., HORTON, M.O., CALDWELL, G.M.: A motor ability test for university women for the classification of entering students into homogeneous groups. Res. Quart. **3**, 85–120 (1932).

AUXTER, D.M.: Proprioception among intellectually typical and differentially diagnosed educable mentally retarded boys. Percept. Mot. Skills **21**, 751–756 (1965).

BASS, R.L.: An analysis of the components of tests of semicircular canal function and of static and dynamic balance. Res. Quart. **10**, 33–52 (1939).

BECK, K.: Untersuchungen über den statischen Apparat von Gesunden und Taubstummen. Z. Psychol. Physiol. Sinnesorg. **46**, 362–378 (1911–1912).

BIRREN, J.E.: Static equilibrium and vestibular function. J. exp. Psychol. **35**, 127–133 (1945).

BRUCK, A.: Über die Beziehungen der Taubstummheit zum sogenannten statischen Sinn. Pflügers Arch. ges. Physiol. **59**, 16–42 (1895).

Callahan, F. E.: A study of the effect of the loss of visual cues and of flat-footedness on locomotor ability in relation to hearing loss. Unpub. Master's Thesis. Lawrence, Kansas: Univ. of Kansas 1958.

Carpenter, M. S.: Astronaut preparation. In: Results of the first United States manned orbital space flight, February 20, 1962. Houston, Texas: Manned Spacecraft Center, National Aeronautics and Space Administration 1962.

Cunningham, D. R.: Normative performance standards for three-hundred children on four subtests of the National Aeronautics and space Administration's floor ataxia test battery. Unpubl. Master's Thesis. Lawrence, Kansas: University of Kansas 1970.

Cunningham, D. R., Goetzinger, C. P.: Floor ataxia test battery. Arch. otolaryng. **96**, 559–564 (1972).

Cureton, T. K.: Physical fitness of champion athletes. Urbana, Ill.: Univ. of Illinois 1951.

Dain, C. A.: The measurement of dynamic balance in boys between ages 13 to 18 with a beam-walking test. Master's Thesis (unpubl.). Springfield, Mass.: Springfield College 1938.

Davey, P. R.: Clinical note: observation on equilibrium in deaf children. J. Laryng. **68**, 329–331 (1954).

Douglas, W. K.: Preparation of the astronaut. Aerospace Med. **34**, 232–235 (1963).

Dusek, E. R.: Standardization of tests of gross motor performance. Tech. Rpt. EP-81. Natick, Mass.: U.S. Army Hdqtrs. Rsch. Engineer. Command 1958.

Fisher, M. B., Birren, J. E., Leggett, A. L.: Standardization of two tests of equilibrium: the railwalking test and the ataxiagraph. J. exp. Psychol. **35**, 321–329 (1945).

Fleishman, E. A.: The structure and measurement of physical fitness. Englewood Cliffs, New Jersey: Prentice-Hall 1964.

Frisina, R.: Motor ability. Hlth. Phys. Educ. Recreat. Rev. **1**, 3–6 (1957).

Goetzinger, C. P.: A re-evaluation of the Heath rail-walking test. J. Educ. Rsch. **54**, 187–191 (1961).

Harris, C. S., von Gierke, H. E.: The effects of high intensity noise on human equilibrium. AMRL-TR-67-41. Wright-Patterson Air Force Base. Ohio: Aerospace Medical Research Laboratories 1967.

Harris, C. S., Sommer, H. S.: Human equilibrium during acoustic stimulation by discrete frequencies. AMRL-TR-67. Wright-Patterson Air Force Base. Ohio: Aerospace Medical Research Laboratories 1967.

Head, H.: The sense of stability and balance in the air. In: The medical problems of flying. Med. Rsch. Council, Spec. Rpt. Series, No. 53, 214–256 (1920).

Heath, S. R.: Rail-walking performance as related to mental age and etiological type among the mentally retarded. Amer. J. Psychol. **55**, 240–247 (1942).

Heath, S. R.: The military use of the rail-walking test as an index of locomotor coordination. Psychol. Bull. **40**, 282–284 (1943).

Heath, S. R.: Clinical significance of motor defect, with military implications. Amer. J. Psychol. **57**, 482–499 (1944).

Hertzberg, O. E.: The relationship of motor ability to the intelligence of kindergarten children. J. Educ. Psychol. **20**, 507–519 (1929).

Hicks, S. A.: The effects of four hours confinement in mobile armored personnel carriers on selected combat relevant skills; a pilot study. Tech. Memo 3–60, Aberdeen Proving Ground, Maryland 1960.

Kreidl, A.: Beiträge zur Physiologie des Ohrlabyrinths auf Grund von Versuchen an Taubstummen. Pflügers Arch. ges. Physiol. **51**, 119–150 (1892).

Leonard, J. A.: Static and mobile balancing performance of blind children. Unpubl. Rpt. Nottingham, England: Med. Rsch. Council, Univ. of Nottingham 1966.

Minners, H. A., Douglas, W. K., Knoblock, E. C., Graybiel, A., Hawkins, W. R.: Aeromedical preparation and results of postflight medical examinations. In: Results of the first United States manned orbital space flight, February 20, 1962. Houston, Texas: Manned Spacecraft Center, National Aeronautics and Space Administration 1962.

Minners, H. A., White, S. C., Douglas, W. K., Knoblock, E. C., Graybiel, A.: Aeromedical studies. Clinical aeromedical observations. In: Results of the second United States manned orbital space flight, May 24, 1962. NASA SP-6. Houston, Texas: Manned Spacecraft Center, National Aeronautics and Space Administration 1962a.

MYKLEBUST, H.R.: Significance of etiology in motor performance of deaf children with special reference to meningitis. Amer. J. Psychol. **59**, 249–258 (1946).

NEWSOM, B.D., BRADY, J.F., GOBLE, G.J.: Equilibrium and walking changes observed at 7 1/2, 10 and 12 RPM in the revolving space station simulator. Aerospace Med. **36**, 322–326 (1965).

NIXON, C.W., HARRIS, C.S., VON GIERKE, H.E.: Rail test to evaluate equilibrium in low-level wideband noise. AMRL-TR-66-85. Wright-Patterson Air Force Base. Ohio: Aerospace Medical Research Laboratories 1966.

PERRIN, F.A.C.: An experimental study of motor ability. J. exp. Psychol. **4**, 24–56 (1921).

SCANLON, S.L., GOETZINGER, C.P.: The Heath rails and Fukuda vestibular tests with deaf and hearing subjects. The Ear, Nose and Throat Monthly **48**, 8–15 (1969).

SEASHORE, H.G.: Some relationships of fine and gross motor abilities. Res. Quart. **13**, 259–274 (1942).

SEASHORE, H.G.: The development of a beam-walking test and its use in measuring development of balance in children. Res. Quart. **18**, 246–259 (1947).

VERNON, J.A., MCGILL, T.E., GULICK, W.I., CANDLAND, D.K.: Effect of sensory deprivation on some perceptual and motor skills. Percept. Mot. Skills **9**, 91–97 (1959).

WHITE, W.J., NYBERG, J.W., WHITE, P.D., GRIMES, R.H., FINNEY, L.M.: Biomedical potential of a centrifuge in an orbiting laboratory. SSD-TDR-64-209 Suppl. Douglas Rpt. SM-48703. Santa Monica, Calif.: Douglas Aircraft Co. 1965.

WHITNEY, E.: A beam-walking test of dynamic balance. Master's Thesis (unpubl.). Springfield, Mass.: Springfield College 1937.

YORK, E., BROWN, K.R., GOLDFIEN, A.: Catecholamine measurements associated with autonomic-labyrinthine responses in man exposed to positive ($+G_z$) acceleration. NADC-MR-6602. Johnsville, Penna.: Naval Air Development Center 1966.

7. Miscellaneous Devices and Techniques Including Force Plates, Electrobasometer, Elevated Platforms, Photographic Methods, Electromyography, Accelerometers, Strain Gauges, Galvanic Methods, and Treadmill

BABSKII, E.B., GURFINKEL, V.S., ROMEL, E.L.: Nova a metodika i nekotorye resul'taty issledovaniia vestibulomotornogo refleksa cheloveska prineadekuatom razdrazhenii vestibulamdgo apparata. Vestn. Oto-rino-laring. **14**, 19–22 (1952).

BÁRÁNY, J.W., ISMAIL, A.H., MANNING, K.R.: A force platform for the study of hemiplegic gait. Amer. Phys. Therapy Assoc. **45**, 693–699 (1965).

BASS, R.I.: An analysis of the components of tests of semicircular canal function and of static and dynamic balance. Res. Quart. **10**, 33–52 (1939).

COERMANN, R.R.: The mechanical impedance of the human body in sitting and standing position at low frequencies. ASD Tech. Rpt. 61-492. Wright-Patterson Air Force Base. Ohio: Aerospace Medical Laboratory 1961.

DAY, M.A.C.: Induced postural reflex reactions as related to the diagnosis of cerebellar and labyrinthine lesions. In: D. BENDERSKY, Ed. Medical application of NASA-developed science and technology. Quart. Prog. Rpt. 4, Jan.–March. Kansas City, Mo.: Medical Research Institute 1967.

DZENDOLET, E.: Sinusoidal electrical stimulation of the human vestibular apparatus. Percept. Mot. Skills **17**, 171–185 (1963).

DZENDOLET, E.: Effect of dramamine on the objective electrical vestibulogram. Percept. Mot. Skills **18**, 465–468 (1964).

EBERHART, H.D., INMAN, V.T.: An evaluation of experimental procedures used in a fundamental study of human locomotion. Ann. N.Y. Acad. Sci. **51**, 1213–1228 (1951).

ELFTMAN, H.: The basic pattern of human locomotion. Ann. N.Y. Acad. Sci. **51**, 1207–1212 (1951).

GALLE, R.R., YEMEL'YANOV, M.D.: Results of physiological studies performed in a slow rotation room. Kosmich. Biol. Med. **1**, 72–79 (1967). Trans. by Joint Pub. Res. Serv. JPRS **44**, 299 (1968).

GOLDBERG, L.: Quantitative studies on alcohol tolerance in man. Acta physiol. scand. **5**, Suppl. 16, 1–128 (1943).

Grieve, D.W., Gear, R.J.: The relationships between length of stride, step frequency, time of swing and speed of walking for children and adults. Ergonomics **5**, 379–399 (1966).

Guignard, J.C.: Effect of vibration of the head and of the whole body on the electromyographic activity of postural muscles in man. Some qualitative observations. FPRC Memo 120. Farnborough: Institute of Aviation Medicine 1959.

Hellebrandt, F.A., Braun, G.I.: Influence of sex and age on the postural sway of man. Amer. J. phys. Anthropol. **24**, 347–360 (1939).

Hellebrandt, F.A., Franseen, E.B.: Physiological study of vertical stance in man. Physiol. Rev. **23**, 220–255 (1943).

Hellebrandt, F.A., Riddle, K.S., Larsen, E.M., Fries, E.C.: Gravitational influences on postural alignment. Physiother. Rev. **22**, 143–149 (1942).

Henriksson, N.G., Johansson, G., Olsson, L.G., Östlund, H.: Electric analysis of the Romberg test. Acta oto-laryng. (Stockh.) Suppl. **224**, 272–279 (1967).

Hinoki, M., Kitahara, M.: An application of strain-gage-type instruments to the analysis of the equilibrium function in human subjects and animals. Acta oto-laryng. (Stockh.) Suppl. **179**, 110–121 (1963).

Hubbard, A.W., Stetson, R.H.: An experimental analysis of human locomotion. Amer. J. Physiol. **124**, 300–313 (1938).

Jonsson, R., Steen, B.: Function of the hip and thigh muscles in Romberg's test and "standing at ease." An electromyographic study. Acta morph. neerl.-scand. **5**, 269–276 (1963).

Joseph, J.: Man's posture. Electromyographic studies. Springfield, Ill.: C.C. Thomas 1960.

Kitahara, M.: Acceleration registrography. A new method of examinations with the labyrinthine righting reflex. Ann. Otol. (St. Louis) **74**, 203–214 (1965).

Morton, D.J.: Human locomotion and body form. Baltimore: Williams & Wilkins 1952.

Nashner, L.M.: Sensory feedback in human posture control. MVT-70-3. Cambridge, Mass.: Massachusetts Institute of Technology 1970.

Pezzoli, J.A., Moore, J.W.: Conditioned vestibular sway as a function of CS-UCS interval. Psychon. Sci. **5**, 461–462 (1966).

Schwartz, R.P., Vaeth, W.: A method for making graphic records of normal and pathological gait. J. Amer. med. Ass. **90**, 86–89 (1928).

Smith, K.U., Greene, D.: Scientific motion study and ageing processes in performance. Ergonomics **5**, 155–164 (1962).

Smith, K.U., McDermid, C.D., Shideman, F.E.: Analysis of the temporal components of motion in human gait. Amer. J. phys. Med. **39**, 142–151 (1960).

Chapter VI.

Arousal and Vestibular Habituation

By

W. E. Collins, Oklahoma City, Oklahoma (USA)

With 2 Figures

That vestibular responses might be affected by arousal, excitement, psychic states, or neural factors was noted as early as 1895 by Bach who stated that relatively weak nystagmus was generally produced in "stupid, indifferent or phlegmatic personalities" while anxious, easily excited individuals gave relatively stronger responses. Ruppert (1906) ascribed low thresholds and high-frequency nystagmus to the "increased nervous irritability" of the subject and Bárány (1907) commented on differences in vestibular responses between neurasthenics (abnormally fatigable patients) and normals. Claude, Baruk and Aubry (1927) reported markedly reduced nystagmus in catatonic (psychologically withdrawn) patients. Guttich (1914) began to approach the general problem of arousal and vestibular reactivity with his report that repeated administration of rotatory stimulation produced decrements in the duration of nystagmus. Rather than attributing the findings to "habituation," Guttich (1914) indicated that the response decline was probably a result of a lessening of nervous tension from the first test through the following series of rotations — a kind of situational or psychological adaptation. Griffith (1920) noted that subjects rotated on a daily basis showed a decline in nystagmus with repeated stimulation, but that an appreciable increase in nystagmus duration, number of eye movements, and duration of apparent movement of the visual field occurred when subjects had been engaging in "violent exercise" just prior to testing.

On the basis of several studies which reported vestibular response reduction (e.g. Dodge, 1923; Fearing, 1926; Griffith, 1920; Mowrer, 1934a), Fearing and Mowrer (1934) examined the effects of anesthesia on habituation of rotation-induced head nystagmus in pigeons in an effort to evaluate the possibility that either a functional change in the central nervous system or a structural modification of the vestibular receptors was involved in the habituation process. They reported no habituation in anesthetized animals and a clear reduction in nystagmus for undrugged birds. From incidental observations made during that study, Mowrer (1934b) became probably the first investigator to attempt to manipulate arousal factors and examine their influence on vestibular responses. Working with pigeons, Mowrer (1934b) differentiated between "excited" and "unexcited" conditions, depending upon how the birds were prepared for rotation trials, and reported longer durations of nystagmus in the "excited" condition. His astute interpretation of the findings, based also on previous studies, was that "excitement" influenced the vestibular reaction but that it could not account completely for the reduction produced by repeated stimulation. Similarly, WENDT (1936, 1951) noted that immobilized animals sometimes went into sleep-like states ("animal hypnosis") and that various types of stimuli (e.g. auditory or tactile) restored alertness and reinstated apparently suppressed nystagmus is some cases. HOOD and PFALTZ (1954), like MOWRER (1934b), reported temporary increases in frequency of nystagmus in rabbits when they appeared excited, and, further, noted that injections of adrenaline in rabbits which had shown substantial response declines to repeated rotation produced a partial recovery of nystagmus. A result identical to the latter was obtained by CRAMPTON and SCHWAM (1961), who used intermittent electric shock and auditory signals as excitatory stimuli during repeated rotation of cats.

WENDT (1951) was apparently the first to attempt a definition of "excitement" or "arousal" in terms of conditions basic to the state of the subject, and to relate these to the problem of habituation. He cited two factors in habituation: in one case, repeated rotatory stimulation under conditions providing opportunities for visual fixation would result in an increasing dominance of the visual stimuli and thereby inhibit nystagmus; in the other case, under conditions of darkness, an "inward orientation of attention" would account for nystagmus reduction while an "environment-directed orientation" would restore nystagmus or prevent its decline.

Primarily on the basis of WENDT's (1951) notions regarding mental or attentional states, COLLINS, CRAMPTON and POSNER (1961) evaluated several instructional procedures aimed at controlling alertness during rotational stimulation of human subjects (tested with eyes open in total darkness) and demonstrated that both quantity and quality of nystagmic output could be manipulated in the same subject by instructions regarding mental activity. If subjects were asked to relax, daydream, and pursue no particular line of thought ("reverie"), relatively weak nystagmic responses were recorded; vigorous nystagmus was obtained when the same subjects performed continuous mental arithmetic (successive division) or signalled turning sensations in 90° intervals (cf. VON BÉKÉSY, 1955; GROEN and JONGKEES, 1948). It is of additional interest that simultaneously recorded EEG alpha activity was not blocked as a result of the angular accelerations and did not appear to be affected by the different instructions, although nystagmus was markedly influenced. These EEG and nystagmus findings were confirmed in a later study (COLLINS and POSNER, 1963) which concluded that, at least under some conditions, EEG monitoring might be a less sensitive indicator of states of alertness than vestibularly-induced eye movements. PENDLETON and PAINE (1961) made a similar observation with newborn infants, and LIDVALL (1962) noted stable alpha activity and lack of blocking during caloric vestibular stimulation. More recently, GOTO, TOKUMASU and COHEN (1968) concluded that (excluding barbiturates or deep sleep) "the frequency and velocity of rapid eye movements are among the most sensitive indices of alertness of any, including the EEG."

Several studies reported that mental tasks or increased alertness produced regular nystagmus in place of dysrhythmic responses (Fig. 1). MAHONEY, HARLAN and BICKFORD (1957) presented electro-oculographic evidence that short periods of arithmetic calculation by subjects given caloric irrigations occasioned brief bursts of nystagmus with eyes closed (a nystagmic response might not otherwise

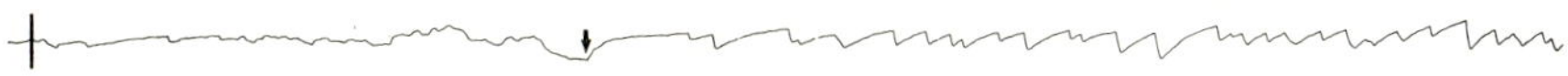

Fig. 1. The effect on caloric nystagmus of alerting a subject. The vertical bar indicates the end of the irrigation; the arrow denotes the point at which the subject (eyes open in darkness) was admonished to "be alert." The tracing represents 42 sec of recording

be evident) and produced higher-frequency, more stable nystagmus when the subjects' eyes were open. LIDVALL (1961) gave an arithmetic problem to a subject with severe nystagmic dysrhythmia (caloric stimulus) and thereby evoked regular nystagmus. GUEDRY, COLLINS and SHEFFEY (1961) noted that inadvertent mental alerting of subjects during repeated rotatory stimulation produced a marked increase in nystagmic activity, while GUEDRY and LAUVER (1961) and COLLINS and GUEDRY (1962) accounted for their own and other data, which indicated declining nystagmus (adaptation) during a period of prolonged angular acceleration, on the basis of tasks assigned to the subjects. If subjects performed mental arithmetic during the prolonged accelerations, there was no decay of nystagmus during the stimulus period.

A series of investigations by COLLINS (1962, 1963, 1964, 1965) has examined in more detail the influence of arousal (to the extent that it is affected by instructions regarding mental activity) on nystagmic reactions. By employing different instructions (continuous mental arithmetic, "reverie," signalling turning sensations, and time estimations of auditory stimuli), it was found that the relaxed state ("reverie") produced significantly less nystagmus than any of the three tasks; mental arithmetic tasks yielded the most nystagmus (COLLINS, 1962). For some subjects, almost no nystagmus was recorded during a "reverie" state even though the subjects were engaged in their first rotatory experience in the laboratory (see Fig. 2). The results also point to the fact that inward- vs. outward-directed orientations probably do not account for the influence of the instructions on nystagmic output since both "reverie" and mental arithmetic may be classified as "inward-directed." What appears to be of importance is that the subject be in a sufficiently aroused or active mental state, whether the arousal arises from attending to his sensations, pursuing a particular line of thought, performing mental calculations, or responding to auditory or other stimuli. It should be noted that not all instructions are effective in this regard. Some tasks, such as counting, may not produce any noticeable effect on nystagmus (LIDVALL, 1962), while others, such as tasks involving timing behavior, appear to require relatively little attention with repetition (COLLINS, 1962).

The influence of instructions is not limited to rotatory conditions. Clear differences occur in the amount of slow-phase eye displacement generated by caloric stimuli, favoring mental arithmetic over "reverie" conditions in total darkness (COLLINS, 1963, 1965; COLLINS, GUEDRY and POSNER, 1962). In addition (1) the duration of nystagmus following caloric irrigations in the light or in the dark is significantly longer, and (2) qualitative ratings of nystagmus observed in the light are higher for mental arithmetic than for "reverie" instructions (COLLINS, GUEDRY and POSNER, 1962).

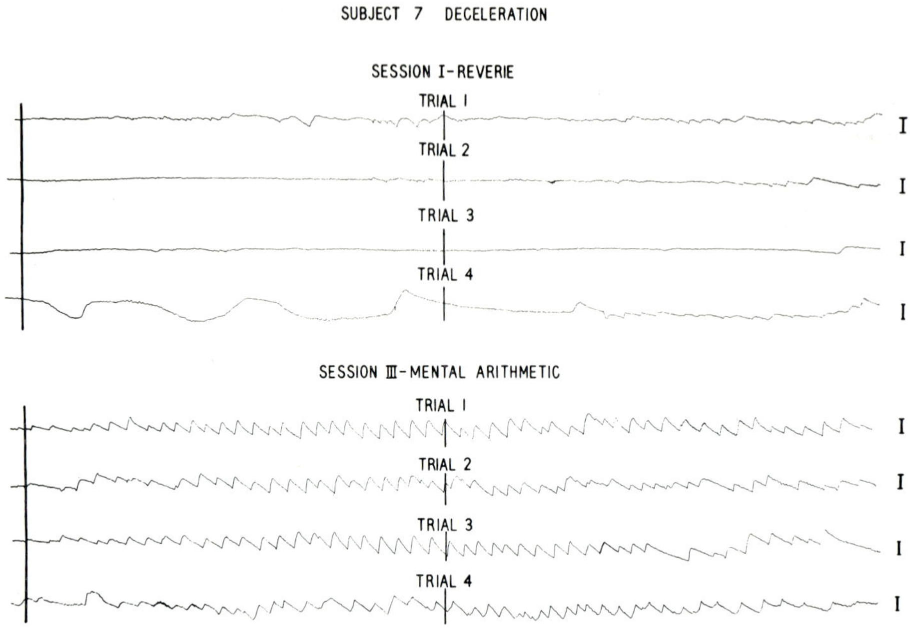

Fig. 2. The influence of instructions on vestibular nystagmus (see text). Vertical bars through the tracings demarcate a 15-sec period of angular deceleration at 4.5°/sec². Markers at the end of each tracing indicate 20° eye calibrations. Recordings were obtained from a subject with eyes open in total darkness. Sessions were held on separate days; trials were consecutive on a given day. The "reverie" task was given to this subject during his first exposure to laboratory vestibular stimulation (Reprinted with permission from the Journal of Experimental Psychology: COLLINS, 1962)

Drugs have also been used to affect alertness. CRAMPTON (1964) introduced the use of d-amphetamine in an effort to maintain arousal levels in the cat; recorded amplitude of nystagmus was increased but the usual rapid reduction of nystagmus occurred with repeated rotation. DOWD (1964) reported an increase in recorded amplitude, but no change in phase relationships of nystagmus during sinusoidal acceleration of cats treated with d-amphetamine; sodium pentobarbital depressed the response. On the other hand, CENACCHI, FENU and GABRIELLI (1964) reported decreased nystagmus in rabbits with various amounts of amphetamine.

WOLFE (1968) has noted that the dosage levels of d-amphetamine that have been used to maintain animal alertness may have some undesirable side effects; some animals become ataxic and appear to have vestibulocerebellar impairment. In addition, the influence of the drug on eye-movement calibrations has been neglected. The importance of the latter was noted by JONGKEES and PHILIPSZOON (1960, 1964) who reported enhancement of rabbit nystagmus with hyoscine and also a slight increase in the (corneoretinal potential) eye-calibration signal. Other drugs such as chlorpromazine and cinnarzine, which have a soporific effect, have been shown to reduce rabbit nystagmus (BERGMANN and GUTMAN, 1962; JONGKEES and PHILIPSZOON, 1960, 1964) without altering the eye-calibration signal (JONGKEES and PHILIPSZOON, 1960, 1964).

The arousal variable which influences the vestibular response does not, however, appear to be simply one of physical tension or drug-enhanced physiological activity. COLLINS and POE (1962) gave subjects mild doses of amphetamine (which significantly increased cardiovascular parameters) and compared the drug and no-drug conditions with both mental arithmetic and "reverie" instructions. There were no statistical differences in total slow-phase eye displacement or duration of nystagmus between the drug and no-drug conditions, but nystagmus was significantly more pronounced during mental arithmetic than in "reverie" trials. Furthermore, HARRIS, GUEDRY and GRAYBIEL (1962) increased positional alcohol nystagmus (PAN) in subjects by means of mental arithmetic problems, but could produce no effect on PAN with a hand-clenching task.

A number of studies (e.g. BARBER and WRIGHT, 1967; BENSON, GOORNEY and REASON, 1966; BRAND, 1968; DOWD, 1966; GILLINGHAM, 1969; LACHMAN, AARONS and ERIKSON, 1968; MARSHALL and BROWN, 1966; SOKOLOVSKI, 1963; TOROK, 1970) have confirmed that assigned tasks or instructions regarding mental activity are important in the maintenance of vigorous nystagmus or the restoration of an attenuated response. Instructions have been effective with drugs (COLLINS and POE, 1962; BENSON and BRAND, 1968), with alcohol (SCHROEDER, 1971, 1972), with positional alcohol nystagmus (HARRIS et al., 1962), and in conjunction with hypnosis (ASCHAN, FINER and HAGBARTH, 1962), although, in one report (JOHNER and PERLMAN, 1968) hypnotized subjects showed suppressed nystagmus (and, frequently, slow pendular eye movements) in spite of assigned tasks. Under some laboratory conditions, mental tasks appeared effective in reducing or preventing motion sickness with unusual vestibular stimulation (CORREIA and GUEDRY, 1964, 1966; GUEDRY, 1964). Further, the absence of alertness or arousal, whatever its neuro-psycho-physiological cause, is probably a major factor in vestibular findings which indicate substantial or total suppression of nystagmic responses in schizophrenic patients (e.g. ANGYAL and BLACKMAN, 1940; CLAUDE et al., 1927; COLBERT, KOEGLER and MARKHAM, 1959; POLLACK and KRIEGER, 1958). Patients who show these subnormal vestibular reactions are frequently characterized as apathetic, indifferent, lacking in initiative, and showing a poverty of mental content. More recent work with autistic children has shown a similar depression of nystagmus (RITVO, ORNITZ, EVIATAR, MARKHAM, BROWN and MASON, 1969). However, the latter deficit has been attributed to vestibular dysfunction in a schema which assigns to the vestibular system the role of regulating the mutual interaction of sensory input and motor output during the waking state and in REM sleep (ORNITZ, 1970).

It is sometimes suggested that the use of mental tasks to maintain arousal level represents an artificial means of preventing or interfering with the habituation process. That is, in the absence of structured mental activity, an overall suppression of nystagmus rapidly appears. It is quite apparent that a decline of nystagmus can occur with relatively few stimulus repetitions in total darkness when subjects are uninstructed regarding arousal. It is equally apparent that any inadvertent alerting of such subjects will result in the reappearance of a vigorous nystagmus (GUEDRY, COLLINS and SHEFFEY, 1961). However, since "reverie" assignments can result in almost no nystagmus to an otherwise adequate rotational stimulus during the first exposure to laboratory angular accelerations (COLLINS,

1962), it seems proper to differentiate between situational or perhaps psychological habituation as opposed to habituation of the vestibular system *per se*. If interest centers around true changes in vestibular functioning as a result of repeated testing, it would appear to be an experimental prerequisite to attempt to effect some control over the mental state of the subject. This is particularly true when subjects are repeatedly tested in total darkness or with their eyes closed; the tendency to doze under such conditions is probably very strong.

References

Angyal, A., Blackman, N.: Vestibular reactivity in schizophrenia. Arch. Neurol. Psychiat. (Chic.) **44**, 611–620 (1940).

Aschan, G., Finer, B.L., Hagbarth, K.E.: The influence of hypnotic suggestion on vestibular nystagmus. Acta oto-laryng. (Stockh.) **55**, 97–110 (1962).

Bach, L.: Über künstlich erzeugten Nystagmus bei normalen Individuen und bei Taubstummen. Arch. Augenheilk. **30**, 10–14 (1895).

Bárány, R.: Weitere Untersuchungen über den vom Vestibularapparat des Ohres reflektorisch ausgelösten Nystagmus und seine Begleiterscheinungen. Mschw. Ohrenheilk. **41**, 477–526 (1907).

Barber, H., Wright, G.: Release of nystagmus suppression in clinical electronystagmography. Laryngoscope (St. Louis) **77**, 1016–1027 (1967).

Békésy, G. von: Subjective cupulometry. Arch. Otolaryng. **61**, 16–28 (1955).

Benson, A.J., Brand, J.J.: Some effects of l-hyascine hydrobromide on post-rotatory sensation and nystagmus in man. Quart. J. exp. Physiol. **53**, 296–311 (1968).

Benson, A.J., Goorney, A.B., Reason, J.T.: The effect of instructions upon post-rotational sensations and nystagmus. Acta oto-laryng. (Stockh.) **62**, 442–452 (1966).

Bergmann, F., Gutman, J.: Effect of Largactil on various forms of nystagmus. Psychopharm. Serv. Cent. Bull. **2**, 57–58 (1962).

Brand, J.J.: The effect of repetition on measurements of post-rotational turning sensation and nystagmus in man. Quart. J. exp. Physiol. **53**, 312–326 (1968).

Cenacchi, V., Fenu, G., Gabrielli, L.: L'azione dell' amfetamina sulla risposta nistagmica da stimoli rotacceleratori. Studio sperimentale condotta sul coniglio. Bull. Soc. ital. Biol. sper. (Napoli) **41**, 527–530 (1964).

Claude, H., Baruk, H., Aubry, M.: Contribution a l'étude de la démence précoce catatonique: Inexcitabilité labyrinthique au cours de la catatonie. Rev. Neurol. **1**, 976–980 (1927).

Colbert, E.G., Koegler, R.R., Markham, C.H.: Vestibular dysfunction in childhood schizophrenia. Arch. gen. Psychiat. **1**, 600–617 (1959).

Collins, W.E.: Effects of mental set upon vestibular nystagmus. J. exp. Psychol. **63**, 191–197 (1962).

Collins, W.E.: Manipulation of arousal and its effects upon human vestibular nystagmus induced by caloric irrigation and angular accelerations. Aerospace Med. **34**, 124–129 (1963).

Collins, W.E.: Task-control of arousal and the effects of repeated unidirectional angular acceleration on human vestibular responses. Acta oto-laryng. (Stockh.) Suppl. **190**, 1–34 (1964).

Collins, W.E.: Subjective responses and nystagmus following repeated unilateral caloric stimulation. Ann. Otol. (St. Louis) **74**, 1034–1054 (1965).

Collins, W.E., Crampton, G.H., Posner, J.B.: Effects of mental activity upon vestibular nystagmus and the electroencephalogram. Nature (Lond.) **190**, 194–195 (1961).

Collins, W.E., Guedry, F.E.: Arousal effects and nystagmus during prolonged constant angular acceleration. Acta oto-laryng. (Stockh.) **54**, 349–362 (1962).

Collins, W.E., Guedry, F.E., Posner, J.B.: Control of caloric nystagmus by manipulating arousal and visual fixation distance. Ann. Otol. (St. Louis) **71**, 187–202 (1962).

Collins, W.E., Poe, R.H.: Amphetamine, arousal, and human vestibular nystagmus. J. Pharmacol. exp. Ther. **138**, 120–125 (1962).

Collins, W.E., Posner, J.B.: Electroencephalogram alpha activity during mild vestibular stimulation. Nature (Lond.) **199**, 933–934 (1963).

CORREIA, M.J., GUEDRY, F.E.: Modification of vestibular responses as a function of rate of rotation about an earth-horizontal axis. Acta oto-laryng. (Stockh.) **62**, 297–308 (1966).

CRAMPTON, G.H.: Habituation of ocular nystagmus of vestibular origin. In: M.B. BENDER, Ed. The Oculomotor System, pp. 332–346. New York: Harper & Row 1964.

CRAMPTON, G.H., SCHWAM, W.J.: Effects of arousal reaction on nystagmus habituation in the cat. Amer. J. Physiol. **200**, 29–33 (1961).

DODGE, R.: Habituation to rotation. J. exp. Psychol. **6**, 1–35 (1923).

DOWD, P.J.: Responses of the habituated vestibulo-ocular reflex arc to drug stress. USAF SAM-TDR-64-72, Brooks AFB, Texas, 1964.

DOWD, P.J.: Factors affecting vestibular nystagmus in coriolis stimulation. Acta oto-laryng. (Stockh.) **61**, 228–236 (1966).

FEARING, F.S.: Post-rotational head nystagmus in adult pigeons. J. comp. Psychol. **6**, 115–131 (1926).

FEARING, F.S., MOWRER, O.H.: The effect of general anesthesia upon the experimental reduction of vestibular nystagmus. J. gen. Psychol. **11**, 133–144 (1934).

GILLINGHAM, K.K.: Mental arithmetic during electronystagmographic testing. Ann. Otol. (St. Louis) **78**, 575–586 (1969).

GOTO, K., TOKUMASU, K., COHEN, B.: Return eye movements, saccadic movements, and the quick phase of nystagmus. Acta oto-laryng. (Stockh.) **65**, 426–440 (1968).

GRIFFITH, C.R.: The organic effects of repeated bodily rotation. J. exp. Psychol. **3**, 15–47 (1920).

GROEN, J.J., JONGKEES, L.B.W.: The turning test with small regulable stimuli. IV. The cupulogram obtained by subjective angle estimation. J. Laryng. **62**, 236–240 (1948).

GUEDRY, F.E.: Visual control of habituation to complex vestibular stimulation in man. Acta oto-laryng. (Stockh.) **58**, 377–389 (1964).

GUEDRY, F.E., COLLINS, W.E., SHEFFEY, P.L.: Perceptual and oculomotor reactions to interacting visual and vestibular stimulation. Percept. Mot. Skills **12**, 307–324 (1961).

GUEDRY, F.E., LAUVER, L.S.: Vestibular reactions during prolonged constant angular acceleration. J. appl. Physiol. **16**, 215–220 (1961).

GUTTICH, A.: Beitrag zur Physiologie des Vestibularapparates. Beitr. Anat. Physiol. **7**, 1–18 (1914).

HARRIS, C.S., GUEDRY, F.E., GRAYBIEL, A.: Positional alcohol nystagmus in relation to labyrinthine function. USNSAM-NASA Jt. Rep. No. 76, Pensacola, Florida, 1962.

HOOD, J.F., PFALTZ, C.R.: Observations upon the effects of repeated stimulation upon rotational and caloric nystagmus. J. Physiol. (Lond.) **124**, 130–144 (1954).

JOHNER, C.H., PERLMAN, H.B.: Hypnosis and vestibular function. Ann. Otol. (St. Louis) **77**, 126–138 (1968).

JONGKEES, L.B.W., PHILIPSZOON, A.J.: Some nystagmographical methods for the investigation of the effect of drugs upon the labyrinth. Acta physiol. pharmacol. neerl. **9**, 240–275 (1960).

JONGKEES, L.B.W., PHILIPSZOON, A.J.: Electronystagmography. Acta oto-laryng. (Stockh.) Suppl. **189**, 1–111 (1964).

LACHMAN, J., AARONS, L., ERIKSON, J.H.: Nystagmus: A parameter of mental function. Percept. Mot. Skills **26**, 943–950 (1968).

LIDVALL, H.F.: Vertigo and nystagmus responses to caloric stimuli repeated at short intervals. Acta oto-laryng. (Stockh.) **53**, 33–44 (1961).

LIDVALL, H.F.: Specific and non-specific traits of habituation in nystagmus responses to caloric stimuli. Acta oto-laryng. (Stockh.) **55**, 315–325 (1962).

MAHONEY, J.L., HARLAN, W.L., BICKFORD, R.G.: Visual and other factors influencing caloric nystagmus in normal subjects. Arch. Otolaryng. **66**, 46–53 (1957).

MARSHALL, J.E., BROWN, J.H.: Visual-arousal interaction and specificity of nystagmic habituation. USAMRL Report No. 688, Ft. Knox, Kentucky, 1966.

MOWRER, O.H.: The modification of vestibular nystagmus by means of repeated elicitation. Comp. psychol. Monog., **9**, (No. 45), 1–48 (1934a).

MOWRER, O.H.: Influence of "excitement" on the duration of post rotational nystagmus. Arch. Otolaryng. **19**, 46–54 (1934b).

Ornitz, E. M.: Vestibular dysfunction in schizophrenia and childhood autism. Comp. Psychiat. **11**, 159–173 (1970).

Pendleton, M. E., Paine, R. S.: Vestibular nystagmus in newborn infants. Neurology **11**, 450–458 (1961).

Pollack, M., Krieger, H. P.: Oculomotor and postural patterns in schizophrenic children. Arch. Neurol. Psychiat. (Chic.) **79**, 720–726 (1958).

Ritvo, E. R., Ornitz, E. M., Eviatar, A., Markham, C. H., Brown, M. B., Mason, A.: Decreased post-rotatory nystagmus in early infantile autism. Neurology **19**, 653–658 (1969).

Ruppert, J.: Untersuchungen über den Drehnystagmus. Zbl. inn. Med. **27**, 465–478 (1906).

Schroeder, D. J.: Influence of alcohol on vestibular responses to angular acceleration. Aerospace Med. **42**, 959–970 (1971).

Schroeder, D. J.: Some effects of alcohol on nystagmus and "vertigo" during caloric and optokinetic stimulation. Ann. Otol. (St. Louis) **81**, 218–230 (1972).

Sokolovski, A.: Factors influencing nystagmus due to rotation in normal subjects. J. Laryng. **77**, 185–201 (1963).

Torok, N.: The effects of arousal upon vestibular nystagmus. Advanc. Oto-Rhino-Laryng. **17**, 76–89 (1970).

Wendt, G. R.: An interpretation of inhibition of conditioned reflexes as competition between reaction systems. Psychol. Rev. **43**, 258–281 (1936).

Wendt, G. R.: Vestibular functions. In: S. S. Stevens, Ed. Handbook of Experimental Psychology. New York: Wiley, 1191–1223, 1951.

Wolfe, J. W.: Evidence for control of nystagmic habituation by foliumtuber vermis and fastigial nuclei. Acta oto-laryng. (Stockh.) Suppl. **231**, 1–48 (1968).

Chapter VII.

Habituation of Vestibular Responses with and without Visual Stimulation

By

W. E. Collins, Oklahoma City, Oklahoma (USA)

With 8 Figures

Contents

I. Introduction

In vestibular physiology, the term "habituation" is frequently used interchangeably with "response reduction" to indicate the effects of repeated stimulation. This phenomenon differs from "fatigue," a temporary state for which brief intervals of rest are usually sufficient for recovery of the response, and from "adaptation," a special type of response decline--one which occurs during a prolonged stimulus. More specifically, "habituation" refers to a relatively long-lasting change; even extended rest periods (48 hours to several weeks) may not be sufficient to restore the response to its original level or form.

The fact that reductions in vestibular responses might occur with repeated stimulation was discussed many years ago. Directional differences in the reactions of experienced dancers were noted by both Ruppert (1906) and Bárány (1907) with reference to nystagmus and by Abels (1906) with reference to dizziness. Responses obtained from such individuals appeared weaker when they were turning in the practiced direction. Abels (1906) apparently borrowed the term "habituation" from Hitzig to describe the gradually acquired ability to inhibit the symptoms of sea sickness. A whole literature on habituation has developed since these early reports. Data and views have at one time or another supported the complete spectrum of possible effects of repeated stimulation on vestibular responses (no change, total suppression, response modification).

II. Vestibular Habituation in Animals

Repeated vestibular stimulation of alert animals produces a suppression of nystagmic reactions (e.g. FERNÁNDEZ and SCHMIDT, 1962a, b; WINGET and SMITH, 1962), but the response reduction is relatively specific to certain conditions of practice. Thus, repeated unidirectional stimulation, whether rotatory or caloric, results in a reduction of nystagmus duration, frequency of eye movement, and slow-phase eye displacement (see Fig. 1). The fast phase of the eye movement may also decline in velocity (see Fig. 2). Responses in the unpracticed direction are, at least initially, relatively unaffected by a unidirectional habituation series (ABELS, 1906; BROWN and MARSHALL, 1967; CAPPS and COLLINS, 1965; COLLINS, 1964a; COLLINS and UPDEGRAFF, 1966, 1970; CRAMPTON, 1962a; HENRIKSSON et al., 1961; MERTENS and COLLINS, 1967; PROCTOR and FERNÁNDEZ, 1963). There may be some tendency for the previously unpracticed direction to decline more rapidly from trial to trial with additional stimulation (CAPPS and COLLINS, 1965; MERTENS and COLLINS, 1967), and it is possible that responses in the un-

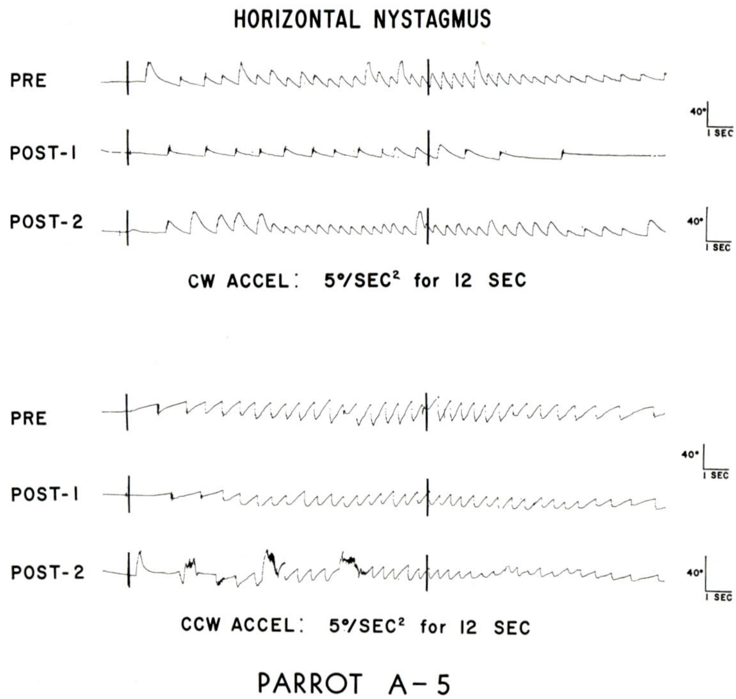

Fig. 1. Directional specificity of habituation of ocular nystagmus in an African parrot. A series of 15 CW angular accelerations (decelerations were subthreshold) was administered between the pre- and post-1 tests. A directionally specific reduction is evident. Post-2 tests, conducted 2 weeks later, show recovery. The bird was rotated under head and body restraint in total darkness. Vertical bars demarcate the stimulus period; optokinetically derived calibration markers are to the right of the tracings. Similar effects are obtained from other animals (Reprinted with permission from Acta oto-laryng. (Stockh.): COLLINS and UPDEGRAFF, 1970)

practiced direction might be affected more if the habituation series comprises a very large number of stimulations. Thus, most of the studies cited above used only 10–20 tests in the habituation series. DUNLAP (1925) obtained a clearly weak nystagmic reaction for the unpracticed direction of response after well over 100 unilateral irrigations in rabbits.

Following habituation, a stronger stimulus will elicit vigorous nystagmic reactions (CAPPS and COLLINS, 1965; GRIFFITH, 1920d; MAXWELL et al., 1922; MERTENS and COLLINS, 1967). However, these responses are lower than the pre-habituation levels (GRIFFITH, 1920d) and may even be reduced to the same level as would have been obtained had the stronger stimulus been used in the habituation series. This appears to be the case at least for caloric stimulation with less than 20 habituation trials (CAPPS and COLLINS, 1965; MERTENS and COLLINS, 1967).

Nystagmic reactions alternately elicited in opposite directions show clear and relatively independent declines for both caloric and rotatory stimulation (CAPPS and COLLINS, 1965; COLLINS, 1967; HENRIKSSON et al., 1961; MERTENS and COLLINS, 1967). That is, driving nystagmus in one direction, after a response in the opposite direction has been elicited, does not seem to alter significantly whatever neurophysiological changes occurred as a result of the first stimulation. Certainly no homeostatic restoration is effected. Nor do succeeding responses in a given direction appear to decline significantly faster as a result of interspersing opposed stimuli than they would if a unidirectional response were repetitively elicited. However, as noted earlier, a number of consecutive unidirectional stimulations may exert some influence on the rate of decline of responses in the opposite direction.

Opportunities for visual still-fixation during and following a vestibular stimulus, or following an angular deceleration during which optokinetic stimulation occurs, results in very brief after-nystagmus (CRAMPTON, 1962b; HENDERSON, 1947; HUDDLESTON, 1930; MOWRER, 1934a, 1935; PILZ, 1926a, 1926b). Such a response can be markedly attenuated or even abolished with repeated stimulation (ABELS, 1906; DUNLAP, 1925; HENDERSON, 1947; HUDDLESTON, 1930; MAXWELL et al., 1922; MOWRER, 1934; PILZ, 1926a). The influence of visual stimulation during habituation on nystagmic reactions in darkness is difficult to assess. MOWRER (1934a) reported different results depending upon whether pigeons' heads were fixed or free and whether still-fixation opportunities or optokinetic stimulation (enhancing or opposing the vestibular response) were available during rotation. CRAMPTON (1962b) found no influence of optokinetic stimulation on nystagmus in cats rotated in darkness during eight habituation trials. A differential effect between the two conditions might require a large number of trials (particularly when habituation is rapidly acquired in darkness), or may best be reflected in retention over long time periods (as with massed and spaced practice), or it may require active attempts to use vision to suppress the vestibular response. Too little information on visual-vestibular interaction during habituation of animals is available for firm conclusions regarding its effects on responses in darkness.

Studies comparing head-fixed and head-free conditions during habituation (KING, 1926; LUMPKIN, 1927; MOWRER, 1934a) are also difficult to assess. The

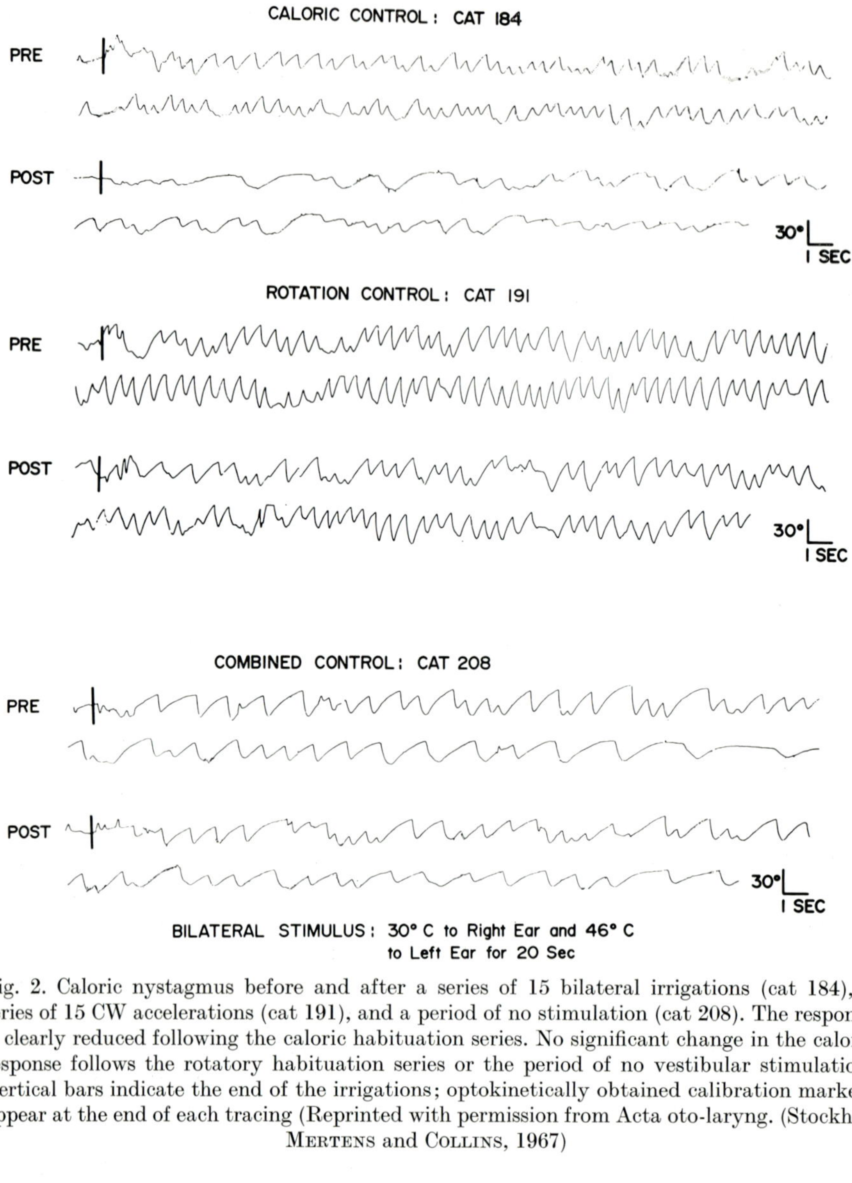

Fig. 2. Caloric nystagmus before and after a series of 15 bilateral irrigations (cat 184), a series of 15 CW accelerations (cat 191), and a period of no stimulation (cat 208). The response is clearly reduced following the caloric habituation series. No significant change in the caloric response follows the rotatory habituation series or the period of no vestibular stimulation. Vertical bars indicate the end of the irrigations; optokinetically obtained calibration markers appear at the end of each tracing (Reprinted with permission from Acta oto-laryng. (Stockh.): MERTENS and COLLINS, 1967)

vestibular stimulus may be effectively weaker in the head-free condition, since during angular acceleration the head of the rabbit (like that of the pigeon) may assume a compensatory position and at the same time produce slow nystagmus, initiated by neck reflexes, opposing the vestibular signal (MAXWELL et al., 1922). Reflex impulses from the neck may be centrally integrated with the vestibular signal and may effectively reduce that signal by cancellation in a way similar to which "double irrigations" (COLLINS, 1965a) can cancel nystagmus and produce no habituation (see SALA, 1965, for another possible explanation). However, other complicating factors were present in these studies; most have already been noted with respect to MOWRER'S (1934a, 1935) findings on the influence of vision. Additional problems include (1) voluntary head movements made by head-free pigeons (HUDDLESTON, 1930) and probably also by rabbits; and (2) the possibility that the plane in which the animal holds its head differs depending upon the visual condition, as well as being different for a head-fixed condition.

Central rather than peripheral mechanisms appear to form the underlying basis of habituation. The following findings support this view: (1) the intervals between stimulations can be as short as several minutes or as long as several days (BROWN, 1965; CRAMPTON, 1964; CRAMPTON and SCHWAM, 1961; HENRIKSSON et al., 1961; HOOD and PFALTZ, 1954); (2) the response does not recover its initial level for several weeks (BROWN, 1965; CAPPS and COLLINS, 1965; COLLINS and UPDEGRAFF, 1966; DUNLAP, 1925; FEARING, 1940, 1941; HALSTEAD, 1935; HALSTEAD et al., 1937; HENRIKSSON et al., 1961; HOOD and PFALTZ, 1954; MERTENS and COLLINS, 1967; PROCTOR and FERNÁNDEZ, 1963); (3) spacing of trials over several days results in greater retention of habituation than massing the trials in a single session (BROWN, 1965; FEARING, 1940, 1941); (4) repeated peripheral stimulation under special conditions (see Fig. 3) fails to produce habituation (anesthetized animals: FEARING and MOWRER, 1934; HENRIKSSON et al., 1961; HOOD and PFALTZ, 1954; "double irrigations": COLLINS, 1965a; interspersing long periods of centrifugation between habituation stimuli: WINGET, SMITH and KELLY, 1962); (5) habituation to unilateral caloric stimulation shows transfer to "equivalent" caloric stimuli (i.e. caloric stimuli which drive nystagmus in the same direction, irrespective of the ear stimulated or the temperature of water used), but not to "nonequivalent" irrigations (CAPPS and COLLINS, 1965; COLLINS, 1964a; HENRIKSSON et al., 1961; PROCTOR and FERNÁNDEZ, 1963); and (6) that habituation is probably specific to the position of the otoliths and other gravireceptors (COLLINS, 1969; COLLINS and UPDEGRAFF, 1970). The latter point may also account for the failure to obtain transfer of habituation from caloric to rotatory (COLLINS, 1964a; MERTENS and COLLINS, 1967) or from rotatory to caloric stimulation (COLLINS, 1964b; HOOD and PFALTZ, 1954; MAXWELL et al., 1922; MERTENS and COLLINS, 1967), since the position of the head (and therefore the pattern of neural signals from specific and nonspecific gravireceptors) differs for the two stimulus conditions. The only study which reported complete transfer of habituation from caloric to rotatory stimulation (DUNLAP, 1925) may have maintained a single head position for both conditions.

A final point with respect to central effects is the conditioned opposed reaction obtained from leghorns by FUKUDA et al. (1958). With vision excluded, repeated angular accelerations not only reduced after-nystagmus of the head, but produced a conditioned reversal of the usual compensatory positioning of the head and body. Since the bodies of the animals were not fixed, the birds had to make active efforts to maintain their position on a perch during stimulation. This situation is similar to studies in which conditioned opposed reactions have also been obtained as a result of human subjects actively attempting to adapt to the disruptive effects of head movements made during rotation (e.g. GUEDRY and GRAYBIEL, 1962; GUEDRY, 1965a).

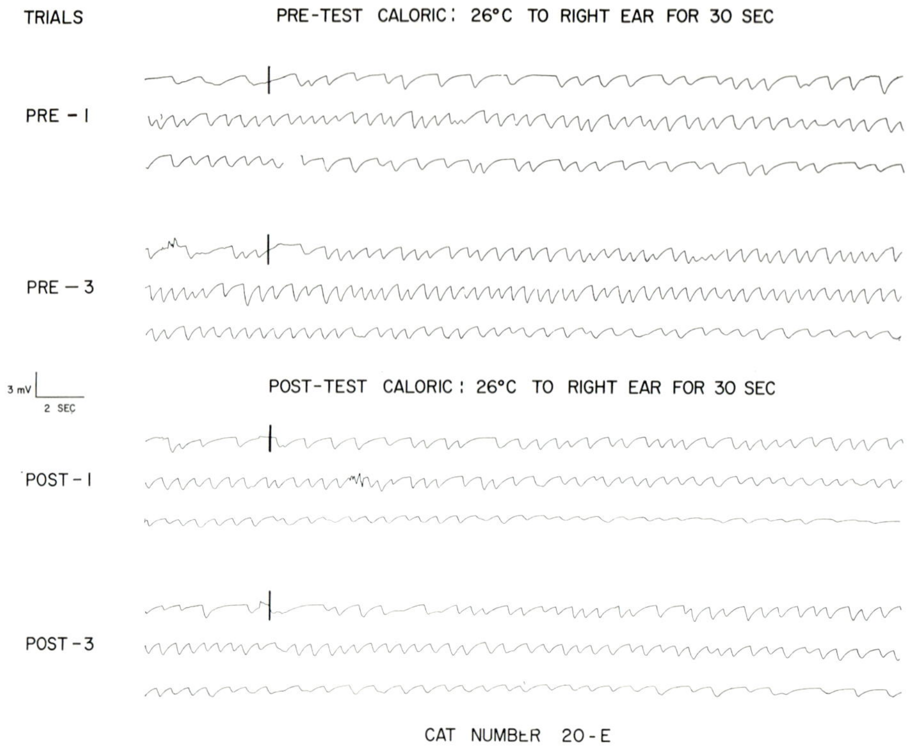

Fig. 3. Repeated peripheral stimulation does not necessarily cause a reduction of vestibular nystagmus. The tracings depicted above were obtained from a cat which received 15 "double irrigations" (administration of 26° C water to both ears simultaneously) between the unilateral pre- and post-tests. Vertical bars denote the end of the irrigation period; all trials were conducted in total darkness (Reprinted with permission from Acta oto-laryng. (Stockh.): Collins, 1965a)

III. Vestibular Habituation in Man

A. Nystagmus

In the absence of techniques designed to keep subjects mentally active and alert, vestibular nystagmus elicited in darkness (1) may exhibit an overall response suppression over the course of only a few trials, (2) may show considerable trial-to-trial variability in output, and (3) may eventually appear to be abolished (Dodge, 1923; Fluur and Mendel, 1962a, 1962b, 1964; Forssman, 1964; Forssman et al., 1963; Lidvall, 1961a, 1961b, 1962a, 1962b; Suzuki and Totsuka, 1960). However, any alerting stimulus (even one mentally generated by the subject) will result in a restoration of vigorous nystagmus (Collins, 1962, 1963, 1964c; Guedry, Collins and Sheffey, 1961; Lidvall, 1961a; Mahoney et al., 1957; Torok, 1970; Wendt, 1951). If subjects are kept alert and mentally active,

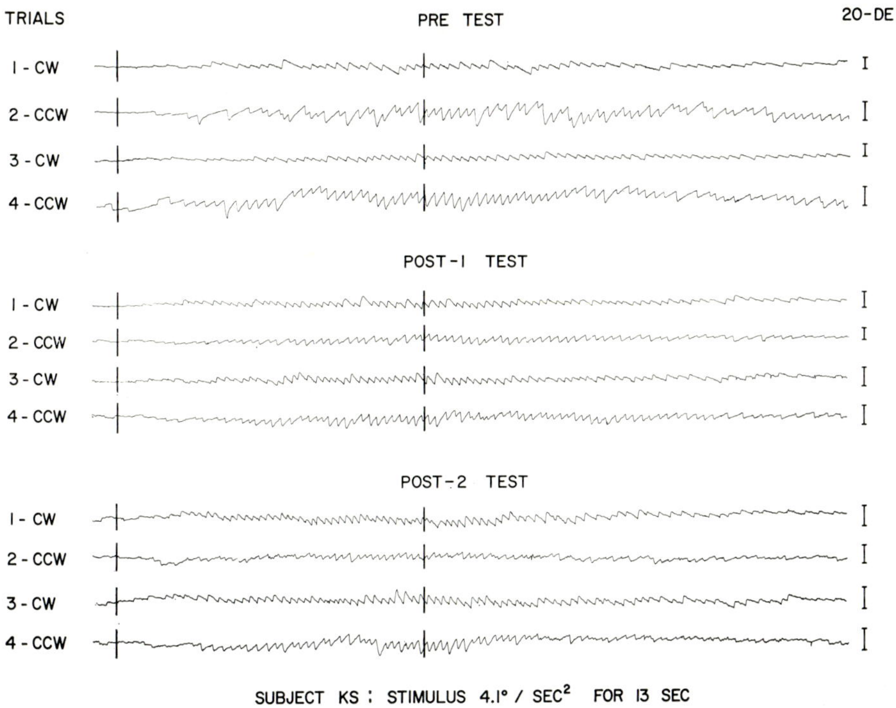

Fig. 4. Tracings of nystagmus obtained from a subject performing mental arithmetic with eyes open in darkness. A 10-day series of 200 CW accelerations (all decelerations were subthreshold) occurred between the pre- and post-1 tests and produced an increase in the frequency of eye movements. Post-2 tests were conducted 1 month later with no intervening trials. Vertical bars demarcate the period of acceleration; calibration markers are at the end of each tracing (Reprinted with permission from Acta oto-laryng. (Stockh.): COLLINS, 1964c)

abolition of nystagmus does not occur following many repetitions of vestibular stimulation in darkness (COLLINS, 1964c, 1965b; GUEDRY, 1965c; WENDT, 1951, 1965). Instead, there may be a change in the form of the response (see Fig. 4); specifically, some reduction of slow-phase eye displacement occurs, but the frequency of fast-phase eye movements appears to increase during (and for a few seconds after) an angular acceleration (COLLINS, 1964c, 1968a; JOHNSON and TOROK, 1970; TOROK, 1969; WENDT, 1965), and may increase (see Fig. 5) throughout a caloric-induced reaction (COLLINS, 1965b). These alterations in the form of nystagmus appear to occur for both directions of the eye-movement response, even though the habituation series may involve unidirectional stimulation (COLLINS, 1964c, 1965b). However, the practiced direction may show somewhat more pronounced changes than the unpracticed direction.

Visual still-fixation during and following a caloric or rotatory vestibular stimulus, or following an angular deceleration during which optokinetic stimuli are present, shortens the nystagmic reaction (COLLINS, 1966; COLLINS et al., 1962; DIX and HOOD, 1969; GRIFFITH, 1920c; MOWRER, 1937; OSTERHAMMEL et al., 1968; WENDT, 1951). Repeated stimulation under these conditions can produce

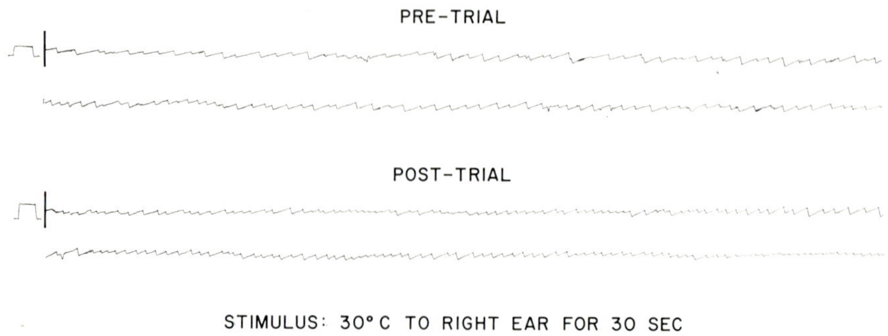

Fig. 5. Caloric nystagmus recorded before and after an habituation series of 40 identical irrigations (all trials in darkness with the subject's eyes open). Dysrhythmia and an overall reduction of nystagmus are not necessary consequences of repeated vestibular stimulation; an increase in the number of eye movements, as depicted above, may occur. Vertical bars indicate the end of the irrigation; 20° calibration markers appear at the beginning of each tracing. Each strip of tracings represents 33 sec of recording

total or almost total suppression of nystagmus (COLLINS, 1966; DIX and HOOD, 1969; FORSSMAN, 1964; FUKUDA et al., 1967; GRIFFITH, 1920a, 1920b, 1924; HOLSOPPLE, 1923a; MARSHALL and BROWN, 1966; MCCABE, 1960; MOWRER, 1937; OSTERHAMMEL et al., 1968), but such a reduction represents visual inhibition of the vestibular response or, as WENDT (1951) has indicated, with repetition "... these (visual) stimuli become increasingly dominant." This visual inhibition (see Fig. 6) is what accounts for suppression of nystagmus during performances by professional figure skaters (COLLINS, 1966) and ballet dancers (DIX and HOOD, 1969; FUKUDA et al., 1967; OSTERHAMMEL et al., 1968).

Repeated exposure to laboratory stimulation with opportunities for active control over one direction of eye movements by visual still-fixation tends to produce a directional imbalance when subjects are subsequently tested in darkness (COLLINS, 1965b; COLLINS et al., 1970; GUEDRY, 1965c), and perhaps also in the light (HOLSOPPLE, 1923a). Aerobatic flying experience which is cited as involving visual control primarily over one direction of vestibular responses is reported to produce a similar imbalance of nystagmus when experienced aerobatic pilots are tested in darkness (ASCHAN, 1954, 1967; CAPORALE and CAMARDA, 1958). However, figure skaters, who effectively use visual still-fixation to inhibit only one direction of vestibular eye movements during on-ice spins (COLLINS, 1966), show no directionally specific effects of their training on nystagmic reactions recorded in the laboratory in darkness (COLLINS, 1968a). Among the possible explanations for the lack of a directional difference in figure skaters are: (1) the extremely high stimulus rates which occur during on-ice spins may be centrally processed in a different manner than the milder laboratory stimuli, (2) the skaters do perform various on-ice turning maneuvers in both directions at rates more closely approximating laboratory stimuli, and (3) visual stimulation may simply selectively (i.e. directionally) speed up the process of change resulting from repeated vestibular experience and, with hundreds of repetitions, both directions may become equally modified.

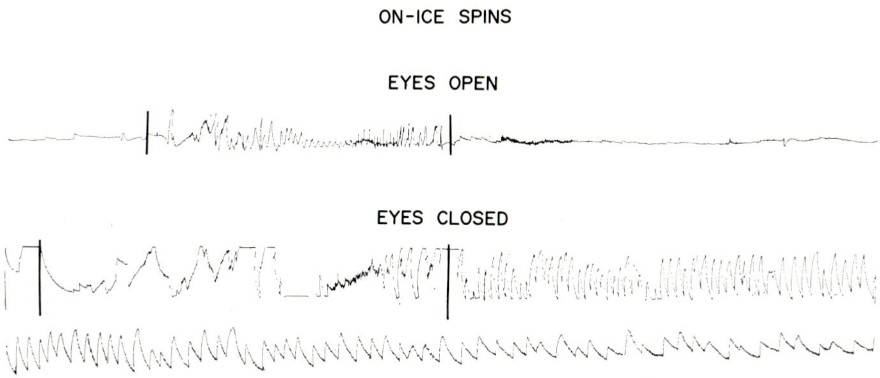

Fig. 6. Eye-movement tracings obtained by means of telemetry during on-ice spins performed by a figure skater. Each strip of tracings represents 33 sec of recording. Vertical bars demarcate the period of spinning. After-nystagmus is markedly suppressed during visual fixation

Laboratory results obtained with professional ballet dancers (OSTERHAMMEL et al., 1968) are similar to those obtained with figure skaters. When deprived of visual stimuli on which to fixate, ballet dancers show vigorous nystagmus (DIX and HOOD, 1969; FUKUDA et al., 1967; OSTERHAMMEL et al., 1968; TSCHIASSNY, 1957) and there is no evidence of directional differences following brake decelerations in the laboratory (OSTERHAMMEL et al., 1968).

Very short series of angular stimulations either in darkness or with opportunities for visual still-fixation produce some reduction in slow-phase eye displacement. However, the decline produced in darkness is relatively specific to that condition, i.e. subjects show no pre- to post-test change in slow-phase nystagmus with visual fixation permitted, following a short series of otherwise identical stimulations in the dark (MARSHALL and BROWN, 1966). Furthermore, a very short series of angular accelerations with vision permitted has no greater reductive effect on nystagmus than does a similar series with vision excluded (BROWN and CRAMPTON, 1966). Perhaps some number of stimulations in excess of 10 is required to produce differential effects between "vision" and "no-vision" conditions.

The nystagmus repetitively produced as a result of head movements during constant rotation in the light shows an overall reduction in both the light and the dark (GUEDRY, 1964; GUEDRY and GRAYBIEL, 1962). If the repeated head movements (Coriolis vestibular stimulation) are restricted to a particular quadrant, nystagmus produced by a head movement in the opposite quadrant is relatively unaffected (DOWD and CRAMER, 1967; GUEDRY, 1964; GUEDRY et al., 1964; GUEDRY et al., 1962). Furthermore, the same number of head movements made in the dark produces only a slight reduction in slow-phase nystagmus for the practiced quadrant (GUEDRY, 1965a). Of considerable significance is the fact that, following habituation to Coriolis stimulation, when subjects are no longer rotating (i.e. in a static situation), head movements which prior to habituation produced no nystagmus, now produce a nystagmus opposite to that provoked by the same

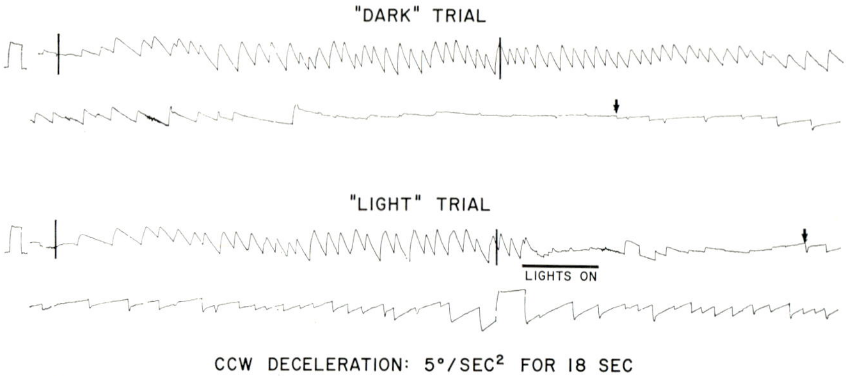

Fig. 7. The influence on nystagmus of a brief period of room illumination immediately after termination of deceleration. Secondary nystagmus (arrows) was vigorous in the "total darkness" trial but appears much earlier and is a stronger response following the period of room lighting with visual still-fixation. Vertical bars demarcate the 18-sec period of deceleration; 15° eye calibrations are at the beginning of each tracing

head movement (during rotation) at the start of the habituation trials (GUEDRY, 1965a; GUEDRY and GRAYBIEL, 1962). This conditioned reaction of opposite sign may be related to the results obtained by FUKUDA et al. (1958) with leghorns, and may also be related to the early onset and vigorous appearance of secondary nystagmus in darkness (see Fig. 7) following brief periods of room illumination (either during or immediately following an angular deceleration), during which time subjects actively attempted to control nystagmus (COLLINS, 1968a, b; SCHROEDER, 1971). An element common to all of these marked opposed reactions is the attempt on the part of the organism to counteract the vestibular input. It is possible that the directional preponderance of nystagmus obtained after repeated unidirectional stimulation (FLUUR and MENDEL, 1964; PFALTZ and ARX, 1967) reflects, in a less pronounced fashion, the development of this opposed process.

B. Subjective Reactions

Repeated stimulation reduces the intensity and duration of subjective vestibular reactions (BENSON, 1962; DEARNALEY et al., 1962; FORSSMAN, 1964; FORSSMAN et al., 1963; GRAYBIEL et al., 1961; GRIFFITH, 1920a, b; GROEN and JONGKEES, 1948a; GUEDRY et al., 1961; GUEDRY and MONTAGUE, 1961; PREBER, 1958). If the habituation series involves only unidirectional stimulation, a directionally specific decline occurs regardless of whether the stimulus is a caloric irrigation, an angular acceleration (see Fig. 8) or a head movement during rotation (COLLINS, 1964c, 1965b; COLLINS and MERTENS, 1968; GUEDRY, 1965a; GUEDRY et al., 1962, 1964; LIDVALL, 1961a).

If visual references fixed with respect to the earth are available during a vestibular response, or for a brief period following an angular deceleration, a

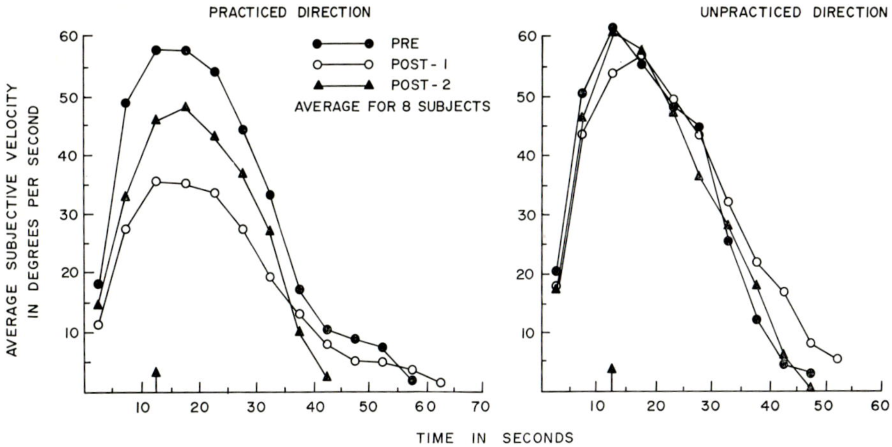

Fig. 8. Subjective velocity estimates made by subjects before (pre-) and after (post-1) a series of 200 CW accelerations (all decelerations were subthreshold). Post-2 tests were conducted 1 month later with no intervening trials. The habituation series produced a clear, directionally-specific reduction in the intensity of the turning sensation (but not in its duration); a month of rest produced considerable recovery (Reprinted with permission from Acta oto-laryng. (Stockh.): Collins, 1964c)

marked curtailment of the vestibular sensation occurs (Brown and Guedry, 1951; Collins, 1965b, 1966, 1968a; Guedry, 1950, 1953a, b, c; Guedry et al., 1961). In addition, a brief period of room illumination following an angular deceleration not only serves to interrupt the sensation of turning, but is effective in preventing any substantial recovery of the primary subjective response during a subsequent period of darkness. That is, unlike nystagmus which shows some (albeit incomplete) recovery in darkness following a brief period of room lighting, the primary subjective reaction is either completely inhibited or very weakly reinstated (Collins, 1968a, b; Guedry et al., 1961; Schroeder, 1971). Room illumination during habituation trials appears to produce a greater reduction of vestibular sensations (or a clearer direction-specific effect) than does a similar habituation series in the dark, irrespective of whether the stimulus is of the caloric, rotatory, or Coriolis type (Brown and Guedry, 1951; Collins, 1965b; Guedry, 1953a, b, c, 1964). Apparent exceptions occur among fighter pilots (Aschan, 1954) and figure skaters (Collins, 1968a). Both groups show a bidirectional reduction of the duration of turning sensations when tested in darkness in the laboratory, although the skaters appear to use visual techniques to inhibit only one direction of turning sensations following on-ice spins, and the pilots demonstrate a unidirectional reduction of nystagmus related to the direction in which they habitually roll their aircraft. However, the rates of turning are much lower in the laboratory situation than in the work activities of these subjects and the skaters do perform a variety of on-ice turning maneuvers in both directions. The fact that the skaters, when compared with ordinary subjects, show proportionally greater attenuation in the duration of their sensations as the rate of angular stimulation is increased (Collins, 1968a), may indicate a different mode for the central processing of vestibular stimuli of "high" or of "low" magnitude, or may reflect the presence of a type of stimulus generalization gradient.

Repeated unilateral irrigation produces a decline in vertiginous sensations (Collins, 1965b; Collins and Mertens, 1968; Forssman, 1964; Forssman et al., 1963; Hinchcliffe, 1967; Lidvall, 1961a, b, 1962, 1963). Moreover, the decline may be relatively specific to the direction of cupula deflection in the repeatedly stimulated ear, i.e. a less pronounced decline or no apparent decline in the intensity of the sensation may be obtained if the opposite ear is irrigated with an "equivalent" stimulus (Collins, 1965b; Collins and Mertens, 1968; Lidvall, 1961a).

C. The Oculogyral Illusion

During rotational stimulation, an object with a minimal visual surround (e.g. a small, dim light source in an otherwise dark room) appears to move in a definite pattern although it and the observer are in fixed positions (Graybiel and Hupp, 1946). This apparent motion, the oculogyral illusion (OGI) has been identified with the sensation of turning rather than with nystagmus (Byford, 1963; van Dishoeck et al., 1954; Vogelsang, 1961; however, see also Clark and Stewart, 1968).

A successive shortening of the duration of the OGI occurs with repeated stimulation (Guedry, 1950), but the declines are more marked when visual stimuli are used in the habituation series (Brown and Guedry, 1951). The vision-induced declines are directionally specific (Guedry, 1953a, b, c) and produce a greater duration-reducing effect on OGI responses to stimuli of lesser intensity and a lesser duration-reducing effect on OGI responses to stimuli of greater intensity (Guedry, 1953b). A more recent study (Brown and Crampton, 1966) showed no differential effects on duration of the OGI of rotating subjects in total darkness, with the OGI, with an illuminated enclosure, or in full-room illumination; however, only six habituation trials were conducted for each group in the direction under consideration.

The OGI has also been used in studies of habituation of Coriolis vestibular responses produced by head movements during constant rotation. The array of effects which occur depends to some extent upon the kind of visual information available during the head movements (Collins, 1968c). The sensations produced (as well as the apparent movement of a target light) are combinations of displacement and acceleration, e.g. tilting the head to the right during CW rotation produces a sensation of tilting backward and accelerating upward (much like a sharp climbing maneuver in an aircraft).

Repeated head movements during rotation in the presence of the OGI produce a reduction in the apparent displacement of the visual target (Guedry and Montague, 1961). Similarly, the magnitude of the illusion has been shown to decline during test intervals throughout a 64-hour period in which subjects made head movements while rotating in a lighted room (Graybiel et al., 1961). In addition, conditioned compensatory OGI reactions occur in static situations (i.e. in the absence of rotation) following repeated Coriolis exposures when the latter are coupled with visual stimulation. That is, following several hours of head movements in a lighted, rotating room, subjects report OGI effects (while at a standstill) which are opposed in direction to those which would have been produced had the same head movement been made during the rotation (GRAYBIEL et al., 1961; GUEDRY et al., 1962, 1964). If head movements during rotation are restricted to a single quadrant, the compensatory OGI in the static situation is relatively specific to that quadrant (GUEDRY, 1964). The effect is absent following Coriolis stimulation in darkness (GUEDRY, 1964). Perhaps related to this compensatory phenomenon is the occurrence in darkness of strong, long-duration, secondary turning sensations following an angular deceleration when room illumination is introduced either during the stimulus or for a brief period immediately after termination of deceleration (COLLINS, 1968b). In these cases and in the Coriolis studies, vigorous opposed reactions appear under conditions in which the organism actively attempts to adapt to unusual stimulation or to process conflicting sensory information.

D. Central Factors

The conditioned compensatory reactions obtained for both nystagmus and the oculogyral illusion, as well as the early appearance of strong secondary reactions following brief exposure to certain types of visual stimulation during a vestibular response, point to the importance of central factors in habituation. The fact that the time course of the nystagmic and subjective reactions can differ during prolonged stimulation (COLLINS and GUEDRY, 1962, 1967; GUEDRY and COLLINS, 1968; GUEDRY and LAUVER, 1961), or as a result of brief periods of visual information (COLLINS, 1968a, b; GUEDRY et al., 1961), supports this view. Other evidence is also available: (1) the modification of the nystagmic response appears different depending upon whether the habituation trials occur in darkness or with opportunities for visual still-fixation (COLLINS, 1964c, 1965b; COLLINS et al., 1970; GUEDRY, 1964, 1965c; MARSHALL and BROWN, 1966); (2) repeated complex vestibular stimulation (head movements in one quadrant) produces clearer directional differences in nystagmus than does the unidirectional repetition of simple vestibular stimulation (GUEDRY, 1964; GUEDRY et al., 1962, 1964); (3) the effects of repeated stimulation on both nystagmus and subjective reactions are maintained for as long as several months, with the subjective response showing a more rapid return to its initial level (COLLINS, 1964c, 1965b; GRIFFITH, 1920a, 1924; GUEDRY, 1965a); (4) the effects of repeated vestibular stimulation are evident regardless of whether the interval between habituation trials is several minutes or several days (LIDVALL, 1961b); (5) habituation fails to show significant transfer from caloric to rotational stimulation (COLLINS et al., 1970); from one quadrant of head movements to another (GUEDRY, 1964; GUEDRY et al., 1962, 1964), from head movements made during one direction of turning to head movements made during rotation in the opposite direction (GUEDRY, 1965a), and from simple to complex (MEDA, 1947) or complex to simple (GUEDRY et al., 1964) stimulation. Perhaps a common feature of the lack of transfer in these cases is the difference in the pattern of stimulation contributed by specific and nonspecific gravireceptors from one condition to the other.

IV. A Modified View of "Habituation"

The term "habituation" has been used throughout this chapter to identify a series of repeated stimulations or to describe the effects of such a series on various responses. Most investigators carefully restrict the meaning of the term to "response reduction" or, considering habituation to represent a valid class of learning, cite THORPE'S (1950) definition ("a tendency merely to drop out responses"). Although vestibular research findings appear to share many of the general characteristics ascribed to other habituation phenomena (DODGE, 1923; HALSTEAD, 1935; RATNER, 1967), such definitions fail to describe adequately the dynamic processes of change which are evident as a result of repeated vestibular stimulation under at least some conditions. For example, repeated exposure to Coriolis stimulation in the light reduces nystagmus and subjective reactions in both light and darkness; an overall suppression of the responses appears to occur. However, closer examination indicates that a conditioned compensatory reaction has developed to oppose these reactions (GUEDRY, 1964; GUEDRY and GRAYBIEL, 1962). There is no simple dropping out of responses; instead there is a gradual inhibition of the original response as the opposed reaction becomes more fully developed. These opposed reactions have appeared most clearly under two non-exclusive conditions: (1) when there is an element of conflict between vestibular and visual signals (and perhaps others of a sensory nature); (2) where the organism is attempting to adapt to an unusual vestibular environment. In darkness, nystagmus repeatedly elicited by simple vestibular stimulation is not simply reduced in alert subjects; the form of the response is changed and the change appears to be due to increased activity of the fast phase of the eye movement, which simultaneously reduces the amount of slow-phase eye excursion (COLLINS, 1964a, 1968a). With very brief responses, such as those elicited by mild turns of short arc, increasingly more frequent fast phases may gradually obliterate the original form of nystagmus (WENDT, 1965). "Active modification" would more closely describe the effects of repeated stimulation on human vestibular responses.

The above suggests the possibility of more than one kind of vestibular "habituation." In the chapter on "Arousal and Vestibular Habituation," elsewhere in this volume, the notion of psychological or situational "habituation" was discussed in terms of arousal factors. In addition, repeated vestibular stimulation of animals produces some effects apparently different from those obtained with human subjects. Cats, for example, show a very rapid reduction of all measures of ocular responses (in darkness or in light), similar to what might occur with a nonalert human subject, even though this overall reduction occurs in animals which seem alert or which have received an analeptic drug and in which various sensory methods of arousal do not significantly restore nystagmus. Thus, in spite of a rich history of research, there remain considerable gaps in our knowledge on specific effects of repeated stimulation on vestibular reactions and, moreover, important questions regarding the extent to which changes in the reaction patterns of animals can be generalized to human response patterns remain unanswered. It is suggested, however, that central processes are activated as a result of repeated vestibular stimulation, and that limiting the term "habituation" to a "simple dropping out of responses" masks dynamic changes and interactions which occur as these responses become modified.

References

Abels, H.: Über Nachempfindung im Gebiete des kinästhetischen und statischen Sinnes. Ein Beitrag zur Lehre vom Bewegungsschwindel (Drehschwindel). Z. Psychol. Physiol. Sinnesorg. **43**, 268–289, 374–422 (1906).

Aschan, G.: Response to rotatory stimuli in fighter pilots. Acta oto-laryng. (Stockh.) Suppl. **116**, 24–31 (1954).

Aschan, G.: Habituation to repeated rotatory stimuli (cupulometry) and the effect of anti-nausea drugs and alcohol on the results. Acta oto-laryng. (Stockh.) **64**, 95–106 (1967).

Bárány, R.: Weitere Untersuchungen über den vom Vestibularapparat des Ohres reflektorisch ausgelösten Nystagmus und seine Begleiterscheinungen. Mschr. Ohrenheilk. **41**, 477–526 (1907).

Benson, A. J.: Modification of labyrinthine after-sensations on shaking the head. FPRC Report 1210. Ministry of Defense (Air), London, 1962.

Brown, J. H.: Acquisition and retention of nystagmic habituation in cats with distributed acceleration experience. J. comp. physiol. Psychol. **60**, 340–343 (1965).

Brown, J. H., Crampton, G. H.: Concomitant visual stimulation does not alter habituation of nystagmic, oculogyral or psychophysical responses to angular acceleration. Acta oto-laryng. (Stockh.) **61**, 80–91 (1961).

Brown, J. H., Marshall, J. E.: Drug control of arousal and nystagmic habituation in the cat. Acta oto-laryng. (Stockh.) **64**, 345–352 (1967).

Brown, R. H., Guedry, F. E.: Influence of visual stimulation on habituation to rotation. J. genet. Psychol. **45**, 151–161 (1951).

Byford, G. H.: Eye movements and the optogyral illusion. Aerospace Med. **34**, 119–123 (1963).

Caporale, R., Camarda, V.: La funzionalita vestibolare di alcuni piloti di pattuglia acrobatica. Riv. Med. aeronaut. **21**, 12–36 (1958).

Capps, M. J., Collins, W. E.: Effects of bilateral caloric habituation on vestibular nystagmus in the cat. Acta oto-laryng. (Stockh.) **59**, 511–530 (1965).

Clark, B., Stewart, J. D.: Comparison of sensitivity for the perception of bodily rotation and the oculogyral illusion. Percep. Psychophys. **3**, 253–256 (1968).

Collins, W. E.: Effects of mental set upon vestibular nystagmus. J. exp. Psychol. **63**, 191–197 (1962).

Collins, W. E.: Manipulation of arousal and its effects upon human vestibular nystagmus induced by caloric irrigation and angular accelerations. Aerospace Med. **34**, 124–129 (1963).

Collins, W. E.: Nystagmus responses of the cat to rotation and to directionally equivalent and non-equivalent stimuli after unilateral caloric habituation. Acta oto-laryng. (Stockh.) **58**, 247–258 (1964a).

Collins, W. E.: Primary, secondary, and caloric nystagmus of the cat following habituation to rotation. J. comp. physiol. Psychol. **57**, 417–421 (1964b).

Collins, W. E.: Task-control of arousal and the effcts of repeated unidirectional angular acceleration on human vestibular responses. Acta oto-laryng. (Stockh.) Suppl. **190**, 1–34 (1964c).

Collins, W. E.: Effects of "double irrigations" on the caloric nystagmus of the cat. Acta oto-laryng. (Stockh.) **59**, 45–54 (1965a).

Collins, W. E.: Subjective responses and nystagmus following repeated unilateral caloric stimulation. Ann. Otol. (St. Louis) **74**, 1034–1054 (1965b).

Collins, W. E.: Vestibular responses from figure skaters. Aerospace Med. **37**, 1098–1104 (1966).

Collins, W. E.: Effects on vestibular habituation of interrupting nystagmic responses with opposing stimuli. J. comp. physiol. Psychol. **64**, 308–312 (1967).

Collins, W.E.: Special effects of brief periods of visual fixation on nystagmus and sensations of turning. Aerospace Med. **39**, 257–266 (1968a).

Collins, W.E.: Modification of vestibular nystagmus and "vertigo" by means of visual stimulation. Trans. Amer. Acad. Ophthal. Otolaryng. **72**, 962–979 (1968b).

Collins, W.E.: Coriolis vestibular stimulation and the influence of different visual surrounds. Aerospace Med. **39**, 125–130 (1968c).

Collins, W.E.: Influence of head position on the habituation of vertical vestibular nystagmus in the cat. J. comp. physiol. Psychol. **67**, 156–159 (1969).

Collins, W.E., Guedry, F.E.: Arousal effects and nystagmus during prolonged constant angular acceleration. Acta oto-laryng. (Stockh.) **54**, 349–362 (1962).

Collins, W.E., Guedry, F.E.: Duration of angular acceleration and ocular nystagmus from cat and man. I. Responses from the lateral and the vertical canals to two stimulus durations. Acta oto-laryng. (Stockh.) **64**, 373–389 (1967).

Collins, W.E., Guedry, F.E., Posner, J.B.: Control of caloric nystagmus by manipulating arousal and visual fixation distance. Ann. Otol. (St. Louis) **71**, 187–202 (1962).

Collins, W.E., Mertens, R.A.: Influence of repeated caloric vestibular stimulation on both caloric and rotation induced vertigo. Preprints of the Annual Meeting of the Aerospace Medical Association, p. 146, 1968.

Collins, W.E., Schroeder, D.J., Mertens, R.A.: Relative specificity of nystagmus reduction to caloric stimuli in humans. Preprints of the Annual Meeting of the Aerospace Medical Association, p. 182, 1970.

Collins, W.E., Updegraff, B.P.: A comparison of nystagmus habituation in the cat and the dog. Acta oto-laryng. (Stockh.) **62**, 19–26 (1966).

Collins, W.E., Updegraff, B.P.: Possible interactions between gravi-receptors and semicircular canals in the habituation of vertical nystagmus in parrots. Acta oto-laryng. (Stockh.) **69**, 257–265 (1970).

Crampton, G.H.: Directional imbalance of vestibular nystagmus in cat following repeated unidirectional angular acceleration. Acta oto-laryng. (Stockh.) **55**, 41–48 (1962a).

Crampton, G.H.: Effects of visual experience on vestibular nystagmus habituation in the cat. Acta oto-laryng. (Stockh.) **55**, 516–526 (1962b).

Crampton, G.H.: Habituation of ocular nystagmus of vestibular origin. In: M.B. Bender, Ed. The Oculomotor System. New York: Harper & Row, 332–346, 1964.

Crampton, G.H., Schwam, W.J.: Effects of arousal reaction on nystagmus habituation in the cat. Amer. J. Physiol. **200**, 29–33 (1961).

Dearnaley, E.J., Reason, J.T., Davies, J.D.: The nature and duration of after-sensations following the cessation of turning in a Chipmunk aircraft. Aerospace Med. **33**, 1224–1229 (1962).

Dishoeck, H.A.E. van, Spoor, A., Nijhoff, P.: The optogyral illusion and its relation to the nystagmus of the eyes. Acta oto-laryng. (Stockh.) **44**, 597–607 (1954).

Dix, M.R., Hood, J.D.: Observations upon the nervous mechanism of vestibular habituation. Acta oto-laryng. (Stockh.) **44**, 310–318 (1969).

Dodge, R.: Habituation to rotation. J. exp. Psychol. **6**, 1–35 (1923).

Dowd, P.J., Cramer, R.L.: Habituation transference in coriolis acceleration. Aerospace Med. **38**, 1103–1107 (1967).

Dunlap, K.: Adaptation of nystagmus to repeated caloric stimulation in rabbits. J. comp. Psychol. **5**, 485–493 (1925).

Fearing, F.S.: The retention of the effects of repeated elicitation of the post-rotational nystagmus in pigeons. I. The retention of the effects of "massed" stimulation. J. comp. Psychol. **30**, 31–40 (1940).

Fearing, F.S.: The retention of the effects of repeated elicitation of the post-rotational nystagmus in pigeons. II. The retention of the effects of "distributed" stimulation. J. comp. Psychol. **31**, 47–56 (1941).

Fearing, F.S., Mowrer, O.H.: The effect of general anesthesia upon the experimental reduction of vestibular nystagmus. J. genet. Psychol. **11**, 133–144 (1934).

FERNÁNDEZ, C., SCHMIDT, R.: Studies on habituation of vestibular reflexes. II. Effect of caloric stimulation in decorticated cats. Ann. Otol. (St. Louis) **71**, 299–321 (1962a).

FERNÁNDEZ, C., SCHMIDT, R.: Studies in habituation of vestibular reflexes. III. A revision. Laryngoscope (St. Louis) **72**, 939–953 (1962b).

FLUUR, E., MENDEL, L.: Habituation, efference and vestibular interplay. I. Monaural caloric habituation. Acta oto-laryng. (Stockh.) **55**, 65–80 (1962a).

FLUUR, E., MENDEL, L.: Habituation, efference and vestibular interplay. II. Combined caloric habituation. Acta oto-laryng. (Stockh.) **55**, 136–144 (1962b).

FLUUR, E., MENDEL, L.: Habituation, efference and vestibular interplay. III. Unidirectional rotatory habituation. Acta oto-laryng. (Stockh.) **57**, 81–88 (1964).

FORSSMAN, B.: Studies on habituation of vestibular reflexes. VII. Habituation in light of calorically induced nystagmus, laterotorsion and vertigo in man. Acta oto-laryng. (Stockh.) **57**, 163–176 (1964).

FORSSMAN, B., HENRIKSSON, N.G., DOLOWITZ, D.A.: Studies on habituation of vestibular reflexes. VI. Habituation in darkness of calorically induced nystagmus, laterotorsion and vertigo in man. Acta oto-laryng. (Stockh.) **56**, 663–674 (1963).

FUKUDA, T., HINOKI, M., TOKITA, T.: Static and kinetic labyrinthine reflex: Functional development of labyrinthine function with rotatory training. Acta oto-laryng. (Stockh.) **49**, 467–477 (1958).

FUKUDA, T., TOKITA, T., AOKIA, S., WATANABE, T., HISHIDA, K., TASHIRO, K., MIYATA, H., MAZUOKA, U.: Study on nystagmus during voluntary acts – observation of rotation in ballet. J. Oto-, Rhino-, Laryng. Soc. Jap. Suppl. **70**, 11–12 (1967).

GRAYBIEL, A., GUEDRY, F.E., JOHNSON, W.H., KENNEDY, R.: Adaptation to bizzarre stimulation of the semicircular canals as indicated by the oculogyral illusion. Aerospace Med. **32**, 321–327 (1961).

GRAYBIEL, A., HUPP, D.: The oculogyral illusion: A form of apparent motion which may be observed following stimulation of the semicircular canals. J. Aviat. Med. **17**, 3–27 (1946).

GRIFFITH, C.R.: The organic effects of repeated bodily rotation. J. exp. Psychol. **3**, 15–47 (1920a).

GRIFFITH, C.R.: The cumulative effects of rotational increments. Ill. State Acad. Sci. Trans. **13**, 122–134 (1920b).

GRIFFITH, C.R.: An experimental study of dizziness. J. exp. Psychol. **3**, 89–125 (1920c).

GRIFFITH, C.R.: The effect upon the white rat of continued bodily rotation. Amer. Naturalist **54**, 524–534 (1920d).

GRIFFITH, C.R.: A note on the persistence of the "practice effect" in rotation experiments. J. comp. Psychol. **4**, 137–149 (1924).

GROEN, J.J., JONGKEES, L.B.W.: The turning test with small regulable stimuli. III. The advantages of cupulometria over the classic technique of Bárány. J. Laryng. **62**, 231–235 (1948a).

GUEDRY, F.E.: The effect of visual stimulation on the duration of post-rotational apparent motion effects. J. genet. Psychol. **43**, 313–322 (1950).

GUEDRY, F.E.: The transfer of habituation to rotation with respect to the directional aspect of the vestibular reaction. USNSAM Jt. Proj. Report No. 35, Pensacola, Florida, 1953a.

GUEDRY, F.E.: The transfer of habituation to rotation with respect to the magnitude of the vestibular stimulus. USNSAM Jt. Proj. Report No. 34, Pensacola, Florida, 1953b.

GUEDRY, F.E.: The retention of effects of "massed" and "distributed" vestibular stimulation as indicated by the duration of the oculogyral illusion. USNSAM Jt. Proj. Report No. 33, Pensacola, Florida, 1953c.

GUEDRY, F.E.: Visual control of habituation to complex vestibular stimulation in man. Acta oto-laryng. (Stockh.) **58**, 377–389 (1964).

GUEDRY, F.E.: Habituation to complex vestibular stimulation in man: Transfer and retention of effects from twelve days of rotation at 10 rpm. Percept. Mot. Skills, Monog. Suppl. **1–V21**, 459–481 (1965a).

GUEDRY, F.E.: Psychophysiological studies of vestibular function. In: W.D. NEFF, Ed. Contributions to Sensory Physiology. New York: Academic Press, 63–135, 1965c.

GUEDRY, F.E., COLLINS, W.E.: Duration of angular acceleration and ocular nystagmus from cat and man. II. Responses from the lateral canals to varied stimulus durations. Acta oto-laryng. (Stockh.) **65**, 257–269 (1968).

GUEDRY, F.E., COLLINS, W.E., GRAYBIEL, A.: Vestibular habituation during repetitive complex stimulation; A study of transfer effects. J. appl. Physiol. **19**, 1005–1015 (1964).

GUEDRY, F.E., COLLINS, W.E., SHEFFEY, P.L.: Perceptual and oculomotor reactions to interacting visual and vestibular stimulation. Percept. Mot. Skills **12**, 307–324 (1961).

GUEDRY, F.E., GRAYBIEL, A.: Compensatory nystagmus conditioned during adaptation to living in a rotating room. J. appl. Physiol. **17**, 398–404 (1962).

GUEDRY, F.E., GRAYBIEL, A., COLLINS, W.E.: Reduction of nystagmus and disorientation in human subjects. Aerospace Med. **33**, 1356–1360 (1962).

GUEDRY, F.E., LAUVER, L.S.: Vestibular reactions during prolonged constant angular acceleration. J. appl. Physiol. **16**, 215–220 (1961).

GUEDRY, F.E., MONTAGUE, E.K.: Quantitative evaluation of the vestibular Coriolis reaction. Aerospace Med. **32**, 487–500 (1961).

HALSTEAD, W.: The effects of cerebellar lesions upon habituation of post-rotational nystagmus. Comp. psychol. Monogr. **12**, 1–130 (1935).

HALSTEAD, W., YACORZYNSKI, G., FEARING, F.: Further evidence of cerebellar influence in the habituation of after-nystagmus in pigeons. Amer. J. Physiol. **120**, 350–355 (1937).

HENDERSON, J.W.: Optokinetic and other factors modifying vestibular nystagmus. Arch. Ophthal. **37**, 459–471 (1947).

HENRIKSSON, N.G., KOHUT, R., FERNÁNDEZ, C.: Studies on habituation of vestibular reflexes. I. Effect of repetitive caloric test. Acta oto-laryng. (Stockh.) **53**, 333–349 (1961).

HINCHCLIFFE, R.: Subjective magnitude of induced vertigo as an index of caloric response. J. Laryng. **81**, 875–885 (1967).

HOLSOPPLE, J.Q.: Factors affecting the duration of post-rotation nystagmus. J. comp. Psychol. **3**, 283–304 (1923a).

HOOD, J.D., PFALTZ, C.R.: Observations upon the effects of repeated stimulation upon rotational and caloric nystagmus. J. Physiol. (Lond.) **124**, 130–144 (1954).

HUDDLESTON, O.L.: The influence of retinal stimuli upon labyrinthine head-nystagmus of pigeons. Amer. J. Physiol. **95**, 465–472 (1930).

JOHNSON, D.D., TOROK, N.: Habituation of nystagmus and sensation of motion after rotation. Acta oto-laryng. (Stockh.) **69**, 206–215 (1970).

KING, B.G.: The influence of repeated rotations on decerebrate and on blinded squabs. J. comp. Psychol. **6**, 399–421 (1926).

LIDVALL, H.F.: Vertigo and nystagmus responses to caloric stimuli repeated at short intervals. Acta oto-laryng. (Stockh.) **53**, 33–44 (1961a).

LIDVALL, H.F.: Vertigo and nystagmus responses to caloric stimuli repeated at short and long intervals. Acta oto-laryng. (Stockh.) **53**, 507–518 (1961b).

LIDVALL, H.F.: Specific and non-specific traits of habituation in nystagmus responses to caloric stimuli. Acta oto-laryng. (Stockh.) **55**, 315–325 (1962a).

LIDVALL, H.F.: Mechanisms of motion sickness as reflected in the vertigo and nystagmus responses to repeated caloric stimuli. Acta oto-laryng. (Stockh.) **55**, 527–536 (1962b).

LIDVALL, H.F.: Neurotic anxiety and vestibular function as reflected in the vertigo and nystagmus responses to repeated caloric stimuli. Acta oto-laryng. (Stockh.) **56**, 445–456 (1963).

LUMPKIN, R.C.: Post-rotation nystagmus in the rabbit with head fixed and head free. J. comp. Psychol. **7**, 181–185 (1927).

MAHONEY, J.L., HARLAN, W.L., BICKFORD, R.G.: Visual and other factors influencing caloric nystagmus in normal subjects. Arch. Otolaryng. **66**, 46–53 (1957).

MARSHALL, J.E., BROWN, J.H.: Visual-arousal interaction and specificity of nystagmic habituation. USAMRL Report No. 688, Ft. Knox, Kentucky, 1966.

MAXWELL, S.S., BURKE, U.L., RESTON, C.: The effect of repeated rotation on the duration of after-nystagmus in the rabbit. Amer. J. Physiol. **58**, 432–438 (1922).

McCABE, B.F.: Vestibular suppression in figure skaters. Trans. Amer. Acad. Ophthal. Otolaryng. **64**, 264–268 (1960).

MEDA, E.: Effetti di repetuti eccitamenti rotatori dell apparato vestibulare sue fenhomeni soggettivi da combiamenta di perizione del capo duranti e dope la rotazione. Riv. Med. aeronaut. **10**, 316–323 (1947).

MERTENS, R.A., COLLINS, W.E.: Unilateral caloric habituation of nystagmus in the cat: Effects on rotational and bilateral caloric responses. Acta oto-laryng. (Stockh.) **64**, 281–297 (1967).

MOWRER, O.H.: The modification of vestibular nystagmus by means of repeated elicitation. Comp. psychol. Monog. **9**, (No. 45), 1–48 (1934a).

MOWRER, O.H.: Some neglected factors which influence the duration of post-rotational nystagmus. Acta oto-laryng. (Stockh.) **22**, 1–23 (1935).

MOWRER, O.H.: The influence of vision during bodily rotation upon the duration of post-rotational vestibular nystagmus. Acta oto-laryng. (Stockh.) **25**, 351–364 (1937).

OSTERHAMMEL, P., TERKILDSEN, K., ZILSTORFF, K.: Vestibular habituation in ballet dancers. Acta oto-laryng. (Stockh.) **66**, 221–228 (1968).

PFALTZ, C.R., ARX, S.V.: Zur Wirkung wiederholter thermischer und rotatorischer Reize auf das normale vestibuläre Endorgan. Acta oto-laryng. (Stockh.) **63**, 191–207 (1967).

PILZ, G.F.: On the relation of the after-nystagmus to rotation nystagmus. I. Direct effects of rotations. Amer. J. Physiol. **77**, 428–442 (1926a).

PILZ, G.F.: On the relation of after-nystagmus to rotation nystagmus. II. Modifying influences. Amer. J. Physiol. **77**, 443–458 (1926b).

PREBER, L.: Vegetative reactions in caloric and rotatory tests. Acta oto-laryng. (Stockh.) Suppl. **144**, 1–119 (1958).

PROCTOR, L.R., FERNÁNDEZ, C.: Studies on habituation of vestibular reflexes. IV. Effect of caloric stimulation in blindfolded cats. Acta oto-laryng. (Stockh.) **56**, 500–508 (1963).

RATNER, S.C.: Annelids and learning: A critical review. In: W.C. CORNING and S.C. RATNER, Eds. Chemistry of Learning. New York: Plenium Press, 391–406, 1967.

RUPPERT, J.: Untersuchungen über den Drehnystagmus. Zbl. inn. Med. **27**, 465–478 (1906).

SALA, O.: The efferent vestibular system. Acta oto-laryng. (Stockh.) Suppl. **197**, 1–34 (1965).

SCHROEDER, D.J.: Influence of alcohol on vestibular responses to angular accelerations. Aerospace Med. **42**, 959–970 (1971).

SUZUKI, J., TOTSUKA, G.: Post rotatory nystagmus: Modifications observed in experiments with repeated rotatory stimulation. Acta oto-laryng. (Stockh.) **51**, 570–578 (1960).

THORPE, W.H.: The concepts of learning and their relation to those of instinct. In: Symp. Soc. Exp. Biol.: Physiological Mechanisms in Animal Behavior. Cambridge: Cambridge Univ. Press, 387–408, 1950.

TOROK, N.: Nystagmus frequency versus slow phase velocity in rotatory and caloric nystagmus. Ann. Otol. (St. Louis) **78**, 625–639 (1969).

TOROK, N.: The effects of arousal upon vestibular nystagmus. Advanc. oto-rhino-laryng. **17**, 76–89 (1970).

TSCHIASSNY, K.: Perrotatory nystagmus in the ballet dancer, pigeon, and blind person. Ann. Otol. (St. Louis) **66**, 641–648 (1957).

VOGELSANG, C.J.: The perception of a visual object during stimulation of the vestibular system. Acta oto-laryng. (Stockh.) **53**, 461–469 (1961).

Wendt, G. R.: Vestibular functions. In: S. S. Stevens, Ed. Handbook of Experimental Psychology. New York: Wiley, 1191–1223, 1951.

Wendt, G. R.: The nature of adaptation to oscillatory rotation. In: The Role of the Vestibular Organs in the Exploration of Space. NASA Report SP-77, NASA, Washington, D. C., 133–139, 1965.

Winget, C. M., Smith, A. H.: Quantitative measurement of the labyrinthine function in the fowl by nystagmography. J. appl. Physiol. **17**, 712–718 (1962).

Winget, C. M., Smith, A. H., Kelly, C. F.: Effects of chronic acceleration on induced nystagmus in the fowl. J. appl. Physiol. **17**, 709–711 (1962).

Chapter VIII.

Motion Sickness

By

W. H. JOHNSON, Toronto (Canada)
and L. B. W. JONGKEES, Amsterdam (Netherlands)

Contents

Part 1. Aetiology and Autonomic Effects

By W. H. JOHNSON

With 5 Figures

I. Introduction

It is sometimes forgotten that the primary cause of motion sickness is motion, although many stimuli (visceral, psychic, visual) may contribute to its incidence. TYLER and BARD (1949) commented in their excellent review that: "The occasional failure to appreciate the fact the fundamental cause of motion sickness is motion has led to some conflict of ideas". As HEMINGWAY (1945) pointed out, "The patient is sick without being aware of the cause and is therefore apt to attribute his troubles to odours, overheated compartments, visceral sensations, disagreeable sights, distasteful foods or anything else unpleasant, unusual or uncomfortable which he experienced shortly before or simultaneously with exposure to motion". Other pertinent reviews on the subject include those by WENDT (1945), NOBLE (1945), McNALLY and STUART (1942), CHINN and SMITH (1955) and MONEY (1970).

The importance of the non-auditory labyrinths as the principal sensory receptors for motion sickness has been well established by the following findings: (a) susceptibility to motion sickness is eliminated in animals by removal of the vestibular organs or by division of the eighth cranial nerve. This was first demonstrated in dogs and subsequently verified in cats (Johnson et al., 1951); (b) ablation of the vestibular tracts in the cerebellum eliminates motion sickness in dogs (Tyler and Bard, 1949); (c) deaf-mutes with congenitally incomplete labyrinths are immune (Tyler and Bard, 1949); (d) patients whose labyrinths have been inactivated by disease are immune (Graybiel, 1956).

II. Aetiology

As indicated above, exposure to linear and angular accelerations can induce nausea. Although there has been some conflict of opinion on the relative importance of these two types of motion in causing sickness (see Part 2), there remains no doubt that they can both result in its development, whether singly or in combination. Laboratory procedures devised to induce nausea have varied accordingly and when assessing their effects on the labyrinth it is essential to ensure that the subject's head not be allowed to move independently of the vehicle (Johnson and Taylor, 1961).

A. Linear Motion

Linear accelerators of one type or another (e.g. the four-pole swing) have been used by various investigators (de Witt, 1953; Manning and Stewart, 1949; Johnson and Taylor, 1961; and others.) The subject sits on the swing platform, which remains almost parallel with the floor, and hence is exposed to minimal angular motion provided the head is fixed to the chair.

An extensive study of the characteristics of vertical linear acceleration required to induce motion sickness in the laboratory was described by Wendt (1945). His wave "machine" consisted of a hydraulically driven elevator allowing vertical excursions of up to eighteen feet in amplitude. He determined the relative effectiveness of different acceleration wave forms by varying the amplitude and frequency. It is perhaps significant that at a cycle rate of sixteen per minute, this device and the motor-driven swing of Noble (1945) produced the highest incidence of motion sickness.

Johnson and Taylor (1964) developed another laboratory method for exposing human subjects to controlled linear acceleration by "orbiting without rotation". The device consisted of a main turntable upon which was mounted a counter-revolving "secondary turntable". For each *rotation* of the main table, the secondary table made one *revolution* in the opposite direction in such a way that a subject seated on the secondary turntable was carried along a circular path around the centre of the main turntable, but always facing in the same direction (i.e. he did not rotate). This situation is shown schematically in Fig. 1. The subject was exposed (besides gravity) only to a horizontal centrifugal force, the direction of which was continuously changing. The magnitude of the above resultant linear acceleration could be controlled by changing either the rate of rotation of the main turntable or the radius of the imposed secondary motion. Disorientation sensations consisted of apparent tilting from side to side in addition to forward and backward.

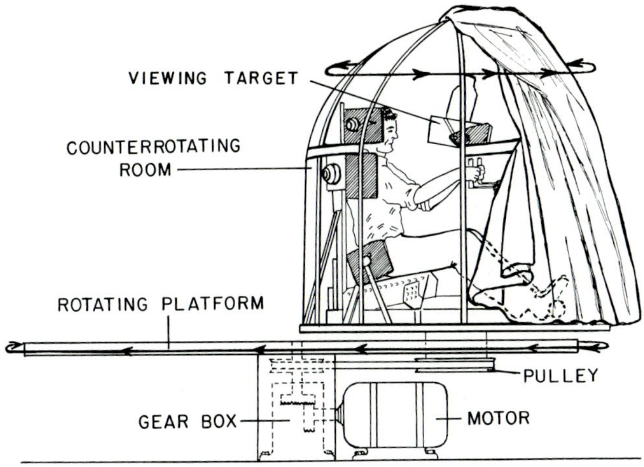

Fig. 1. Laboratory apparatus used to stimulate the otoliths by orbiting motion without rotation. Ann. Otol. (St. Louis) **72**, 1 (1963)

Although the incidence of motion sickness in subjects exposed to such orbital motion was low, it is apparent that stimulation of the otoliths in the horizontal plane can constitute an appropriate stimulus. However, Money (1966) has demonstrated on this device that strong centrifugal force applied to the head can induce nystagmus, indicating that the semicircular canals may be involved. Similar observations have been noted by Niven et al. (1967), who used a similar device with a larger radius and a slower rate of revolution.

Most of the controversy about the nature of the stimulus has resulted from failure to realize that unless the head is supported or restrained it moves in a somewhat different way from the vehicle, thus exposing the non-auditory labyrinth to accelerations which are not only additional to those of the vehicle, but may differ from person to person. As examples of opposing conclusions in this regard, Manning (1943) was unable to cause motion sickness in an elevator when the heads of his test subjects were fixed to the chair, while Wendt (1945) and McEachern et al. (1942) were able to make their subjects sick by similar vertical accelerations without head fixation. From these and other findings it is apparent that linear accelerations can result in motion sickness, although the relative roles of the otolithic receptors and the canals is not always apparent.

B. Angular Motion

Several types of laboratory devices involving appreciable angular movements have also been used in motion-sickness research. These consist of the simple two-pole swing, the human centrifuge and different types of multi-planar angular acceleration devices.

The simple two-pole swing has been used extensively by Nobel (1945), Cipriani (1942), Tyler and Bard (1949), Johnson et al. (1951) and others in studies involving both the basic physiology and the drug therapy of motion sickness. In order to determine the optimum specifications required, Noble (1945) compared the relative effectiveness of this device with different dimensions, and came to the conclusion that the most suitable should have an arc of 70°, a radius of 15 feet (from axis to subject's head) and a period of 16 complete cycles per minute.

Undoubtedly, the most effective stimulation for motion sickness results from multi-planer angular acceleration applied simultaneously, as has been established by SPIEGEL et al. (1944), JOHNSON et al. (1951) and GRAYBIEL et al. (1965). SPIEGEL found that head movements in the coronal plane during rotation of the seated subject around the vertical axis readily induced nausea. JOHNSON has repeatedly shown (1951, 1953, 1954, 1961, etc.) how significant any voluntary or involuntary head movements can be in any motion situation insofar as stimulation of the labyrinth is concerned. By superimposing specific head movements in the sagittal plane upon rotation of the trunk around the vertical axis (Fig. 2), it has been possible to produce disorientation effects which apparently result from stimulation of both the semicircular canals and the otoliths (vertigo and tilting sensations) together with the rapid onset of motion sickness in most individuals. These physiologic responses are the result of both angular and linear motions (including Coriolis accelerations), which have been well described from the aspect of the physics involved (MEDA, 1952; WEAVER, 1965).

The human centrifuge has often been used to investigate the effects of centrifugal force on the cardiovascular system. Its adaptability to motion-sickness research has been well demonstrated by GRAYBIEL (1960, 1965, etc.) since both angular and linear accelerations can be precisely administered. By attaching a circular laboratory, he constructed the "Slow-Rotating Room" by means of which our knowledge of motion sickness has been greatly increased. A standardized pattern of head movement superimposed on a constant rate of rotation of the room has made it possible to study various associated physiological and psychological problems (adaptation, drug therapy etc.). The effectiveness of this rotating room as a means of inducing sickness is indicated by the fact that a rate of only two rotations per minute has proved affective when combined with specific voluntary head movements.

Other recently developed laboratory procedures for the study of motion sickness involve a constant rate of rotation about off-vertical axes and have proved very effective (CORREIA and GUEDRY, 1964; GUEDRY, 1965). It should be noted that with this device (including that producing orbital motion without rotation), the stimulus varies (direction of gravity relative to the subject's head or direction of centripetal acceleration relative to subject). Thus the resultant vector presenting the subject's head movement must change with time for the motion to cause sickness.

III. Autonomic Effects

The objective signs of motion sickness (skin colour changes, cold perspiration, yawning, vomiting) must be external signs of extensive internal physiologic effects resulting in a generalized feeling of "malaise". Such disturbances of the normal physiology, in addition to vomiting *per se*, can cause serious incapacity which would certainly be of great significance in aerospace travel (YUGANOV et al., 1966; BERRY, 1970). Although much remains to be determined about these effects, some significant physiologic changes have been correlated.

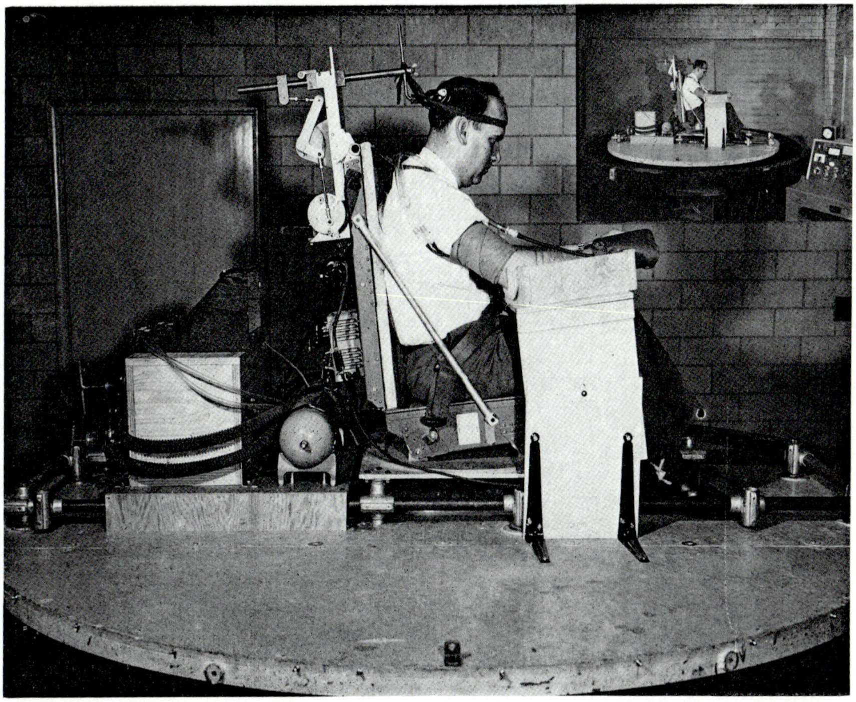

Fig. 2. The turntable, showing arrangements for moving the head and the plethysmograph. (Inset: general view of turntable. Canad. J. Physiol. Pharmacol. **42**, 200 (1964))

A. Vascular Changes

Various authors have attempted to correlate susceptibility to motion sickness with characteristic alterations in blood pressure and cardiac action, but have not been able to show consistent relationships (Tyler and Bard, 1949; Taylor et al., 1960).

One consistent physiologic effect, however, is that of skin pallor, the degree of which is dependent upon the severity of the motion sickness. In order to determine the significance of this autonomic response, Sunahara et al. (1964) made quantitative determinations of the blood volume redistributions occurring in specific parts of the body and concluded that serious detrimental effects could ensue. Their studies involved monitoring changes in blood flow through the skeletal muscles as an important parameter. Healthy young men acted as subjects and strong vestibular stimulation was induced by applying multiplanar accelerations. Because of the apparent significance of these findings, the results will be described in some detail.

The subjects were rotated around the vertical axis in the normal sitting position. Attached to the back of the seat was a motor-driven head holder designed to effect controlled oscillation of the head in its saggital plane. From its normal upright position, the head was rotated forward and downward through an angle of 45° in 6 sec, held in this position for 6 sec, returned to the original position over the next 6 sec and allowed to remain at rest for 6 sec before the cycle was repeated. When the turntable was in motion, this square-wave cyclic superimposed motion of the head resulted in the rapid development of disturbing vestibular stimulation with nausea in all but the most resistant subjects.

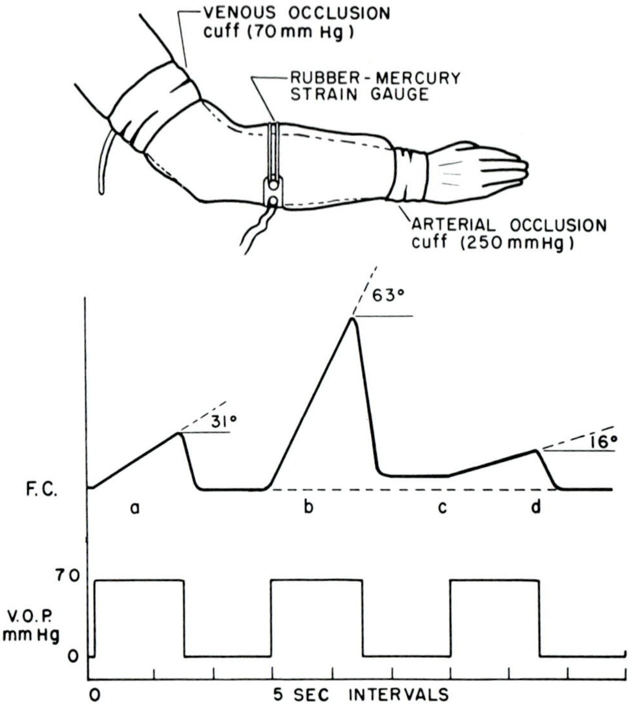

Fig. 3. Measurement of forearm blood flow, schema of the apparatus, procedure and results. *F.C.* forearm circumference. The angles indicated are the forearm blood flows shown in Fig. 5. *(a)* Prestimulus (control); *(b)* response in a subject sensitive to vestibular stimulation; *(c)* failure of the circumference of the forearm of a sensitive subject to return to baseline when venous occlusion pressure released; *(d)* poststimulus response. *V.O.P.*, venous occlusion pressure (Canad. J. Physiol. Pharmacol. **42**, 201 (1964))

Forearm blood flow was measured with the aid of a venous occlusion plethysmograph. An arterial occlusion cuff was placed around the wrist and a venous occlusion cuff around the arm above the elbow. Changes in the circumference of the forearm were measured by a strain gauge. The rate of swelling of the arm is represented by the slope of the record, which was used as an index of blood flow. Blood flow readings were obtained every 15 sec by a system that inflated the venous occlusion cuff to 60 or to 70 mm Hg, allowed it to deflate, and then repeated the cycle automatically. For further technical details, the reader is referred to the original publication.

In a few experiments, the blood pressure was measured directly by arterial puncture and recorded continuously. In other tests it was estimated by means of sphygmomanometry and auscultation before and after rotation. The heart rate was recorded by either an electrocardiogram or a cardiotachometer. Movements of the head were begun as soon as a stable blood flow was established and the subject was requested to signal verbally when his nausea became so severe that he believed further stimulation would cause vomiting.

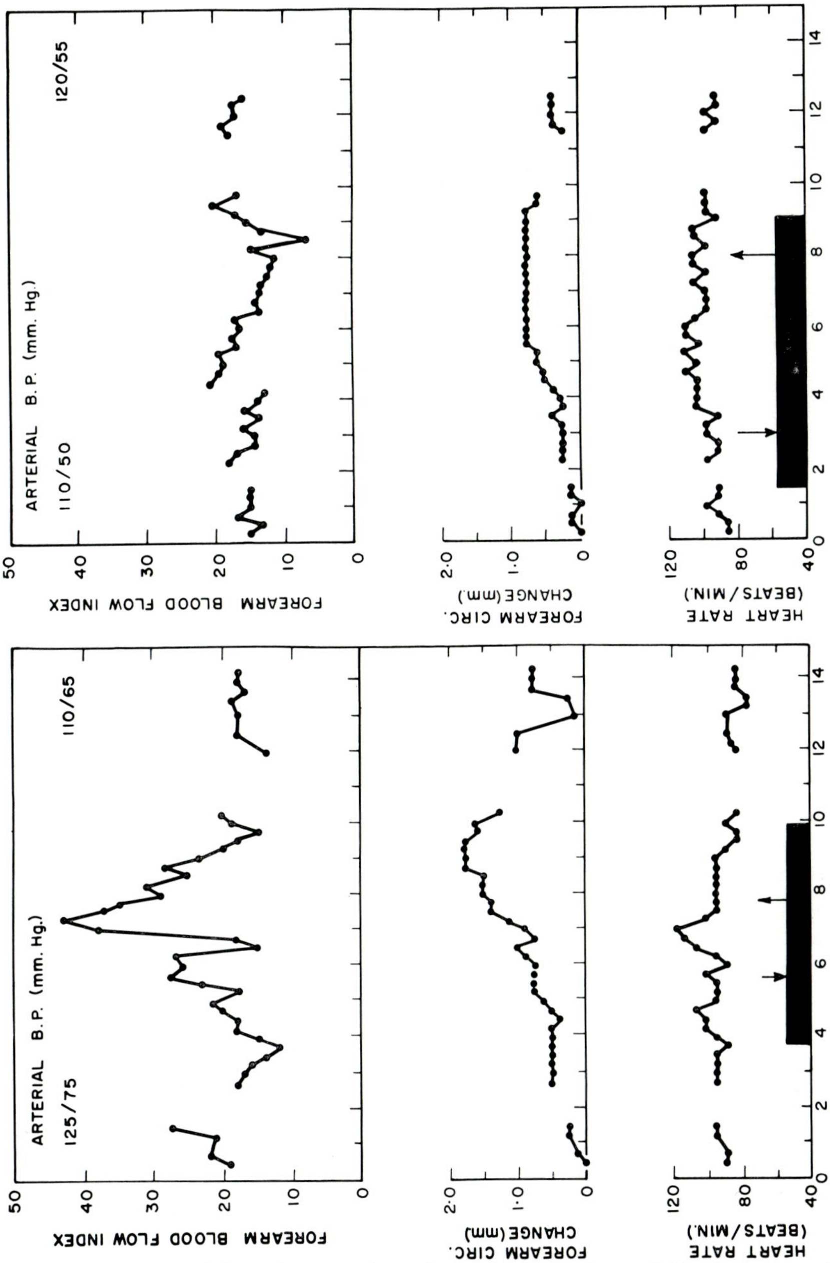

Fig. 4. Forearm blood flow, forearm circumference, heart rate, and blood pressure during vestibular stimulation. Turntable in motion (30 r.p.m.); ↑, start of head movement; ↓, end of head movement. (a) Sensitive subject, motion-sick after 2 min of vestibular stimulation; (b) resistant subject, not motion-sick after 5 min of vestibular stimulation (Canad. J. Physiol. Pharmacol. **42**, 203 (1964))

Figure 4 shows the forearm blood flow, forearm circumference and heart rate responses of both a susceptible and a resistant subject before, during and after two and five minutes of vestibular stimulation. In a subject with a low tolerance to vestibular stimulation (nausea to limit of tolerance after two minutes of head movement) forearm blood flow immediately rose to two or three times the previous level. As the head movement continued, there was also an increase in the circumference of the arm between the periods of venous occlusion (interim arm circumference) and this was taken to indicate an increase in blood volume. The heart rate increased sharply, but immediately returned to normal levels even though the forearm blood flow and interim arm circumference remained above normal. There was a slight drop in arterial blood pressure (124/75 to 110/65). In the subject with a high tolerance to vestibular stimulation (not nauseated after 5 min of head movement) there were no important changes in the forearm blood flow, interim arm circumference or heart rate. Subjects in whom blood pressure was recorded continuously through a needle inserted into the brachial artery showed no significant changes in blood pressure or heart rate, although both subjects were definitely nauseated.

Figure 5 shows the blood flow responses of four subjects who tolerated head movement for 3 to 5 min. These responses are representative of those observed throughout the series. During the 5-min control rotation at 30 revolutions per minute without head movement, no increase in forearm blood flow was recorded in any subject, nor were there any complaints of nausea. Subjects WHR and AIK, who were nauseated to their tolerance limits, each showed a marked increase in forearm blood flow. Subjects MBD and JCB denied having any sensation of nausea after 5 min of superimposed head movement. In subject NBD, the forearm blood flow increased gradually throughout the period of superimposed head movement. Although this subject admitted no symptoms of nausea, sweating of the forehead was observed. In subject JCB the forearm blood flow remained constant within the limits of the method and he exhibited no signs of motion sickness.

The sensation described by the subjects exposed to this potent vestibular stimulation varied from mild vertigo to severe vertiginous disorientation and nausea, and occasionally culminated in emesis. There was a recognizable correlation between the extent of the changes in forearm blood flow and the severity of the symptoms, and it was often possible to predict from the blood flow recordings when a subject would signal that he would vomit if the stimulation continued. Simultaneous measurements have shown increases of blood flow in both forearms and one calf during vestibular stimulation of subjects susceptible to motion sickness. This indicates that the effects are not confined to one limb. Similarly, when three strain gauges were used on one forearm (one at the wrist, one at the point of maximum circumference and one midway between these two) vestibular stimulation in subjects susceptible to motion sickness caused an increase in the circumference of the forearm at all three sites, whereas deliberate clenching of the fist to cause a shifting of the muscle mass of the forearm and simulate changes in muscle tension such as might reasonably be expected to result from vestibular postural reflexes invariably resulted in a decrease in circumference of one or two of the strain gauges. It may, therefore, be assumed that changes in blood flow

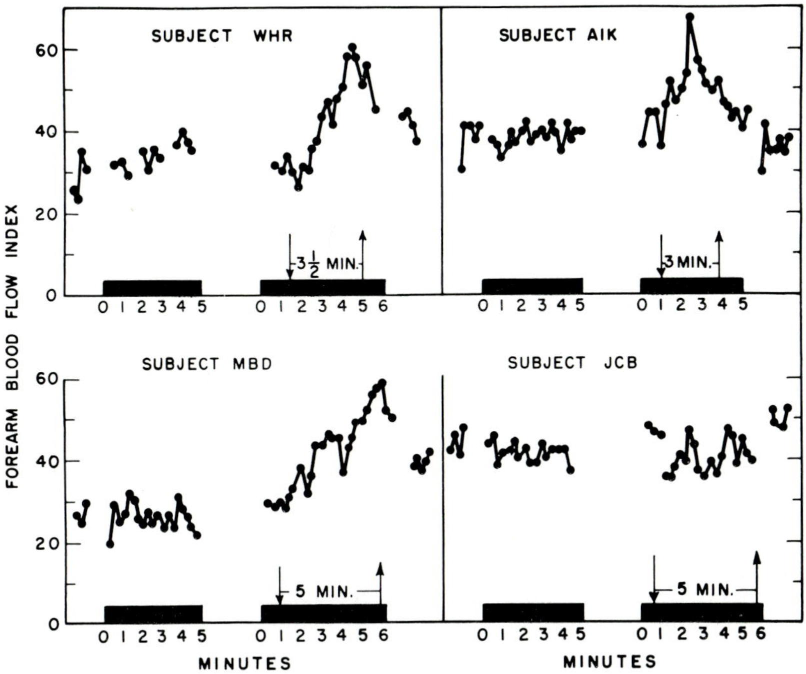

Fig. 5. Forearm blood flow. Subjects representative of the series – see text. Turntable in motion; ↓, start of head movement; ↓, end of head movement (Canad. J. Physiol. Pharmacol. **42**, 204 (1964))

occurred in all extremities and probably most skeletal muscles; moreover, the changes in the limb volume (or circumference) were not due to the artefact of shifting muscle mass caused by changes in muscle tension.

The results do not establish the mechanism of the increase in blood flow or limb blood volume. It appears unlikely that increase in adrenaline output is significant because there is no consistent change in heart rate or blood pressure. In a few experiments where increased heart rate was evident, the increase was transient and the heart rate returned to normal while the blood flow remained elevated. It is unlikely that these responses are attributable to the results of hyperventilation (Rushmer, 1942), because although subsequent experiments have revealed that increased respiratory minute volume is a regular concomitant of vestibular stimulation of this type, the increase in peripheral blood flow and the increase in respiratory minute volume occur simultaneously, often within seconds of the onset of the vestibular stimuli. From this evidence it can be concluded that, although the two phenomena may have a common cause, the increased peripheral blood flow is not caused by hypocapnoea because it is increased before the increased respiratory minute volume could have resulted in lowered CO_2 content.

Taylor et al. have demonstrated a marked antidiuretic response due to motion sickness; it is similar to the antidiuretic response to vasovagal syncope (Brun et al., 1946; Noble and Taylor, 1953). Barcroft and Edholm (1945) have shown that there is a marked increase in forearm blood flow and concomitant vasoconstriction of the hand during fainting as a result of haemorrhage. They concluded that the increased forearm flow blood was in the muscle. Intravenous injection of pitressin to the human subject caused muscle vasodilatation and skin vasoconstriction with no consistent change in arterial blood pressure. Collectively, these findings indicate a close similarity between the signs and symptoms of the vasovagal syndrome and those of motion sickness resulting from vestibular stimulation.

In general terms, an increase in blood flow in one part of the body must either be compensated by decreased flow elsewhere or by an increase in cardiac output or result in reduced arterial blood pressure. The human forearm is 85% muscle by volume, and the skeletal muscle represents about 50% of the total body mass. By calculation, blood flow in the muscle represents about 15—16% of the cardiac output. If we assume that blood flow in the forearm and calf is representative of the total body skeletal body muscle blood flow, a slight increase in flow in these muscles must be compensated by a prompt substantial cardiovascular adjustment if normal blood pressure is to be maintained. The increase in blood flow is obviously considerable. Since there is little or no apparent change in blood pressure or heart rate concomitant with increased blood flow, in order to maintain the blood pressure one or both of the following adjustments must occur:

a) an immediate increase in the cardiac output effected by an increase in stroke volume (because heart rate does not change significantly);

b) increased vasoconstriction in other regions of the body.

The latter is certainly evident in the marked pallor observed in sick subjects. Skin blood flow is — 13 ml/100 ml tissue per minute, according to which of the various reported values is accepted. By calculation, as skin is about 5% of the total body mass, the total skin blood flow would be equal to some 30–50% of the total muscle blood flow under resting conditions. Even the total cessation of skin blood flow could compensate for only a small part of the observed two-to three-fold increase.

These findings would undoubtedly have a bearing on aerospace flight during manoeuvres that cause vestibular stimulation and increased g. In some subjects under certain conditions, failure of one or more of the compensatory mechanisms could cause the peripheral resistance to fall below an already critical level. This would result in a decrease in arterial blood pressure, and among other effects a decrease in g tolerance and possibly a loss of consciousness due to cerebral anaemia. This is another factor to be added to the list of physiological stresses that can lead to flying accidents, and is also applicable to vestibular stimulation during space flight. Medical hazards of prolonged space flight include motion sickness and decreased tolerance to orthostatic hypotension (BERRY, 1970). Since orthostatic hypotension can easily result from a combination of weightlessness and general inactivity, any concomitant motion sickness may well contribute to a physiologic emergency because of the autonomic effects discussed above. Similar effects might be applicable to pathologic states involving the labyrinth.

Although motion sickness is not considered to be a development of the autonomic effects of vestibular stimulation (Borison and Wang, 1953), the reverse is true to the extent that nausea-inducing vestibular stimulation results in some specific functional changes controlled by the autonomic division of the nervous system. As already discussed, some of these involve the vascular system, effecting not only changes in the surface arteries but more extensive changes in blood flow elsewhere. Because of the general feeling of "malaise" which is such a significant feature of motion sickness, it seems only reasonable to assume that widespread physiologic changes are induced, some of which are not yet known. As far as the autonomic nervous system is concerned, skin pallor is simply one obvious entity of visceral effector innervation activity; others should be considered. Furthermore, McClure (1971) has demonstrated that flushing of the skin is an even earlier sign of the onset of nausea, with skin pallor being an indication of more advanced motion sickness associated with vomiting.

B. Perspiration

Marked activity of the sweat glands during motion sickness is another consistent manifestation of its onset, a fact which has been well documented by numerous authors (e.g. Hemingway, 1944; Clark and Graybiel, 1961; Money, 1970). In fact, its onset can be detected prior to any noticeable awareness of nausea and can thus be considered an early symptom. This finding was recently confirmed by Ackerman et al. (1968) as a result of the development of an extremely sensitive detector which indicates that sweating occurs as soon as five seconds after the onset of appropriate motion under controlled conditions in the laboratory. Recordings showed simultaneous sweat outbreak on both the forehead and the back of the hand, and the authors recommend the latter as the more suitable location for such measurements (forehead sweating could also be induced by apprehension).

Since the sweat glands are also concerned in the maintenance of thermic equilibrium, being controlled for this purpose by the visceral motor neurons of the autonomic nervous system (as is also the case for the cutaneous blood vessels), laboratory studies of motion sickness should be carried out under appropriate conditions of temperature and humidity when these responses are being used to indicate the onset of sickness. McClure and Fregly (1971) have further emphasized the importance of differentiating between motion-sickness sweating and that due to temperature and anxiety.

C. Salivation

As reported by McEachern et al. (1942): "Hypersalivation and frequent swallowing are common in the early stages of sea sickness. Later the tongue is apt to be dried and furred".

Intense salivation is particularly conspicuous in susceptible animals. This can be readily demonstrated in dogs (Money and Freidberg, 1964) and in squirrel monkeys (Johnson et al., 1962). It is accompanied by chewing movements and precedes vomiting, should it occur. It is significant to note that apprehension has the reverse effect, namely dryness of the mouth.

Although the salivary glands are innervated by both divisions of the autonomic system, the copious outflow symptomatic of motion sickness possibly implicates the sympathetic nerves, although there may be species differences in the innervation (Rawlinson, 1933; Babkin, et al., 1942). Each of the major glands has both sympathetic and parasympathetic innervation in man and the relative importance of the two in motion sickness has not yet been clarified.

D. Respiration

Although there have been some reports to the contrary (McEachern et al., 1942), exposure to nausea-inducing motion generally results in hyperventilation (Colehour and Graybiel, 1966) as can also be the case when anxiety is present. When the two circumstances occur together (as in aviation or space flight), the resulting hyperventilation can be sufficiently severe to result in lowering of the blood CO_2 level. The physiologic effects of acapnia are well know, i.e. lowering of the tonic activity of the vasoconstrictor centre with arteriolar dilatation and a resultant fall in blood pressure. This effect may be further augmented by interference with the venous return resulting from forced expiratory movements (Best and Taylor, 1966). This could result in sufficient pooling of blood in the lower parts of the body (when in the upright position) to cause syncope from decreased cerebral blood flow. Although such extreme physiologic effects seldom occur in cases of sea sickness, car sickness or air sickness, the result could be catastrophic during prolonged and extreme stress.

E. Gastrointestinal Effects

It is well known that people suffering from motion sickness have a complete lack of interest in food, so much so that even the sight or smell of it is usually obnoxious. Consequently, interference with normal digestive processes can be expected.

Babkin and Bornstein (1943) studied several physiologic effects of motion sickness in susceptible dogs and reported a resultant reduction in gastric motility. This effect has also been reported in humans by Crampton (1955), who found it was inconsistent. Defaecation is a common manifestation in animals, even when they are otherwise house-trained (Money and Freidberg, 1964).

In regard to afferent visceral effects, it has been suggested that gross movements of the abdominal organ may induce nausea, an opinion derived from the observation that traction applied to the mesentery during surgery under local anaesthesia induces nausea (Leggenhager, 1936). Abdominal belts have been claimed to prevent this effect (Maitland, 1932).

F. Yawning and Sleepiness

These symptoms are early in onset and prolonged, persisting even after the incapacitating motion has ceased (Babkin, 1942; Money and Freidberg, 1964). Yawning is a response to a wide variety of stimuli, including sleepiness and intracranial disturbances as described by Proctor (1964) who also points out that "it is an effective way of fully expanding the lungs and increasing venous return to the heart". It is possible, therefore, that in motion sickness it results in compensation for diminished intracranial circulation (Johnson, 1967).

G. Vision

It is known that visual disturbances in the absence of actual motion can induce nausea (STEELE, 1963). Blind subjectes, however, are susceptible to motion sickness (MONEY, 1970). An observation of dilated pupils during emesis has been reported (MCEACHERN et al., 1942), but the reverse has also been claimed (SCHWAB, 1954). GRAYBIEL et al. (1965) found no significant change of ocular imbalance with motion sickness during a twelve-day exposure in the slow-rotating room.

DICHGANS and his associates (1972) have demonstrated very significant relationships between optokinetic stimulation and responses formerly thought to be specific to the labyrinth. These investigators found that visually induced pseudocoriolis effects could be developed by tilting the head during optokinetic stimulation alone (without body rotation), and that it was impossible to distinguish these effects from the well known Coriolis effect produced by superimposing head motion upon body rotation. Furthermore, the nausea normally induced by oculomotor activity fails to develop in labyrinthectomized subjects. These highly significant findings indicate interaction between vestibular responses and the oculomotor system, a matter of considerable importance for the determination of the stimuli involved in any situation resulting in motion sickness.

H. Chemical Aspects Including Space Flight

Blood and urine have been studied in attempts to determine signs of autonomic and other stress effects associated with motion sickness. These findings have been reviewed by MONEY (1970) and include blood acetylcholine, carbon dioxide, glucose, dehydrogenase, eosinophils, ketones, lactate, phosphorus and oxygen content; plasma alkali reserve, calcium, proteins, potassium and serum; serum and urinary 17 hydroxy-corticosteroids, urinary catecholamines and dehydrogenase.

Although such determinations have, for the most part, shown inconsistent changes, oliguria with its associated constituent concentration changes has proved to be a reliable indicator of the degree of motion sickness (e.g. TAYLOR et al., 1957; CLARK and GRAYBIEL, 1961; COLEHOUR, 1965). The precise aetiology of the antidiuresis has not been established, although there is suggestive evidence. The specific gravity of the urine was consistently increased in the motion sick subjects, and the concentration of urinary chlorides was appreciably increased, whereas the total amount of chlorides excreted per unit of time remained relatively constant. These findings are indicative of increased renal resorption of water. The signs accompanying motion sickness are similar to the effects that would be expected to result from the liberation of a neurophypophyseal hormone known to cause prolonged antidiuresis, which is characterized by increased chloride concentration and the presence of an antidiuretic substance (ADH) in the urine. The release of ADH has been suggested for this effect, its presence having been conclusively demonstrated by a bio-assay procedure. Although it may be released from the neurohypophysis, its central nervous control remains to be established. Such effects are not confined only to motion sickness, however, but also occur as the result of a variety of stresses including pain and fainting.

An adequate understanding of the supression of motion sickness by chemical means may well clarify the relative activity of the two divisions of the autonomic nervous system in this malady; the incidence of motion sickness during space flight

(BERRY, 1970) has prompted a critical evaluation of the therapeutic value of different compounds. The findings have indicated that only drugs with a parasympatholytic or a sympathomimetic action and some of the antihistamines are effective. The studies by WOOD (1968) indicate a preference either for cyclizine or for scopolamine taken with either amphetamine or ephedrin. However, no drug has yet been found to be completely protective and it may well be that for space travellers the procedure of choice is careful selection together with development of a high degree of resistance obtained by in-flight adaptation exercises involving incremental head movements (GRAYBIEL and WOOD, 1969). In this connecion, it is interesting to note that some space travellers have experienced dizziness and nausea during the early stages of orbital space flight, the severity of which increased with sharp head movements. Some of the Soviet cosmonauts have also experienced incapacity due to "vestibulo-vegetative" disorders. This was reported to have occurred in the first manned orbital flight when cosmonaut Titov executed head movements after several hours in the weightless state. Some of the other cosmonauts (Foekistov and Yegerov) in later space flights also noted similar reactions, describing them as autonomic and unpleasant sensory reactions (YUGANOV et al., 1966). It has been suggested that this space sickness results from increased labyrinthine sensitivity due to the absence of stimulation of the otoliths (normally the result of the earth's gravitational pull) and the time characteristics of the stimulus (BERRY, 1970).

Although "space" or "cosmos" sickness did not develop during the Mercury and Gemini flights, there were nine definite cases during the Apollo missions, ranging from stomach awareness to nausea and vomiting. As reported by BERRY and HOMICK (1973)[1], "The first clear-cut case of motion sickness in American space flight was experienced by the Apollo 8 astronauts. All three crew members experienced symptoms ranging from stomach awareness to vomiting lasting for up to 5 days in the case of one crewman. Motion sickness drugs were taken with mixed results".

A similar high incidence of motion sickness was experienced during the first few days of the second Skylab mission of 1973 when astronaut activity was considerably limited until adaptation to weightlessness developed. It seems apparent, therefore, that when man's physiologic responses to motion in the strange environment of weightless space are understood, we shall attain a better appreciation of the complexities of various autonomic changes characteristic of motion sickness.

References

ACKERMAN, U., JOHNSON, W. H., THOMAS, E. L.: A detector for the outbreak of sweating. Report of Institute of Biomedical Electronics, University of Toronto, 1968.

BABKIN, B. P., BORNSTEIN, M. B.: The effect of swinging on the motility of the stomach in dogs. N.R.C. Canada, Report C 4030, October, 1943.

BABKIN, B. P., DIVORKIN, S.: Experimental studies of motion sickness. N.R.C. Canada, Comm. Med. Res. Rep. No. C 736, 1942.

BARCROFT, H., EDHOLM, O. G.: On the vasodilation in human skeletal muscle. J. Physiol. (Lond.) **104**, 161 (1945).

---

1 BERRY, C. A., HOMICK, G. L.: Findings on astronauts bearing on artifical gravity. Aerospace Med. **44**, 163 (1973).

Berry, C.: Recent advances in aerospace. Med. Proc. 18th Int. Cong. Aviation and Space Med., Amsterdam, 1969. D. Ridel. Dordrecht, Netherlands, 1970.

Best, C.H., Taylor, N.B.: The physiological basis of medical practice, 8th ed. Baltimore: Williams and Wilkins 1966.

Borison, H.L., Wang, S.C.: Physiology and pharmacology of vomiting. Pharmacol. Rev. **5**, 193 (1953).

Brun, E., Knudson, E., Raaschov, F.: Kidney function and circulatory collapse. J. clin. Invest. **25**, 568 (1946).

Chinn, H., Smith, P.: Motion sickness. Pharmacol. Rev. **7**, 33 (1955).

Cipriani, A.: An analysis of the forces encountered on the simple swing used in the study of motion sickness. N.R.C. Canada, Comm. on Sea Sickness, Nov., 1942.

Clark, B., Graybiel, A.: Human performance during adaptation to stress in Pensacola slow rotation room. Aerospace Med. **32**, 93 (1961).

Colehour, J.K., Graybiel, A.: Biochemical changes occurring with adaptation to accelerative forces during rotation. Aerospace Med. **37**, 1205 (1966).

Correia, M.J., Guedry, F.E.: Influence of labyrinth orientation relative to gravity on response elicited by stimulation of the horizontal semicircular canals. Naval School Aviation Med. Pensacola, Florida. Report No. 100, 1964.

Crampton, G.H.: Studies of motion sickness XVII: Psychological changes accompanying sickness in man. J. appl. Physiol. **7**, 501 (1955).

De Witt, G.: Sea sickness (Motion Sickness): a labyrinthological study. Acta Otol. Suppl. **108** (1953).

Dichgans, J., Brandt, Th.: Visual-vestibular integration and motion perception. In: E. Bizzi and F. Dichgans, Eds. "Cerebral Control of Eye Movements and Motion Perception". Basel-New York: S. Karger 1972.

Graybiel, A.: The importance of the otolith in man. Ann. Otol. (St. Louis) **65**, 470 (1956).

Graybiel, A.: Vestibular sickness and some of its implications for space flight. Chap, XI in Neurological Aspects of Auditory and Vestibular Disorders. Springfield, Ill.: C. C. Thomas 1964.

Graybiel, A., Clark, B., Zarriello, J.J.: Observations on human subjects living in slow rotating room for periods of two days. Amer. Med. Ass. Arch. Neurol. **3**, 55 (1960).

Graybiel, A. et al.: Effect of exposure to a rotating environment (10 rev/min) on four aviators for a period of twelve days. Aerospace Med. **36**, 733 (1965).

Graybiel, A., Wood, C.D.: Rapid vestibular adaptation in a rotating environment by means of controlled head movements. Aerospace Med. **40**, No. 6: 638 (1969).

Guedry, F.E.: Orientation of the rotation axis relative to gravity. Acta oto-laryng. (Stockh.) **60**, 30 (1965).

Hemingway, A.: Cold sweating in motion sickness. Amer. J. Physiol. **141**, 172 (1944).

Hemingway, A.: Cardiovascular changes in motion sickness. J. Aviat. Med. **16**, 417 (1945).

Johnson, W.H.: Head movements and motion sickness. Int. Rec. Med. gen. Practice Clin. **167**, 638 (1954).

Johnson, W.H.: The importance of the otoliths in disorientation. Aerospace Med. **35**, 874–877 (1964).

Johnson, W.H.: Physiologic responses to unusual vestibular stimulation. Third N.A.S.A. Symposium on the Role of the Vestibular Organs in Space Exploration, Pensacola, Florida, Jan., 1967.

Johnson, W.H., Mayne, J.W.: Stimulus required to produce motion sickness 11. J. Aviat. Med. **24**, (1953).

Johnson, W.H., Meek, J.C., Graybiel, A.: Effects of labyrinthectomy on canal sickness in squirrel monkeys. Ann. Otol. (St. Louis) **71**, 289 (1962).

Johnson, W.H., Stubbs, R.A., Kelk, G.F., Franks, W.R.: Stimulus required to produce motion sickness. J. Aviat. Med. **22**, 362 (1951).

Johnson, W.H., Taylor, N.B.J.: Some experiments on the relative effectiveness of various types of accelerations in motion sickness. Aerospace Med. **32**, 205 (1961).

Leggenhager, K.: Schweiz. med. Wschr. **66**, 354 (1936).

Maitland, T.G.: Practitioner **129**, 251 (1932).

MANNING, G.: Failure of a vertical accelerator to produce motion sickness. N.R.C., Canada, Report C, 2649, Dec., 1943.

MANNING, G.W., STEWART, W.G.: Effect of body position on incidence of motion sickness. J. appl. Physiol. **1**, 619 (1949).

McCLURE, J.A., FREGLY, A.R., MOLINA, E., GRAYBIEL, A.: Responses from arousal and thermal sweat areas during motion sickness. Aerospace Med. **43**, 2: 176 (1972).

McCLURE, J.A.: Personal communication, 1971.

McEACHERN, D., MORTON, G., LEHMAN, P.: Seasickness and other forms of motion sickness. War Med. (Chic.) **2**, 410 (1942).

McNALLY, W.H., STUART, G.: Physiology of the labyrinth reviewed in relation to seasickness and other forms of motion sickness. War Med. (Chic.) **2**, 683 (1942).

MEDA, E.: A research on the threshold for the coriolis and purkinje phenomenon of excitation of the semicircular canals. Arch. Fisiol. **52**, 116 (1952). (Eng. Transl. by E. R. Hope, Defence Research Board, Canada, T 171, Sept., 1954).

MONEY, K.E.: Third N.A.S.A. symposium on the role of the vestibular organs in space exploration, Pensacola, Florida, Jan., 1966.

MONEY, K.E.: Motion sickness. Physiol. Rev. **50**, 1:1–39 (1970).

MONEY, K.E., FREIDBERG, J.: The role of the semicircular canals in causation of motion sickness and nystagmus in the dog. Canad. J. Physiol. Pharmacol. **42**, 793 (1964).

NIVEN, J.I., HIXSON, W.C., CORREIA, M.J.: Elicitation of horizontal nystagmus by periodic linear acceleration. Acta oto-laryng. (Stockh.) **62**, 429 (1967).

NOBLE, R.L.: Observations on various types of motion causing vomiting in animals. Canad. J. Res., E **23**, 226 (1945).

NOBLE, R.L., TAYLOR, N.B.J.: Antidiuretic substances in human urine after haemorrhage, fainting, dehydration and acceleration. J. Physiol. (Lond.) **122**, 220 (1953).

PROCTOR, D.F.: Physiology of the upper airway, Handbook Physiol. 1:309. Washington, D. C.: Amer. Physiol. Soc. 1964.

RAWLINSON, H.E.: Cytological changes after autonomic and adrenalin stimulation of the cat's submaxillary gland. Anat. Rec. **57**, 289 (1933).

RUSHMER, R.F.: Overventilation in subjects during the swing test. Comm. Av. Med. Rep. No. 157, N.R.C., U.S.A., May, 1942.

SCHWAB, R.S.: The nonlabyrinthine causes of motion sickness. Int. Rec. Med. **167**, 631 (1954).

SPIEGEL, E.A.: Effect of labyrinthine reflexes on the vegetative nervous system. Arch. Otolaryng. **44**, 61 (1946).

SPIEGEL, E.A. et al.: Experimental production of motion sickness. War Med. (Chic.) **6**, 283 (1944).

STEELE, J.E.: Motion sickness and spatial perception – A theoretical study. In: Symposium on Motion Sickness with Special References to Weightlessness. USA Wright-Patterson Air Force Base, Ohio. ASD. Technical Report No. 61–530, 1963.

SUNAHARA, F.A., JOHNSON, W.H., TAYLOR, N.B.G.: Vestibular stimulation and forearm blood flow. Canad. J. Physiol. Biochem. **42**, 199 (1964).

TAYLOR, N.B.J., HUNTER, J., JOHNSON, W.H.: Antidiuresis as a measurement of laboratory induced motion sickness. Canad. J. Biochem. Physiol. **35**, 1017 (1957).

TAYLOR, W.J.R., JOHNSON, W.H., SELLERS, E.A.: Cardiovascular stimulation with vestibular stimulation. J. Aerospace Med. **31**, 627 (1960).

TYLER, D.B., BARD, P.: Motion sickness. Physiol. Rev. **29**, 311 (1949).

WENDT, G.R.: "Final report", N.R.C., U.S.A., Dec., 1945.

WEAVER, R.S.: Theoretical aspects of the role of angular acceleration in vestibular stimulation. Acta oto-laryng. (Stockh.) Suppl. **205** (1965).

WOOD, C.D.: Use of drugs in the prevention of motion sickness. Fourth Symp. on Role of Vest. Organs in Space Exploration, Pensacola, Florida, N.A.S.A. 1968.

YUGANOV, E.M. et al.: Vestibular reactions of cosmonauts during the flight in the "voskhod" spaceship. Aerospace Med. **37**, 691 (1966).

Part 2. Some Sensory Aspects

By

L. B. W. Jongkees

With 4 Figures

Any vestibular stimulation applied repeatedly is said to cause vegetative collapse characterized by depression of the circulation and blood pressure, a slower heart beat, respiration with prolonged expiration, myosis, stomach contraction, quicker peristalsis, nausea, and vomiting (Montandon, 1952). This is what we observe in motion-sick (the word was introduced by Irwin, 1881) people.

Of all forms of motion sickness (from camel riding to space exploration) seasickness has been investigated most extensively. It not only affects humans, but also many animals. Some, such as guinea pigs and pigeons, seem to be insensible to it (van Maanen, 1965). It appears to be provoked by the clash of misleading information reaching the body from visual, proprioceptive, and especially vestibular receptors which are subjected to stimuli outside the normal pattern of everyday life. Flourens (1830) was the first to suspect the vestibular labyrinth as the cause. Deaf-mutes with non-functioning vestibular organs are not susceptible to seasickness (James, 1882; Pollak, 1893; Sjoberg, 1931). Destruction of the labyrinth or section of the VIIIth nerve on both sides made the sensitivity to seasickness disappear in experimental animals (Kreidl, 1893). Seasick people never show nystagmus, and the linear accelerations to which people on board ship on a turbulent sea are exposed are much greater (compared by their respective thresholds) than the rotatory ones. These facts led Wojatschek (1909), Bárány (1910) and Quix (1922) to the conclusion that the origin of seasickness has to be sought in the otoliths and not in the semicircular canals.

According to Nieuwenhuysen (1958) (Fig. 1), who examined his test persons during a sea voyage, the percentage of people that become seasick is more or less proportional to the level of the vertical linear accelerations to which they are exposed. Van Maanen reports the data of an investigation of the British fleet which clearly show the speed with which people habituate to the movements of the ship (Table 1). Not everybody is equally susceptible to motion sickness. Young

Table 1.

Duration of the journey, days	Percentage of seasick people
1	22
2	20
3	16
4	13
5	4

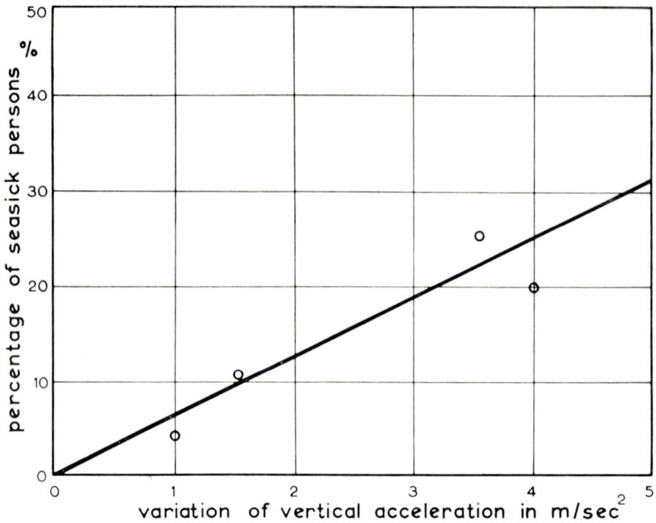

Fig. 1. Percentage of seasick passengers as a function of the variation of the vertical acceleration. Pitching period 7 sec. From Experimental investigations on seasickness. Academic Thesis, Utrecht 1958. J. H. NIEUWENHUYSEN

children are especially liable to become seasick; old people (over 60) are less prone to it. In certain positions (lying in bed) people are better able to tolerate a rough sea. According to QUIX (1922), this is due to the fact that in this situation the otoliths do not give much information. In this position (turned through more than 90° from the vertical position), man can hardly orientate himself relative to the gravitational vertical in the absence of vision. On the other hand, there are people who never become seasick and others who get seasick whenever the sea becomes a little rough (Lord Nelson). DE WIT (1953) investigated this problem and found that among those who are prone to seasickness, there is a group who seem to lack the ability to adapt themselves, i.e. to build a pattern copy (for further details see chapter on the pathology of vestibular sensation). He examined these subjects and found that the inclination of the sensation curves in the cupulograms was remarkably steep and nearly or completely parallel to the nystagmus curves, which might indicate that this curve was not influenced by adaptation (Fig. 2).

In these sensation cupulograms the π/Δ value (i.e. the inclination) appears to be approx. 25 sec. In normal people, however, this value was found to be much smaller (HULK and JONGKEES, 1948; SCHIERBEEK, 1953). It seems likely that vestibular sensation to rotational stimuli is diminished in people not susceptible to motion sickness (VAN WULFFTEN PALTHE, 1922; BRUNS, 1926; DE WIT, 1953; KRIJGER, 1954; ASCHAN, 1954; PREBER, 1958; VAN MAANEN. 1965; LIDVALL, 1967) and it is probable that the capacity for adaptation in the vestibular field plays an important part in motion sickness.

As stated in Chapter F.IX., this capacity can be measured from the steepness of the sensation cupulogram. In expert seamen it can be very low ($<$ 4 sec), in

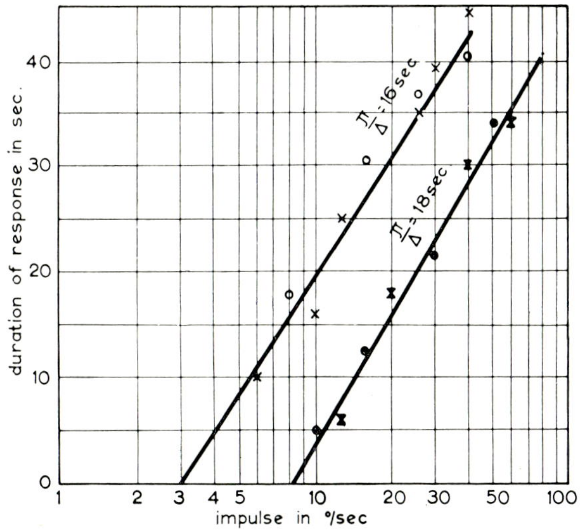

Fig. 2. Case of hypersensitivity to motion sickness. Parallelism between sensation (16 sec) and nystagmus (18 sec). The thresholds are normal. From Experimental investigations on seasickness. Academic Thesis, Utrecht 1958. J. H. Nieuwenhuysen

normal people about 6 sec, and in the chronically seasick it can be as high as 25 sec or more. In expert seamen and test pilots the sensation threshold rises to a higher level. The susceptibility to adaptation is measured for the semicircular canals in the cupulogram. This does not prove, however, that these canals are the organs responsible for the genesis of motion sickness. It may be that the entire labyrinth has this susceptibility and even that the otoliths are the main sub-organs responsible.

The experiments of Money and Friedberg (1964), who found that "discreet surgical inactivation of all six semicircular canals eliminates motion sickness in dogs", do not prove that the semicircular canals cause seasickness. Their investigation of otolithic function by means of a variation of de Kleyn and Versteegh's (1927) "Sprungbereitschaft" (readiness to jump) is not enough to prove the otoliths intact since this reaction is still present when the otoliths are thrown from their maculae by centrifugal force. The discreet surgery consisted of opening the canals with a burr and letting the loose bone dust enter the labyrinthine space. This, of course, can also damage utricular function.

It appears that neither the semicircular canals nor the otoliths alone provoke motion sickness. Other sense organs can provoke symptoms quite similar to it, e.g. if a sensitive person watches clouds driven by the wind, especially while standing on top of a high building or moutain; misinformation due to mirror effects or pseudomotions can produce strong sensations in sensitive persons, and the clash of contradicting information from various sense organs or from sub-organs seems to be of paramount importance here. It is possible to produce motion sickness by rhythmically changing linear accelerations in both vertical and horizontal directions, but it is still easier to provoke motion sickness together with its vasovagal reactions by the so-called (wrongly) "Coriolis forces" (de Wit, 1957; Sunahara et al., 1964).

The sensation of falling over when a person bends his head up or down during rotation at constant speed, and the strong sensation of nausea that accompanies this exercise, were already known to Purkinje (1820) (for the forces acting in the labyrinth see Groen, 1961).

Van Rossum (1908) used the sensations provoked by Coriolis forces for threshold measurements. Tschermak (1921) describes complete disorientation and Fernández and Lindsay (1964) agree with him. But Delage (1888) was the first to give a more exact description. Apart from very severe nausea ("a more severe nausea can hardly be imagined"), he finds that a quick bending of the head onto the left shoulder during clockwise rotation provokes a sensation of vertical rotation backwards together with horizonatal counterclockwise rotation of longer duration but smaller intensity. When the head is moved back to the original position, vertical rotation forward, again with counterclockwise horizontal rotation is felt. The movement can be made so slowly, however, that no sensation is observed. Schubert (1935) describes the Coriolis effects during stunt flying and attributes various flying accidents to Coriolis sensations. Downward movements of the head during clockwise rotation provoke an illusion of falling backward to the left. Upward movements lead to a spiraling sensation upward and forward to the right.

In a glass model Groen (1961a) saw the fluid movements caused by inertia entering the semicircular canals that were not originally in the plane of rotation. This happens abruptly and with comparatively strong force dependent on the movement's size and the speed of the extra rotation.

The author and his associates also performed some experiments on glass models, and were especially struck by the turbulences that originated in the utricle; this suggested that the utricle would also be stimulated. The strong sensation of falling or rising incorporated in the spiral sensations could be provoked by otolith stimulation. However, caution is necessary in drawing conclusions from experiments with enlarged models.

Some people are very sensitive to vestibular stimulation and easily react with vegetative reactions. They are said to have hypersensitive vestibular organs. The author does not think that this is correct. These persons very often do not show particularly low thresholds for vestibular stimulation (rotatory or caloric). In these cases one should set vegetative hypersensitivity against vegetative hyposensitivity. Different pathway and connections in the central nervous system are involved (Karbowski, 1961) for sensation and vegetative reactions. Many people will be seasick, but a large percentage will adapt and be able to withstand the burdens of a sea voyage, while others will never adapt (the chronically seasick). Not all of them have a steep sensation cupulogram (the genuine seasick according to de Wit). Other deviations in vestibular examinations have been mentioned, but the results are contradictory. De Wit finds steepness of the sensation cupulograms a reason for seasickness, van Maanen does not. Krijger implicates different reactions for clockwise and anticlockwise sensation cupulograms, but

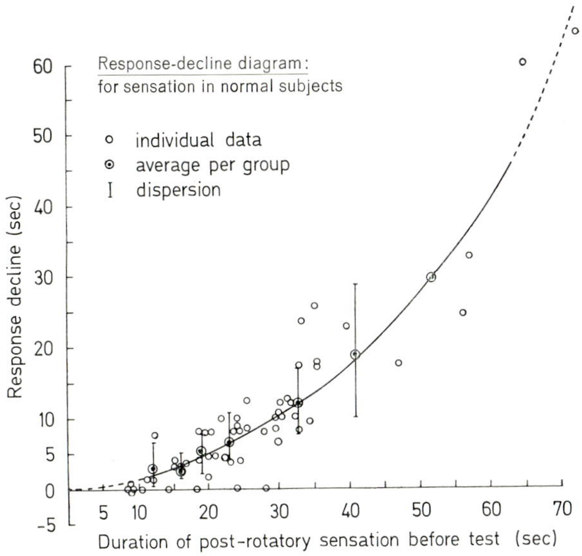

Fig. 3

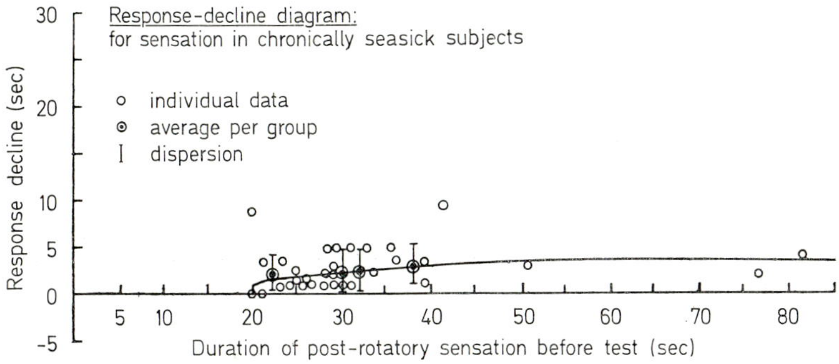

Fig. 4

Fig. 3. — Fig. 4. From J. C. D. van Maanen Chronic Seasickness. Academic Thesis, Utrecht 1965. After provocation tests the duration of postrotatory sensations (in a sensation cupulogram) gets smaller than before the test but there is a striking difference between healthy (Fig. 3) and chronically seasick sailors (Fig. 4) (see text)

Aschan finds the phenomenon in expert test pilots. Van Maanen (1965) proposed a provocation test and examined both healthy and chronically seasick sailors by measuring their sensation cupulograms before and after the test (Figs. 3 and 4), which consisted of active head movements during a rotation at a constant speed of 100°/sec for 3 min. Thereafter, the duration of the after-sensations was measured again. The difference between the results was striking when the groups of seasick and normal seamen were compared. The response decline is very much more significant in the normal than in the seasick group (and much more intense for sensation than for nystagmus). The adaptability is not always equal in both directions, and this might also be a reason for chronic seasickness. In the caloric test LIDVALL (1967) found that habituation curves for seamen who were often seasick were parallel to those for expert sailors who were never seasick. This seems to prove again that habituation is a very specifically directed phenomenon, not identical in the caloric and in the acceleration field.

It is clear enough that psychological, visual and other factors are of importance for motion sickness, but it would be outside the field of this short survey to discuss them here. A few words about the treatment might be valuable for the understanding of the problem. Antihistaminics (Cinnarizine, Dramamine) have an important depressive effect on the vestibular organ (PHILIPSZOON, 1959; BOS and PHILIPSZOON, 1963) and are very good drugs for the prevention of seasickness, but less useful if the patient is already sick. The central adaptation system in the substantia reticularis and its connections with the thalamus and the cortex are activated by adrenaline and acetylcholine, but depressed by atropine and parasympatholytic drugs. The last group is said to have a good effect in cases of seasickness. Some people can diminish their sick feeling by intense fixation of a stationary point (especially the horizon), while others are helped by lying down in the dark. In the last instance the number of incoming signals, and therefore of conflicting information, is strongly reduced. As soon as these persons get up and walk around they often become severely seasick again. Many other treatments are purely psychological though not unimportant (fresh air, avoidance of the presence of others who are seasick, 1001 mixtures, pills, powders, etc.).

References

AUBERT, H., DELAGE, Y.: Physiologische Studien über die Orientierung. Tübingen: Laupp 1888.

ASCHAN, G.: Response to rotatory stimuli in fighter pilots. Acta oto-laryng. (Stockh.) Suppl. **116**, 24–31 (1954).

BÁRÁNY, R.: Weitere Untersuchungen über den vom Vestibularapparat des Ohres reflektorisch ausgelösten rhythmischen Nystagmus und seine Begleiterscheinungen. Mschr. Ohrenheilk. **41**, 477–523 (1907).

BÁRÁNY, R.: Über Seekrankheit. Mschr. Ohrenheilk. **44**, 723–732 (1910).

BOS, J. H., PHILIPSZOON, A. J.: Some forms of nystagmus provoked by stimuli other than accelerations. Pract. oto-rhino-laryng. (Basel) **25**, 108–118 (1963).

BRUNS, O.: Münch. med. Wschr. **73**, 977 (1926).

FERNÁNDEZ, C., LINDSAY, J. R.: The vestibular Coriolis reaction. Arch. Otolaryng. **88**, 469–472 (1964).

FLOURENS, P.: Experiences sur les canaux semicirculaires de l'oreille dans les mammifères. Acad. roy. Sci. Paris **9**, 467–477 (1830).

GROEN, J. J.: Vestibular stimulation and its effect from the view of theoretical physics. Confin. neurol. (Basel) **21**, 380–381 (1961a).

GROEN, J. J.: The problems of the spinning to applied top the semicircular canals. Confin. neurol. (Basel) **21**, 454–455 (1961b).

HULK, J., JONGKEES, L. B. W.: The normal cupulogram. J. Laryng. **62**, 70–75 (1948).

IRWIN, J. A.: On the pathology of seasickness. Lancet **11**, 907 (1881).

JAMES, W.: The sense of dizziness in deaf-mutes. Amer. J. Otol. **4**, 239–254 (1882).

KARBOWSKI, K.: Über die von den Labyrinthbogengängen ausgelösten Reaktionen. Pract. oto-rhino-laryng. (Basel) **23**, 289–297 (1961).

KLEYN, A. DE, VERSTEEGH, C.: Present position of the physiology of the labyrinth. J. Laryng. **42**, 649–655 (1927).

KREIDL, A.: Weitere Beiträge zur Physiologie des Ohrlabyrinthes. (1893).

KRIJGER, R.: De betekenis van het evenwichtszintuig voor de vlieger. Academic thesis, Utrecht 1954.

LIDVALL, H.F.: Mechanism of motionsickness as reflected in the vertigo and nystagmus responses to repeated caloric stimuli. Acta oto-laryng. (Stockh.) **55**, 527–536 (1967).

MAANEN, J.C.D. VAN: Chronic seasickness. Academic thesis, Utrecht 1965.

MONEY, K.E., FRIEDBERG, J.: The role of the semicircular canals in causation of motion sickness and nystagmus in the dog. Canad. J. Physiol. Pharmacol. **42**, 793–801 (1964).

MONTANDON, W.: Le reflex de depression d'origine vestibulaire. Pract. oto-rhino-laryng. (Basel) **14**, 257–260 (1952).

NIEUWENHUYSEN, J.H.: Experimental investigations on seasickness. Academic thesis, Utrecht 1958.

PHILIPSZOON, A.J.: The effect of some drugs on the labyrinth. Academic thesis, Amsterdam 1959.

POLLAK, J.: Über den galvanischen Schwindel bei Taubstummen und seine Beziehungen zur Funktion des Ohrlabyrinthes. Pflügers Arch. ges. Physiol. **54**, 188–208 (1893).

PREBER, L.: Vegetative reactions in caloric and rotation tests. Acta oto-laryng. (Stockh.) Suppl. **144** (1958).

PURKINJE, J.E.: Beyträge zur nähernen Kenntnis des Schwindels aus heautognostischen Daten. Med. Jahrb. K. K. Österr. Staates **VI**, 79–125 (1820).

QUIX, F.H.: Le mal de mer, le mal des aviateurs. Monogr. otorhinolaryng. Internat. 8th ed. Legrand, Paris 1922.

ROSSUM, A. VAN: Gewaarwordingen en reflexen opgewekt vanuit de halfcirkelvormige kanalen. Academic thesis, Utrecht 1908.

SCHIERBEEK, P.: Vestibular turning test by means of weak-stimuli. Pract. oto-rhino-laryng. (Basel) **15**, 73–87 (1953).

SCHUBERT, G.: Physiologie des Menschen im Flugzeug. Berlin-Göttingen-Heidelberg: Springer 1953.

SJOBERG, A.A.: Experimentelle Studien über den Auslösungsmechanismus der Seekrankheit. Acta oto-laryng. (Stockh.) Suppl. **14** (1931).

SUNAHARA, F.A., JOHNSON, W.H., TAYLOR, N.B.G.: Vestibular stimulation and forearm bloodflow. Canad. J. Physiol. Pharmacol. **42**, 199–207 (1964).

TSCHERMAK, A.: Der exacte Subjektivismus in der neuen Sinnesphysiologie. Pflügers Arch. ges. Physiol. **180**, 1–35 (1921).

WIT, G. DE: Seasickness. Acta oto-laryng. (Stockh.) Suppl. **108** (1953).

WIT, G. DE: Some animal experiments on motion sickness. Acta oto-laryng. (Stockh.) **47**, 172–175 (1957).

WOJATSCHEK, W.: Einige neue Erwägungen über das Wesen der Seekrankheit. Beitr. Anat. etc., Ohr. **2**, 336–345 (1909).

WULFFTEN PALTHE, P.M. VAN: Functions of the deeper sensibility and of vestibular organs in flying. Acta oto-laryng. (Stockh.) **4**, 415–449 (1922).

Chapter IX.

Pathology of Vestibular Sensation

By

L. B. W. Jongkees, Amsterdam (Holland)

With 16 Figures

Contents

I. Introduction

A survey of the pathology of vestibular sensation must start with a definition of the normal way in which the vestibular organ causes sensations. Leiri (1927a) and Muskens (1934) attributed sensations of change in position or movements to muscular sense. According to these authors the vestibular organ is not a sense organ, but only a reflex organ. It is recognized that definitions are difficult to compare and vulnerable. An organ of sense can be defined as one that reacts to a specific external stimulus with specific effects. One could object to this definition on the grounds that unspecific stimuli such as electric stimuli to the cochlear nerve, mechanical stimuli to the eye, or caloric stimuli to the vestibular organ can produce the specific reactions of sound, sight, or sensation of movement, but on the whole it is serviceable, and if it is accepted the vestibular apparatus must be included amongst the organs of sense (Jongkees, 1952).

In normal life the vestibular organ informs man with great precision about what happens to his position relative to his environment. It may not be a sensation that generally attracts his attention, but as soon as something happens, if he slips or actually falls, not only will the reflexes from this organ help him restore his balance, but he will feel exactly what is going on. The fact that the sensations provoked by stimuli acting upon the vestibular organ often do not reach consciousness has been used as an argument in support of the idea that the vestibular organ is not a real sense organ. As with all the other senses, however, perception of stimulation of the vestibular organ only becomes conscious when changes take place which disturb a continuous "white noise" pattern. In the same way we do not consciously perceive all the visual stimuli that reach our eyes, neither do we consciously hear all the sounds, nor smell all the smells that stimulate our peripheral senses in their specific fields.

Some special difficulties arise in the field of vestibular perception, however. The vestibular organ is only one of the organs that inform us about our position in space. It cooperates with vision and kinesthetic sensations from muscles, joints, etc. As long as the information from these various sources is the same, we are well informed about our position and our movements and everything is "balanced"; but as soon as they do not agree our balance is lost and we are subject to the frightening sensation of having lost contact with the world around us. It can be compared to an earthquake. We lose the feeling of having two steady feet on the earth (KITAHARA and UNO, 1967). Even living in a house that is tilted only very slightly by such an event can lead to nausea, headache, anorexia and insomnia.

The structure of the vestibular organ is such that abnormal stimuli easily provoke sensations which are misleading. Nevertheless, it is not rational to state that the sensation caused by stimulation of the vestibular organ is vertigo and that therefore the vestibular sensation is always pathologic. These abnormal sensations are caused by unphysiological stimulation.

Man has been familar with motion sickness since the days when the first lazy king or fierce soldier took a camel to bring him to his destination in a shorter time and with less effort (FERRERI, 1956). And the opportunities to become seasick, carsick, airsick, or spacesick have increased at an enormous speed. The unnatural reactions of this organ are not only encountered in motion sickness, however, but also in the clinical methods routinely used to examine patients, to test pilots, or to extend our knowledge of the function of the vestibular organ. In all these cases both the reflexes and the sensations are inappropriate. They give us wrong information about our surroundings. They are provoked by unphysiological stimuli. Vestibular nystagmus and sensations that do not reflect reality are abnormal, i.e. pathologic.

II. The Specific Stimuli of the Vestibular Organ

According to BISCHOF (1966) the definition of an appropriate stimulus can be found in various fields. Psychologically a stimulus is appropriate if the conscious perception it provokes can be interpreted as its effect. Biologically a stimulus is appropriate if the stimulation of the sense organ provokes reactions that can be interpreted as its significant answer. Physiologically, a stimulus is appropriate if the filtering properties of the sense organ are specifically laid out for its selective relay. The stimulus can be inappropriate for qualitative, but also for quantitative reasons, in the latter case both for intensity and for duration.

For the vestibular organ we have to consider two parts: the semicircular canals and the otoliths. MACH (1875) and BREUER (1874) pointed out, and many proofs have been described since then, that accelerations provoke a stimulation of both these suborgans. The semicircular canals are stimulated by rotatory accelerations and the otoliths by linear accelerations (JONGKEES, 1944; PHILIPSZOON, 1964).

However, problems arise when we try to apply the above definitions. The cupulae and the otoliths, the sensing elements, are inertia-dependent. *The mechanical behavior of the cupula-endolymph system* can be described in terms of a highly damped torsion pendulum (STEINHAUSEN, 1933).

A differential equation (VAN EGMOND et al., 1949b; GROEN et al., 1952) has been described from which the mechanical behavior of the cupula-endolymph apparatus can be computed. Sensations provoked by various types of stimulation have even been used to find the constants of the equation.

For clinical use the equation has proved to be of value in the genesis of cupulometry, but these sensations cannot be interpreted as the significant answer of the canal system. In normal daily life the canals act as speedometers. For physiological movements, i.e. rotations with a fairly abrupt beginning, a duration of not more than about 3 sec, and a fairly abrupt ending, e.g. a turn of the head, or a fall, it is a most appropriate instrument because it performs an integration in time of the angular acceleration to which it is exposed.

Excitation of the canals gives rise to a very accurate subjective estimation of the angle of turning, provided that the movement lasts not more than 3 sec. Within that period acceleration multiplied by time is constant ($a\tau = k$; MULDER's law, 1908). If a turn lasts longer or contains a period of constant velocity, the cupula no longer acts as a speedometer, but is forced back to equilibrium by its own directional property (stiffness of the cupula, which fits hermetically in its ampulla like a swing-door). A decelerative phase following one of constant velocity annihilates the last traces of a deviation provoked by the forces used to attain the constant velocity. It also, however, drives it past the point of equilibrium in the opposite direction, from which the cupula will slowly return, provoking an after-reaction. (In the rotation tests of BÁRÁNY, 1907; BUYS, 1928; VEITS, 1931; VAN EGMOND et al., 1948; etc. this phenomenon is used by clinicians).

The integration described by MULDER only takes place during the short movements common in daily life; it gives perfect information about what "really happens" even though the accelerations are generally not constant.

In conclusion: the appropriate stimulus for the semicircular canals is a brief rotation. In the three-dimensional apparatus of the 3 pairs of canals (2 lateral, left anterior and right posterior vertical canals, right anterior and left posterior vertical canals), both the extent and the direction of absolute angular displacement are sensed, by integration of the acceleration of the skull relative to the environment. All other stimuli, even in the domain of rotatory acceleration, lead to reactions beyond the range of normal and do not give rise to significant answers. In motion sickness they lead to the well-known symptoms, but even without sickness they could be disastrous, e.g. if the pilot of a fast plane tried to fly it guided by his sensation of position or movement (JONES, 1960). Totally different patterns of movement are encountered in flight and space, and serious mismatching occurs between the sensory system and the new environment.

On the other hand, if rightly adapted, this pathologic functioning can be exploited in examination of the function of the cupula organs.

The stimulation of the otolithic organs by linear accelerations leads to other difficulties. Linear accelerations present in three forms: acceleration of gravity, centrifugal acceleration during rotations outside the axis of rotation (such as in a centrifuge), and linear accelerations during linear movements with changing speed. If a linear accelerations acts on the labyrinth in a direction other than the vertical, the direction of the resultant from the parallel of forces of gravity and the other acceleration will be felt as "the vertical" and the surrounding world will be felt to have an oblique position (MACH, 1875; BREUER, 1889).

This situation can be provoked in a human centrifuge and on the parallel swing. Under the influence of linear accelerations inertia makes the heavy otoliths (statoliths is a better name) move in relation to their maculae. It seems fairly certain that shearing forces are responsible for the stimulation of the nerve endings and lead to the appropriate sensation (BREUER, 1874; VON HOLST and MITTELSTAEDT, 1950; BÉKÉSY, 1966).

In this situation the appropriate stimulus is the acceleration of gravity which gives the significant answer about the position in space of the person subjected to the stimulation.

It indicates the direction and the alterations in direction of the constant gravitational force during the movements in daily life. This is also one of the difficulties the investigator of otolithic function is confronted with. It is very difficult to investigate the function of the labyrinth without stimulation by gravity. This is only possible during a fall (a jump and a parabolic flight are essentially identical to a fall).

The acceleration of gravity acts on each mass particle in the same way (GROEN, 1953). In the case of the otolith, gravity pulls on the otolith as well as on the macula. The macula, being supported by the underlying tissues, remains in its place, bearing the otoliths. In this way stimulation of the end-organs will result.

The two otolithic maculae, being nearly perpendicular to each other, are well suited to sense the direction of the forces acting upon them. If the body is submitted to an acceleration other than gravity (e.g. on a parallel swing) the acceleration is transmitted to every part of the body. Each suspension system undergoes a force equal to the product of the acceleration and of the mass to be accelerated. In this case, the macula feels a force equal to the mass of the otolith times the acceleration. Here again the sensations will not reflect reality. According to VON WEIZSÄCKER (1947) "in the world space and time are in the objects and not the objects in space and time. Our metric-physical projection of space should not be appreciated as a constant reference system for perception. It is continuously built up from senso-motoric perceptions." Perception does not comprise movements of the eye as a causative factor but is this movement. Subjective space is not a simple reflection of physical space. Vestibular and extravestibular perception are of equal importance and form one space. If this space is built on misinterpretations, the whole relation between subject and world is changed. This is also the basis for interesting phenomena like oculogyral and oculogravic illusions (GRAYBIEL et al., 1956). These symptoms have no causal connections with eye movements produced by vestibular reflexes, but are an expression of the lack of matching between perceptive and physical space (TSCHERMAK, 1921). In a fine series of experiments, VAN DISHOECK et al. (1954) proved the parallelism between oculogyral illusion and rotatory sensations and their complete independence from the movements of the eyes. Oculogravic illusions surpass largely the angle of counterrotation of the eyes (BRANDT and FLUUR, 1967). In the same way, other senses fit into the apparent perceptive world e.g. hearing (audiogyral phenomena, see also DITTLER, 1921).

But the perception of linear acceleration by all the parts of the body where a "suspension systems" is submitted to a linear acceleration is also and inseparably bound up wich otolithic stimulation. It is no wonder therefore, that a person without labyrinths still has a fairly good impression of his position in space (FISCHER, 1928; JONGKEES and GROEN, 1950). Nevertheless, the otoliths have the filtering system specifically laid out for its selective relay. Experiments with a human centrifuge, and a parallel swing gave sensations that could be compared

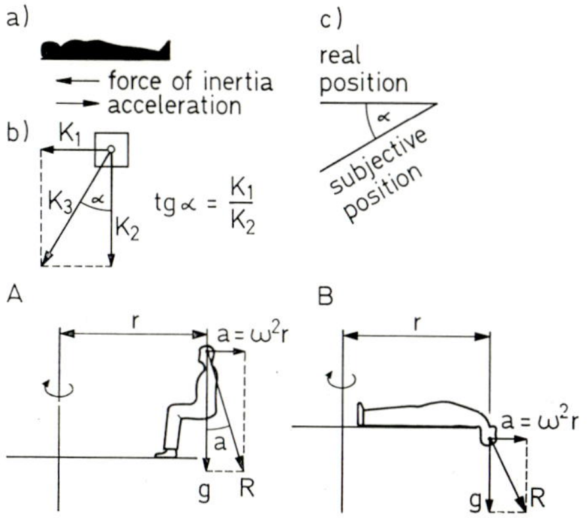

Fig. 1. Scheme of the forces acting on an otolith organ in the case of a combination (resultant force k_3) of gravity (k_2) and centrifugal force (k_1). (*a*) acceleration and force of inertia acting on the test person. (*b*) composition of forces. (*c*) effect on the position sense. A. The sensation depends on the direction of the resultant force R. In B, however, R acts in the direction of the blind spot of the otoliths

Table 1. Comparison of Sensation Caused by Centrifugal Acceleration and Gravitational Acceleration

I Time of revolution T. sec	II Angular velocity ωrad./sec	III Centrifugal force ω^2R rad./sec^2	IV Sensation of leaning backwards *a* degrees	V Same sensation at an inclination of the position chair *a* degree	VI Calculated tg *a*	VII sensation *a*°
8.2	0.77	65	10°	5°	65/981	3.9°
6.0	1.05	127	30°	10°	127/981	7.5°
3.5	1.79	368	45°	20°	368/981	20.0°

Table 2. Comparison of Sensation Caused by Centrifugal Accelerations and Gravitational Acceleration Acting in the Direction of the Blind Spot of the Labyrinths

I Time of revolution T. sec	II Angular velocity ω rad./sec^2	III Centrifugal force ω^2R rad./sec^2	IV Sensation of leaning backwards *a* degree	V Same sensation at an inclination of the position chair *a* degree	VI Calculated tg *a*	VII sensation a °
4.5	1.4	254	0°	0°	254/981	14.5°
3.5	1.8	520	14°	5°	520/981	28.0°

to the sensation of position on a positioning apparatus. Only when the labyrinths were intact was there quantitative conformity (Table 1 and 2, Fig. 1). On a parallel swing a subject without labyrinths has a vague feeling of moving to and fro but the threshold is about double the threshold for subjects with intact labyrinths (6 as against 12 cm/sec^2), who feel a sinusoidal rotation about a horizontal axis perpendicular to the movements of the swing (Jongkees and Groen, 1946b).

As measures against stimulation of the sensitivity of the skin become more efficient, the apparent to-and-fro movements become smaller compared to the rotations (Aubert and Delage, 1888).

At this point another difficulty becomes evident. A sensation of rotation can be induced by purely linear acceleration and stimulation of the otoliths if the direction of the resultant "g" is changing rhythmically (Fig. 2). On the other hand

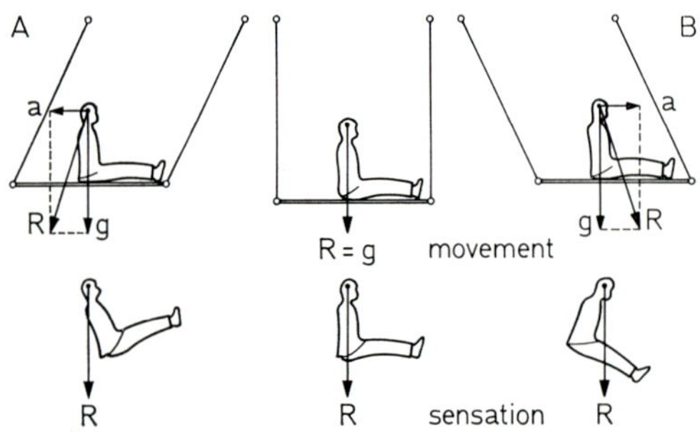

Fig. 2. Movements and sensations on the parallel swing

Fischer and Veits (1927) found that bilateral caloric stimulation of the semicircular canals leads to sensation of linear movements and of change of position relative to gravity. Great caution is necessary in the inference of conclusions from the character of the sensation and their use in establishment of its origin.

From stimulation to conscious perception. Bárány (1907), Buys (1913), and later Dodge (1923) found that test subjects submitted to an angular acceleration of long duration felt a rotation phasically changing from one direction to the other when the acceleration was changed into a rotation with constant speed. They concluded that this "seemed to indicate the interplay of some central neural agency, whose nature we do not know". Fischer (1928) gives an extensive description of the sensations that Wodak (1922) and he had when they submitted themselves to the Bárány rotation test (10 rotations in 20 sec). They had the same series of phasic sensations of rotation in alternating directions. He also described the difference between the first after-sensation and the later ones. A movement of the head in a plane perpendicular to the plane of the foregoing rotation greatly influenced the sensation as it changed the direction of the plane in which the subjective rotation takes place. In later phases these movements of the head no longer influence the sensation of rotation (Fig. 3). This can be explained by the fact that the first after-sensation is caused by a movement of the endolymph-cupula system following all the laws of physical mechanics as, for

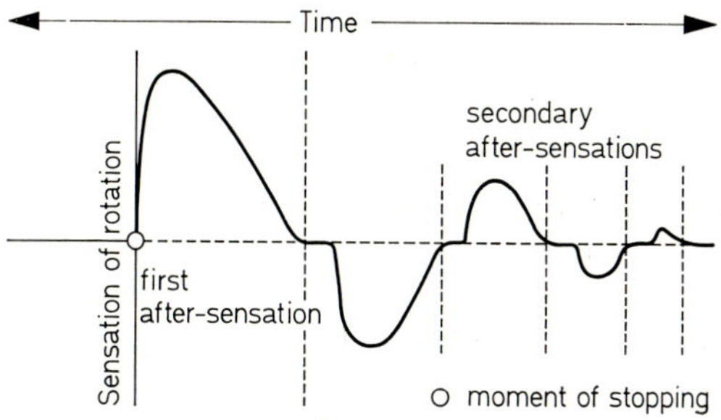

Fig. 3. Primary and secondary sensations after a stop of rotation with high speed

instance, the production of an endolymph-flow in canals other than those originally stimulated; and the secondary after-sensation by a rhythmic and alternating discharge of vestibular nuclei (SCHMALZ, 1932). During secondary after-sensations a difference between those in the plane of the horizontal canals and those in the planes of the vertical canals appears. Their temporal development is different. The horizontal sensations persist longer than the vertical ones. Only when rotation takes place in the plane of two coupled canals (see earlier) is this disintegration absent (AUBERT and DELAGE, 1888).

According to JONGKEES and GROEN (1946a), there is no proof that this central origin is the only reason for secondary after-sensations. A peripheral causation is not impossible. Certainly the hypothesis that rhythmic after-sensations arise from oscillations of a periodically damped cupula can be excluded. However, many other peripheral causes are conceivable, e.g. chemical processes such as are known in the retina and are held to be responsible for the formation of after-images, electrical phenomena, and finally phenomena of hysteresis in the cupula, which is not only deviated after a deflection from the state of equilibrium, but whose internal structure is also distorted (see also GROEN, 1961a). This process of recovery may, no doubt, last for several minutes and there is no reason why there might not be pauses between successive phases of the after-sensation. The fact that secondary after-sensations do not always have alternating directions, but are sometimes observed in the same direction a few times in succession, and that changes of the position of the head do not influence the direction of the turning sensation can be readily understood from this standpoint. We have never stated that central influences do not exist (the fact that after-effects are found after optokinetic stimuli proves the existence of nonmechanical, probably central influences) (ASCHAN and BERGSTEDT, 1955), but we wish to stress that peripheral factors may play a part in the formation of secondary after-sensations if the stimulus is sufficiently pronounced. After normal movements of the head there are no after-sensations, and after small stimuli such as are used in cupulometry (stopping impulses of 60°/sec and less), there is only one primary after-sensation. If the impulse lies above 60°/sec the afore-mentioned distortion might develop (see also ASCHAN, 1955; HOOD, 1967).

On the other hand it seems quite certain that the central vestibular system, its pathways, centers, and connections have an important influence on the final effect of the stimulation of the peripheral organ. The intensities of stimuli passing through the brain are inhibited or enhanced by different influences (DOLOWITZ, 1965).

A clear indication is found in cupulometry. By this rotating test VAN EGMOND et al. (1948) tried to achieve a quantitative examination of the function of the cupula-endolymph system in the semicircular canals and at the same time to record the results of this investigation in a curve. A patient is placed in a rotating chair, to which a subthreshold acceleration is applied until a certain angular velocity is attained. Then the chair is brought to a standstill in about 1–2 sec. This is repeated for velocities of different magnitude and the duration of both after-sensation and after-nystagmus is determined for each given stimulus. As the equation of the movements in the cupula-endolymph system suggests, large impulses provoke deviations of the cupula that last longer than the ones provoked by smaller stimuli, and the duration of a deviation is proportional to the logarithm of the impulse. This is the reason the cupulogram is on a logarithmic scale for the impulse. In normal cases a straight line is obtained.

In the semicircular canal the differential equation of a torsion pendulum when there are no external forces is $\theta\ddot{\xi} + \pi\dot{\xi} + \Delta\xi = 0$, where

θ = moment of inertia of the cupula,
π = moment of friction at unit angular velocity,
Δ = directional momentum at unit angle,
ξ = angular deviation of the cupula-endolymph relative to the skull,
$\dot{\xi}$ = angular velocity of the cupula-endolymph relative to the skull,
$\ddot{\xi}$ = angular acceleration of the cupula endolymph relative to the skull,
π/Δ = is given by the inclination of the ideal (peripheral) cupulogram,
Δ/θ = can be found from the latent natural period on the torsion swing,
π/θ = can be calculated from the size of the canals and viscosity and density of the endolymph.

From the fact that the cupulogram conforms to the theoretical expectation it seems justifiable to conclude that the after-reaction does depend on the deviation of the cupula, at least in normal cases.

HULK and JONGKEES (1948) found that the curves for sensation of rotation and nystagmus are not identical in normals. This is confirmed by many workers in the vestibular field (Fig. 4).

As far as I know only HENNEBERT (1961) expresses a different opinion when he states: "I can ascertain, as MONTANDON, that the nystagmus and the sensation are always concomitant."

The threshold and the inclination of the sensation curve are both lower than the threshold and the inclination of the nystagmus curve (Fig. 5). This proves that, though both answers to vestibular stimulation seem to depend on the mechanical behavior of the cupula, their pathway through the central vestibular field is differently influenced. This observation corroborates BUYS' (1913) statement that nystagmus and deviations in walking, pastpointing etc. have a different threshold. Therefore it seems inevitable to assume that if nystagmus and rotatory sensation are indeed caused by a deviation of the cupula in the semicircular canal, at any rate a completely different mode of accomplishment exists in both cases. This finishing touch must be sought in central vestibular influences. If the largest

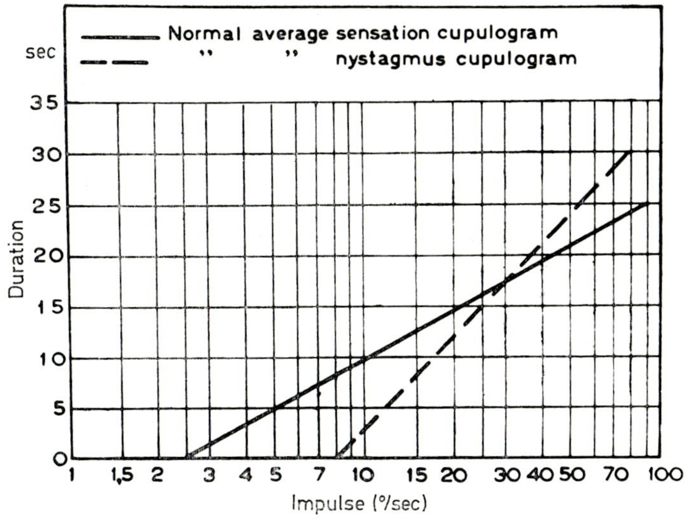

Fig. 4. The average nystagmus- and sensation-cupulogram of normal subjects constructed with the normal average threshold and inclination of fifty subjects

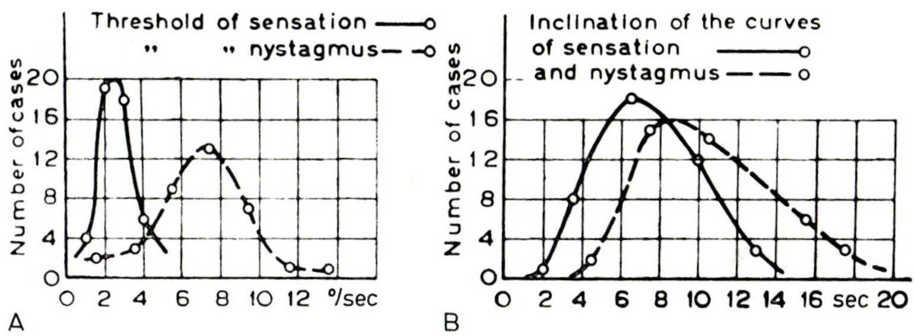

Fig. 5. A. Distribution of the threshold of the stopping impulse for sensation and nystagmus in 50 normal subjects. B. Idem for the inclination

impulse is not over 60°/sec the cupulogram is identical at various repetitions and can even be found in another way, i.e. by following the subjective angular velocity of the rotated person during the after-sensation period by asking him to indicate as far as possible when he thinks he has rotated through 360°, 180° or 90° until he stops (GROEN and JONGKEES, 1948b, c). This subjective cupulogram also appears to determine the magnitude of the stimulating impulse with satisfactory certainty (see below) (Fig. 6, 7).

The application of strong impulses (e.g. BÁRÁNY's test, i.e. 180°/sec), however, changes the cupulogram (Fig. 8). The sensation curve is displaced toward a higher threshold and a lower inclination and sometimes the curves for clockwise and anti-clockwise rotation diverge. FEARING (1926) has shown that repeated turning

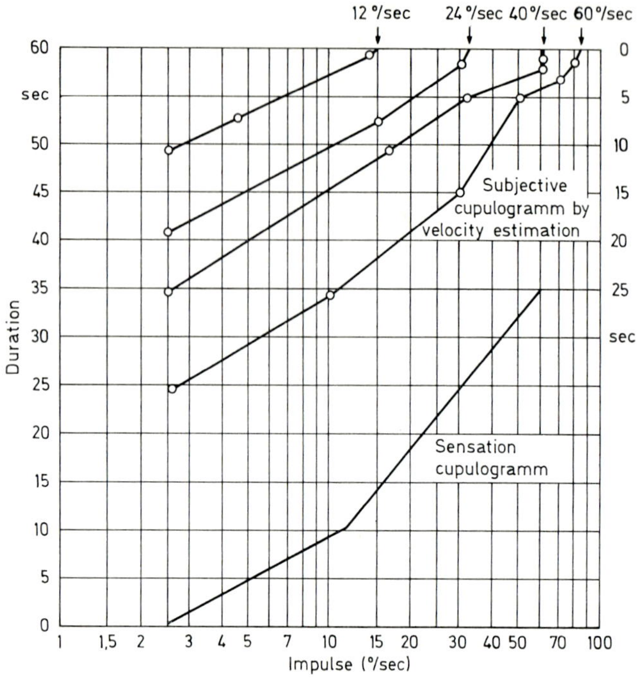

Fig. 6. In one person the sensation cupulogram (lower curve) and the subjective cupulogram by angular velocity estimation are compared. The stimulus used to take the subjective cupulogram and its strength are indicated by an arrow at the zero point of the diagram

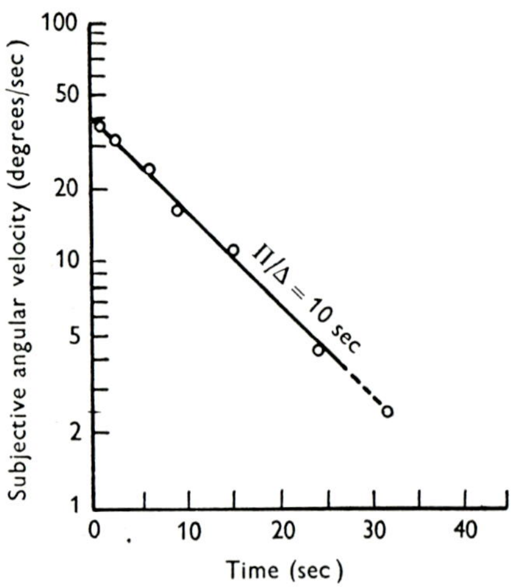

Fig. 7. Subjective angular velocity against time. The impulse administered was 40°/sec, as is the extrapolated subjective velocity. The slope gives $\Pi/\triangle = 10$ sec

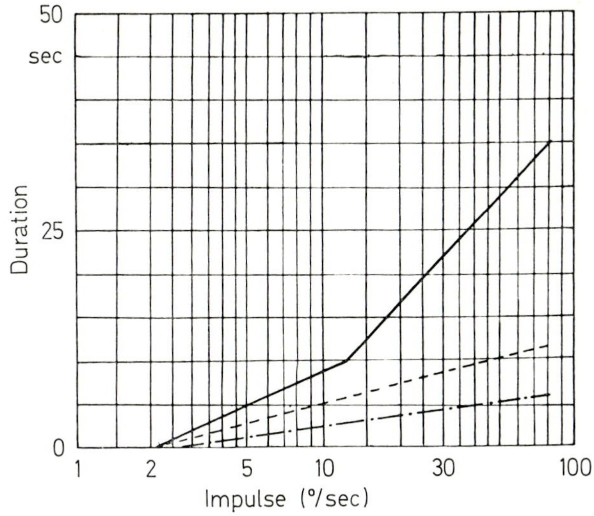

Fig. 8. Sensation cupulogram before (——), and hour (–.–.–.), and four days (- - - - -) after a Bárány test

tests with strong stimuli in one direction diminish the after-reactions after turning in this direction, but do not influence the reactions after turning in the opposite direction.

It seems to be fairly certain that adaptation is not found in the peripheral vestibular suborgans (Adrian, 1943; Groen et al., 1952).

Beerens (1968) did not find any change in the frequency of spontaneous discharges in the peripheral utricular nerve of the cat even when a certain oblique position which had caused an increase or decrease of the original frequency at zero position was maintained for 45 min.

The "adaptation" in the vestibular domain must be of central origin. After strong rotatory stimuli the inclination of the sensation cupulogram curves changes. This again proves that normals do not react to semicircular-canal stimulation in accordance with the mechanical laws laid down in the differential equation of the movements of the cupula-endolymph system. This is also evident from the investigations of Ek et al. (1960) on a rotating device which can give a very constant acceleration from 0.5–6°/sec^2 up to a final speed of 360°/sec. The speed can then be maintained at a constant level for an arbitrarily long time and finally the chair can be decelerated within the same limits. It goes without saying that the patient has to be fixed to his chair with the greatest care lest he should be thrown from it, or even make movements (Coriolis force).

In orientating experiments van Egmond et al., when using constant small accelerations found that the sensation of rotation was greatest in their subjects after about 40 sec. Ek et al. found under stricter conditions that the subject who is submitted to an acceleration (of say 1°/sec^2) feels an increasing rotatory speed for about 30 sec (Fig. 9).[1]

1 Collins and Guedry (1967) found a nystagmus peak at 27 sec for both horizontal and vertical canals.

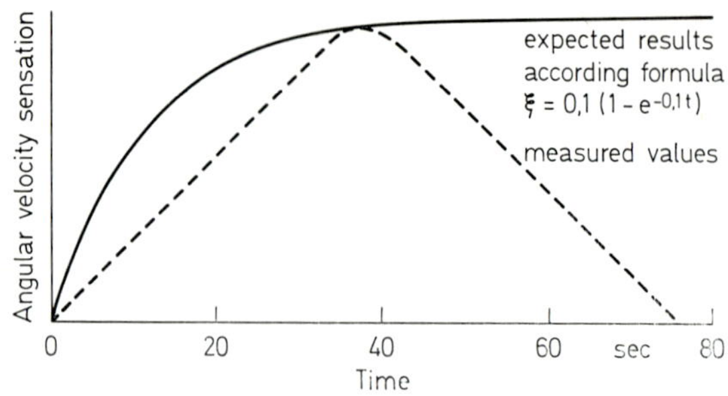

Fig. 9. According to the formula discussed, constant angular acceleration acting upon a test subject should cause a sensation of angular velocity as described by the drawn line. The measured results (dotted line), however, are different

Thereafter it remains constant for a short period of time, but very soon the sensation of rotation decreases again, i.e. the subject has the impression that the speed of rotation is diminishing and eventually he will have the impression of being at a standstill. The sensation can be measured in the way described above (subjective angle estimation). The sensation of being at a standstill is present while the acceleration is still acting upon him and the cupula must therefore still be deflected. If the acceleration is now stopped, and the rotation therefore continued at a constant speed, the subject immediately has the sensation of a strong counterrotation which slowly decreases. As soon as deceleration begins he will have a new countersensation. From this the conclusion is clear: a sensation of counterrotation may exist even while the cupula is still deflected towards a side which usually causes the sensation of a reversed rotation.

Processes in the brain (adaptation) make it impossible to read the position of the cupula from a "recording instrument" such as sensation of rotation. Pichler (1966) suggests that the stimulation of the otoliths causes the disappearance of the sensation of rotation during continuous acceleration. The existence of an influence of the various parts of the labyrinths on each other seems to be quite certain, but to prove it in a specific case is difficult.

Whatever the cause, "the mere conception of a simple reflex chain of unconnected particular reactions happening each time "*de novo*" seems to be too narrow" (Trincker, 1961).

III. Adaptation and Pattern-Building

As stated above, space around us is built up continuously from the information we receive. The many sense organs that constitute the elaborate and complicated system which provides man and animal with this information, "hearing, equilibrium, vision, touch, smell and taste," convey a large number of messages to its brain where they are integrated to form a manifold picture of the momentaneous relationship between the animal's self and the outer world (Groen, 1957).

As long as a certain kind of information does not change, it does not constitute an important factor, since the living being has learnt that an unchanging source of information and even changes which follow a certain pattern are not dangerous and not interesting (GROEN's description is very fascinating and should be read in the original). The result is that not all the stimulations of all the sense organs become messages that reach consciousness or lead to reflexes. Only the abrupt or new stimuli will pass because they change the pattern and cause alarm. A situation called adaptation has come about.

It goes without saying that a complicated systematic apparatus is necessary for this selective action and that the apparatus must have all the information at its disposal. This kind of adaptation, which is perhaps better called habituation, and which also comprises the learning and training processes and the compensation of losses of certain sense organs, must be localized in the brain. (I intend to use the name adaptation in a general sense and habituation for central processes only.)

Messages reaching the sense organ can be suppressed or even completely stopped. Stimuli from one sense organ can influence the information coming from other sense organs. The vestibular organ gives some very clear examples of this kind of habituation, e.g. in motion-sickness, but also in rhythmic stimulations used in clinical practice (torsion swing).

Adaptation was mentioned as early as 1889 by BREUER. It is not a phenomenon which depends on one sense organ. Adaptation takes place in the field of balance, and since our equilibrium is mainly based on visual, kinesthetic, and vestibular information, these sources of information are also involved in the process of adaptation (SINGLETON, 1967).

It is possible to achieve adaptation in various ways, however, and by different kinds of stimulation. It appears that this adaptation phenomenon is rather selective. It is more or less bound to the situation that provokes it. Rotatory stimulations give an adaptation that does not show very much in caloric or galvanic stimulation. Stimuli, in one direction cause homolateral adaptation and much slighter heterolateral adaptation (COLLINS, 1964). The phenomenon has been extensively described in clinical examinations (VAN EGMOND et al., 1949; FISCHER, 1928; DOLOWITZ, 1965; GROEN, 1957, 1965; HALLPIKE and HOOD, 1953; HAMERSMA, 1957; EK et al., 1960), but examples that prove the great value of adaptation are also found in normal life e. g. in special jobs (ballet dancers, ice-skaters, testpilots, aeronauts, dancing dervishes) (BREUER, 1874; ABELS, 1906; VAN WULFTEN PALTHE, 1922; COLLINS, 1964; ASCHAN, 1954, 1967; KRIJGER, 1954). They prove that the normal individual not only reduces the coupling between vegetative centers, but also suppresses nystagmus and sensation, the latter being the easier to control (GROEN, 1962). But not only specific movements belonging to unusual motion patterns provoke adaptation. The normal movements of everyday life also lead to adaptation. This was clearly proved by GROEN (1965), who examined newborn babies and puppies and compared them to adult humans and dogs.

If therefore seems that the phenomenon of adaptation is provoked regularly by the movements of everyday life. Adaptation to stimulations given during sleep or narcosis does not take place (ASCHAN, 1967; SINGLETON, 1967), and the phenomenon sometimes disappears under certain conditions (alcohol intoxication, light anesthesia, ASCHAN, 1967). Sensations and nystagmus do not behave in the same manner (ASCHAN, 1967). Even the TULLIO effect seems to provoke response decline.

For the influence of the direction of "g" (be it pure or presenting itself as a resultant force with other forms of linear acceleration), habituation seems to be absent (GRAYBIEL, 1956; BRANDT, 1962).

The anatomical substrates for response decline are still little known to date. It seems fairly certain that the cerebellum contains elements which play an important part in it. The flocculonodular lobe (LANGELAAN, 1919) has an inhibiting effect on vestibular function. According to MCCABE and GILLINGHAM (1964), there is no response decline after repeated rotation when the lateral and superior vestibular nuclei are extirpated.

According to WENDT (1951) decerebration and decerebellation do not completely prevent habituation. According to GERNANDT (1967), the formatio reticularis in the brainstem influences the relay of the sensory signals in the vestibular nuclei. Generally the response decline of sensation is much more important than that of nystagmus (VAN MAANEN, 1965). FORSSMAN pointed to the similarity of the labyrinthine reactivity pattern in cases of congenital nystagmus and blindness to that in normals habituated by repeated calorizations. He discusses the hypothesis that habituation might cause the special reactivity pattern in these pathologic cases (1963).

It is even contradicted that vestibular habituation should be a normal process. WENDT (1964) points out that people like himself (BUYS and DOHLMAN) have investigated rotational stimulation over many years by submitting themselves to rotatory stimuli without any decrease in their reactions, and others are of the opinion that visual stimuli are much more important than vestibular ones (WENDT, 1951).

Whatever the case, inhibitory tendencies are present whenever a vestibular stimulus lasts too long (be it a constant or a periodic stimulus). In newborns (GROEN, 1965) this tendency is apparent within the first week. If the vestibular system is stimulated with long-lasting stimuli it will adapt itself by inhibition, suppression, and a reduction in duration, but for new stimuli it will show practically the same sensitivity as the unadapted system. "Fundamental principles of a cybernetic character with afferent and efferent pathways make these organs into self-adapting systems which adjust themselves to whatever circumstances demand." However, the responses to new and unknown stimulations that might prophesy dangers or attractive situations to the being in its natural state find an unadapted sense system.

In case of complicated rhythmic stimulations (VON HOLST and MITTELSTAEDT, 1950) which can be looked upon as a certain pattern of vestibular stimuli, the brain builds up a pattern-copy which counteracts the stimuli acting upon the person or animal subjected to it. This counterpart of a periodic or quasiperiodic stimulation reduces or even abolishes the influx of signals to the cortical area where the sensations are presumably located (GROEN, 1957; NIEUWENHUYSEN, 1958).

After the pattern disappears the counterpattern built up in the central nervous system remains active for some hours or even days.

This is why people who have left a ship after a tumultuous sea voyage go on feeling the movements of the ship, skaters still have the sensation of a swinging motion in the evening after a long spell of skating, and even after a torsion-swing experiment the after-sensation can be discovered some hours later (KLIJN and EK, 1959). Pattern-copy formation seems to be merely a complicated form of adaptation.

Pattern building is also found in secondary postrotational reactions and on the torsion swing. Near the threshold the alternating stimulations are sometimes covered by the pattern-copy. This may be why in some instances the sensations in one direction are not felt, though those in the other direction are still above threshold (VON BÉKÉSY, 1955). The pattern-copy anticipates the movement to come and adjusts the body to meet it or as TRINCKER (1961) puts it, the vestibular system "learns to extrapolate from the past into the future." MALECKI (1965) ascribes it to the working of a functional circuit of which the pathways and effects are determined mainly by feedback in agreement with the laws of biological regulation and equilibrium.

The pattern proves to be specific. One who has adapted himself to a big ship will become seasick again on a small one, and a good ocean-sailor is not always able to stand a lot of wind on a lake.

Motion sickness (IRWIN, 1881) indicates the vegetative collapse characterized by depression of the circulation and the blood pressure, a slower heart beat, and prolonged expiration, myosis, stomach contraction, nausea and vomiting. It appears to be provoked by a repetition of vestibular stimuli such as we find during travelling in various ways, not only in man but also in animals (e.g. chimpanzees, squirrel monkeys (MEEK et al., 1962). It is discussed in the chapter Motion sickness in this volume, by W. JOHNSON and L. B. W. JONGKEES.

IV. The Sensation and its Clinical Value in Rotation Tests

The old-type rotatory tests were not very suitable for the examination of sensations of rotation. First of all the stimulus was so pronounced that many people subjected to it became nausous, the dizziness masking any slight or strong rotatory sensation. Secondly the BÁRÁNY test begins with a marked acceleration, followed by 10 rotations in 20 sec and then an abrupt stop. When rotation stops the stimulation of the canals by the initial acceleration is not yet finished and the stopping impulse is applied to a cupula which is still deflected. A quantitative estimation of a cupular stimulus was possible when VEITS (1931) made the acceleration at the start so low as to stay below the threshold of perception; after this the rotation is kept at constant speed until any influence of the first stimulus which might have surpassed the threshold, however slightly, has definitely disappeared.

Only then is the braking impulse given. This stop has an effect which is almost certainly attributable wholly to the braking. VEITS, however, used rotations of 180°/sec and the stimulus was still very strong. The reaction is the answer of the canals to an unphysiologic stimulus leading to deflections of the cupula that are many times bigger than those obtained in daily life. In normal stimuli an acceleration (which may be very high) is immediately followed by a contralateral acceleration (equally high) so that only small deviations result.

Various authors (BRUNNER, 1943; LORENTE DE NÓ, 1935) used less pronounced stimuli, i.e. stopped after slower rotational speeds, and MITTERMAIER (1934) even used different stimuli. The last author concluded that the responses after less pronounced stimuli were more similar in repetition than those after intense stimuli. It was only when VAN EGMOND et al. (1948) introduced cupulometry, that genuinely quantitative rotatory examination of the canal system became possible and at the same time the results were recorded in a curve. In this curve the duration of the reaction after the stop is noted down as a function of the stopping impulse, the latter plotted on a logarithmic scale.

As predicted by VAN EGMOND et al. (1943), the responses to various stimuli lie on a straight line in normal subjects (Fig. 10, Fig. 11).

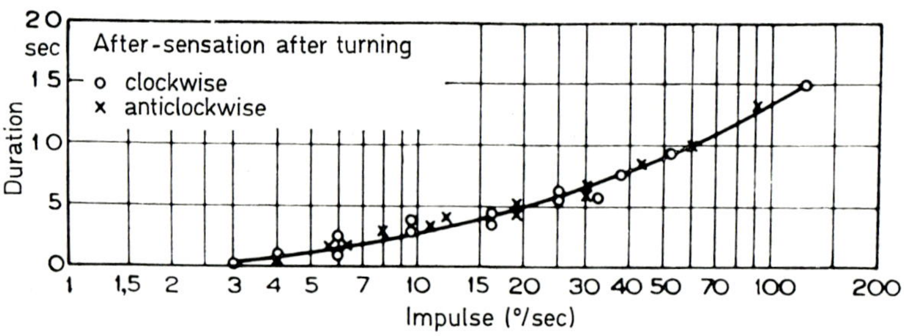

Fig. 10. An example of a sensation-cupulogram with very small dispersion. Abscissa: impulse (degrees per second). Ordinate: duration of the after-sensation (seconds)

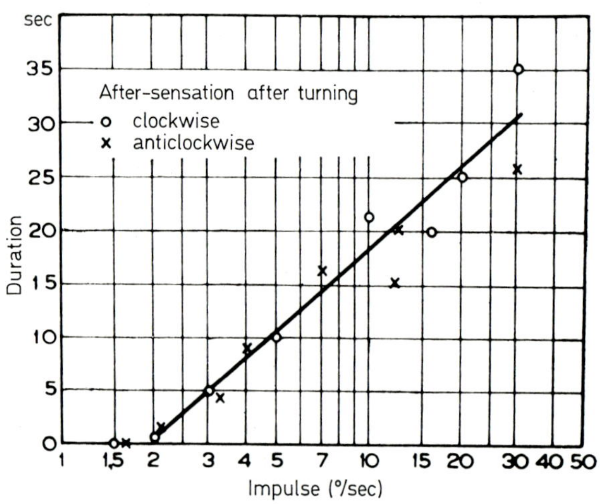

Fig. 11. An example of a sensation-cupulogram with moderately strong dispersion

There are two kinds of answers, however, which are not directly dependent on each other: a nystagmus curve and a sensation curve (see also JONES et al., 1964). The nystagmus curve will not be discussed in detail, but the latter needs some comment.

First of all the rotation should be very smooth (ballbearings, very well regulated acceleration). Other influences should be excluded e.g. the rotation should take place in the dark and the patient should close his eyes. Stimuli such as wind or sounds should be avoided (talking, motor in action). When the after-sensation cupulogram was determined the good results obtained from patients with no experience were particularly striking. The question was a very simple one: "Are you rotating or not? If in doubt, the answer is no!."

Intelligent people, especially those who know something about the vestibular problems, give the least reliable answers. The more sophisticated people seem to feel inclined to extract more information than is really justified. They do not seem to be able to free themselves from their own interpretations. This is also the reason why some of the conclusions on sensations of rotations and movement expressed by people who call themselves very well-trained in self-observation, should be looked upon with a certain reserve. They do not always want what they feel, and therefore feel what they want.

The advantages of the cupulogram method are that the stimulus is known, can be regulated, and does not lead to appreciable adaptation. The cupulogram gives an impression of the action of the semicircular canals at various levels of stimulation and opens a new field of quantitative examination (i.e. sensation) to the clinician. MACH (1875), VAN ROSSUM (1908), and FISCHER and WODAK (1922) had already introduced the quantitative use of sensations into physiological experiments. VAN ROSSUM warned against the hallucinations of rotation felt by his patients, especially near to the threshold. VON BÉKÉSY (1955) gives a very thorough survey of problems pertaining to sensation cupulometry, e.g. the sensations of displacement that often accompany the sensations of rotation even though the head of the patient is very carefully fixed. Postrotatory sensations become gradually slighter when the stimuli are repeated, especially with stimuli greater than 60°/sec. This was established by subjective angle estimation following the stimuli. Stimuli of physiological size also led to some kind of adaptation if the author repeated the stimulus frequently in alternating directions with a fixed interval. Even near the threshold, BÉKÉSY found adaptation in this way. This experiment does not indicate, however, that cupulometry leads to adaptation. Repetition of cupulometry during which the stimuli are not greater than 60°/sec normally does not produce adaptation. The explanation seems very simple. The stimulus in cupulometry takes the labyrinth by surprise (GROEN, 1955; TRINCKER, 1961). During alternating, sinusoidal stimulation, however, pattern building takes place, which quickly leads to response decline (torsion swing).

ASCHAN et al. (1952) and HALLPIKE et al. (1952) were able to confirm the value of sensations for obtaining quantitative data, but HALLPIKE and HOOD (1953) found response decline when they used GRAYBIEL's oculo-gyral illusion. The subject had to look fixedly at a dimly lighted point during the investigations. SOKOLOVSKI (1966) later found that oculogryal illusions suppress vestibular reactions and TSUIKI (1965), who is convinced of the usefulness of sensations for the clinician, states that light, even of the lowest intensity, reduces the reliability of the tests. SCHIERBEEK (1953) finds a wide distribution in the results of the sensation cupulogram and doubts its practical value.

ASCHAN et al. (1952) have the same doubts, but DE WIT's (1953) result in the examination of seasickness seems to have proved its value. In order to estimate the quantitative changes of the sensation cupulogram in various pathologic circumstances it is necessary to know its inclination and the threshold. The normal dispersion of the responses must also be taken into account (HULK and JONGKEES, 1948) (Fig. 4).

The sensation threshold lies between 1 and 4°/sec (average 2.5°/sec), the inclination of the curves lies between 2 and 14 sec (average 7 sec). In general the sensation curves after clockwise and counterclockwise turning are identical. In cases of disturbed labyrinthine function the inclinations of the two curves are sometimes found to be different. At the same time a difference in threshold is found (intersecting lines). Parallel curves with identical inclination were never found by VAN EGMOND et al. (1949), though this type of pathology is not rare in nystagmus cupulograms. In cases of long-standing unilateral loss of vestibular function, VAN EGMOND et al. (1949a) did not find EWALD's law helped them in establishing which side was affected, but in acute cases (e.g. after fenestration operations, JONGKEES and HULK, 1949, Fig. 12) it proved that generally the stop

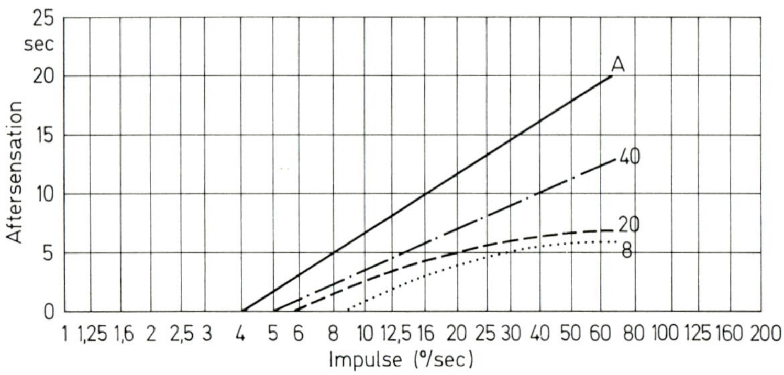

Fig. 12. The sensation-cupulogram of a patient before (graph —— A) and after fenestration of the labyrinth. . . . . 8: this graph was made 8 days after the operation. — — — — — 20: made 20 days after the operation, and ——.——. 40: made 40 days after the operation. The duration of the after-sensation is plotted as a function of the magnitude of the stopping impulse

from counter-clockwise rotation resulted in the stronger (lower threshold, steeper curve) sensation when the right labyrinth was affected and the stop from clockwise rotation was the more powerful stimulus when the left labyrinth was non- or subfunctional. GROEN (1949) found that the subjective angle estimation was increased in persons in whom one labyrinth had stopped functioning a long time before. HULK and JONGKEES (1950) examined a group of patients suffering from otosclerosis by cupulometry and compared them to normals. On average the threshold of after-sensation is found to be raised (average 5°/sec) (Fig. 13), though the inclination remains within normal bounds. Patients with vestibular symptoms due to incipient streptomycin intoxication often show a typical pathologic pattern in the sensation cupulogram, viz. plateau formation, which generally coincides with a directional preponderance in the nystagmus curves (Fig. 14) (JONGKEES and HULK, 1950). Plateau formation results when the sensation after stimuli above a certain strength do not increase in duration. This is generally a transient symptom. When medication is not stopped the reactions slowly disappear, the

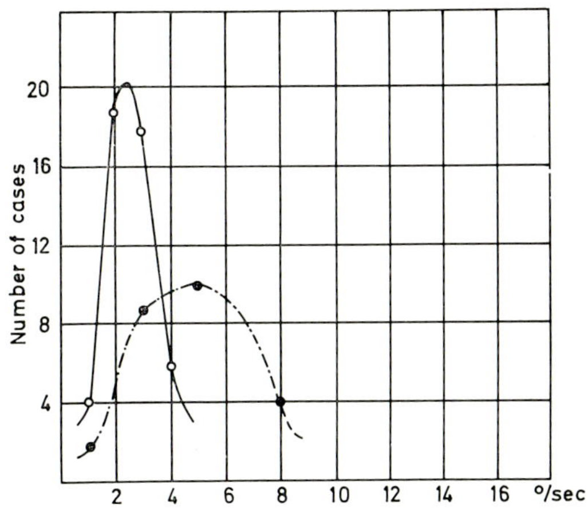

Fig. 13. ○—— threshold of the sensation in normal cases, °/sec ●.–.–.–. idem in cases of otosclerosis

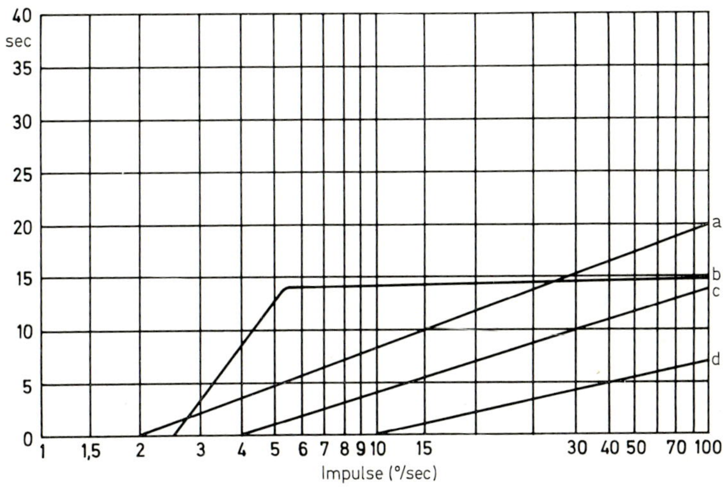

Fig. 14. Sensation cupulogram before (a) and during streptomycine treatment after 10 days (b), after 1 month (c), and after 3 months (d)

nystagmus sometimes prior to the sensation. Plateau formation is also observed in patients with diabetes, local processes in the base of the skull (basal meningitis, arachnoiditis), head injury, and some central lesions.

The *threshold for the perception* of acceleration is a very difficult parameter to measure. Theoretically the cupula system is "thresholdless" in the resting discharge (EK et al., 1959; TRINCKER, 1961). DE VRIES (1949) gave a very detailed account of the difficulties involved in finding the minimum perceptible angular acceleration. He concludes that well-defined acceleration for which the fraction of stimuli perceived by the observer jumps from 100% to zero does not exist. The fraction of perceived stimuli gradually decreases with decreasing acceleration. The relation between the fraction of perceived stimuli and the value of the acceleration can merely be represented by a straight line that seems to go through the origin (0 point), which would mean that no threshold exists. One of the greatest difficulties proved to be the existence of "spurious accelerations," or "hallucinations" (VAN ROSSUM, 1908), sensations of rotation without a causative real acceleration. DE VRIES worked out a way to measure these by starting every test either negative (i.e. no physical stimulus) or positive (acceleration), with a signal. Near the threshold, 20% of the negative stimuli were evaluated as positive. This makes it possible to calculate the fraction of really positive stimuli. As a method of determining pathology of the vestibular organ the measuring of the threshold for rotatory sensation does not seem promising, especially since the threshold for pure rotation of some observers rises with unexpected rapidity in repeated experiments (VON BÉKÉSY, 1955). This is especially true for sinusoidally rotatory oscillations ("the kind that make babies sleepy"). Irregularly applied stimulation may have the opposite effect.

Rotatory oscillations of the kind mentioned here may elicit data on the presence or absence of rotatory directional preponderance of nystagmus. As a means of obtaining information in the field of sensation this tool is of limited value outside the research into normal physiological function of the cupula-endolymph system. VAN EGMOND et al. (1949b) used it to establish a constant of the differential equation of this system, i.e. its latent natural frequency indicated by the coincidence between the real physical change in direction and the sensation of change in direction. This simultaneity indicates a phase difference of 90° between the swing and the cupula. In the investigation mentioned, the natural period proved to be about 6 sec. For investigation of individual cases the sensations provoked on the torsion swing are generally much too vague, even if optic or acoustic sensations (oculogyral; audio-gyral illusion) are added, which according to TRINCKER can improve the perception of the coincidence of real and subjective turning points indicating 90° phase differences.

It may be that sudden phase reversals of the oscillations of the chair will make this method of investigation useful. According to VON BÉKÉSY, these sudden reversals are precisely reproduced by the sensation which indicates that the damping of the cupular movement is very high. The extrapolation towards individual usefulness, however, is pure speculation.

Vertical canals. HULK and JONGKEES (1948), and VAN DER VIS (1958) found in cupulograms that the threshold and the steepness of the sensation curves are equal when the rotation takes place in the plane of one of the 3 pairs of canals

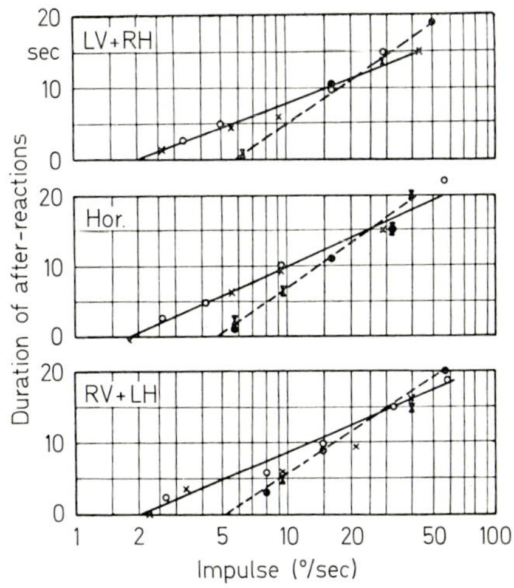

Fig. 15. Cupulograms of one subject made in the plane of the two lateral semicircular canals (Hor), of left anterior and right posterior (LV+RH), and of left posterior and right anterior (RV+LH) semicircular canals. The three curves are nearly identical

(Fig. 15). If the rotation takes place in a plane other than one of the three indicated here, the duration of the after-sensations is much shorter. In the earlier literature one often finds that the reactions of the vertical canals are shorter. This is true in the case of rotation with the head forward or bent on the shoulder. As stated earlier, the phasic secondary after-sensations do not behave identically, but separately in the three planes of the paired semicircular canals (Tschermak, 1921). Up to now pathology of sensations provoked by stimulation of the vertical canals has not been studied thoroughly enough for its importance, to be discussed.

The pathology of secondary phasic after-sensations is given particular emphasis in the German literature as a way of diagnosing central vestibular deviations. The fact that they cannot be caused by oscillations of a periodically damped cupula leads investigators to the conclusion that central vestibular function can be deducted from the individual secondary (and even third, fourth, etc.) after-sensations. According to Mittermaier (1952, 1967) even very slight stimuli should give rise to reactions of this kind. It is a pity that he only states that accelerations of 3°/sec^2 are enough to cause perrotatory after-reactions and that "therefore" the secondary after-reactions are not due to an unphysiologically strong stimulus. Accelerations, however, is not the dimension which can be used for this conclusion.

In cupulometry after-reactions are not normally found as long as the stopping impulse is not greater than 60°/sec. Whether secondary after-sensations are due to unphysiologically powerful stimuli or to normal stimuli does not seem to be very important. It is more important that spontaneous hallucinations of rotatory movements are so frequent (de Vries, 1949) that it is very difficult to be sure of the character of the sensation in the postrotatory period.

According to Aubert and Delage (1888), the secondary after-sensations take the form of a vague feeling of rotation, with no sense of direction. Fischer and

Wodak (1926) do not agree with this, stating that during secondary aftersensation neither speed nor displacement can be felt. And secondly, it seems a difficulty to me that the central origin of the secondary after-sensations may be probable, but is not proved. As explained in § III of this chapter, the causes may also be peripheral. Conclusions inferred from phenomena whose origin is not definitely known are still dangerous. The periodically oscillating after-reactions are said to be due to a lack of central damping (Mittermaier, 1967) and to reflect a predominance of function of one side of the vestibular system or a directional preponderance even more often and more clearly than the first after-reactions. Dodge (1923) speaks about "faint illusions of rotation," but they were without regularity or compelling clearness. Graybiel and his co-workers state that they never found more than one secondary after-sensation of rotation.

Caloric stimulation. Though the present author appreciates the value and usefulness of sensations provoked by stimulation of the vestibular organ, e.g. in cupulometry, he must differ as to the value of the sensations provoked by calorization (1948a, b, 1949). In the case of caloric stimulation, the sensation failed to yield any valuable information. Many patients, even those who were used to self-observation, had no turning sensation whatsoever; others needed strong stimuli before any sensation resulted. In most cases the sensation appeared long after the nystagmus and disappeared long before the nystagmus ceased. Tokita (1965) states that caloric stimulation only provokes unsteadiness. This is in clear contradiction to the experiments of Fischer and Wodak (1922), which indicated that in the caloric test sensation is a much more sensitive basis for examination than nystagmus. They experimented only with themselves as subjects, and their extensive training in self-observation may explain their results. The sensations are not useful for clinical investigation (Mittermaier, 1967). The sensation depends upon the temperature of the water, the position of the patient, on whether unilateral or bilateral irrigation is used, and on the duration of the irrigation.

Usually the patient lying on his back will have a sensation of rotation away from cold and towards hot stimuli. Often a sensation of changed position is found, viz. one of lying on the side contralateral to cold, homolateral to warm calorization (Grahe, 1927).

This may be explained by stimulation of the otolithic nerve by the temperature stimulus (Gernandt et al., 1966). After long-lasting cold stimulation the sensation disappears (Jongkees, 1948).

This may be due either to efferent influences or to cooling of the entire labyrinth, which changes the temperature distribution and in this way the endolymph movements. That the caloric stimulus even reaches the cochlea is proved by experiments of Voogd (1946). She was able to find a clearly perceptible effect of caloric stimulation on her capacity to determine pitch; calorization led to dysacousis.

This deep penetration of the temperature wave (Schmalz, 1932) may even provoke the secondary phenomena found by Hamersma (1957). According to this author, a sensation of a change in the position of the body always preceded the actual turning sensation. He very carefully investigated 36 patients who showed postcaloric sensation. In all of them the sensation of turning was stronger with cold (30° C) than with hot (44° C) water[2]. They found the beginning easy to determine, but the end more difficult.

The mean latency for sensation was 32.6 (both for left and right 30° and 44° C), the mean duration 75.5 sec, for nystagmus these values were 25.5 sec and about 200 sec.

His conclusion is that although sometimes fairly accurate, the postcaloric sensations are in general not accurate enough for clinical use. The type of turning sensation varied. About 50% turned in a horizontal plane about an axis through the umbilicus, the rest turned about their body-length axis in the direction of the quick phase of the nystagmus.

The rotation axis often changed in the same person and also in the same test.

Four patients had secondary after-sensations in the opposite direction.

An interesting phenomenon is the sensation that can be provoked by irrigation of the two ears with identical quantities of water at the same (cold or hot) temperature (equal bilateral irrigations after RUTTIN, 1926). In normal subjects a cold stimulation provokes a sensation of "retropulsion" when the head is bent forwards, propulsion when the head is bent backwards and lateropulsion when the head is turned on the shoulder.

According to QUIX, the combined action of the vertical canals from both sides can explain these sensations. Small imbalances between the two sides are said to be more easily found by bilateral than by monolateral irrigations (FISCHER and VEITS, 1927).

It is true that galvanic tests can provoke rotatory sensations, and especially a sensation of falling and of linear movements (TOKITA, 1965), but as galvanic stimulation has gone out of favor these sensations have not attracted much attention.

Linear accelerations. As stated before, a linear acceleration acting on the otoliths provokes a sensation of verticality in the subject. The tilt chair and the centrifuge have clearly proved this point. If more than one linear acceleration is acting on the subject it is the direction of the resultant force which is perceived. Increase in size of this resultant force does not change this direction. Even after elimination of visual (darkness) and tactile (under-water) stimuli, the perception of position remains unchanged. This indicates that in the situation investigated the perception of position is almost exclusively determined by the activity of the otoliths (SCHÖNE, 1964). A practical difficulty, however, is the fact that people in whom both labyrinths are deficient are still able to indicate their position in space fairly well, even with their eyes closed (ALEXANDER and BÁRÁNY, 1904; FISCHER, 1928). The only instrument that could give some information about the pathology of sensation and might have some practical use is the parallel swing. On this apparatus the patient can be submitted to a sinusoidally alternating linear acceleration in a horizontal plane. The cooperation with gravity will cause a changing direction of the resultant force. This leads to a sensation of to-and-fro or up-and-down rotation depending on the direction of the movement of the swing and little or no sensation of linear displacement appears when the examination is conducted in the dark (MACH, 1875).

---

2 HINCHCLIFFE (1967) found a stronger rotatory sensation with hot than cold stimulation.

JONGKEES and GROEN (1946b) gave a detailed description, analyzed the movements and sensations, and used the parallel swing to determine the threshold of perception (Fig. 16). It appeared to be about 2–6 cm/sec^2, and to be considerably higher in patients in whom both labyrinths were deficient (JONGKEES and GROEN, 1950), but normal if only one labyrinth is still functioning. WALSH (1966) found the threshold was not noticeably influenced when the subject was immersed in water or more viscous fluids. The sensations are disturbed when the patient's head is brought into the position of QUIX's "blind spot of the otoliths," i.e. head-down position. High thresholds were also found in deaf children with nonfunctioning vestibular labyrinths (up to 20 cm/sec^2). Hereditary deafness with intact pars superior labyrinthi also led to a higher threshold, but not as much as the dead labyrinths did. The threshold appeared to be normal in patients with one labyrinth destroyed as long as they were lying in the supine position, but the sensitivity was consistently reduced when the patient lay with the defective side down, and the threshold was lower when he lay with the defective side up.

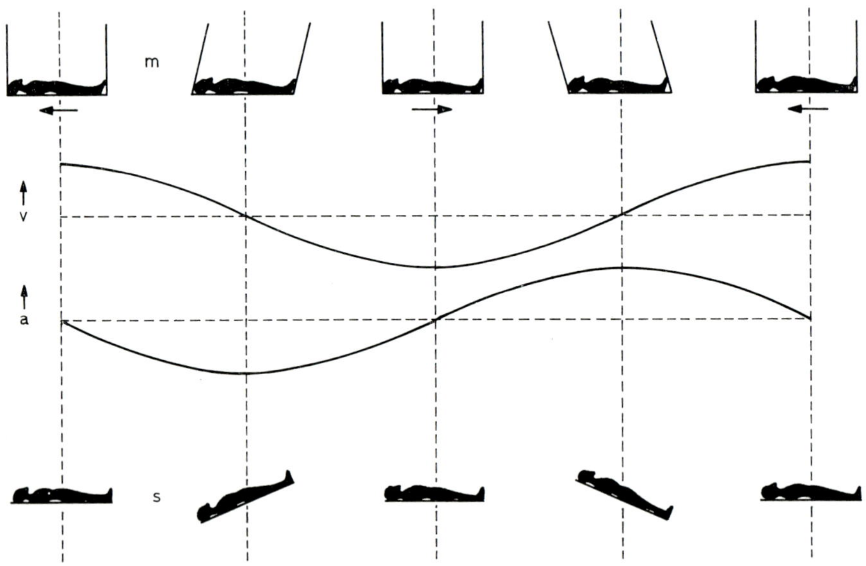

Fig. 16. Scheme of the place, movement, and acceleration of the parallel swing with the subjective position of the test person. (*m*) movement. (*v*) velocity. (*a*) acceleration. (*s*) sensation

The present author was able to corroborate these findings (JONGKEES, 1967). At present, however, the use of sensation for routine examinations seems too difficult for untrained subjects and the recording of eye movements seems to be a much safer way.

Cervical vertigo. DE JONG (1967), in his study on cervical nystagmus, gives an extensive survey of the problem of the spinovestibular connections and on spinovestibular interaction. In a series of experiments he extends the findings of BARRÉ

(1926), who recorded that injection of 10–30 ml 1% procain solution on one side of the nuchal vertebrae provokes rotatory vertigo, nystagmus to the heterolateral side and other vestibular symptoms. GÜTTICH (1939), BOS (1962), and BOS and PHILIPSZOON (1963) provoked nystagmus in normals and in patients with two dead labyrinths by torsion of the neck relative to the head. HINOKI and KUROSAWA (1964) describe swaying vertigo, nausea, and vomiting resulting from injection of 1% procain solution into the deep nape muscles, and attribute this effect to the abolition of the normal impulses from these muscles towards the vestibular nuclei. DE JONG, using positional nystagmus as an indicator, concluded from his systematic surgical investigations that the elimination of information from the deep neck ligaments, the intravertebral joints, and perhaps from the muscles, is very important in the genesis of the "vestibular" phenomena. He proposes that they depend on changes in the same receptors that produce the afferent impulses for the tonic neck reflexes of MAGNUS and DE KLEYN. He also found that acute unilateral resection of neck nerves and ipsilateral labyrinthectomy produce the same effect. Labyrinthectomy, however, produces more marked effects. The fact that rotation of the neck provokes vertigo in some patients (whiplash in judo) with an extremely short latent period seems to support the view that this phenomenon is not due to vascular influences, as is often suggested (BOS and PHILIPSZOON, 1963). DE JONG also found that cooling of one side of the neck led to dizziness, lateropulsion, and deviations from a straight course in walking. Galvanic stimulation of the neck muscles gave similar results.

The influence of torsion of the neck must be taken into account when so-called *positional vertigo* is found. In the cases described by CITRON and HALLPIKE (1956) under the name benign paroxysmal positional nystagmus, this stimulation of the neck is not avoided and cervical nerve stimulation can play a part in the genesis of the symptoms.

V. Positional and Positioning Vertigo

STENGER (1966) differentiated clearly between vestibular symptoms provoked by a certain position (Lage-Nystagmus, positional nystagmus) and those that develop during the act of being brought into a certain position (Lagerungs-nystagmus, positioning nystagmus). In the latter case it is rather common for vertigo to develop both during positioning and again during return to the normal position. In the former vertigo is rare, though it may occur during intoxications (e.g. alcohol). Positioning symptoms may occur in cases of a labyrinthine fistula, but also after traumas to the head, in patients with low or high bloodpressure, anaemia e.a. The dizziness is not always of a typical vertiginous type, generally of short duration and develops when the patient bends forward, lies down, gets up, often accompanied by more or less severe nausea and a feeling of fright. The cause is not yet quite clear, but is is certainly not true that positioning vertigo is always benign (DIX and HALLPIKE, 1952; CAWTHORNE and HALLPIKE, 1957).

VI. Spontaneous Vertigo

Vertigo in the literal sense implies a sensation of rotation, but WILLIAMS (1967) states that there is no basic physiological difference between this experience and any sense of disequilibrium whatever the subject's symptoms. According to the same author, vertigo or disequilibrium is always labyrinthine in origin, i.e. caused by some disorder of the peripheral labyrinth or its central connections. Unfortunately, it seems to me that although this is a practical standpoint, it is not entirely true, or is at least to some extent a play upon words. Vertigo can be provoked by certain stimulations to cervical nerve roots and also by visual stimuli (to give some examples). If it can be proved that some of their pathways cross vestibular nuclei or pathways, are we then free to call this labyrinthine in origin? I shall leave the question unanswered.

A second question remains when we read this statement. When the patient has a sensation of movement forwards, or backwards, up or down, when he feels uncertain and is afraid to fall, feels tipsy, his knees give way or his head feels funny and light, when it sometimes goes dark before his eyes (FRENZEL, 1961), do all those complaints prove the presence of a labyrinthine disorder, and if not, where is the dividing line?

I am afraid that it must be accepted that vertigo and dizziness cannot be so easily explained by one malefactor, but originate from lack of coordination of the information from various sense organs, above all optic, vestibular, tactile, and proprioceptive. This clash of information generally leads to reactions orginating in the autonomic nervous system: nausea, anguish, vomiting, sweating, etc. As an orientating classification of the causes of vertigo, I proposed (1953):

Vertigo caused by direct disorders of the vestibular system:

Labyrinth (inflammation, bleeding, trauma, hydrops, etc.);
Vestibular nerve (syphilis, meningitis, tumors, etc.);
Centers and *Pathways* in the central nervous system (tumors, inflammation, concussion, systemic disease, etc.).

Vertigo caused by deviations of the vestibular function due to general disorders:

Vascular disturbances (artherosclerosis, anemia, high or low blood pressure, etc.);
Infectious diseases (typhus, gastritis, etc.);
Endogenous and exogenous intoxications (diabetes, uremia, alcohol, streptomycin etc.);
Avitaminosis (concentration-camp vertigo, Gerlier's disease, etc.);
Reflectory (intestinal worms, gastric ulcer, pregnancy, etc.).

Nonvestibular vertigo:

ocular (diplopia, myopy, bifocal glasses, etc.);
somesthetic (tabes dorsalis);
psychogenic (claustrophobia, agoraphobia).

It can also be classified in another way: The brain may be receiving conflicting information on account of misleading messages from sense organs, or from wrong perception relay or transmission in sense organs, the nuclei or the pathways. Faulty appreciation or interpretation of normal signals reaching the brain is also a possible cause of vertigo.

Electrical stimulation of the cortex in the neighbourhood of HESCHL's gyrus provokes dizziness, while in the parietal cortex it causes sensations of rotation and other movements (PENFIELD, 1957).

I agree with WILLIAMS' statement that "there is nothing about the clinical description of vertigo as such which will help the examiner to locate its cause, and he must rely upon associated phenomena." The first cause may be in the ear, in the brainstem, in its connections or in the cerebrum, especially the temporal lobe, but the effects on the subject are the same; the circumstances in which the episodes of vertigo occur may differ and the accompanying symptoms may be of supreme importance in diagnosis.

Paroxysmal vertigo (type Ménière), chronic vertigo, acute-onset, slowly decreasing vertigo (type labyrinth trauma), chronic vertigo with changing intensity (type encephalitis), positional or positioning vertigo (Hallpike's benign paroxysmal positional nystagmus) are distinguished by the German school (Frenzel, 1961; Kornhuber, 1966) and form a good basis for specification. A further thorough examination, however, will be necessary for a definite diagnosis. Slight vertigo can be caused by some very serious disease and strong vertigo can be due to a benign disorder, but patients who complain about it have the right to be carefully examined.

There is one more very typical type of symptom in the field of equilibrium (Dandy, 1941; Jatho, 1959), which consists of disorders in visual perception when a patient with loss of vestibular function moves about too abruptly.

It is called jumbling and seems to be provoked by the absence of feedback information from the vestibular organ to the nuclei for the eye muscles. The patient senses apparent movements of his surroundings because the corrective eye movements are not brought into action, or not fast enough. The patient learns to suppress them by moving around as quietly as possible.

VII. Nosology of Vertigo

In many diseases vertigo or dizziness is a symptom of more or less importance. Quite frequently the case history will give enough information for a tentative diagnosis to be possible (Ménière's disease, benign paroxysmal positional nystagmus, orthostatic or epileptic vertigo). In other cases the case history suggests the necessary examinations, which can help to unravel diagnostic puzzles. The combination of deafness, tinnitus, sensitivity to loud noises, and vertigo points to peripheral disorders.

In the case of headache, paralyses of cranial nerves other than the VIII, pathologic reflexes, loss of consciousness, etc., central disturbances are more probable. In still other cases sensations in the equilibrium field may be absent though there are obviously disorders in the peripheral or central vestibular system, e.g. when the progress of the disease is so slow as to allow compensation to cover the appearance of these sensations (e.g. chronic labyrinthitis, VIII nerve tumors).

Vertigo (and dizziness) can be differentiated as:

I. paroxysmal vertigo: attacks of vertigo separated by free intervals;

II. acute vertigo, starting abruptly and thereafter slowly decreasing in intensity;

III. chronic vertigo, less severe, but continuing over a long period, often periodic or showing changes in intensity. In some cases the position of the patient plays a part in the appearance of the symptoms.

Ad. I. Paroxysmal vertigo

A. Ménière's syndrome

the combination of hearing loss and tinnitus with attacks of vertigo together with nystagmus and other objective signs of labyrinthine disorder and with autonomic symptoms like nausea, cold sweat, vomiting, fright etc.

1. *Ménière's disease* is characterized by attacks of the syndrome of Ménière and strong recruitment. The attacks are often preceeded or accompanied by stronger tinnitus, a sensation of fullness or tension deep in the affected ear and changes in acuity of hearing (generally worse, sometimes better: Lermoyez). The nystagmus is nearly always horizontal rotatory towards the sound ear. There is neither loss of consciousness nor any other neurologic symptoms. The anatomical substratum is a hydrops of the endolymphatic spaces of the labyrinth.

2. In rare cases *labyrinthitis* complicating otitis media may present as paroxysmal vertigo. The eardrum should be examined in every case of Ménière's syndrome.

3. *VIII nerve tumors* may also present, though rarely, by attacks of Ménière's syndrome. The Békésy continuous audiometry shows an audiogram according to Jerger type III or IV.

4. *Brain tumors* may give rise to paroxysmal vertigo. Medial cerebellar tumors, for instance, can cause attacks of severe vertigo together with headache, serious ataxia, nystagmus, vomiting, and tinnitus. Paralyses of cranial nerves and contralateral hemiplegia support the diagnosis. Nystagmus is mostly a gaze nystagmus. X-rays of the skull, especially ventriculography, are of great aid in diagnosis. Significant hearing losses make brain tumors unlikely.

5. *Cerebellopontile arachnoiditis*, a cystic inflammation of the cerebello pontile angle, can mimic Ménière's disease but is generally attended by headache, facial and abducent paralyses, trigeminal neuralgia, and severe vomiting. Differentiation from Ménière's disease is sometimes very difficult.

6. Intermittent *ischemic disorders* of the domain *of the vertebrobasillary circulation* can provoke attacks of dizziness and even of real vertigo. This vertigo is not usually rotatory but rather a sensation of instability, a faint feeling, or actual blacking out. Equilibrium disturbances are uncommonly seen alone when their cause is arterial insufficiency. Thick speech, hazy vision, Babinski reflex, weakness of the limbs are much more common. Beside labyrinthine reflex disorders one finds gaze nystagmus, disorders in vibration sense, and optokinetic nystagmus. The disease is very uncommon in patients under the age of 50.

7. *Cogan's syndrome:* Ménière's syndrome in young people, combined with non-syphilitic interstitial keratitis. It starts acutely with photophobia pains in the eyeball, blepharospasm, and hazy vision.

B. Very brief attacks of vertigo

1. *Vertige de l'enfance* (childhood vertigo), attacks of a pure vestibular disorder (partial or complete absence of caloric responses) without cochlear symptoms; genuine rotatory vertigo starting very abruptly and of short duration (in general less than 1 minute); no loss of consciousness. Except for nystagmus in some instances, no objective symptoms are found. The basic process is unknown.

2. *Gerlier's syndrome* is characterized by paroxysmal serious vertigo, pain in the muscles of neck and back, weakness of these muscles and of these of the upper eyelids. It may be provoked by avitaminosis or virus infections.

3. *Epileptic vertigo* starts very abruptly and often lasts only seconds. It is generally combined with loss of consciousness. The differential diagnosis may be difficult, especially as vestibular disorders can provoke epileptic insults.

4. *Migraine attacks* can also be combined with vertigo. Conversely, attacks of vertigo can appear as equivalents of migraine attacks. Hearing is not affected.

5. Attacks of vertigo without loss of hearing are also found in patients suffering from diseases of the stomach and the bladder, hypoglycemia, colitis, helminthiasis, etc.

C. Positional and positioning vertigo

In the forms, the attacks of vertigo are provoked by a certain position of the head or only by the act of bringing the head into that position.

1. *Benign paroxysmal positional nystagmus* is a typical positioning nystagmus, a vertigo together with nystagmus provoked by quick changes in position-bending forward or standing up again. The vertigo appears after a latent period of some seconds. The nystagmus is generally of the frontal type, but may also show horizontal or vertical components. It is directed towards the side on which the patient is lying. The symptoms disappear in a relatively short time (<1 min) and when the movements are repeated. Its origin is still dubious.

2. *Permanent positional nystagmus* is not accompanied by (severe) vertigo (except in some cases of cerebellar tumors). It is provoked either by tumors of the brain or by intoxications (e.g. alcohol, barbiturates). The nystagmus is often directed away from the lower side and continues as long as the position that provokes it remains unchanged.

3. *Orthostatic vertigo* is caused by standing up. In serious cases it may be followed by fainting. No nystagmus is present. It appears to be the result of hypotension. Cervical disorders can sometimes lead to attacks of vertigo, tinnitus and even hearing loss. Nystagmus is only found or is increased when the neck is rotated. Movements provoke the vertiginous attacks.

Ad. II. Vertigo which begins abruptly and decreases slowly in intensity can be A. accompanied by hearing impairment, or B. not accompanied by hearing impairment.

A. With hearing impairment.

1. *Labyrinthitis* either as a complication of otitis media, meningitis, etc., or via the blood circulation, leads to a complete Ménière's syndrome.

In case of very slow development, vertigo and nystagmus may be absent, but the caloric reactions are weak or absent. Cerebral or cerebellar complications may change the picture.

2. One single Ménière's attack is also found in cases of *neuritis of the VIII nerve* (viral or syphilitic infection). Nystagmus is generally influenced by position and not very marked, the caloric reaction is decreased on the diseased side.

3. *Ramsay-Hunt syndrome* is very easily discovered if the typical vesicles are found or if trigeminal, facial, and other paralyses are present. It may be very

difficult to diagnose it if vertigo is the only symptom. Determination of viral reactions may settle the matter.

B. Without hearing disorders

1. *Vestibular neuronitis* as defined by Hallpike is a purely vestibular syndrome without hearing loss, showing 3rd-degree horizontal rotatory nystagmus and a harmonic group of deviations in walking, pointing, and standing. The symptoms disappear within a few weeks, but some remnants persist much longer when the patient closes his eyes. The caloric excitability is decreased and often remains so. The vertigo is generally very severe. The cause might be either vascular or infectious (viral).

In some cases deviations in the electroencephalogram seem to indicate that encephalitis can provoke an identical syndrome. In some epidemics of influenza the syndrome is very frequent but of short duration.

2. In about 5% of the sufferers from *disseminated sclerosis* the first symptom may be an attack of vertigo, nystagmus, vestibular deviation, and severe vomiting. Quite often there is a discrepancy between the slight vertigo and the vomiting. If the nystagmus is purely rotatory or vertical the diagnosis is not too difficult. In the same manner, Babinski reflexes, asymmetry of the optokinetic nystagmus or other neurological symptoms are convenient for the doctor who is trying to find the diagnosis, but not uncommonly the syndrome seems to be purely peripheral and only later developments make the diagnosis possible.

3. *Cerebrovascular accidents* can also lead to this type of vertigo. *Wallenberg's syndrome* is one of them. It is caused by arteriosclerosis, syphilitic processus or embolism in the posterior inferior cerebellar artery. Headache in the back of the head and homolateral trigeminal disorders, difficulties in swallowing, and hiccoughs are observed, together with the acute vestibular disturbances. In the event of a block of the superior cerebellar artery, symptoms of acute vertigo, slowly de creasing over the course of time, can also occur. In this case homolatera cerebellar symptoms and contralateral sensitivity disorders, and occasionally even hearing loss may be found.

4. *Posttraumatic vertigo*, though often of the peripheral type with concomitant hearing disorders, can also be caused by concussional lesions of the vestibular centers. The variations in the vertiginous symptoms, but also in the objective signs of vestibular disturbances, are practically unlimited. The duration of the posttraumatic symptoms may be months or years. The differentiation between a purely physical and a psychogenic basis of the complaints may be very difficult. In general the absence of objective signs of active vestibular defects can be accepted as an indication of healing of the posttraumatic disease.

Ad. III. A. Chronic vertigo over a long period, generally not very severe, is found in *chronic processes in the ear*, like chronic otitis media or labyrinthitis. In these cases of chronic vertigo, examination of the eardrum is always necessary.

B. When *the drums are normal* chronic vertigo can be found in cases of

1. *Tumors of the VIII nerve* showing a picture of a combination of a type III or IV Jerger audiogram according to BÉKÉSY, strong tone decay, decreased or absent caloric reactions, not many vertiginous symptoms, and X-ray findings indicating a tumor in the cerebello pontile angle.

2. *Tuberculous meningitis* can lead to very slowly developing labyrinthitis. The symptoms of the labyrinthitis are extremely few. A slow loss of hearing, some deviations from a straight course in walking in the dark, Dandy's symptom, and loss of caloric reactions. Differentiation from iatrogenic streptomycin intoxication can be extremely difficult.

3. *Luetic meningoencephalitis* is notorious for the disharmonic and discordant symptomatology, e.g. rotatory reactions decreased and caloric ones normal, horizontal rotatory nystagmus, but negative Romberg and Unterberger tests.

Nocturnal headache, Argyll Robertson sign, and serological examination in blood and cerebrospinal fluid can generally help to diagnose the cause of the chronic vertigo.

4. *Syringobulbia* gives rise to slight dizziness. Pathognomonic is the frontal nystagmus together with dissociated disorders of sensation, corneal areflexia and atrophy of the tongue.

5. The *chronic vertigo in elderly people* is attributed to cerebral arteriosclerosis. It comes in spasms and is described as a feeling of being drunk and unsure, especially during walking. Headache, tinnitus, and "drop attacks" are not unusual. The optokinetic nystagmus is often more pathologic than spontaneous or positional nystagmus. The entire picture of arteriosclerosis is so variable that I must abstain from more details.

6. Chronic vertigo is also found in various *disseminated disorders of the brain*, (disseminated sclerosis, diffuse encephalitis, avitaminosis, e.g. concentration-camp dizziness, postconcussional) characterized by paroxysmal illusions of movement; sometimes strong vestibular reactions are found in the caloric tests and sometimes decreased ones.

7. *Fainting fits* are sometimes described as dizziness; no vestibular symptoms are found. This is also true in cases of hysterical origin.

References

Abels, H.: Über Nachempfindungen im Gebiete des kinästhetischen und statischen Sinnes. Z. Psychol. **43**, 269–324 (1906).

Adrian, E.D.: Discharges from vestibular receptors in the cat. J. Physiol. (Lond.) **101**, 389–407 (1943).

Alexander, G., Bárány, R.: Psycho-physiologische Untersuchungen über die Bedeutungen des Statolithenapparates für die Orientierung im Raume an Normalen und Taubstummen. Z. Psychol. **37**, 321–362 (1904).

Aschan, G.: Response to rotatory stimuli in fighter pilots. Acta oto-laryng. (Stockh.) Suppl. **116**, 24–31 (1954).

Aschan, G.: The mechanism of the cupula ampullaris in man. Acta Soc. Med. upsalien. **60**, 77–88 (1955).

Aschan, G.: Habituation to repeated rotatory stimuli and the effect of antinausea drugs and alcohol on the results. Acta oto-laryng. (Stockh.) **64**, 95–106 (1967).

Aschan, G., Bergstedt, M.: The genesis of secondary nystagmus induced by vestibular stimuli. Acta Soc. Med. upsalien. **60**, 113–122 (1955).

Aschan, G., Nylén, C.O., Stahle, J., Wersäll, R.: The rotation test. Acta oto-laryng. (Stockh.) **42**, 451–459 (1952).

Aubert, H., Delage, Y.: Physiologische Studien über die Orientierung. Tübingen: Laupp 1888.

Bárány, R.: Weitere Untersuchungen über den vom Vestibularapparat des Ohres reflektorisch ausgelösten rhythmischen Nystagmus und seine Begleiterscheinungen. Mschr. Ohrenheilk. **41**, 477–523 (1907).

Barré, J. A.: Sur un syndrome sympatique cervical et sa cause fréquente: l'arthrite cervicale. Rev. neurol. **1**, 1246–1248 (1926).

Beerens, A. J. J.: Recording from primary afferents in the utricular nerve in the cat. Amsterdam: Academic thesis 1968.

Behr, K., Preber, L., Silfverskiold, D. F.: Recording of skin resistance in thermal and rotatory stimulation of the labyrinth. Acta psychiat. scand. **30**, 741–748 (1955).

Von Békésy, G.: Subjective cupulometry. Arch. Otolaryng. **61**, 16–28 (1955).

Von Békésy, G.: Pressure and shearing forces as stimuli of labyrinthine epithelium. Arch. Otolaryng. **84**, 122–130 (1966).

Bischof, N.: Stellungs-, Spannungs- und Lagewahrnehmung. In: W. Metzger, Ed. Handbuch der Psychologie, Bd. I, S. 409–497. Göttingen: Hogrefe 1966.

Bos, J. H.: On vestibular nystagmus without causative endolymph displacement. Amsterdam: Academic thesis 1962.

Bos, J. H., Philipszoon, A. J.: Some forms of nystagmus provoked by stimuli other than accelerations. Pract. oto-rhino-laryng. (Basel) **25**, 108–118 (1963).

Brandt, U.: Reorientation and vestibular function. Acta oto-laryng. (Stockh.) **54**, 543–552 (1961).

Brandt, U., Fluur, E.: Postural perception and eye displacements produced by a resultant vector acting in the medial sagittal plane of the head. Acta oto-laryng. (Stockh.) **65**, 489–512 (1967).

Breuer, J.: Ueber die Funktion der Bogengänge des Ohrlabyrinthes. Med. Jahrbuch (Wien) **4**, 72–124 (1874).

Breuer, J.: Neue Versuche an den Ohrenbogengängen. Pflügers Arch. ges. Physiol. **44**, 135–152 (1889).

Brunner, H.: Neurology in otolaryngology. Laryngoscope (St. Louis) **53**, 117–137 (1943).

Bruns, O.: Wesen und Bekämpfung der See- und Luftkrankheit. Münch. med. Wschr. **73**, 977–979 (1926).

Buys, E.: Du fonctionnement des centres du nystagmus. Bull Soc. belge Otol. Lar. Rhin. **4**, 156–167 (1913).

Buys, E.: Contribution à l'étude de la physiologie vestibulaire. Bull Acad. roy. Méd. Belg. **6**, 510 (1928).

Cawthorne, T., Hallpike, C. S.: A study of the clinical features and pathological changes within the temporal bones, brainstem and cerebellum of an early case of positional nystagmus of the socalled benign paroxysmal type. Acta oto-laryng. (Stockh.) **48**, 89–105 (1957).

Citron, C., Hallpike, C. S.: Observations upon the mechanism of positional nystagmus of the socalled benign paroxysmal type. J. Laryng. **70**, 253–259 (1956).

Collins, W. E.: Nystagmus responses of the cat to rotation and to directionally equivalent and non-equivalent stimuli after unilateral caloric habituation. Acta oto-laryng. (Stockh.) **58**, 247–258 (1964).

Collins, W. E.: Problems in spatial orientation-vestibular studies of figure skaters. Trans. Amer. Acad. Ophthal. Otolaryng. **70**, 575–578 (1966).

Collins, W. E., Guedry, F. E.: Arousal effects and nystagmus during prolonged constant angular acceleration. Acta oto-laryng. (Stockh.) **54**, 349–362 (1962).

Collins, W. E., Guedry, F. E.: Duration of an angular acceleration and ocular nystagmus from cat and man. Acta oto-laryng. (Stockh.) **64**, 373–387 (1967).

Dandy, W. E.: The surgical treatment of Ménière's disease. Surg. Gynec. Obstet. **72**, 421–425 (1941).

Van Dishoeck, H. A. E., Spoor, A., Nijhoff, P.: The opto-gyral illusion and its relation to the nystagmus of the eye. Acta oto-laryng. (Stockh.) **44**, 597–607 (1954).

Dittler, R.: Ueber die Raumfunktion der Netzhaut in ihrer Abhängigkeit vom Lagegefühl der Augen und vom Labyrinth. Z. Sinnesphysiol. **52**, 274–310 (1921).

Dix, M. R., Hallpike, C. S.: The Pathology, symptomatology, and diagnosis of certain common disorders of the vestibular system. Proc. roy. Soc. Med. **45**, 341–354 (1952).

DODGE, R.: Habituation to rotation. J. exp. Psychol. **6**, 1 (1923).

DODGE, R.: Thresholds of rotation. J. exp. Psychol. **6**, 107–137 (1923).

DOLOWITZ, D.A.: Vertigo. Laryngoscope (St. Louis) **75**, 805–819 (1965).

VAN EGMOND, A.A.J., GROEN, J.J., HULK, J., JONGKEES, L.B.W.: The turning test with small regulable stimuli. VI. Deviations in the cupulogram. J. Laryng. **63**, 306–310 (1949a).

VAN EGMOND, A.A.J., GROEN, J.J., JONGKEES, L.B.W.: The turning test with small regulable stimuli. I. Cupulometria. J. Laryng. **62**, 63–69 (1948).

VAN EGMOND, A.A.J., GROEN, J.J., JONGKEES, L.B.W.: The mechanism of the semicircular canal. J. Physiol. (Lond.) **110**, 1–17 (1949b).

VAN EGMOND, A.A.J., JONGKEES, L.B.W., GROEN, J.J.: Welke sensaties en reflexen gaan er uit van het vestibulaire orgaan bij prikkeling door rechtlijnige versnellingen. Ned. T. Geneesk. **87**, 1791–1792 (1943).

EK, J., JONGKEES, L.B.W., KLIJN, J.A.J.: The threshold of the vestibular organ. Acta oto-laryng. (Stockh.) **50**, 292–300 (1959).

EK, J., JONGKEES, L.B.W., KLIJN, J.A.J.: On the effect of continuous acceleration. Acta oto-laryng. (Stockh.) **51**, 416–419 (1960).

FEARING, F.: Post-rotational head nystagmus in adult pigeons. J. comp. Psychol. **6**, 115–131 (1926).

FELDMANN, H.: Das Labyrinth als quantitativ arbeitendes Sinnesorgan. Arch. Ohr.-, Nas.-, u. Kehlk.-Heilk. **187**, 631–636 (1966).

FERNÁNDEZ, C., LINDSAY, J.R.: The vestibular Coriolis reaction. Arch. Otolaryng. **88**, 469–472 (1964).

FERRERI, G.: Le mal de mer. In: A. AUBIN, L'appareil vestibulaire. Paris: Presses Universitaires de France 1956.

FISCHER, M.H.: Die Regulationsfunktionen des menschlichen Labyrinthes und die Zusammenhänge mit verwandten Funktionen. Ergebn. Physiol. **27**, 209–379 (1928).

FISCHER, M.H., VEITS, C.: Beiträge zur Physiologie des menschlichen Vestibularapparates. VII. Die Pulsionsreflexe. Pflügers Arch. ges. Physiol. **217**, 357–388 (1927).

FISCHER, M.H., WODAK, E.: Experimentelle Untersuchungen über Vestibularisreaktionen. Z. Hals.-, Nas.-, u. Ohrenheilk. **3**, 198–215 (1922).

FISCHER, M.H., WODAK, E.: Prinzipielle Betrachtungen zum Problem des Zeigeversuches. Acta oto-laryng. (Stockh.) **10**, 24–51 (1926).

FLOURENS, P.: Expériences sur les canaux semicirculaires de l'oreille dans les mammifères. Acad. roy. Soc. Paris **9**, 467–477 (1830).

FORSSMAN, B.: Studies of congenital nystagmus and vestibular reactivity. Lund: Academic thesis 1963.

FRENZEL, H.: Zur Systematik, Klinik und Untersuchungsmethodik der Vestibularisstörungen. Arch. Ohr.-, Nas.-, u. Kehlk.-Heilk. **177**, 353–395 (1961).

GERNANDT, B.: Central regulation of the vestibular system. Arch. Otolaryng. **85**, 521–528 (1967).

GERNANDT, B., IGARASHI, E.M., ADES, H.W.: Effects of prolonged caloric stimulation upon oculomotor, vestibulospinal, and segmental spinal activity. Exp. Neurol. **14**, 249–263 (1966)

GRAHE, K.: Die Vertikalempfindung auf dem Vestibulartische bei kalorischer Reizung des normalen und labyrinthlosen Ohres und des Halses. Acta oto-laryng. (Stockh.) **11**, 158–168 (1927).

GRAYBIEL, A.: The importance of the otolith organs in man based upon a specific test for utricular function. Ann. Otol. (St. Louis) **65**, 470–487 (1956).

GRAYBIEL, A., NIVEN, J.I., MACCORQUODALE, K.: The effect of linear acceleration on the oculogravic illusion, U.S. school Av. Med. rep; Pensacola, Nr. 42, 1956.

GROEN, J.J.: De evenwichtszintuigen. In: H. C. BURGER, G. C. E. BURGER, Eds. Medische physica, p. 510–561. Amsterdam: Noord Hollandse Uitgevers 1949.

GROEN, J. J.: The mechanics of the labyrinth. International course in vestibular examination, p. 15–33. Utrecht: Schotanus en Jens 1953.

GROEN, J. J.: Adaptation. Pract. oto-rhino-laryng. (Basel) **19**, 524–530 (1957).

GROEN, J. J.: Vestibular stimulation and its effects from the point of view of theoretical physics. Confin. neurol. (Basel) **21**, 380–381 (1961a).

GROEN, J. J.: The problems of the spinning to applied to the semicircular canals. Confin. neurol. (Basel) **21**, 454–455 (1961b).

GROEN, J. J.: Inhibitory mechanism of the vestibular system in man in comparison with hearing. J. acoust. Soc. Amer. **34**, 1497–1503 (1962).

GROEN, J. J.: Central regulation of the vestibular system. Acta oto-laryng. (Stockh.) **59**, 211–218 (1965).

GROEN, J. J., JONGKEES, L. B. W.: The threshold of angular-acceleration perception. J. Physiol. (Lond.) **107**, 1–7 (1948a).

GROEN, J. J., JONGKEES, L. B. W.: The turning test with small regulable stimuli. III. The advantage of cupulometry over the classic technique of BÁRÁNY. J. Laryng. **62**, 231–235 (1948b).

GROEN, J. J., JONGKEES, L. B. W.: The turningtest with small regulable stimuli. IV. The cupulogram obtained by subjective angle estimation. J. Laryng. **62**, 236–240 (1948c).

GROEN, J. J., LOWENSTEIN, O., VENDRIK, A. J. H.: The mechanical analysis of the responses from the end organs of the horizontal semicircular canal in the elasmobranch labyrinth. J. Physiol. (Lond.) **117**, 329–346 (1952).

GUEDRY, F. E.: Orientation of rotation axis relative to gravity. Its influence on nystagmus and sensation of rotation. Acta oto-laryng. (Stockh.) **60**, 30–48 (1965).

GÜTTICH, A.: Ueber den Antagonismus der Hals- und Bogengangsreflexe bei der Bewegung des menschlichen Auges. Arch. Ohr.-, Nas.-, u. Kehlk.-Heilk. **147**, 1–4 (1939).

HALLPIKE, C. S., HOOD, J. D.: Fatigue and adaptation of the cupular mechanism of the human horizontal semicircular canal. Proc. roy. Soc. B **141**, 542–561 (1953).

HALLPIKE, C. S., HOOD, J. D., BYFORD, G. H.: The design, construction, and performance of a new type of revolving chair. Some experimental results and their application to the physical theory of the cupular mechanism. Acta oto-laryng. (Stockh.) **42**, 511–538 (1952).

HAMERSMA, H.: The caloric test. Academic thesis, Amsterdam 1957.

HENNEBERT, P.: Discussion. Confin. neurol. (Basel) **21**, 399 (1961).

HINCHCLIFFE, R.: Normal values for the caloric tests using electric oculographic recordings. J. Laryng. **81**, 221–228 (1967).

HINOKI, M., KUROSAWA, R.: Studies on vertigo provoked by neck and nape muscles. Rep. oto-rhino-laryng. Clin. (Kyoto) **57**, 10–11 (1964).

VON HOLST, E., MITTELSTAEDT, H.: Das Reafferenzprinzip. Naturwissenschaften **37**, 464 (1950).

HOOD, J. D.: Discussion. In: A. V. S. DE REUCK, J. KNIGHT, Eds. Myotatic, kinesthetic, and vestibular mechanisms, Ciba Symp. London: Churchill 1967.

HULK, J., HENKES, H. E.: Meetbare vegetatieve reacties van vestibulaire oorsprong. Ned. T. Geneesk. **93**, 783–791 (1949).

HULK, J., JONGKEES, L. B. W.: The normal cupulogram. J. Laryng. **62**, 70–75 (1948).

HULK, J., JONGKEES, L. B. W.: Vestibular examination in cases of otosclerosis. J. Laryng. **64**, 126–130 (1950).

IRWIN, J. A.: On the pathology of seasickness. Lancet **1881** II, 907.

JAMES, W.: The sense of dizziness in deaf-mutes. Amer. J. Otol. **4**, 239–254 (1882).

JATHO, K.: Ueber die Bedeutung des Dandyschen Symptoms bei einseitigem Verlust der vestibularen Funktion. Arch. Ohr.- Nas.-, u. Kehlk.-Heilk. **172**, 543–552 (1959).

JONES, G.M.: Vestibular inaptitude in the environments of flight and space. J. Laryng. **80**, 207–221 (1966).

JONES, G.M., BORRY, W., KOWALSKY, W.: Dynamics of the semicircular canals compared in yaw, pitch, and roll. Aerospace Med. **35**, 984–989 (1964).

DE JONG, J.M.V.B.: Over cervicale nystagmus en aanverwante verschijnselen. Amsterdam: Academic thesis 1967.

JONGKEES, L.B.W.: De physiologische prikkel voor het evenwichtsorgaan. Ned. T. Geneesk. **88**, 198–199 (1944).

JONGKEES, L.B.W.: Value of the caloric test of the labyrinth. Arch. Otolaryng. **48**, 402–417 (1948a).

JONGKEES, L.B.W.: Origin of the caloric test of the labyrinth. Arch. Otolaryng. **48**, 645–657 (1948b).

JONGKEES, L.B.W.: Which is the preferable method of performing the caloric test? Arch. Otolaryng. **49**, 594–608 (1949).

JONGKEES, L.B.W.: Some remarks on the function of the vestibular organ. Rep. Inst. Laryng. Otol. (Lond.) **2**, 1–10 (1952).

JONGKEES, L.B.W.: Ueber die Untersuchungsmethoden des Gleichgewichtsorganes. Fortschr. Hals-Nas.-Ohrenheilk. **1**, 1–165 (1953).

JONGKEES, L.B.W.: The parallel-swing test. In: WOLFSON, Eds. The vestibular system and its disorders, p. 218–228. Philadelphia: Univ. Penns. Press 1966.

JONGKEES, L.B.W.: The function of the otoliths. NASA Symposium, Pensacola 1967.

JONGKEES, L.B.W., GROEN, J.J.: Consideration regarding the secondary aftersensations caused by a stimulation of the semicircular-canal system. J. Laryng. **61**, 241–244 (1946a).

JONGKEES, L.B.W., GROEN, J.J.: The nature of the vestibular stimulus. J. Laryng. **61**, 529–541 (1946b).

JONGKEES, L.B.W., GROEN, J.J.: A quantitative analysis of the reactions of a person after loss of the function of both inner ears. J. Laryng. **64**, 135–140 (1950).

JONGKEES, L.B.W., HULK, J.: Changes in vestibular reactions after the fenestration operation J. Laryng. **63**, 125–130 (1949).

JONGKEES, L.B.W., HULK, J.: The action of streptomycin on vestibular function. Acta oto-laryng. (Stockh.) **38**, 225–232 (1950).

JONGKEES, L.B.W., KLIJN, J.A.J.: On per- and post-rotatory reactions. Acta oto-laryng. (Stockh.) **46**, 314–318 (1956).

JONGKEES, L.B.W., PHILIPSZOON, A.J.: Electronystagmography. Acta oto-laryng. (Stockh.) Suppl. **189**, (1962).

KARBOWSKI, K.: Ueber die von den Labyrinthbogengängen ausgelösten Reaktionen. Pract. oto-rhino-laryng. (Basel) **23**, 289–297 (1961).

KITAHARA, M., UNO, R.: Equilibrium and vertigo in a tilting environment. Ann. Otol. (St. Louis) **76**, 166–178 (1967).

DE KLEIJN, A., VERSTEEGH, C.: Present position of the physiology of the labyrinth. J. Laryng. **42**, 649–655 (1927).

KLIJN, J.A.J., EK, J.: A case of aftereffects in vestibular stimulation. Pract. oto-rhino-laryng. (Basel) **21**, 391–393 (1959).

KORNHUBER, H.: Physiologie und Klinik des zentralvestibulären Systems. In: BERENDES, LINK, ZÖLLNER. Hals-, Nasen-, Ohrenheilkunde, Vol. III, **1**, p. 2150–2351. Stuttgart: Thieme 1966.

KREIDL, A.: Weitere Beiträge zur Physiologie des Ohrlabyrinthes, Sitzungsber. Akad. Wissensch. Math.-Natur. **102**, 149 (1893).

Krijger, R.: De betekenis van het evenwichtszintuig voor de vlieger. Utrecht: Academic thesis 1954.

Langelaan, J.W.: On the development of the external form of the human cerebellum. Brain **42**, 130–170 (1919).

Leiri, E.: Ueber den Schwindel. Z. Hals-, Nas.- u. Ohrenheilk. **17**, 392–402 (1927).

Lidvall, H.F.: Mechanism of motionsickness as reflected in the vertigo and nystagmus responses to repeated caloric stimuli. Acta oto-laryng. (Stockh.) **55**, 527–536 (1967).

Lorente de Nó, R.: Observations on nystagmus. Acta oto-laryng. (Stockh.) **21**, 416–437 (1934).

Lowenstein, O.: Peripheral mechanism of equilibrium. Brit. med. Bull. **12**, 114–118 (1956).

Van Maanen, J.C.D.: Chronic seasickness. Utrecht: Academic thesis 1965.

Mach, E.: Grundlinien der Lehre von den Bewegungsempfindungen. Leipzig: W. Engelmann 1875.

Malecki, J.: The problem of habituation in the light of the information theory. Ann. Otol. (St. Louis) **74**, 970–977 (1965).

McCabe, B.F.: Vestibular suppression in figure skaters. Trans. Amer. Acad. Ophthal. Otolaryng. **64**, 264–268 (1960).

McCabe, B.F., Gillingham, K.: Mechanism of vestibular suppression. Trans. Amer. otol. Soc. **51**, 226–228 (1964).

Meek, J.C., Graybiel, A., Beischer, D.E., Riopelle, A.J.: Observations of canalsickness and adaptation in chimpanzees and squirrel monkeys. Aerospace Med. **33**, 571–580 (1962).

Mittermaier, R.: Gleichgewichtsprüfungen mit verschiedener Drehgeschwindigkeit. Arch. Ohrenheilk. **143**, 339–362 (1937).

Mittermaier, R.: Neuere Ansichten über die Wirkungsweise des Vestibularapparates. Wien. klin. Wschr. **64**, 893–897 (1952).

Mittermaier, R.: Die experimentellen Gleichgewichtsprüfungen. In: Berendes, Link, Zöllner. Hals-, Nasen-, Ohrenheilkunde, Vol. III, 1, p. 581–642. Stuttgart: Thieme 1967.

Money, K.E., Friedberg, J.: The role of the semicircular canals in causation of motionsickness. Canad. J. Physiol. Pharmacol. **42**, 793–801 (1964).

Montandon, W.: Le réflex de dépression de origine vestibulaire. Pract. oto-rhino-laryng. (Basel) **14**, 257–260 (1952).

Mulder, W.: Quantitatieve betrekking tusschen prikkel en effect bij het statisch orgaan. Utrecht: Acad. Thesis 1908.

Muskens, L.: Das supravestibulare System bei den Tieren und beim Menschen. Amsterdam: Noord Hollandsche Uitgevers 1934.

Nieuwenhuyzen, J.H.: Experimental investigations on seasickness. Utrecht: Acad. Thesis 1958.

Penfield, W.: Vestibular sensations and the cerebral cortex. Ann. Otol. (St. Louis) **66**, 691–698 (1957).

Philipszoon, A.J.: The effect of some drugs on the labyrinth. Amsterdam: Acad. Thesis 1959.

Pichler, H.J.: Klinische Vestibularprüfmethoden in der Darstellung des Gravogramms. Mschr. Ohrenheilk. **100**, 264–271 (1966).

Pollak, J.: Über den galvanischen Schwindel bei Taubstummen und seine Beziehungen zur Funktion des Ohrlabyrinthes. Pflügers Arch. ges. Physiol. **54**, 188–208 (1893).

Preber, L.: Vegetative reactions in caloric and rotation tests. Acta oto-laryng. (Stockh.) Suppl. **144**, (1958).

PURKINJÉ, J.E.: Beyträge zur näheren Kentniss des Schwindels aus heautognostischen Daten. Med. Jahrb. K. K. Österr. Staates VI, 79–125 (1820).

QUIX, F.H.: Le mal de mer, le mal des aviateurs. Monogr. otorhinolaryng. Internat., 8. Paris: A. Legrand 1922.

VAN ROSSUM, A.: Gewaarwordingen en reflexen opgewekt vanuit de halfcirkelvormige kanalen. Utrecht: Acad. Thesis 1908.

RUTTIN, E.: Equal bilateral irrigations. In: DENKER, KAHLER. Handbuch Hals-, Nas.-, Ohrenheilk. Vol. VI. Berlin: Springer 1926.

SCHIERBEEK, P.: Vestibular turning test by means of weak-stimuli. Pract. oto-rhino-laryng. (Basel) **15**, 73–87 (1953).

SCHMALTZ, G.: The physical phenomena occurring in the semicircular canals during rotatory and thermic stimulation. Proc. roy. Soc. Med. **25**, 359–381 (1932).

SCHÖNE, H.: On the role of gravity in human spacial orientation. Aerospace Med. **35**, 764–772 (1964).

SCHUBERT, G.: Physiologie des Menschen im Flugzeug. Berlin: Springer 1935.

SINGLETON, G.T.: Relationship of the cerebellar modulus to vestibular function: a study of the effects of nodulectomy on habituation. Laryngoscope (St. Louis) **77**, 1579–1620 (1967).

SJÖBERG, A.A.: Experimentelle Studien über den Auslösungsmechanismus der Seekrankheit. Acta oto-laryng. (Stockh.) Suppl. **14** (1931).

SOKOLOWSKI, A.: The influence of mental activity and visual fixation upon caloricinduced nystagmus in normal subjects. Acta oto-laryng. (Stockh.) **61**, 209–220 (1966).

STEINHAUSEN, W.: Ueber die Beobachtung der Cupula in den Bogengangsampullen des Labyrinthes des lebenden Hechtes. Pflügers Arch. ges. Physiol. **232**, 500–512 (1933).

STENGER, H.H.: Schwindelanalyse. In: BERENDES, LINK, ZÖLLNER; Hals-, Nas.- u. Ohrenheilk. Vol. III, 1, p. 540–546. Stuttgart: Thieme 1966.

SUNAHARA, F.A., JOHNSON, W.H., TAYLOR, N.B.G.: Vestibular stimulation and forearm bloodflow. Canad. J. Physiol. Pharmacol. **42**, 199–207 (1964).

TOKITA, T.: Objective evidence of experimental vertigo. J. Otorhinolaryng. Soc. Japan **68**, 837–844 (1965).

TRINCKER, D.: Analysis of the physical and neurophysiological principles underlying vestibular stimulation. Confin. neurol. (Basel) **21**, 372–379 (1961).

TSCHERMAK, A.: Der exacte Subjektivismus in der neuen Sinnesphysiologie. Pflügers Arch. ges. Physiol. **180**, 1–35 (1921).

TSUIKI, Y.: Rep. Dpt. Otorhinolaryng. Tohuku Univ. School Med., Japan 1965.

VEITS, C.: Zur Drehprüfung. Z. Hals-, Nas.- u. Ohrenheilk. **29**, 368–376 (1931).

VEITS, C.: Quantitative Untersuchungen über die Pulsionsreflexe nach äqualen Doppelspülungen. Arch. Ohr.-, Nas.-, u. Kehlk.-Heilk. **142**, 316–324 (1937).

VAN DER VIS, K.: Cupulometry of the vertical semicircular canals. Pract. oto-rhino-laryng. (Basel) **20**, 250–260 (1958).

VOOGD, J.: Experimentelle displacusie. Rap. Nederl. Keel-, neus-, oorheelk. Verh. 1946.

DE VRIES, H.: The minimum perceptible angular acceleration. Acta oto-laryng. (Stockh.) **37**, 218–229 (1949).

WALSCH, E.G.: The use of impulsive mechanical stimuli of variable duration of the indication time of the otolith organs. J. Laryng. **30**, 1218–1223 (1966).

VON WEIZSÄCKER, V.: Der Gestaltkreis. Stuttgart: Thieme 1947.

WENDT, G.R.: Vestibular function. In: STEVENS, Handb. Exp. Psychol., S. 1191–1223. New York: J. Wiley 1951.

Wendt, G. R.: Man and motion. In: Hill, Adolph, Wilber, Handbook of Physiology. Washington: Amer. Physiol. Soc. 1964.

Williams, D. J.: Vertigo. Proc. roy. Soc. Med. **60**, 961–964 (1967).

De Wit, G.: Seasickness. Acta oto-laryng. (Stockh.) Suppl. **108** (1953).

De Wit, G.: Some animal experiments on motion sickness. Acta oto-laryng. (Stockh.) **47**, 172–175 (1957).

Wodak, E.: Neue Beiträge zur Funktionsprüfung des Labyrinthes. Mschr. Ohrenheilk. **56**, 826–860 (1922).

Wodak, E.: Physiopathologische Probleme des menschlichen Vestibularapparatus. Fortschr. Hals-, Nas.-, u. Ohrenheilk. **1**, 166–268 (1953).

Wojatschek, W.: Einige neue Erwägungen über das Wesen der Seekrankheit. Beitr. Anat. etc., Ohr. **2**, 336–345 (1909).

Van Wulfften Palthe, P. M.: Functions of the deeper sensibility and of the vestibular organs in flying. Acta oto-laryng. (Stockh.) **4**, 415–449 (1922).

Chapter X.

Characteristics of Vestibular Neurons after Acute and Chronic Labyrinthine Destruction

By

W. Precht, Frankfurt a. M.

With 4 Figures

Contents

I. Introduction

Effects of labyrinthectomy or neurotomy of the VIII nerve have been studied by numerous investigators, and a variety of hypotheses have been proposed to explain the long-term postoperative changes (Bechterew, 1883; Ewald, 1892; Bárány, 1907; Magnus, 1924; Spiegel and Dèmètriades, 1925; Spiegel and Sato, 1926; Lorente de Nó, 1928; Dohlman, 1929; Cawthorne et al., 1942; Mittermaier, 1950; van Eyck, 1954; Stenger, 1959; Fluur, 1960; Pfaltz, 1971). Details of the behavioral disturbances following uni- and bilateral labyrinthectomy are fully described in Chapters F.I. and F.XI. and only a few major points related to eye movements will be repeated here.

The fact that most of the disturbances following *acute labyrinthectomy* undergo significant changes with advancing time after injury, and that the recovery of vestibularly controlled eye movements in particular is accessible to quantitative analysis, has indeed made detailed microphysiological studies of this process which tends to restore the "normal function" a most attractive prospect. In this Chapter single neuron studies performed during the process of vestibular compensation will be briefly summarized. The classic term "*compensation*," i.e. partial or complete restoration of a normal function after injury of some related structures, has always been used in the past to describe this process. Moreover, the studies of equilibrium disturbances resulting from lesions in the vestibular system have proved to be a very important source of better understanding of normal vestibular function.

II. Neuronal Activity in Bilateral Intact Animals: Vestibular Tone

EWALD's (1892) experiments were the first to indicate a *tonic action* of the labyrinthine organs on the muscular system of the body. Slackness of muscles in various parts of the body resulted from a bilateral labyrinthectomy. Since then many investigators have obtained direct proof of the tonic activity of the end-organs by recording from *single nerve fibers* in the vestibular nerve. Most of the otolithic and semicircular canal afferents fire at rest with a frequency in the range of 2–90 impulses per sec or more (MOWER, 1935; ROSS, 1936; LOWENSTEIN and SAND, 1936, 1940; GERNANDT, 1949; LEDOUX, 1949; RUPERT et al., 1962; TRINCKER, 1965; GUALTIEROTTI and ALLTUCKER, 1967; PRECHT et al., 1971; GOLDBERG and FERNÁNDEZ, 1971). Similarly, many of the second-order neurons in the vestibular nuclei (for details see Chapter D.II.) exhibit a fairly regular resting activity (ADRIAN, 1943; GERNANDT and THULIN, 1952; ECKEL, 1954; SCHÖN, 1957; DUENSING and SCHAEFER, 1958; SHIMAZU and PRECHT, 1965; PETERSON, 1967; FUJITA et al., 1968). This tonic activity of central vestibular neurons in turn provides much of the background tone of related motor systems, i.e. ocular and spinal motoneurons. Given that in the resting condition the neuronal activity on both sides is equal, it can be concluded that at rest the vestibular and related motor systems are in equilibrium. Stimulation or surgical interference on one side will result in a disturbance of this equilibrium, and the influence from one labyrinth will thus become dominant.

III. Neuronal Activity during the Acute Postoperative Stage

Following surgical removal of *one* labyrinth, the balance between the two sides will be upset as a consequence of unilateral withdrawal of the tonic excitatory input to the brain stem. Since eye movement disturbances (nystagmus) can be easily observed and measured, in most studies they have been used as the main parameter to define the various stages of compensation after labyrinthine lesion. Neurons belonging to the semicircular canal system have been selected for experiments on single neurons. Due to the influence from the remaining intact labyrinth, the eyes rhythmically deviate towards the injured side and quickly return to the normal side, i.e. the well-known *vestibular nystagmus* can be observed and recorded for the first three to four days (acute stage) after the operation (Fig. 1A). The frequency and amplitude of this lesion-evoked nystagmus are greatly enhanced by utriculofugal stimulation (Fig. 1A). Thus, at this acute postoperative stage, *directional predominance* of nystagmus similar to that observed in man (FLUUR, 1960) (compare Fig. 2A and B) was also observed in cats (PRECHT et al., 1966).

Microphysiological studies in decerebrate and unanesthetized animals have shown that during the acute postoperative stage the spontaneous activity of neurons in the deafferented vestibular nuclei is significantly reduced, while it is still present or even enhanced on the intact side (GERNANDT and THULIN, 1952; TRINCKER, 1965; SHIMAZU and PRECHT, 1966). It appears that in animals with

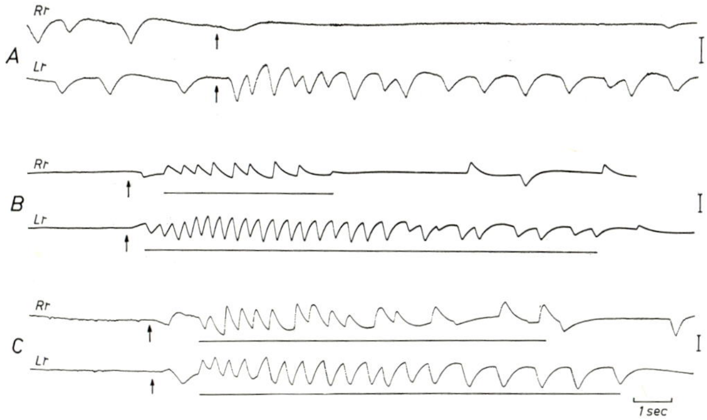

Fig. 1. Postrotatory nystagmus recorded at different stages following left hemilabyrinthectomy in cat. A: 2 days, B: 3 days, C: 33 days after operation. Rr = clockwise rotation (toward the intact labyrinth), Lr = counter clockwise rotation (toward operated side). Velocity of constant rotation maintained for 2 min before stop: 70°/sec in A; 200°/sec in B; and 150°/sec in C. Arrows indicate the time of sudden arrest of the turntable. Horizontal lines in B and C indicate the whole period of postrotatory nystagmus. Upward or downward deflections after these periods represent spontaneous eye movements. Downward deflection in each record indicates the movement of the pupil toward right. Amplitude calibration: 1 mV (PRECHT et al., 1966)

intact cerebellum the shutdown of resting activity of vestibular neurons occurs on the deafferented as well as on the intact side (McCABE et al., 1972). The effect on neurons on the intact side is explained by cerebellar inhibition acting on these neurons since removal of the cerebellum reveals resting activity in previously silent medial vestibular nucleus neurons (McGABE et al., 1972), but the occurrence of vestibular nystagmus during the acute postoperative stage indicates that only some vestibular neurons on the intact side are affected by cerebellar inhibition and that others (not located in the medial nucleus) may account for the observed imbalance of vestibulo-oculomotor innervation.

It is important to emphasize that the deafferented nuclei also contain neurons whose resting discharge frequency is still in the range of 0–30/sec (PRECHT et al., 1966). The frequency of these neurons increases following *utriculopetal* and decreases after *utricolofugal* endolymph flow induced in the intact *contralateral* horizontal canal by horizontal angular acceleration. Units responding with this pattern to horizontal rotation have been referred to as *type-II* vestibular neurons (DUENSING and SCHAEFER, 1958; SHIMAZU and PRECHT, 1965, 1966). Since these units are found in the completely deafferented nucleus, type-II responses from the nucleus on that side must be caused by influences arising from the horizontal canal on the intact side. Furthermore, all type-II neurons recorded from the destroyed side are excited by electrical stimulation of the contralateral intact vestibular nerve.

The *thresholds for electrical excitation* of type-II neurons tested with 50/sec stimulation are 1.57 ± 0.41 times the threshold for evoking N_1 potentials on the ipsilateral side (PRECHT et al., 1966). These values are very close to those for type-II neurons (1.52 ± 0.17), which were exclusively related to the commissural system in normal control animals (SHIMAZU and PRECHT, 1966), there being no statistically significant differences between them. Similarly, the *thresholds for frequency response* of type-II neurons recorded on the chronically deafferented side to horizontal angular acceleration varied from 1.7 to 10°/sec^2 or more. These values are almost the same as those obtained with both labyrinths intact (SHIMAZU and PRECHT, 1966).

Thus the lack or decrease of spontaneous discharge and the failure of a rotational response of neurons on the deafferented side, as reported by GERNANDT and THULIN (1952) and TRINCKER (1965) does not include type-II neurons in these nuclei. Unilateral labyrinthectomy, however, has a pronounced effect on type I neurons; their frequency is increased by utriculopetal endolymph flow in the ipsilateral horizontal canals and decreased by utriculofugal currents. These *type-I* neurons are the main *second-order vestibular neurons* of the horizontal canals, showing the same type of response as the primary afferent fibers (ADRIAN, 1943; GERNANDT, 1949; ECKEL, 1954; DUENSING and SCHAEFER, 1958; SHIMAZU and PRECHT, 1965). It was very unusual to find type-I neurons in the vestibular nuclei ipsilateral to the acute labyrinthine destruction, and the few neurons reacting in a type-I pattern needed enormously high accelerations before showing a modest frequency increase (PRECHT et al., 1966). On the intact side, however, spontaneous type-I neurons could be easily recorded while no type-II responses connected with the contralateral labyrinth were found.

Thus a distinct difference in neuronal activity is apparent between the vestibular nuclei on both sides following unilateral labyrinthectomy. The lack of spontaneous type-I neurons on the side of the lesion causes a disturbance of the tonic symmetric control of the oculomotor effectors at rest because spontaneous activity of type-I neurons in the intact nuclei becomes clearly dominant in the influence on the corresponding eye muscles leading to the well-known slow *conjugate deviation* towards the affected side. Other mechanisms responsible for *nystagmic reflexes* rapidly move the eyes back to the unaffected side. This sequence of slow and rapid eye movements continues for about 3 to 4 days following labyrinthectomy in cats (PRECHT et al., 1966), and nystagmus was seen to persist in human patients for about 2 weeks or more when recorded while the subjects had their eyes closed (CAWTHORNE et al., 1942; FRENZEL, 1955; FLUUR, 1960; LANGE and KORNHUBER, 1962). Recordings of *spontaneous nystagmus* are shown in Fig. 1A. When a utriculofugal endolymph flow is generated in the remaining horizontal canal, either by contralateral rotation or by irrigation with cold water (FLUUR, 1960), the spontaneous nystagmus is completely suppressed (Fig. 1A upper record) (PRECHT et al., 1966). As mentioned above, utriculofugal endolymph movements in the horizontal semicircular canals cause a *decrease* or abolition of the *spontaneous activity* of type-I neurons in the ipsilateral nerve as well as in the nuclei. This decrease of activity on the intact side causes a transient equilibrium (zero discharge) between both sides, resulting in the disappearance of the spontaneous nystagmus. Soon after stimulation, the spontaneous ocular rhythm starts again.

IV. Neuronal Activity during the Course of Recovery

Before the neuronal activity is described, the time course of the functional recovery of symmetric control of eye movements will be analyzed. Soon after the disappearance of spontaneous vestibular nystagmus, the afore-mentioned directional predominance of postrotatory nystagmus is still remarkable, as shown in Fig. 1B. Figure 2B shows the relation between *duration* of postrotatory nystagmus and *speed of rotation* in both directions, tested *3–4 days after operation* (PRECHT et al., 1966). The *duration* is approximately proportional to the *logarithm* of the angular velocity in both right and left rotations, as described also by VAN EGMOND et al. (1949). It was found that postrotatory nystagmus did not persist as long after rotation toward the intact side as after rotation toward the treated side; the difference was highly significant. The *amplitude* also shows a clear difference in magnitude. As can be seen from the *control experiments* in normal cats (Fig. 2A), the duration and the amplitude of nystagmus are usually almost the same

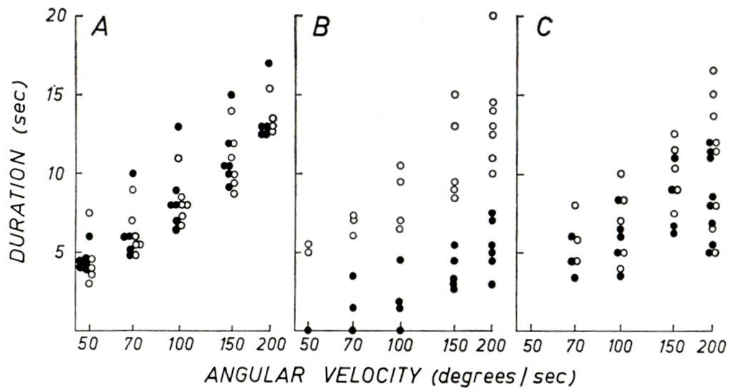

Fig. 2. Relation between duration of postrotatory nystagmus (ordinate) and velocity of rotation before the sudden arrest of the turntable. Abscissa in logarithmic scale. A: control with three normal cats; B: 3–4 days after left labyrinthectomy with five cats; C: 30–45 days after the operation, six cats. Filled circles: after clockwise rotation; open circles: after counterclockwise rotation (PRECHT et al., 1966)

in both directions. When recorded about *40 days after operation*, the duration of postrotatory nystagmus after rotation to the intact side is much longer than in the acute stage and approaches that obtained after rotation to the treated side (Figs. 1C and 2C). As shown in Fig. 2C, the duration of nystagmus after left and right rotations is very similar, though slight differences are still present. Asymmetry of the amplitudes of electronystagmograms is usually also much reduced.

It may be concluded from these results (PRECHT et al., 1966) that the asymmetry in vestibular influences on the oculomotor nuclei of both sides following labyrinthectomy is much reduced by about 40 days after operation, though not completely abolished. Apparently in the *stage of compensation*, utriculofugal endolymph flow in the intact horizontal semicircular canal can produce eye movements of a similar duration but in the reverse direction and of a smaller amplitude, as compared to the eye movements generated by utriculopetal stimulation. By increasing and decreasing its spontaneous resting activity, only *one semicircular canal* can now cause conjugate eye movements in both directions such that the oculomotor system is nearly in balance, as is the case when both labyrinths are intact.

The mechanisms involved in this process have been studied mainly by means of operative interference with structures related to the vestibular system. BECHTEREW (1883) found that after disappearance of spontaneous nystagmus following unilateral labyrinthectomy, destruction of the contralateral labyrinth produces distinct nystagmus whose quick component is directed toward the labyrinth *first* destroyed as if it were still intact. This phenomenon is called *Bechterew's compensatory nystagmus*. The Bechterew phenomenon is preserved in the decerebrate animal as well as after decerebellation (MAGNUS, 1924; SPIEGEL and DÈMÈTRIADES, 1925). SPIEGEL and DÈMÈTRIADES (1925) concluded that the integrity of the vestibular nuclei on the side labyrinthectomized first is essential for the compensation of vestibular function. They assumed that after isolating the vestibular nuclei from the ipsilateral labyrinth, these nuclei become gradually *hyperexcitable* and balance the activity of the contralateral vestibular nuclei, thus leading to a compensated state.

PRECHT et al. (1966) recorded single unit activity in the vestibular nuclei of the chronically deafferented side and studied their response to horizontal angular acceleration. The results obtained in acutely deafferented animals have been described above. In contrast to the situation in the acute postoperative state, in the compensated stage it is very easy to record spontaneously active neurons which increase their discharge frequency exponentially during ipsi-

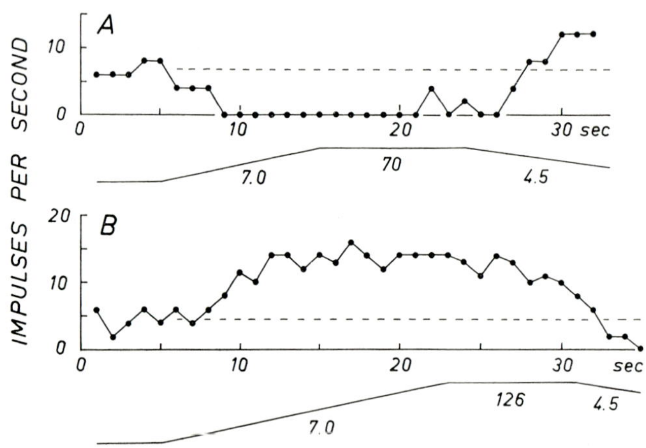

Fig. 3. Frequency diagrams of discharges of a tonic type-I vestibular neuron in response to contralateral (A) and ipsilateral (B) horizontal angular acceleration and deceleration. Ipsilateral labyrinth was destroyed 30 days before recording. In each diagram, the ordinate represents spikes per second of single unit discharges measured in each second. Horizontal broken line in each diagram represents the average frequency over 10 sec before rotation. Curve below each frequency diagram indicates the velocity of rotation. Numbers below the rotation curve indicate (left to right) the magnitude of acceleration (degree/sec²), velocity of constant rotation (degree/sec), and deceleration magnitude (PRECHT et al., 1966)

lateral angular acceleration and cease to fire during contralateral rotation, thus showing a *type-I response* to rotation (Figs. 3 and 4). Since the horizontal semicircular canal on the intact side is the only receptor organ being stimulated, the type-I responses must be caused by influences arising from these receptors. As already noted above, type-II neurons receiving an excitatory influence from the contralateral labyrinth were shown to be present in all stages after unilateral labyrinthectomy. It has been found that some *type-II* neurons are *inhibitory* interneurons mediating influences from the contralateral horizontal canal via the *commissural fibers* and inhibiting the main sensory neurons (type-I) on the same side (SHIMAZU and PRECHT, 1966, see also Chapter D.II.). Thus utriculofugal endolymph flow in the intact contralateral canal results in a *decreasing excitatory influence*, not only on type-I on the same side but also on type-II on the deafferented side. This means that type-I neurons on that side receive *less inhibition* and hence increase their firing rate. On the other hand, *utriculopetal* flow in the intact horizontal canal *increases* the crossed inhibition on type-I discharge frequency by activating the inhibitory type-II neurons. In the stage of compensation this mechanism is for the most part responsible for the type-I response of neurons on the deafferented side, which is at least *qualitatively* similar to the type-I pattern on the intact side. However, some important differences with respect to the bilaterally intact animals deserve mention (PRECHT et al., 1966). The frequency of spontaneous activity of type-I neurons on the labyrinthectomized side were never found to be higher than 10/sec. High-frequency discharges of 30/sec or more, as obtained from the intact side, were not observed. Many type-I neurons on the operated side show no spontaneous discharges, and their *thresholds* to angular acceleration are higher (2.0–8.0°/sec^2) than those of *tonic type-I* neurons in the intact nuclei (0.23–1.0°/sec^2) (SHIMAZU and PRECHT, 1965). However, their characteristics during rotation did not allow them to be classified as *kinetic type-I* neurons as described by SHIMAZU and PRECHT (1965). This may indicate that the type-I neurons without tonic discharges found on the operated side were originally tonic in nature but are still depressed in their activity, due to elimination of the excitatory influence arising from the ipsilateral receptors. *Kinetic* type-I neurons were not identified in chronic preparations, possibly because their high thresholds to acceleratory stimulation were still further elevated by the ipsilateral operation.

The *maximum discharge* frequency of type-I units on the deafferented side during ipsilateral angular acceleration is about 25/sec, which is much lower than the type-I frequency increase obtained with the same stimulus amplitude on the intact side, but almost the same value as maximum spontaneous activity obtained by *cutting the commissural fibers*. This may indicate that *maximum increase* in discharge frequency of *type-I* neurons on the deafferented side during ipsilateral rotation is produced by *minimal inhibition* from the intact contralateral horizontal canal, thus resulting in the same effect as section of the commissural fibers. It is reasonable to expect that in the compensated stage following unilateral labyrinthectomy, destruction of the *second* labyrinth or interruption of the commissural system releases type-I activity of the first operated side from commissural inhibition, thus producing *Bechterew's compensatory nystagmus*. Similarly, release of tonic inhibition from the contralateral nuclei would give an

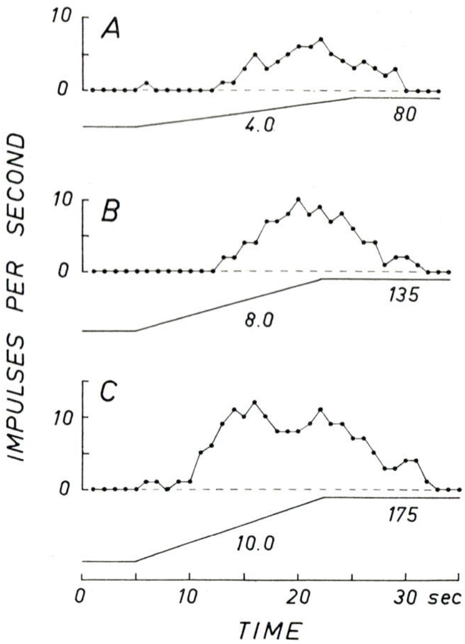

Fig. 4. Frequency diagrams of discharges of a type-I vestibular neuron in response to different magnitudes of ipsilateral constant angular accelerations. Ipsilateral labyrinth was destroyed 30 days before recording. In each diagram impulses per second of a single unit are plotted along the ordinate and the time in seconds along the abscissa. The curve below each diagram shows the velocity of rotation. Numbers below each rotation curve in A to C indicate (left to right) the magnitude of acceleration (degree/sec^2) and velocity of constant rotation (degree/sec) (PRECHT et al., 1966)

explanation for SPIEGEL and SATO's (1926) findings that even after acute bilateral labyrinthectomy additional destruction of the vestibular nuclei on one side produces nystagmus and slow ocular deviations. In man the symptoms of peripheral labyrinthine deficit often disappear due to a slow recovery of the *peripheral* function and are replaced by nystagmus in the opposite direction to that occurring after acute lesions (STENGER, 1959). Apparently the reappearance of spontaneous activity in the nerve summates with the increased central activity in the ipsilateral vestibular nuclei, resulting in a new disequilibrium.

Since type-I vestibular neurons can be assumed to transmit excitatory influence to the contralateral abducens motoneurons (SCHAEFER, 1965; PRECHT et al., 1967; PRECHT et al., 1969; BAKER et al., 1969) and ipsilateral medial rectus motoneurons of the oculomotor nucleus (SASAKI, 1963), the *bilateral* reappearance of this type of unitary response in the compensated stage seems to be essential for the gradually subsiding directional predominance of postrotatory nystagmus during the course of compensation (as shown in Figs. 1 and 2). The absence of type-I responses in the *acutely* deafferented nucleus might appear curious since the commissural inhibitory pathway is also functionally active in this kind of preparation. One important reason for their absence is certainly the very low level of spontaneous discharge frequencies of type-I neurons in the acute stage.

In addition, it has been found that the *threshold* of electrical vestibular nerve stimulation for producing the *contralateral inhibition* of type-I vestibular neurons is significantly *lower* in the stage of compensation following unilateral labyrinthectomy than that in animals with both labyrinths *intact* (SHIMAZU and PRECHT, 1965; PRECHT et al., 1966). In the stage of compensation the commissural inhibition may therefore be able to inhibit the resting activity of type-I neurons more powerfully, thus leading to the distinct bidirectional response pattern.

Any part along the above pathway might be responsible for lowering the thresholds for contralateral inhibition of type-I neurons. However, the contralaterally evoked initial positive *field potentials* and the later slow negative waves in the vestibular nuclei on the deafferented side do not show any significant differences from those in the acute preparation (SHIMAZU and PRECHT, 1966; PRECHT et al., 1966). Furthermore, the threshold for contralateral activation of type-II neurons in the deafferented nuclei are almost the same as are obtained in normal cats. These results indicate that no significant functional alteration occurred either in commissural fibers from the intact side or in type-II neurons on the chronically deafferented side. It is likely, therefore, that remarkable *functional changes* occur *mainly in type-I neurons* on the labyrinthectomized side. These neurons receive *primary afferent fibers* (PRECHT and SHIMAZU, 1965) from the ipsilateral labyrinth, which were shown to be *degenerated* after labyrinthine destruction (PRECHT et al., 1966), whereas *type-II* neurons are innervated by the commissural fibers originating on the *intact* contralateral side.

It is well known that functional changes in central neurons after long-term injury of related structures are produced by degeneration of synaptic endings terminating at the neurons. The degeneration of some afferent fibers causes *increased sensitivity* of postsynaptic membrane to chemical influences (CANNON and HAIMOVICI, 1939; DRAKE and STAVRAKY, 1948; CANNON and ROSENBLUETH, 1949), as well as collateral *sprouting* of neighboring presynaptic fibers (LIU and CHAMBERS, 1955; MCCOUCH et al., 1958). One possible explanation of the lowered threshold for contralateral inhibition of type-I neurons is that degeneration of primary afferents stimulates sprouting of neighboring presynaptic fibers from type-II neurons, thus increasing the inhibitory synaptic action on type-I neurons. *Hypersensitivity* of type-I neurons to the inhibitory impingement might be another reason for the lowered threshold. The reappearance of spontaneous discharges of type-I neurons after degeneration of the main excitatory sensory input may be caused by biochemical sensitization of deafferented type-I neurons or by sprouting of other afferent fibers such as reticulo-vestibular fibers, which have been shown to be excitatory on type-I neurons (MARKHAM et al., 1966; SHIMAZU and PRECHT, 1966). This possibility appears unlikely, however, since lesions of large parts of the reticular formation did not abolish the new resting activity of vestibular neurons in the deafferented nucleus (MCCABE et al., 1972). Furthermore, these results suggest that the cerebellum, the cerebrum, the contralateral vestibular nuclei, the ipsilateral superior and lateral vestibular nuclei and the spinal cord do not make any major contribution to the regeneration of resting activity of vestibular neurons (MCCABE et al., 1972). Possibly these neurons become truly spontaneously active during the regeneration phase.

These statements, however, do not exclude the possibility that the *cerebellum*, or other systems such as the *visual* system, or the spinal cord (AZZENA, 1969) may also play a role in establishing central compensation of vestibular function after labyrinthine lesion. The data obtained from operative interference with the vestibular system and that gained from a single unit analysis combine to demonstrate the importance of the vestibular nuclei in the process of compensation. Finally it should be pointed out that these studies are only a first step towards a better understanding of central compensation of vestibular function. In particular, microphysiological recovery studies of the otolith system are needed for a more complete concept of the neuronal mechanisms involved in central compensation.

References

ADRIAN, E.D.: Discharges from vestibular receptors in the cat. J. Physiol. (Lond.) **101**, 389–407 (1943).

AZZENA, G.B.: Role of the spinal cord in compensating the effects of hemilabyrinthectomy. Arch. ital. Biol. **107**, 43–53 (1969).

BAKER, R.G., MANO, N., SHIMAZU, H.: Postsynaptic potentials in abducens motoneurons induced by vestibular stimulation. Brain Res. **15**, 577–580 (1969).

BÁRÁNY, R.: Physiologie und Pathologie des Bogengangsapparates beim Menschen. Wien: Franz Deuticke 1907.

BECHTEREW, W. VON: Ergebnisse der Durchschneidung des N. acusticus, nebst Erörterung der Bedeutung der semicirculären Canäle für das Körpergleichgewicht. Pflügers Arch. ges. Physiol. **30**, 312–347 (1883).

CANNON, W.B., HAIMOVICI, H.: The sensitization of motoneurons by partial "Denervation". Amer. J. Physiol. **126**, 731–740 (1939).

CANNON, W.B., ROSENBLUETH, A.: The Supersensitivity of Denervated Structures. New York: Macmillan 1949.

CAWTHORNE, T.E., FITZGERALD, G., HALLPIKE, C.S.: Studies in human vestibular function. II. Observations on the directional preponderance of caloric nystagmus (Nystagmusbereitschaft) resulting from unilateral labyrinthectomy. Brain **65**, 138–160 (1942).

DOHLMAN, G.: Experimentelle Untersuchungen über die galvanische Vestibularisreaktion. Acta oto-laryng. (Stockh.) Suppl. **8**, 1–48 (1929).

DRAKE, C.G., STAVRAKY, G.W.: An extension of the "law of denervation" to afferent neurons. J. Neurophysiol. **11**, 229–238 (1948).

DUENSING, F., SCHAEFER, K.P.: Die Aktivität einzelner Neurone im Bereich der Vestibulariskerne bei Horizontalbeschleunigungen unter besonderer Berücksichtigung des vestibulären Nystagmus. Arch. Psychiat. Nervenkr. **198**, 225–252 (1958).

ECKEL, W.: Elektrophysiologische und histologische Untersuchungen im Vestibulariskerngebiet bei Drehreizen. Z. Hals-, Nas.-, u. Ohrenheilk. **164**, 487–513 (1954).

EWALD, J.R.: Physiologische Untersuchungen über das Endorgan des N. Oktavus. Wiesbaden: Bergmann 1892.

FLUUR, E.: Vestibular compensation after labyrinthine destruction. Acta oto-laryng. (Stockh.) **52**, 367–375 (1960).

FRENZEL, H.: Spontan- und Provokations-Nystagmus als Krankheitssymptom. Berlin-Göttingen-Heidelberg: Springer 1955.

FUJITA, Y., ROSENBERG, J., SEGUNDO, J.P.: Activity of cells in the lateral vestibular nucleus as a function of head position. J. Physiol. (Lond.) **196**, 1–18 (1968).

GERNANDT, B.E.: Response of mammalian vestibular neurons to horizontal rotation and caloric stimulation. J. Neurophysiol. **12**, 173–184 (1949).

GERNANDT, B.E., THULIN, C.A.: Vestibular connections of the brain stem. Amer. J. Physiol. **171**, 121–127 (1952).

GOLDBERG, J.M., FERNÁNDEZ, C.: Physiology of peripheral neurons innervating semicircular canals of the squirrel monkey. Resting discharge and response to constant angular accelerations. J. Neurophysiol. **34**, 635–660 (1971).

GUALTIEROTTI, T., ALLTUCKER, D.S.: Prolonged recording from single vestibular units in the frog during plane and space flight, its significance and technique. Aerospace Med. **38**, 513–517 (1967).

LANGE, G., KORNHUBER, H.H.: Zur Bedeutung peripher- und zentral-vestibulärer Störungen nach Kopftraumen. Arch. Ohr.-, Nas.-, u. Kehlk.-Heilk. **179**, 366–385 (1962).

LEDOUX, A.: Activité électrique des nerfs des canaux semicirculaires du saccule et de l'utricle chez la grenouille. Acta oto-rhino-laryng. belg. **3**, 335–349 (1949).

LIU, C.N., CHAMBERS, W.W.: Intraspinal sprouting elicited from intact spinal sensory neurons by adjacent posterior root sections. Amer. J. Physiol. **183**, 640–641 (1955).

LORENTE DE NÓ, R.: Die Labyrinthreflexe auf die Augenmuskeln nach einseitiger Labyrinthexstirpation nebst einer kurzen Angabe über den Nervenmechanismus der vestibulären Augenbewegungen. Berlin, Wien: Urban und Schwarzenberg 1928.

LOWENSTEIN, O., SAND, A.: The activity of the horizontal semicircular canals of the dog fish. J. exp. Biol. **13**, 416–428 (1936).

LOWENSTEIN, O., SAND, A.: The individual and integrated activity of the semicircular canals of the elasmobranch labyrinth. J. Physiol. (Lond.) **99**, 89–101 (1940).

LOWENSTEIN, O., SAND, A.: The mechanism of the semicircular canals. A study of the responses of single-fibre preparations to angular accelerations and rotation at constant speed. Proc. roy. Soc. Biol. **129**, 256–275 (1940).

MAGNUS, R.: Körperstellung. Berlin: Springer 1924.

MARKHAM, C.H., PRECHT, W., SHIMAZU, H.: Effect of stimulation of interstitial nucleus of Cajal on vestibular unit activity in the cat. J. Neurophysiol. **29**, 493–507 (1966).

MCCABE, B.F., RYU, I.H., SEKITANI, T.: Further experiments on vestibular compensation. Laryngoscope (St. Louis) **82**, 381–396 (1972).

MCCOUCH, G.P., AUSTIN, G.M., LIU, C.N., LIU, C.Y.: Sprouting as a cause of spasticity. J. Neurophysiol. **21**, 205–216 (1958).

MITTERMAIER, R.: Über die Ausgleichsvorgänge im Vestibularapparat. Z. Laryng. Rhinol. **29**, 487–585 (1950).

MOWRER, O.H.: The electrical response of the vestibular nerve during adequate stimulation. Science **81**, 180–181 (1935).

PETERSON, B.W.: Effect of tilting on the activity of neurons in the vestibular nuclei of the cat. Brain Res. **6**, 606–609 (1967).

PFALTZ, C.R., KAMATH, R.: The problems of central compensation on peripheral vestibular dysfunction. Acta oto-laryng. (Stockh.) **71**, 266 (1971).

PRECHT, W., SHIMAZU, H.: Functional connections of tonic and kinetic vestibular neurons with primary vestibular afferents. J. Neurophysiol. **28**, 1014–1028 (1965).

PRECHT, W., SHIMAZU, H., MARKHAM, C.H.: A mechanism of central compensation of vestibular function following hemilabyrinthectomy. J. Neurophysiol. **29**, 996–1010 (1966).

PRECHT, W., GRIPPO, J., RICHTER, A.: Effect of horizontal angular acceleration on neurons in the abducens nucleus. Brain Res. **5**, 527–531 (1967).

PRECHT, W., RICHTER, A., GRIPPO, J.: Responses of neurones in cat's abducens nuclei to horizontal angular acceleration. Pflügers Arch. ges. Physiol. **309**, 285–309 (1969).

PRECHT, W., LLINÁS, R., CLARKE, M.: Physiological responses of frog vestibular fibers to horizontal angular rotation. Exp. Brain Res. **13**, 378–407 (1971).

ROSS, J.A.: Electrical studies on the frog's labyrinth. J. Physiol. (Lond.) **86**, 117–146 (1936).

RUPERT, A., MOUSHEGIAN, G., GALAMBOS, R.: Microelectrode studies of primary vestibular neurons in cat. Exp. Neurol. **5**, 100–109 (1962).

SASAKI, K.: Electrophysiological studies on oculomotor neurons of the cat. Jap. J. Physiol. **13**, 287–302 (1963).

SCHAEFER, K.P.: Die Erregungsmuster einzelner Neurone des Abducens-Kernes beim Kaninchen. Pflügers Arch. ges. Physiol. **284**, 31–52 (1965).

SCHOEN, L.: Mikroableitungen einzelner zentraler Vestibularisneurone von Knochenfischen bei Statolithenreizen. Z. vergl. Physiol. **39**, 399–417 (1957).

SHIMAZU, H., PRECHT, W.: Tonic and kinetic responses of cat's vestibular neurons to horizontal angular acceleration. J. Neurophysiol. **28**, 991–1013 (1965).

SHIMAZU, H., PRECHT, W.: Inhibition of central vestibular neurons from the contralateral labyrinth and its mediating pathway. J. Neurophysiol. **29**, 467–492 (1966).

SPIEGEL, E.A., DÈMÈTRIADES, T.D.: Die zentrale Kompensation des Labyrinthverlustes. Pflügers Arch. ges. Physiol. **210**, 215–222 (1925).

SPIEGEL, E.A., SATO, G.: Experimentalstudien am Nervensystem. V. Über den Erregungszustand der medullären Zentren nach doppelseitiger Labyrinthausschaltung. Pflügers Arch. ges. Physiol. **215**, 106–119 (1926).

STENGER, H.H.: Erholungsnystagmus nach einseitigem Vestibularisausfall, ein dem BECHTEREW-nystagmus verwandter Vorgang. Arch. Ohr.-, Nas.-, u. Kehlk.-Heilk. **175**, 545–549 (1959).

TRINCKER, D.: Physiologie des Gleichgewichtsorgans. In: Hals-Nasen-Ohren-Heilkunde, Vol. III, Part 1. J. BERENDES, R. LINK, F. ZÖLLNER, Eds. Stuttgart: Georg Thieme 1965.

VAN EGMOND, A.A.J., GROEN, J.J., JONGKEES, L.B.W.: The mechanism of the semicircular canal. J. Physiol. (Lond.) **110**, 1–17 (1949).

VAN EYCK, M.: Recherches sur le phénomène de compensation après labyrinthectomie. Acta oto-laryng. (Stockh.) **44**, 456–461 (1954).

Chapter XI.

Compensation of Vestibular Lesions

By

K.P. Schaefer and D. L. Meyer, Goettingen (West-Germany)

With 4 Figures

Contents

I. Introduction

Significant knowledge about vestibular functions was already available before the turn of the century. After the first investigations on the semicircular canals of the inner ear by Flourens (1824), Goltz (1870) initiated further research when he demonstrated the effects of labyrinthine injury in pigeons. The impressive clinical picture of Ménière's disease has also caused several authors to direct their attention to labyrinthine physiology (e.g. Cyon, 1874; Bornhardt, 1876; Spamer, 1880; Lee, 1894, 1894–1895). Most of them sectioned or partially removed the membranous semicircular canals and thus gained some insight into labyrinthine pathophysiology. A comprehensive list of this early literature can be found in Ewald (1892).

These investigations revealed that a labyrinthine lesion induces a torsion of the animal about its longitudinal bodyaxis towards the side of the injury, that considerable uncertainty of gait is caused and that birds lose the ability to fly. The observers differentiated between symptoms seen immediately after surgery and symptoms still present days or even months after the lesion. However, few workers have undertaken chronic investigations on the mechanisms that partially compensate for the symptoms of labyrinthine lesions. In a paper still well worth reading, Bechterew (1883) reported experiments in which the two labyrinths of an animal were successively destroyed at intervals of up to several days. He observed a reversal of the direction of the compulsive movements due to the second lesion if the interval between the lesions was sufficiently long. In the recent literature this phenomenon is called Bechterew compensation and is one of the most interesting points to be discussed here.

In the early periods of vestibular research two contradictory hypotheses existed to explain the occurrence of the symptoms after unilateral labyrinthectomy: they could be due either to an irritation, or to a defect. Goltz (1870) and Bechterew (1883) were firm supporters of the defect theory and considered the loss of centripetal impulses from the labyrinth to cause the movement disturbances that occurred. The irritation theory was unlikely to be correct, since the reactions to irritation by electrical stimulation of the semicircular canals differ from the symptoms after the destruction of the canals. Spamer (1880) was one of the first to prove that the destruction of one labyrinth results in a rotation of the body towards the injured side, whereas electrical irritation causes a rotation of the body to the opposite side. Among other arguments, the fact that the most intense symptoms resulting from a labyrinthine lesion are the ones which disappear after some time was interpreted by the defenders of the irritation theory as indicating that an irritation rather than a defect is caused by the lesion. The defect theory was based on two suppositions:

1. In the normal position of the animal a continuous centripetal impulse-flow from the labyrinths maintains a resting level of excitation in the vestibular nuclei.
2. The symptoms of labyrinthine lesions are due to a loss of this resting activity and can be partially compensated by other sense organs and CNS structures.

Labyrinth tonus. The continuous influence of the labyrinths on the muscle tone and several brain centers made Ewald (1892) coin the often misunderstood term "Tonus-Labyrinth." *By affecting the labyrinths this influence can be increased or decreased.* This interpretation coincides, to a large degree, with the theory von Holst (1950) developed some 50 years later. He suggested that the labyrinthine posture receptors are automatically active; rotatory tendency and asymmetrical body posture after unilateral labyrinthectomy or utriculus elimination were thought to result from changes of the afferent-activity rather than being caused by a "reflex" from the statoliths.

Since then, direct evidence has been obtained for the existence of a spontaneous activity in vestibular nerve fibers and in the vestibular nuclei (Mowrer, 1935; Lowenstein and Sand, 1936; Adrian, 1943; Gernandt and Thulin, 1952; Eckel, 1954; Schoen, 1957; Duensing and Schaefer, 1957, 1958, 1960; Shimazu and Precht, 1965, 1966; Gualtierotti and Alltucker, 1967). Assuming that at the resting position the spontaneous level of activity on both sides is equal, a lesion on one side will create a dominance of the influence from the contralateral side.

Compensation. As mentioned above, the symptoms resulting from the elimination of one labyrinth may be compensated for partially. The following chapters will describe the dependence of this compensation on vestibular mechanisms, as well as on other CNS functions and sense organs. Kornhuber (1966) differentiates between a specific vestibular process, called compensation (Mittermaier, 1950), and a substitute mechanism by other sensory functions for which the term 'adjustment' is used. In the recent literature, however, both 'compensation' and 'adjustment' are often used to mean the first of these two mechanisms.

Ewald (1892), Magnus (1922, 1924) and others recognized the importance of optic, somato-sensory, cortical, and spinal influences on the compensation of labyrinthine lesions. Several authors have since sought to clarify the question of how far these multiple influences differ from species to species (see Fischer, 1930; Magnus and De Kleijn, 1930). They attempted to solve this problem by unilateral and bilateral elimination of the labyrinth combined with hemispherectomy, transsection of the spinal cord, cerebellectomy, or microrecordings from single nerve cells.

II. Unilateral Labyrinthine Lesions

The symptoms resulting from unilateral labyrinthectomy are basically identical in all vertebrates (see FISCHER 1930; MAGNUS and DE KLEIJN, 1930). However, depending on the species, the pattern of movement induced may vary in time-course and strength. Compensatory mechanisms were also found in all animals examined. Little attention has yet been paid to the exact time-courses of compensation of the different symptoms.

The following sections will give a comparative description of compensatory mechanisms in the most intensively studied vertebrates. Similar processes in invertebrates, compensating for unilateral posture-receptor lesions or blinding (DOLLEY, 1916; BUDDENBROCK 1930; CLARK, 1931; LÜDTKE, 1935; MITTELSTAEDT, 1950; SCHÖNE, 1950 and others), cannot be discussed here. Nor will experiments based on microrecordings from the vestibular nuclei of labyrinthectomized animals be considered here (a detailed description is given by PRECHT, this volume). For historical reasons the experiments on birds will be reported first.

Pigeons. In 1824 FLOURENS showed that section of one semicircular canal in pigeons induces head movements in the plane of the destroyed semicircular canal; the head movements were found to cease after some time. GOLTZ (1870), CYON (1874), BORNHARDT (1876), SPAMER (1880), BECHTEREW (1883), EWALD (1892), GROEBBELS (1926/1928) and HUIZINGA (1931, 1932) have confirmed FLOURENS' findings and extended them in several respects.

The irritation resulting from opening one of the bony semicircular canals diminishes the intention to fly or run. During running the birds are somewhat insecure on the leg ipsilateral to the operation. The symptoms are more distinct after all three bony canals on one side have been opened, but all disturbances diminish after about 15 min. After additional section of one membranous semicircular canal no attempts to fly are made for several hours.

Destruction of all membranous canals on one side causes complete loss of the ability to fly and the animals fall to the ground clumsily when thrown into the air; spontaneous movements are rare. Nystagmus-like eye movements in these birds have been described by CYON (1874). The animals start moving again after about 24 hours, but the gait is uncertain for a long time and flying remains permanently restricted. During sitting and running the head is held in an asymmetrical position towards the injured side. Fits of rotatory movements occur and make the animals seek the proximity of walls to obtain security through tactile stimuli. Considering these disturbances, it is quite striking how quickly the birds regain the ability to sit on a branch, even after serious lesions. The importance of tactile and proprioceptive afferents for birds balancing on the branch of a tree can hardly be demonstrated more obviously (see FISCHER 1930).

Compensation of symptoms resulting from bilateral elimination of homologous canals was found to be significantly slower than compensation after total destruction of all canals on one side (FLOURENS, 1824; SPAMER, 1880). Bilateral labyrinthine defects particularly reduce the ability to fly. Violent pendulous movements of the head occur, which make running and feeding difficult. A certain security in standing is regained after hours, in running after weeks or months.

Fish. At the end of the last century, LOEB (1891) and BETHE (1899) showed that dissection of the right VIII nerve of sharks causes an oblique swimming position, rolling movements of the animals about their longitudinal axis to the right, circular movements to the right, and an eye deviation towards the right side. Rolling and circular movements disappear within a few days; the oblique swimming position is compensated more slowly and may increase or decrease from one moment to the next. "Emotional stimuli," such as feeding the fish or threatening him may cause a striking reappearance of already compensated symptoms (LOEB, 1891; BETHE, 1899; LOWENSTEIN, 1932; VON HOLST, 1935, 1948, 1950; SCHÖN, 1950).

According to VON HOLST (1935, 1948, 1950) the swimming position of fish is determined by vestibular afferents, as well as by the direction of light. An oblique posture was induced if the light penetrated into the tank from the side. No adaptation was observed under these conditions. In contrast, an oblique swimming position resulting from the removal of one utricle was found to be compensated by the animals after some time. After removal of the utricle the fish continually roll about their longitudinal axis; sometimes they come to rest on the bottom of the tank and then lie down on the injured side. If compensation has progressed for days or weeks, the oblique swimming position diminishes, and can be even further reduced by an increase of "gravity" when the animals are centrifuged. The oblique posture induced by the lesion decreases rapidly during the first few days, and then more and more slowly. Species differences in compensation have been intensively studied in different fishes by SCHÖN (1950). After unilateral utricle ablation, compensation of the oblique swimming position takes approximately 36 days under normal gravitational conditions, but may be accomplished more quickly if gravity is increased by centrifugation of the fish. With doubled gravity only one third the normal time is required. This is not a consequence of accelerated compensation, but is rather due to lower starting values; i.e. the oblique posture is already reduced by increased gravity, as mentioned before. According to VON HOLST'S (1935, 1948, 1950) and SCHÖN'S (1950) observations, a lability of postural control is still present even if the asymmetrical swimming position and the movement disturbances have already disappeared. In diffuse light and after diminution of gravity to its normal strength, animals already free of symptoms in the increased gravitational field start to roll slowly about the longitudinal axis again.

Frogs. Numerous investigations on the vestibular system of frog have been published, but most reports give no exact details on compensation of vestibular defects. GOLTZ (1870), BECHTEREW (1883), EWALD (1892), MCNALLY and TAIT (1925), THAUER and PETERS (1935), and KOLB (1955) revealed in their experiments that elimination of one labyrinth causes temporary disturbances in balance and turning of the head about the longitudinal axis towards the ipsilateral side. As a consequence of the low degree of head mobility there are marked effects on the body in addition; the contralateral extremities are extended and the vertebral column appears to curve slightly (Fig. 1). In a comparative study involving jackdaws, cockatoos, salamanders, rabbits, and dogs, EWALD (1892) reported that the disturbances mentioned are considerably more pronounced in water.

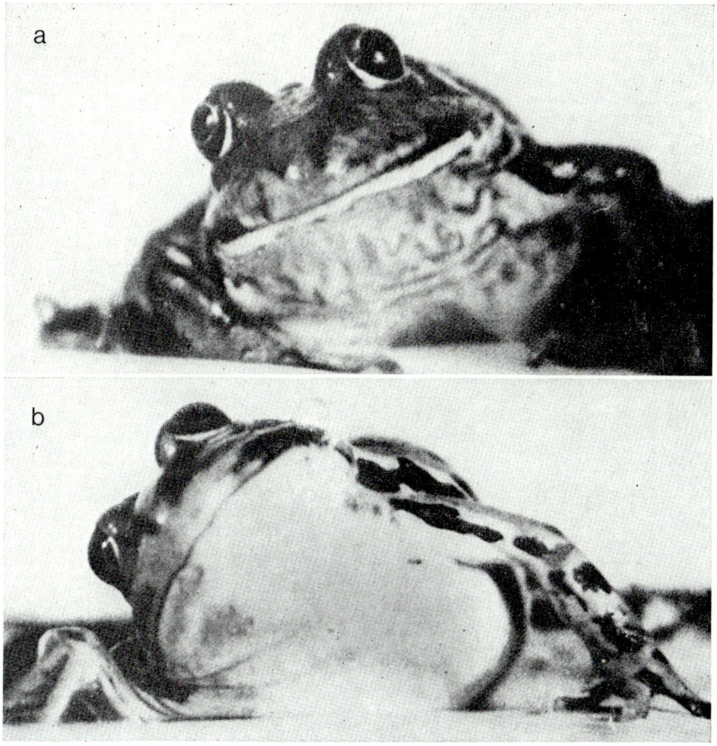

Fig. 1. Postural asymmetry in a frog (Rana esculenta) shortly after labyrinthectomy on the right side (a), and 3 hours after additional removal of the forebrain (b) (After KOLB, 1955)

The symptoms of the unilateral labyrinthine lesions disappear after some time, the security in prey catching is regained, and swimming movements in water become symmetrical again. KOLB (1955) carried out investigations under quantitative conditions, measuring the position of the oral cleft, and thereby determining the degree of compensation already accomplished after certain time intervals (Fig. 2). As in fish, an exponential time course of compensation was found in water frogs (*Rana esculenta*) and grass frogs (*Rana temporaria*).

According to KOLB's (1955) report, water frogs hold their heads in the normal position after about 6 months, whereas grass frogs compensate unilateral labyrinthectomy somewhat faster. *Rana esculenta* is obviously more dependent on the labyrinths, and therefore compensates more slowly, than the grass frog. In the latter, tactile and optical stimulation appear to be more involved in compensating processes after vestibular lesions. After section of the optic nerve, transection of the spinal cord or removal of the forebrain, the speed of compensation is retarted.

An interesting observation has been described by THAUER and PETERS (1935) after unilateral labyrinthectomy: the symptoms of the labyrinthectomy did not occur immediately, but were delayed for some time. A similar observation had been made in pigeons by EWALD (1892). THAUER and PETERS (1935) interpreted this as due to an irritation after the operation, which masks the defect symptoms for a short period.

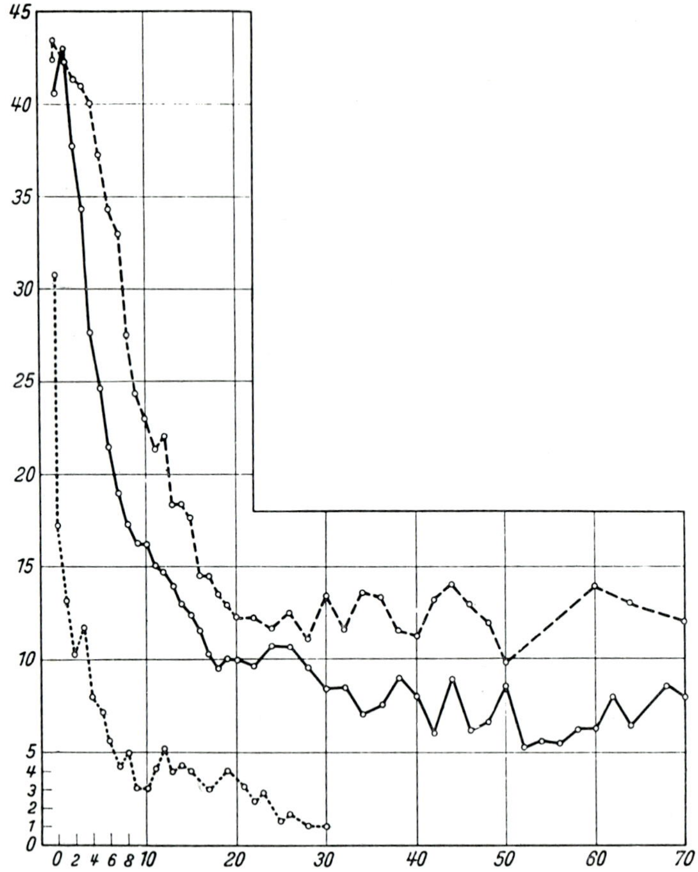

Fig. 2. Time course of compensation after destruction of one labyrinth in Rana esculenta. Angle of head deviation (ordinate) plotted against days after the lesion. (— — — —) time course of compensation after unilateral labyrinthine lesion, (- - - - - - - - - -) after unilateral labyrinthine lesion with additional blinding of the animal, and (. . . . .) after unilateral labyrinthine lesion combined with transection of the spinal cord (After KOLB, 1955)

Rabbits. Observations on rabbits with unilateral labyrinthine lesions have been reported by BECHTEREW (1883), BORNHARDT (1876), EWALD (1892), and WILSON and PIKE (1913); more detailed descriptions of compensatory processes were given by WINKLER (1907), MAGNUS (1922, 1924) and DE KLEYN (1914, 1925). Consequences of labyrinthectomy in rabbits are nystagmus with its fast phase directed towards the intact side, head turning towards the destroyed labyrinth, and rolling movements about the longitudinal body axis. EWALD (1892) emphasized that rolling movements after unilateral vestibular lesions are particularly marked in rabbits, compared with other animals like dogs and cats. Most of the symptoms of the lesion abate quickly and disappear after 1–2 days. The spontaneous nystagmus observed in all head positions immediately after the lesion is present later only when the animal is lying on the treated side. Complete disappearance of the spontaneous nystagmus in rabbits takes up to twelve months. In man even longer periods may be required, as will be described below. A permanent symptom of the vestibular defect is a deviation of the eyes: the eye on the treated side deviates forward and downward, and the eye on the intact side upward and to the rear. Torsion of head and trunk about the longitudinal body axis towards the treated side also persists: this was called "Grunddrehung" by MAGNUS (1924); it can best be observed when the animal is in a position with the head hanging downwards. Another permanent consequence of the unilateral lesion is a decreased tone in the extremities ipsilateral to the destroyed labyrinth. The experiments of MAGNUS (1922, 1924) revealed that the head turning due to the lesion induces neck reflexes which then indirectly cause most of the other postural abnormalities. In sitting positions the animals gradually compensated for the torsion about the longitudinal axis; this observation is consistent with KOLB'S (1955) findings in frogs. Optic postural reflexes do not significantly influence compensatory processes, and accordingly, the position of the head is more or less the same whether the eyes are open or closed.

LORENTE DE NÓ (1928) presented a summary of labyrinthine reflexes in the rabbit and recognized the importance of an intact reticular formation for the generation of the fast phase of nystagmus after unilateral labyrinthectomy. In 1957 DUENSING and SCHAEFER found neurons in this area of the brainstem which discharged synchronously with the fast nystagmus phase.

Guinea pigs. Detailed description of symptoms after unilateral labyrinthectomy and of compensatory processes in guinea pigs have been given by DREYFUSS (1900), MAGNUS (1922, 1924) and SCHAEFER and MEYER (1973). Immediate consequences of the lesion are vigorous ocular nystagmus, head nystagmus, turning of head and body towards the side of the destroyed labyrinth (Fig. 3), circular movements, and turning of head and body about the longitudinal body axis, which sometimes amounts to about 90° when the animal is in a hanging position; while the animal is sitting it is distinctly diminished. The turning of the head towards the injured side disappears within 2 to 5 days according to MAGNUS. The permanent symptoms that persist after compensation are deviation of the eyes, torsion of head and body about the longitudinal axis and a slight extension of the contralateral foreleg.

To study compensatory processes after unilateral labyrinthectomy under quantitative conditions SCHAEFER and MEYER (1973) destroyed one labyrinth in a large number of animals, by injecting chloroform into the middle ear. Shortly after induction of the lesion the ocular nystagmus had a frequency of 150–180 beats/min. This frequency declined to half within 3 to 4 hours, and the nystagmus disappeared after about 9 hours. The frequency plot of the decrease ran linearly on a semilogarithmic scale. The speed of compensation was again independent of the animals' ages. But differences in compensation were found in light and darkness.

Three to four hours after the operation, head turning had asymptotically decreased to half its initial value, and it disappeared completely within 8–12 hours. The rate of compensation per hour was independent of the animals' ages, but

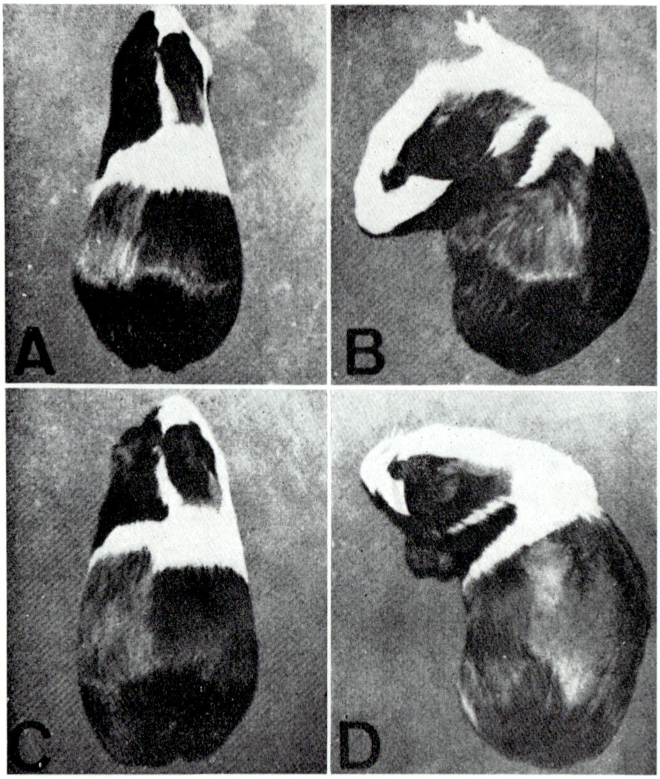

Fig. 3. Guinea pig after unilateral labyrinthine lesion and reappearence of compensated symptoms after transsection of the spinal cord. A = normal situation, B = 30 min, C = 55 days after destruction of the left labyrinth. D = hemisection of the spinal cord causes already compensated symptoms to reappear (After AZZENA, 1969)

owing to higher starting values, compensation took longer in older animals. In this connection it is of interest that labyrinthine lesions are more quickly compensated for by children than by adults in human subjects too (TEUBER, 1959).

Cats. Labyrinthectomized cats have been examined by KREIDL (1906) and CAMIS (1912, 1930), and in greater detail by MAGNUS (1924). In contrast to that in guinea pigs and rabbits, the eye deviation is slight and of short duration. In addition, the ocular nystagmus immediately resulting from the operation usually disappears after 24 hours, the animals learn to sit upright again within a few hours, and the head turning is diminished within 2 to 3 days. As soon as an animal in which compensation is incomplete touches the ground, its head is held in a normal position. This has also been observed in decerebrated cats, in which compensation is even accelerated. In cats the postural reflexes of head and body seem to account for the fast compensation of asymmetrical body postures.

In view of the previously described results on rabbits, it is remarkable that the disturbances of unilateral labyrinthine lesions in cats are essentially milder if the tonic neck reflexes are abolished by severance of the three upper cervical dorsal roots.

Dogs. Dogs with unilateral vestibular lesions have been examined by BECHTEREW (1883), EWALD (1892) and CAMIS (1912) after severance of the VIII nerve, and by MAGNUS and DE KLEYN (see MAGNUS, 1924) after labyrinthectomy. Although a little faster, the time course of compensation is quite similar to that in cats. Ocular nystagmus and turning of the head towards the injured side disappear after a few days. A tendency to run in circles is present shortly after the lesion and diminishes within 2 days. The ability to run is regained after about 4–6 days, and after 14 days the animals have completely recovered the ability to climb stairs and jump. A permanent consequence of unilateral vestibular lesion is torsion of head and body about the longitudinal axis when the animal is in a position with its head hanging downwards. This torsion usually increases during the first 2 days after the operation and then amounts to 20°–40° when the animals are standing. As in other species, the head turning about the longitudinal axis causes a difference in tone in the extremities, due to neck reflexes.

In dogs, postural reflexes of the body (somato-sensory and proprioceptive afferents) are involved in the compensatory processes, as in all animals, but in dogs optic postural reflexes also play an important role. In contrast to rabbits and guinea pigs, blindfolding may cause an already compensated asymmetrical head position to reappear.

Monkeys. Temporal eye deviation and nystagmus are also present in monkeys after labyrinthectomy (MAGNUS and DE KLEYN, see MAGNUS, 1924). The initial turning of the head towards the side of the lesion is relatively slight and is quickly compensated for by postural reflexes of the head, as well as by optic postural reflexes. Torsion of the head about the longitudinal axis can be observed when the animal is in a position with the head hanging downwards. This head torsion induces neck reflexes which cause asymmetries of muscular tone in the extremities. The postural reflexes of the body are quite strong in monkeys and take an effective part in the compensation process. Moreover, afferents from the hands seem to accelerate compensation after unilateral vestibular lesions in monkeys, and therefore the animals regain security in climbing very quickly.

NORTHINGTON and BARRERA (1934) emphasize that compensation is achieved more quickly in monkeys than in rabbits, cats and dogs (although not as fast as stated by MAGNUS, 1922, 1924). They also report that the duration of the vestibular after-nystagmus in both directions differs for about 1 month after the lesion and that even after 6 months a slightly asymmetric head posture was still observed.

The permanent symptoms of labyrinthectomy are relatively slight in higher mammals and may therefore be overcome more easily. According to MAGNUS (1922, 1924) the importance of the labyrinths in achieving postural control decreases with the increase of brain development. Correspondingly, the postural reflexes and somatosensory and proprioceptive afferents from the extremities increase in importance. Furthermore, optic posture reflexes take part in compensatory processes in higher mammals, especially cats, dogs, and monkeys (see FISCHER 1930); MAGNUS and DE KLEIJN, 1930). This development in phylogenesis can be followed up to Man. Nevertheless vestibular afferents are of such importance, even in Man, that abolition of them leads to insecurity in standing nystagmus and vertigo (KORNHUBER, 1966).

Further investigations. Several studies have concentrated exclusively on the nystagmus of animals and humans after unilateral labyrinthectomy. The results contributed to the discussion about whether or not Ewald's law is correct and, accordingly, whether rotatory stimulation towards the ipsilateral side is the optimal stimulus for the horizontal canals of each labyrinth (see: Laurens and Miles, 1927; Cawthorne, Fitzgerald and Hallpike, 1942; van Egmond, Groen and Jongkees, 1952; Niven and Graybiel, 1953, 1954). The directional preponderance of caloric and rotational nystagmus after unilateral labyrinthectomy was interpreted as supporting Ewald's hypothesis, but other authors considered this a consequence of the asymmetry of tonus due to the lesion. There was general agreement, however, on the observation that the directional preponderance disappears during the course of compensation (Ruttin compensation), or remains if compensatory processes do not progress (Ruttin, 1926; Escher, 1948; Meyer zum Gottesberge and Maurer, 1950).

III. Bilateral Labyrinthine Lesions

Bilateral labyrinthine lesions can be induced by eliminating both labyrinths simultaneously or by destroying one after the other, with varying time intervals in between.

After simultaneous removal of both labyrinths no asymmetrical symptoms are induced, as is to be expected. Postural reflexes are at first seriously impaired, but not completely abolished. The investigations of Ewald (1892) on pigeons, of Bechterew (1883) and Ewald (1892) in dogs, of Magnus (1922, 1924) on cats, dogs and monkeys and of Northington and Barrera (1934) and Dow (1938) on monkeys revealed that the loss of both labyrinths is also compensated to a large degree by other mechanisms, particularly by body postural reflexes and optic postural reflexes (see Fischer, 1930; Magnus and De Kleijn, 1930).

A quite different experimental situation arises if, after removal of the first labyrinth, the second one is destroyed during, or even after, compensation for the first lesion has been achieved. Under these circumstances the second lesion causes symptoms which are the mirror-image of those of the previous operation. This symptomatology, known as "Bechterew compensation", consists of head turning, body and head torsion about the longitudinal axis, and an eye deviation, all towards the side of the last-removed labyrinth. Furthermore, there is ocular nystagmus with its fast phase directed towards to the opposite side. The time needed for these symptoms to disappear, and also their severity, is dependent on the time interval between the two labyrinthine lesions.

Of particular interest is the fact that the second lesion also induces a torsion of head and body about the longitudinal axis; as already mentioned, this torsion is not completely compensated in animals with unilateral labyrinthine lesions and remains as a permanent consequence which can always be seen when these animals are in a position with the head hanging downwards. In view of the lack of compensation of this symptom, one might expect the second labyrinthine lesion to just eliminate the torsion caused by the first operation, but not to induce a torsion itself. Nevertheless, a torsion about the longitudinal axis towards the opposite side can be observed for some time; one probably has to interpret this as evidence for the existence of a "latent compensation" for the torsion of head and body about the longitudinal axis in animals with a unilateral vestibular lesion.

Few authors have systematically changed the interval between the removal of the first and the second labyrinth and carried out quantitative examinations on the Bechterew compensation. The knowledge gained by these studies has given some insight into what mechanisms achieve the consolidation of the new equilibrium after unilateral vestibular lesions.

Fish. Löwenstein (1932) and Schön (1950) subsequently removed both statoliths in fish. The second operation was performed after compensation of the asymmetry symptoms resulting from the first lesion had been attained. The compensation curve of the new asymmetric swimming position is more or less comparable to the compensation curve after the first statolith elimination, and approaches the zero value asymptotically. After a few days the strong visual component in postural control diminishes the oblique swimming position. Under diffuse overhead illumination, fish which are guided largely by vision show a less oblique swimming position than fish which have attained an identical degree of compensation but are less dependent on vision. The regained equilibrium is less stable than in terrestrial animals. Shaking, changes in illumination, or active turning movements may cause asymmetry symptoms to reappear.

Frogs. Thauer and Peters (1935) have reported experiments on Bechterew compensation with various intervals between the two lesions in amphibia. When the two operations were performed at least 5 minutes apart, early indications of compensation of the first lesion were found before the second was induced. An insight into the dynamics of compensatory mechanisms is provided by the quantitative examinations of Kolb (1955). As in fish, the turning tendency after the second lesion is about as distinct as that after the first operation; compensation after the second lesion, however, often takes place more slowly. According to Kolb (1955) this can be attributed to the cessation of "loaded" afferents from the second labyrinth.

Kolb (1955) discussed the influence of other sense organs in compensation after the vestibular lesions, and suggested that compensation-promoting actions seemed to be limited to the sense organs that contribute to spatial orientation. Von Holst (1950) differentiated between stimulus-dependent and self-generated excitations of receptors. This concept explains why compensation in frogs was found to be hardly influenced by darkness (removal of stimulus-dependent excitation), but can be delayed by cutting the animals' optic nerves (elimination of self-generated activity).

Rabbits. Bechterew compensation in rabbits was studied by Magnus (1924). An interval of 5 days between the two operations was found sufficient to cause Bechterew symptoms. Of all mammals so far examined, unilateral labyrinthectomy has the most pronounced immediate consequences in rabbits. This observation is also true for Bechterew compensation.

Guinea pigs. Schaefer and Meyer's (1973) experiments on Bechterew compensation in guinea pigs revealed that 3 days after the first lesion the asymmetry of tone in the vestibular system was not yet equalized. This was evident from the fact that the second operation induced only slight symptoms. With a time interval of 3 days between induction of the two lesions head deviation and body rotation did not show Bechterew symptoms. The eyes, however, showed Bechterew nystagmus even with this interval. This result may be evidence that eye nystagmus and head deviation are compensated at different rates. In animals in which the second labyrinth was destroyed 7 days after the first, eye nystagmus and body rotation were both directed towards the same side, i.e. the side of the second lesions. When the interval between the two vestibular lesions was increased from a few days to 6 weeks the symptoms of the second operation were more pronounced. Figure 4 shows the Bechterew compensation of ocular nystagmus when intervals of 7 days and 6 weeks have elapsed between induction of the first and of the second lesion; the nystagmus frequency is found to be higher, if the intervals between the operations are longer.

Cats. In cats (MAGNUS, 1922, 1924) extirpation of the second labyrinth 4 days after the first has the same effect as when both labyrinths are removed at the same time. When the interval between the operations is longer than 11 days distinct Bechterew nystagmus with its fast phase directed towards the side of the first operation results, but no asymmetrical head posture is observed. When an interval

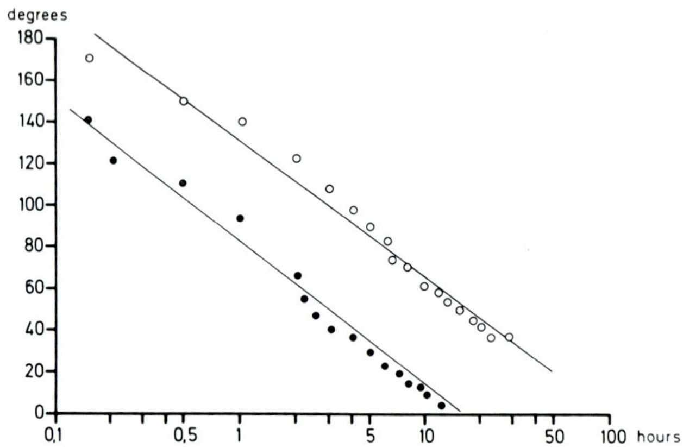

Fig. 4. Bechterew compensation of head deviation in guinea pigs. Intervals of 7 days (•–•) and 6 weeks (○—○) between induction of the two labyrinthine lesions. Angle of head deviation plotted against time after the second lesion. Mean values, n = 10 (After SCHAEFER and MEYER, 1973)

of 3 weeks elapses between the operations head deviation always occurs. This head deviation, and also torsion about the longitudinal axis, can be elicited with induction of the second lesion only 3 days after the first if the cerebrum has previously been removed. The importance of the cerebrum for compensation of vestibular lesions will be discussed below.

Monkeys. MAGNUS (1922, 1924) destroyed both labyrinths in monkeys with relatively long time intervals (22–38 days) between the operations and demonstrated Bechterew compensation in these animals; for a few days he saw an eye deviation in the horizontal plane towards the side ipsilateral to the second lesion, decreased muscle tone in the extremities of the same side and ocular nystagmus.

In the investigations on the effects of unilateral labyrinthectomy it became evident that compensation develops at different speeds in different species. In rabbits and guinea pigs the symptoms are of longer duration than in dogs or monkeys (MAGNUS, 1922, 1924). Consideration of the minimum time intervals in different species which have to elapse between two labyrinthine lesions in order to let compensation of the first lesion progress so far that the second lesion can elicit Bechterew nystagmus, reveals a mirror-like situation: according to MAGNUS (1922, 1924), the necessary intervals between the two operations becomes shorter as the animal's position on the phylogenetic scale rises.

Further investigations. An attempt to understand what mechanisms achieve compensation after unilateral vestibular lesions raises the question of whether or not the vestibular system alone can induce Bechterew symptoms. Several authors have attempted to solve this problem by ablation experiments. First of all MAGNUS (1922, 1924) emphazised that Bechterew compensation still occurs after removal of the cerebrum, after exclusion of optic influences and after section of the upper cervical dorsal roots. Apart from the fact that several CNS structures may influence compensation of vestibular lesions, even an intact medulla oblongata is sufficient for compensation to take place.

According to SPIEGEL and DÉMÉTRIADES (1925) Bechterew compensation is also present in cerebellar deficiency. Bechterew nystagmus due to a second labyrinthine lesion is not abolished by ablation of the cerebellum, extirpation of cerebrum and diencephalon, injury of the corpora quadrigemina or destruction of the vestibular nucleus on the side of the second operation. But existing Bechterew nystagmus can be eliminated by destruction of the vestibular nuclei on the side of the first operation. These experiments support the view that only an intact vestibular system on the side of the first lesion is necessary for the occurrence of the Bechterew symptoms.

The experimental evidence seems to suggest that the activity in a vestibular nucleus that has lost its afferents due to labyrinthectomy is "regenerated" and after some time counterbalances the activity of the opposite side again. In favor of this interpretation is the fact that unilateral lesions, in the vestibular nuclei cause nystagmus and head turning persisting for some time in previously labyrinthectomized animals (UEMURA and COHEN, 1972). Microrecordings from the vestibular nuclei have directly proved the regaining of activity in deafferented vestibular nuclei during the course of compensation (PRECHT, SHIMAZU and MARKHAM, 1966; MCCABE and RYU, 1969).

IV. Influence of the Cerebral Cortex

The cerebral cortex can influence vestibular, visual and postural functions, mainly via the reticular formation and the cerebellum. Although direct connections to the vestibular nuclei have not been conclusively proved (SZENTÁGOTHAI and RAJKOVITS, 1958; DI GIORGIO and MANNI, 1963) electrical stimulation of the cortex, especially in the region of so called nystagmogenic zones, leads to changes of the neural activity within the vestibular nuclei (ARSLAN and MOLINARI, 1965; AZZENA, GIRETTI and DERIU, 1967; MANNI and GIRETTI, 1968; GILDENBERG and HASSLER, 1971). The significance of cortical functions for the compensation of unilateral vestibular lesions has been investigated with cortical ablation experiments in which hemispherectomy was performed either before or after labyrinthectomy. The results obtained under these experimental conditions depend on the significance of the cerebral cortex in the species of animal on which the studies are performed.

Frogs. Unilateral forebrain extirpation in frogs causes no postural asymmetries (KOLB, 1955). In animals with completely removed forebrains, unilateral labyrinthectomy induces extreme postural abnormalities, which are compensated more slowly than in normal animals (Fig. 1). Combination of extirpation of one or both forebrain hemispheres with unilateral labyrinthectomy revealed that the most pronounced effects of forebrain lesions are obtained if the labyrinth ipsilateral to the removed forebrain hemisphere is destroyed. Ablation of the forebrain in frogs that have already completed compensation for a previous labyrinthectomy causes an oblique posture of about 20° to appear again.

According to the findings of KOLB (1955), the forebrain exerts an inhibiting effect on the vestibular tonus asymmetries after unilateral labyrinthine lesions and also seems to accelerate the compensatory process.

Guinea pigs. Detailed examination of effects of hemispherectomy on symptoms of labyrinthectomy have been performed by MENZIO (1949), GIRETTI (1971) and SCHAEFER and MEYER (1973). It was shown to be of importance whether hemispherectomy is performed before or after the labyrinthine lesion is inflicted.

GIRETTI (1971) and SCHAEFER and MEYER (1973) described the asymmetrical posture of head and body after unilateral lesions of frontal and parietal cortical areas. The postural abnormalities were found to be very similar to the symptoms resulting from removal of the contralateral labyrinth; compensation for the cortical lesions occurred within a few days. Ablation of one hemisphere following a bilateral labyrinthectomy caused strong head and ocular nystagmus. In this case, at first, deviation of the head into the direction ipsilateral to the missing hemisphere was observed, which changed to the opposite direction after about 3 days.

If one labyrinth is destroyed in an animal that has previously lost one hemisphere, the symptoms occurring after the vestibular lesion are dependent on whether the labyrinth ipsilateral or contralateral to the ablated hemisphere is destroyed. SCHAEFER and MEYER (1973) reported that the removal of the contralateral labyrinth leads to very strong asymmetry effects which are compensated very slowly. In contrast to this, compensation of the ocular nystagmus resulting from the vestibular lesion is only slightly affected by hemispherectomy. Extirpation of the labyrinth homolateral to the ablated hemisphere induces approximately the same effects as are obtained if no cortical lesion is present. But under these conditions Bechterew compensation is distinctly retarded when the second labyrinth (ipsilateral to the extirpated hemisphere) is destroyed after compensation for the first vestibular lesion is complete.

These findings underline the significance of the contralateral hemisphere for compensation of unilateral vestibular lesions; of particular interest is the observation, mentioned above, that the cortex seems to be less important for the compensation of the permanent ocular nystagmus than for the compensation of the asymmetrical head position.

DI GIORGIO (1939, 1950) and MENZIO (1949) carried out hemispherectomy in animals that had previously lost one labyrinth and had already compensated for the resulting symptoms. In these animals bilateral destruction of the cerebral cortex was found to cause partial reappearence of the symptoms observed after labyrinthectomy.

Cats. Immediately after hemispherectomy, an asymmetrical body posture towards the contralateral side and often circular movements into the same direction can be observed. 2–3 days after induction of the lesion the postural asymmetries and circular movements change direction. SCHALTENBRANDT and COBB

(1929) used the term "Umkehrphänomen" (reversal phenomenon) for this. Blindfolding these animals induces a situation similar to that present immediately after the operation.

Spiegel and Aronson (1934) examined the influence of cortical stimulation on vestibular nystagmus and on Bechterew nystagmus. Cortical stimulation in animals previously subjected to unilateral labyrinthectomy increases the already existing permanent nystagmus if the electrical stimulation is carried out on the hemisphere ipsilateral to the eliminated labyrinth; contralateral cortical stimulation diminishes the nystagmus. The observation that cortical stimulation in animals which have attained complete compensation after unilateral labyrinthectomy induces effects similar to those obtained in normal animals seems to be of importance. It can accordingly be assumed that the integration of cortical and vestibular impulses occurs normally in animals that have compensated for unilateral labyrinthine lesions.

Although no extensive investigations on the effects of hemispherectomy on compensatory processes after unilateral vestibular lesions in cats are available, the findings reported so far indicate close connections between the cortex and postural mechanisms. These connections are further demonstrated by cortical stimulation experiments (Spiegel and Teschler, 1929; Spiegel, 1934, 1966). According to the observations in animals that have lost only one hemisphere, vision can also be assumed to be of great importance for compensation of vestibular lesions in cats.

V. Influence of the Cerebellum

It is well known that phylogenetically the cerebellum has close connections with the vestibular apparatus. Vestibular fibers project to the so-called vestibulocerebellum, and the cerebellar Purkinje cells have direct inhibitory effects on the large neurons of Deiters' nucleus. After removal of the cerebellum the vestibular nystagmus is more violent and there is a long-lasting impairment of body-postural reflexes (Luciani, 1891; Magnus, 1924). It may therefore be assumed that removal of the cerebellum also disturbs the compensatory processes after unilateral labyrinthine lesions. Relevant investigations on pigeons, guinea pigs and cats have been reported.

Pigeons. Löwenberg (1873) and Spamer (1880) reported that labyrinthine reflexes are not dependent on the cerebellum. In 1891 Lange reported that if one labyrinth is removed in the chronic state after cerebellar extirpation the same kind of symptoms are observed as if labyrinthectomy is performed in an animal without cerebellar lesions. Nevertheless the symptoms develop more rapidly and are more pronounced in animals which have previously been deprived of their cerebellum.

Removal of the cerebellum in animals which are in the state of compensation after unilateral or bilateral labyrinthectomy does not lead to a reappearance of the typical labyrinthectomy symptoms such as may be observed after cerebral injury. Under these conditions only those symptoms occur which are also induced if only the cerebellum is extirpated; they are, however, distinctly more pronounced.

As early as 1891, LANGE rejected the hypothesis that the compensated symptoms of the previous vestibular lesion simply reappear after cerebellectomy. The symptoms resulting from removal of the cerebellum and the consequences of labyrinthectomy are different, and overlap only to some extent. However, cerebellum and labyrinths influence each other in the compensation of the consequences of deficits. No quantitative investigations of this aspect in pigeons have been published.

Guinea pigs. Cerebellectomy in guinea pigs results in a marked disturbance of central nervous function, which lasts about 5 days. A delayed compensation of labyrinthectomy symptoms during this period may therefore be caused primarily by unspecific trauma effects (SCHAEFER and MEYER, 1973). The same was suggested by BATINI et al. (1956, 1957) on the basis of their work on cats. Judging by the animals' general condition the trauma is probably overcome approximately 2 weeks after cerebellectomy. According to SCHAEFER and MEYER (1973) it takes 14 days for the body-postural reflexes to become manifest again after ablation of the cerebellum. Consequently it is to be expected that the time at which labyrinthectomy is carrried out in relation to the previous cerebellar lesion needs to be taken into consideration in the interpretation of these experiments.

SCHAEFER and MEYER (1973) described the compensation of unilateral labyrinthine lesions in cerebellectomized guinea pigs and reported a different effect of the cerebellar lesion on the compensation of ocular nystagmus and head turning. Compensation of ocular nystagmus was retarted only if the vestibular lesion was performed during the first 5 days after cerebellectomy. This delay is probably a consequence of general trauma. Compensation of the asymmetrical head position was found to be perceptibly slower in animals with no cerebellum, even if the labyrinth was destroyed as long as 9 months after the ablation of the cerebellum. It must therefore be assumed that compensation of the head deviation resulting from unilateral labyrinthectomy is mediated by the cerebellum. The extent of the involvement of cerebrum and spinal cord in these phenomena is of interest. As shown above, the cerebral influence in compensation of vestibular lesions obviously takes place via the cerebellum. The elicitation of cerebral release phenomena by cooling of the cerebellum (GIRETTI, 1971) also suggests close interactions of cerebellum and cerebrum in compensatory processes.

Cats. Several authors have described cerebellar ablation experiments which clarify the functional connections between the cerebellum and the vestibular nuclei and postural mechanisms in general (MAGNUS, 1924; BATINI et al., 1957; BATINI and POMPEIANO, 1957; SPRAGUE and CHAMBERS, 1959). According to SPRAGUE and CHAMBERS (1959) extirpation of the cerebellum in cats causes pronounced opisthotonus with extensor rigidity of the legs, absence of "placing reactions," and other symptoms. The symptoms abate quite rapidly, and within 2 weeks a steady state with hypokinesia, disturbances during standing and walking, and impaired coordination of the legs is reached. Several authors have shown that this symptomatology can also be obtained after bilateral lesions of the roof nuclei (LINDSLEY et al., 1949; CHAMBERS and SPRAGUE, 1951, 1952; BATINI et al., 1956, 1957; BATINI and POMPEIANO, 1957). These effects are probably a consequence of the loss of inhibitory influences to several brainstem centers. These influences interact with inhibitory afferents from the spinal cord which can be demonstrated after postbrachial spinal transection. Such spinal cord lesions cause an increase of forelimb reflex activity (Schiff-Sherrington phenomenon). It can be assumed that both cerebellar and Schiff-Sherrington inhibition influence the mechanisms compensating vestibular defects.

Carpenter et al. (1959) have eliminated the labyrinths and the fastigial nuclei and reported a summation of both defect symptoms, for which compensation is very much retarded. These authors also observed that when compensation of labyrinthectomy symptoms has already been attained it can be abolished by lesions in the fastigial nuclei.

McCabe and Ryu (1969) recorded from the medial vestibular nuclei of cats after unilateral labyrinthectomy and found an almost complete loss of resting activity in the nuclei of both sides during the first days after the lesion. In experiments during which recordings were taken after extirpation of the cerebellum, it was found that only the activity in the medial vestibular nucleus ipsilateral to the labyrinthine lesion was decreased. These results were interpreted as evidence for a cerebellar "shutdown" of the activity of the "intact" nucleus which may help to decrease the asymmetries of tonus after unilateral labyrinthine lesions until compensation has taken place. During the course of compensation the activity in both vestibular nuclei increases and finally normal values are reached (Precht et al., 1966; McCabe and Ryu, 1969).

VI. Influences of the Spinal Cord and Somato-Sensory Afferents

Vestibular impulses which reach the spinal cord ipsilaterally via the tractus vestibulo-spinalis and via the contralateral reticular formation exert distinct influences on gamma-motoneurons. Commands from the vestibular organs are fed through these pathways into the gamma-spindle loops, during postural reflexes as well as in the resting position. Recordings from single dorsal root filaments during changes of the head position have proved the existence of interactions of vestibular organs, neck proprioception, and spinal cord mechanisms. In view of the close association between the vestibular organs and the motor system, it is understandable that unilateral labyrinthectomy causes postural asymmetries of the trunk and the extremities. Conversely, damage of the spinal cord or changes of somato-sensory afferents exert influences on vestibular functions and have a marked effect on the compensation of lesions in the vestibular system.

Goltz reported in 1870 that some symptoms of labyrinthectomy in pigeons disappear when the birds are being handled. Similar observations were made by Bechterew (1883) in dogs and by Dal Ri and Schaefer (1956, 1957) in guinea pigs. In order to study the spinal influence on compensatory processes after vestibular lesions, several authors have combined labyrinthectomy and dissection of the spinal cord; some of these investigations will be mentioned briefly.

Pigeons. During investigations on patterns of movement in pigeons after dissection of dorsal roots, experiments with additional labyrinthectomy were also carried out (Trendelenburg, 1906). Unilateral and bilateral labyrinthectomy following the section of dorsal roots from the wings did not increase or change the symptoms already caused by the spinal cord lesion. Additional blindfolding had no obvious influence on the animals' behavior. However, labyrinthectomy after section of the dorsal roots of the leg segments resulted in intense disturbances. Unilateral labyrinthectomy 2 to 3 weeks after dorsal root section caused a distinct impairment of the security of movements even during standing. The insecurity was especially noticeable when the animals changed direction while walking (see FISCHER, 1930).

Extirpation of both labyrinths combined with an additional dissection of the dorsal roots from the legs resulted in a long-lasting insecurity in standing and walking; it was several weeks before the birds could stand freely again. Thus under these conditions, recovery of the ability to stand seems to be independent of visual cues.

Frogs. In his search for the mechanisms that achieve adaptation of central tone after vestibular lesions, KOLB (1955) sectioned the lumbar plexus of frogs and also examined the consequences of combined and separate lesions of the dorsal and ventral spinal roots. Dissection of the VIII to X spinal nerves in *Rana esculenta* reduced the asymmetry of the body posture and accelerated the mechanisms compensating for the labyrinthectomy. Reduction of the abnormal body posture and faster compensation of the vestibular lesion were also found if only the ventral spinal roots had been cut. Section of the dorsal sensory roots accentuated the abnormal body posture and delayed compensation of the labyrinthine defect. These observations were only made on *Rana esculenta* and could not be reproduced on *Rana temporaria*; differences between water frogs and grass frogs have already been discussed above. After dissection of the lower segments of the spinal cord in a *Rana esculenta* with a unilateral labyrinthine lesion the oblique posture is also relatively moderate, and the time necessary for compensation is shortened from 6–8 months to about 4 weeks (Fig. 2). Under these experimental conditions grass frogs compensate for the vestibular defect somewhat faster. The asymmetrical position of the head in relation to the body can be completely eliminated if the spinal cord is cut at the cranial segments. Similar findings have been mentioned by THAUER and PETERS (1935).

These investigations demonstrate that the abnormal posture after labyrinthectomy is not only a consequence of a labyrinthine tonus difference, but according to KOLB (1955) is due to mechanisms normally coordinating the positions of head, trunk and extremities. Nowadays such findings can be explained by the neurophysiology of the spinal cord and of the relationship between the vestibular organs and the gamma- spindle loop.

Guinea pigs. The role of the spinal cord and somato-sensory afferents in mechanisms compensating for labyrinthine lesions has been extensively studied in guinea pigs. SCHAEFER and MEYER (1973) removed the animals' contact to the ground by suspending the animals in the air. Under these conditions compensation was delayed. If the animals were put down on the ground several hours after labyrinthectomy, head turning was observed to about the same degree as was normally present immediately after the labyrinthine injury; compensation proceeded at its normal rate from this moment. The normalization of the ocular nystagmus was only slightly delayed when the animals were suspended.

Similar results were obtained when unilateral labyrinthectomy was combined with transection of the spinal cord at Th 5. Compensation of the ocular nystagmus was only slightly affected under these conditions too, whereas compensation of the asymmetrical head position was distinctly delayed (SCHAEFER and MEYER, 1973); the delay is probably caused by the loss of spinocerebellar connections rather than by the lack of spinoreticular afferents. This interpretation fits well with the data obtained in the experiments with cerebellectomized animals described above; the spinoreticular tracts remaining intact after removal of the cerebellum were found to be insufficient to achieve compensation of the head deviation within the normal space of time.

Influences of the spinal cord can also de demonstrated in completely compensated animals. SCHAEFER and MEYER (1973) produced reappearance of the asymmetrical tone when the animals were lifted off the floor. AZZENA (1969) observed in guinea pigs that the symptoms of the previous unilateral labyrinthectomy reappeared 20–60 days after the vestibular lesion in some cases in which the spinal cord was dissected at Th 6 or Th 7 or deafferentation of the cord was subsequently performed (Fig. 3). Under these experimental conditions ocular nystagmus was also precipitated.

The studies provide evidence for the involvement of the spinal cord in compensatory processes after labyrinthine as well as after cerebral and cerebellar injury. As mentioned before, BATINI et al. (1956, 1957) considered the disappearance of the release syndrome after cerebellectomy as a compensatory mechanism achieved by Schiff-Sherrington inhibition of labyrinthine reflexes and forelimb extensor tonus. The evidence reported by AZZENA (1969) suggests that such an explanation could also be accepted for the phenomena induced by unilateral labyrinthectomy.

VII. Pharmacological Investigations

Since MAGNUS (1922, 1924) and his collaborators reported basic observations on how several specific poisons affect particular vestibular functions, intense work has been devoted to this important clinical field. MAGNUS' work revealed that the postural reflexes of both head and neck are less resistant to general anesthetics than rotatory ocular nystagmus. Drugs that may cause convulsions, such as strychnine, picrotoxin and caffein, lead in small doses to an increase of postural reflexes. When high doses are used paralysis of most of the labyrinthine reflexes is observed, while postural reflexes of the body remain intact. Accordingly, compensatory processes after unilateral labyrinthectomy were expected to be influenced differently by different drugs. So far it is mainly the acute effects of several drugs on symptoms resulting from vestibular lesions that have been the subject of pharmacological investigations (DAL RI and SCHAEFER, 1956). Apart from a recent study on guinea pigs (SCHAEFER and MEYER, 1973), however, the influence of drugs on the long-term compensation processes described has received little attention.

Drugs delaying compensation. Phenobarbital (50 mg/kg i.p.) administrated shortly after the destruction of one labyrinth resulted in a marked inhibition of the compensatory processes. Repeated administration of a sufficiently large dose of phenobarbital delayed the compensation by 3 days or more. Chlorpromazine, as well as other drugs which have a high sedative effect, slow down compensation in guinea pigs at doses which have little effect on vestibular functions. Neuroleptic drugs with good neuroleptic potencies combined with strong antipsychotic effects (e.g. butyryperazine, clopenthixol and perphenazine), exerted only a slight influence on compensation (SCHAEFER and MEYER, 1973).

The observation that already compensated symptoms of vestibular lesions may reappear during narcosis is of importance for the understanding of compensatory mechanisms (RUSSEL, 1894, 1895; SCHAEFER and MEYER, 1973). According to RUSSEL, the reappearance of head displacement and nystagmus confirms the view that after removal of part of one hemisphere, the cerebellum, or one labyrinth the nervous arrangements for certain functions are lost forever. The ideas developed by RUSSEL (1894, 1895) are in agreement with the earlier hypothesis of EWALD (1892) on the nature of the compensatory CNS mechanisms after unilateral labyrinthectomy. In other experiments, MAGNUS (1922, 1924), KOLB (1955) and SCHAEFER and MEYER (1973) have demonstrated that the loss of somato-sensory afferents after transection of the spinal cord or the loss of contact with the ground also causes the asymmetrical body posture to reappear.

Since alcohol affects postural reflexes in roughly the same manner as some of the narcotics previously mentioned, it might well be expected that alcohol also exerts comparable influences on compensatory processes. It can accordingly be assumed that compensation of vestibular and other brain lesions can be abolished by alcoholic beverages and that abnormal reactions can be caused by even small amounts of alcohol in patients with long-standing brain damage.

Drugs accelerating compensation. Metamphetamine, pentetrazole, strychnine, paraoxon (E 600) and Risatarun®, a glutama-containing substance, accelerate the compensation of unilateral labyrinthine lesions (SCHAEFER and WEHNER, 1966); the head deviation was found to be more strongly affected than the spontaneous ocular nystagmus.

Of particular interest is the influence of these drugs on the body rotation about the longitudinal axis; this symptom of vestibular lesions is not completely compensated by the CNS. The body rotation about the longitudinal axis was slightly affected by caffein and more strongly by strychnine and cardiazole. The body rotation was completely eliminated by E 600, a cholinesterase inhibitor, and could not be elicited again by lifting the animals off the ground; the compensatory effect of the drug diminished after 1 or 2 days. Risatarun®, which is known to accelerate anabolic processes, had a particularly pronounced and long-lasting effect; the body rotation did not reappear until 8 to 14 days after the repeated application of the drug had been discontinued.

SCHAEFER and MEYER (1973) assumed that these drugs have two basic effects. Firstly a nonspecific generalized arousal effect, accelerating compensation processes, and secondly a pharmacological activation of synapses and pathways. The drugs mentioned above which accelerate compensation are also known to influence other learning and adaptation processes (e.g. HUDSPATH, 1964).

Much attention has been directed towards RNA and proteins as a form of chemical information storage (see UNGAR, 1965; DOMAGK and ZIPPEL, 1970). The findings of HAMBURGER and HYDÉN (1949) in cytochemical investigations are of importance for the problems under discussion here. They revealed a change in nucleoproteins within the vestibular ganglions and Deiters' nucleus after a moderate angular acceleration treatment of the rabbit. The amount of these specific nucleic acids which are influenced by vestibular afferents can also be changed by anesthetics. Anesthetics can induce a specific protease that leads to a disintegration of such proteins (UNGAR, 1965). The fact that anesthetics and continuous vestibular stimulation both influence these proteins may provide some hints for the basis of long-term compensatory processes. In this context it is worth noting that the vestibular paralysis resulting from streptomycin therapy is interpreted as due to an inhibition of intracellular reproduction of nucleic acids (LEVIN, 1939; CHUSID and DE GUTIERRY-MAHONEY, 1946; WINSTON, 1948; FLOBERG et al., 1949; NORTHINGTON, 1950).

The pharmacological experiments described suggest that unspecific alerting or arousal effects, cytochemical changes, and an activation of synaptic pathways may be of importance for the processes of compensation after labyrinthectomy. This corresponds to CRAMPTON'S (1964) proposals for mechanisms responsible for habituation to repeated vestibular stimuli.

VIII. Labyrinthine Lesions in Humans

After partial or total functional loss of one vestibular nerve, recovery in Man runs through several stages characterized by spontaneous ocular nystagmus (see JUNG, 1953; FRENZEL, 1955; JUNG and KORNHUBER, 1964; STENGER, 1965; KORNHUBER, 1966). Often the initial symptoms of inflammation, vascular lesions or other diseases of the peripheral vestibular apparatus are either permanent spontaneous horizontal nystagmus or combined horizontal and rotatory nystagmus directed towards the damaged side; because of its direction this nystagmus is interpreted as due to an irritation of a still-functioning vestibular nerve. With the progression of the disease the irritated labyrinth may be even further damaged and lose its function. This results in a change of the direction of the spontaneous nystagmus (STENGER, 1965). The stage of functional loss is characterized by nystagmus towards the intact side, an increase of the threshold of the damaged labyrinth to caloric stimulation and continous dizziness. The severity of the clinical symptoms is directly proportional to the rapidity with which the functional loss occurs.

A sudden loss of one vestibular apparatus is often due to particular types of skull fractures. A rapid onset of the "irritation" and the "loss syndrome" can be found with attacks of Ménière's disease. Ipsilateral nystagmus is frequently observed during the initial phase of the attack, resembling irritation of the peripheral vestibular apparatus. This may then be succeeded by contralateral spontaneous nystagmus at the end of the attack, a result of functional loss.

As shown in animal experiments, a loss of one peripheral vestibular apparatus immediately brings central compensation mechanisms into action, which cause the permanent nystagmus and several other symptoms to diminish within less than about 7 days. Similar mechanisms compensating for unilateral vestibular lesions also exist in Man. The directional preponderance of rotational nystagmus after unilateral labyrinthine lesion also diminishes after some time due to the equalization of tonus asymmetries in the CNS (RUTTIN, 1926; CAWTHORNE et al., 1942; VAN EGMOND et al., 1952; NIVEN and GRAYBIEL, 1953–1954; MEYER ZUM GOTTESBERGE et al., 1950). Nevertheless, careful clinical examination with Frenzel glasses often still reveals positional nystagmus weeks or even months after the injury. Nystagmography has revealed that slight spontaneous nystagmus can still be present years after labyrinthine lesions (FRENZEL, 1955; LANGE and KORNHUBER, 1962).

Caloric testing of these patients shows that excitability is decreased or totally absent on the damaged side; it is remarkable that an increased threshold for the elicitation of nystagmus on the intact side is frequently noted in addition. According to MITTERMAIER (1950), this indicates that the vestibular centers on the undamaged side are now operating at a lower level of excitation in order to give some relief from the attack symptoms. This hypothesis has gained particular interest since McCABE and RYU (1969) found direct experimental evidence for it by recording from cats' vestibular nuclei after unilateral labyrinthectomy. After extirpation of one labyrinth only, McCABE and RYU (1969) found a lack of resting activity in virtually all neurons of both the ipsilateral and the contralateral medial vestibular nuclei. As mentioned above, the authors showed that the cerebellum imposes a "shutdown" of the intact side, to rebalance the asymmetry at a lower level.

Bechterew nystagmus, with its classic symptoms, has rarely been seen in humans (JUNG and KORNHUBER, 1964), since few patients lose one labyrinth and subsequently also the second. Nevertheless a change in the direction of nystagmus during vestibular disorders is described by several authors (BÁRÁNY, 1907;

Uffenorde, 1924; Vogel, 1932, 1955). Vogel (1932, 1955) considers this phenomenon to be a central event due to changes of tonus asymmetries in the vestibular system, and therefore uses the term "Bechterew-Nystagmus." This definition is weak, since the second labyrinth is not destroyed in these cases as it is in Bechterew's classic experiments. The change in the direction of nystagmus is induced when a damaged labyrinth recovers and its regained activity disturbs the equilibrium already accomplished by compensatory mechanisms (Stenger, 1959). Stenger therefore calls this nystagmus "Erholungsnystagmus" (recovery nystagmus) rather than Bechterew nystagmus.

As in animals, the nystagmus resulting from lesions in different brain regions in Man disappears after some time due to the development of compensatory mechanisms (Jung and Kornhuber, 1964). Bulbar lesions in Man (Wallenberg's syndrome, syringobulbia etc.) cause either horizontal or rotatory nystagmus, which is partially compensated within some weeks or months. Vascular lesions in the thalamus or the cerebral hemispheres may not cause permanent nystagmus but do induce a directional preponderance of the vestibular nystagmus and disturbances of the optokinetic nystagmus. The directional preponderance decreases and the optokinetic nystagmus improves with a characteristic time course (Lange and Kornhuber, 1962). Vertical optokinetic nystagmus in particular may be diminished after tegmental lesions ("lamina quadrigemina syndrome"); compensation also occurs in these patients after some time. Duensing, Schaefer and Trevisan (1963) found neurons in these brainstem structures, which responded with vertical and rotational nystagmus.

References

Adrian, E.D.: Discharges from vestibular receptors in the cat. J. Physiol. (Lond.) **101**, 389–407 (1943).

Arslan, M., Molinari, G.A.: Modifications of the activity of the vestibular nuclei in the cat, following stimulation of the temporal lobe. Acta oto-laryng. (Stockh.) **59**, 338–344 (1965).

Azzena, G.B.: Role of the spinal cord in compensating the effects of hemilabyrinthectomy. Arch. ital. Biol. **107**, 43–53 (1969).

Azzena, G.B., Giretti, M.L., Deriu, P.L.: Convergence of labyrinthine and cerebral nystagmogenic impulses on brainstem units. Exp. Neurol. **19**, 401–411 (1967).

Bárány, R.: Physiologie und Pathologie des Bogengangsapparates beim Menschen. Wien: Franz Deuticke 1907.

Batini, C., Pompeiano, O.: Chronic fastigial lesions and their compensation in the cat. Arch. ital. Biol. **95**, 147–165 (1957).

Batini, C., Moruzzi, G., Pompeiano, O.: The release phenomena following cerebellectomy. Proc. XX. int. physiol. Congress, Bruxelles, 70–71, 1956.

Batini, C., Moruzzi, G., Pompeiano, O.: Cerebellar release phenomena. Arch. ital. Biol. **95**, 71–95 (1957).

Bechterew, W. von: Ergebnisse der Durchschneidung des N. acusticus, nebst Erörterung der Bedeutung der semicirculären Canäle für das Körpergleichgewicht. Pflügers Arch. ges. Physiol. **30**, 312–347 (1883).

Bethe, A.: Die Lokomotion des Haifisches und ihre Beziehungen zu den einzelnen Gehirnteilen und zum Labyrinth. Pflügers Arch. ges. Physiol. **76**, 470–493 (1899).

Bornhardt, A.: Experimentelle Beiträge zur Physiologie der Bogengänge des Ohrlabyrinthes. Arch. Physiol. (Pflügers Archiv) **12**, 471–521 (1876).

Buddenbrock, W. v.: Körperhaltung und Körperstellung bei wirbellosen Tieren. In: Hb. norm. pathol. Physiol. Vol. 15,1, p. 88–96. Berlin: Springer 1930.

Camis, M.: Contributi alla fisiologia del labirinto. III. Effetti della labirintectomia nel cane particolarmente sulla innervazione vasomotoria. Folia Neurobiologica **6**, 138–165 (1912).

CAMIS, M.: The physiology of the vestibular apparatus, translated by R. S. CREED. New York: Oxford University Press 1930.

CARPENTER, M.B., FABREGA, H., GLINSMANN, W.: Physiological deficits occuring with lesions of labyrinth and fastigial nuclei. J. Neurophysiol. **22**, 222–234 (1959).

CAWTHORNE, T.E., FITZGERALD, G., HALLPIKE, C.S.: Studies in human vestibular function. II. Observations on the directional preponderance of caloric nystagmus (Nystagmusbereitschaft) resulting from unilateral labyrinthectomy. Brain **65**, 138–160 (1942).

CHAMBERS, W.W., SPRAGUE, J.M.: Differential effects of cerebellar anterior lobe cortex and fastigial nuclei on postural tonus in the cat. Science **114**, 324–325 (1951).

CHAMBERS, W.W., SPRAGUE, J.M.: Role of the cerebellum in regulation of decerebrate spasticity in the cat. Fed. Proc. **11**, 23–24 (1952).

CHUSID, J.G., GUTIÉRRY-MAHONEY, G.G. DE: The syndrom of bilateral vestibular paralysis. J. nerv. ment. Dis. **103**, 172–180 (1946).

CLARK, L.B.: Some factors involved in the reaction of insects to changes in luminous intensity. Shock reactions in *Dineutes assimilis*. J. exp. Zool. **58**, 31–41 (1931).

CRAMPTON, G.H.: Habituation of ocular nystagmus of vestibular origin. In: B. MORRIS, M. D. BENDER, Ed. The oculomotor system. New York, Evanston and London: Harper and Row 1964.

CYON, E.: Über die Funktion der halbzirkelförmigen Kanäle. Pflügers Arch. ges. Physiol. **8**, 306–340 (1874).

DAL RI, H., SCHAEFER, K.-P.: Pharmakologische Untersuchungen am artifiziellen Dauernystagmus des Meerschweinchens. Naunyn-Schmiedeberg's Arch. exp. Path. Pharmak. **234**, 79–90 (1956).

DAL RI, H., SCHAEFER, K.-P.: Beeinflussung des Nystagmus durch Stell- und Haltereflexe am nichtfixierten Meerschweinchen. Pflügers Arch. ges. Physiol. **265**, 125–137 (1957).

DI GIORGIO, A.M.: Effetti di lesioni unilaterali della corteccia cerebrale sui fenomeni di compenso da hemislabirintazione. Atti Acc. fisiol. Fac. Med. Siena, Ser. XI **2**, 382–384 (1939).

DI GIORGIO, A.M.: Comportamento della reazioni oculari labirintiche nelle lesioni di una metá laterale del cerveletto. Boll. Soc. ital. Biol. sper. **26**, 31–32 (1950).

DI GIORGIO, A.M., MANNI, E.: Anatomical and functional relationships of the cerebral nystagmogenic area to some subcortical centers. Arch. ital. Biol. **101**, 48–58 (1963).

DOLLEY, W.L.: Reactions to light in Vanessa antiopa, with special reference to circus movements. J. exp. Zool. **20**, 357–420 (1916).

DOMAGK, G.F., ZIPPEL, H.P.: Biochemie der Gedächtnisspeicherung. Naturwissenschaften **57**, 152–162 (1970).

DOW, R.S.: The effects of unilateral and bilateral labyrinthectomy in monkey, baboon and chimpanzee. Amer. J. Physiol. **121**, 392–399 (1938).

DREYFUSS, R.: Experimenteller Beitrag zur Lehre in den nicht-akustischen Funktionen des Ohrlabyrinths. Pflügers Arch. ges. Physiol. **81**, 604–633 (1900).

DUENSING, F., SCHAEFER, K.-P.: Die Neuronenaktivität in der Formatio reticularis des Rhombencephalons beim vestibulären Nystagmus. Arch. Psychiat. Nervenkr. **196**, 265–290 (1957).

DUENSING, F., SCHAEFER, K.-P.: Die Aktivität einzelner Neurone im Bereich der Vestibulariskerne bei Horizontalbeschleunigung unter besonderer Berücksichtigung des vestibulären Nystagmus. Arch. Psychiat. Nervenkr. **198**, 225–252 (1958).

DUENSING, F., SCHAEFER, K.-P.: Die Aktivität einzelner Neurone der Formatio reticularis des nicht gefesselten Kaninchens bei Kopfwendung und vestibulären Reizen. Arch. Psychiat. Nervenkr. **201**, 97–122 (1960).

Duensing, F., Schaefer, K.-P., Trevisan, C.: Die Raddrehung vermittelnden Neurone in der zentralen Funktionsstruktur der Labyrinthstellreflexe auf Kopf und Augen. Arch. Psychiat. Nervenkr. **204**, 113–132 (1963).

Eckel, W.: Elektrophysiologische und histologische Untersuchungen im Vestibulariskerngebiet bei Drehreizen. Arch. Ohr.-, Nas.-, Kehlk.-Heilk. ver. Z. Hals-, Nas.-, u. Ohrenheilk. **164**, 487–513 (1954).

Egmond, A. A. van, Groen, J. J., Jongkees, L. B. W.: The function of the vestibular organ. Pract. oto-rhino-laryng. (Basel) **14**, Suppl. 2 (1952).

Escher, F.: Die otologische Beurteilung des Schädeltraumatikers. Pract. oto-rhino-laryng. (Basel) **10**, Suppl. 1. Basel, New York: Karger 1948.

Ewald, J. R.: Physiologische Untersuchungen über das Endorgan des N. Oktavus. Wiesbaden: Bergmann 1892.

Fischer, M. H.: Körperstellung und Körperhaltung bei Fischen, Amphibien, Reptilien und Vögeln. In: Hb. norm. pathol. Physiol. Vol. 15,1, p. 97–159. Berlin: Springer 1930.

Floberg, I. E., Hamburger, C. A., Hydén, H.: Inhibition of nucleic acid production in vestibular nerve cells by Streptomycin. Acta oto-laryng. (Stockh.) **75**, 36 (1949).

Flourens, M.: Recherches experimentales sur les propriétés et les fonctions du système nerveux dans les animaux vertébrés. Paris: Crevot 1824.

Fluur, E.: Vestibular compensation after labyrinthine destruction. Acta oto-laryng. (Stockh.) **52**, 367–375 (1960).

Frenzel, H.: Spontan- und Provokationsnystagmus als Krankheitssymptom. Berlin-Göttingen-Heidelberg: Springer 1955.

Gernandt, B. E., Thulin, C. A.: Vestibular connections of the brain stem. Amer. J. Physiol. **171**, 121–127 (1952).

Gildenberg, P. L., Hassler, R.: Influence of stimulation of the cerebral cortex on vestibular nuclei units in the cat. Exp. Brain Res. **14**, 77–94 (1971).

Giretti, M. L.: Spinal compensation of the cerebral release phenomena. Exp. Neurol. **30**, 459–466 (1971).

Goltz, F.: Über die physiologische Bedeutung der Bogengänge des Ohrlabyrinthes. Pflügers Arch. ges. Physiol. **3**, 172–193 (1870).

Groebbels, F.: Die Lage- und Bewegungsreflexe bei Vögeln. III. Mitteilung. Der Effekt der operativen Entfernung der Bogengänge und Ampullen auf die Lage- und Bewegungsreflexe der Haustaube. Pflügers Arch. ges. Physiol. **114**, 721–743 (1926).

Groebbels, F.: Die Lage- und Bewegungsreflexe bei Vögeln. IX. Die Wirkung von Kleinhirnläsionen und ihre anatomisch-physiologische Analyse. Arch. ges. Physiol. **221**, 15–40 (1928).

Gualtierotti, T., Alltucker, D. S.: Prolonged recording from single vestibular units in the frog during plane and space flight, its significance and technique. Aerospace Med. 513–517 (1967).

Güttich, A.: Neurologie des Ohrlabyrinthes. Leipzig: Thieme 1944.

Hamburger, C. A., Hydén, H.: Production of nucleoproteins in the vestibular ganglion. Acta oto-laryng. (Stockh.) **75**, 53–81 (1949).

Holst, E. von: Die Gleichgewichtssinne der Fische. Verh. dtsch. zool. Ges. **37**, 108–114 (1935).

Holst, E. von: Quantitative Untersuchungen über Umstimmungsvorgänge im Zentralnervensystem. Z. vergl. Physiol. **31**, 134–148 (1948).

Holst, E. von: Die Arbeitsweise des Statolithenapparates bei Fischen. Z. vergl. Physiol. **32**, 60–120 (1950).

HUDSPATH, W.J.: Strychnine. Its facilitating effects on the solution of a simple oddity problem by the rat. Science **145**, 1331–1333 (1964).

HUIZINGA, E.: Über die galvanische Vestibularisreaktion und über die Folgen der Extirpation des Scarpaschen Ganglions bei der Taube. Pflügers Arch. ges. Physiol. **226**, 709–722 (1931).

HUIZINGA, E.: Teilweise Entfernung der Pars superior labyrinthii bei der Taube. Pflügers Arch. ges. Physiol. **229**, 441–446 (1932).

JUNG, R.: Nystagmographie: Zur Physiologie und Pathologie des optisch-vestibulären Systems beim Menschen. In: Hb. inner. Med. Vol. V, p. 1325–1379. Berlin-Göttingen-Heidelberg: Springer 1953.

JUNG, R., KORNHUBER, H.H.: Results of electronystagmography in man: The value of optokinetic, vestibular and spontaneous nystagmus for neurologic diagnosis and research. In: M. B. BENDER, Ed. The oculomotor system, p. 423–482. New York: Harper and Row 1964.

DE KLEIJN, A.: Zur Analyse der Folgezustände einseitiger Labyrinthextirpation beim Frosch. Pflügers Arch. ges. Physiol. **159**, 218–223 (1914).

DE KLEIJN, A.: Die reziproke Innervation der Augenmuskeln des Kaninchens bei calorischer Reizung nach totaler Cerebellumextirpation. Acta oto-laryng. (Stockh.) **8**, 195–198 (1925).

KOLB, G.: Untersuchungen über zentrale Kompensation und Kompensationsbewegungen einseitig entstateter Frösche. Z. vergl. Physiol. **37**, 136–160 (1955).

KORNHUBER, H.H.: Physiologie und Klinik des zentralvestibulären Systems (Blick- und Stützmotorik). Hals-, Nasen-, Ohrenheilk. Vol. III, pt. 3, p. 2150–2351. Stuttgart: Georg Thieme 1966.

KREIDL, A.: Die Funktion des Vestibularapparates. Ergebn. Physiol. **5**, 572 (1906).

LANGE, B.: In wieweit sind die Symptome, welche nach Zerstörung des Kleinhirns beobachtet werden, auf Verletzungen des Acusticus zurückzuführen? Pflügers Arch. ges. Physiol. **50**, 612–625 (1891).

LANGE, G., KORNHUBER, H.H.: Zur Bedeutung peripher- und zentral-vestibulärer Störungen nach Kopftraumen. Arch. Ohr.-, Nas.-, u. Kehlk.-Heilk. **179**, 366–385 (1962).

LAURENS, H., MILES, A.: The effect of unilateral labyrinthectomy on rotational nystagmus. Amer. J. Physiol. **80**, 150–156 (1927).

LEE, F.S.: A study of the sense of equilibrium in fishes. I. J. Physiol. (Lond.) **15**, 311–348 (1894).

LEE, F.S.: A study of the sense of equilibrium in fishes. II. J. Physiol. (Lond.) **17**, 192–210 (1894–1895).

LEVIN, P.M.: The syndrome of vestibular paralysis in man. J. nerv. ment. Dis. **89**, 335 (1939).

LINDSLEY, D.B., SCHREINER, L.H., MAGOUN, H.W.: An electromyographic study of spasticity. J. Neurophysiol. **12**, 197–205 (1949).

LOEB, J.: Über den Antheil der Hörnerven an den nach Gehirnverletzungen auftretenden Zwangsbewegungen, Zwangslagen und assoziierten Stellungsänderungen der Bulbi und Extremitäten. Pflügers Arch. ges. Physiol. **50**, 66–83 (1891).

LORENTE DE NÓ, R.: Die Labyrinthreflexe auf die Augenmuskeln nach einseitiger Labyrinthextirpation nebst einer kurzen Angabe über den Nervenmechanismus der vestibulären Augenbewegungen. Berlin, Wien: Urban und Schwarzenberg 1928.

LÖWENBERG, D.: Über die nach Durchschneidung der Bogengänge des Ohrlabyrinths auftretenden Bewegungsstörungen. Arch. Augen- u. Ohrenheilk. **3**, 1–12 (1873).

LÖWENSTEIN, O.: Experimentelle Untersuchungen über den Gleichgewichtssinn der Elritze. Z. vergl. Physiol. **17**, 806–854 (1932).

LOWENSTEIN, O., SAND, A.: The activity of the horizontal semicircular canals of the dog fish. J. exp. Biol. **13**, 416–428 (1936).

Luciani, K.: Il cervelletto. Nuovi studi di fisiologia normale e patologica. Le Monnier: Firenze 1891.

Lüdtke, H.: Die Funktion waagerecht liegender Augenteile des Rückenschwimmers und ihr ganzheitliches Verhalten nach Teillackierung. Z. vergl. Physiol. **22**, 67–118 (1935).

Magnus, R.: Körper-Stellung und Labyrinthreflexe beim Affen. Arch. ges. Physiol. **193**, 396 (1922).

Magnus, R.: Körperstellung. Berlin: Springer 1924.

Magnus, R., De Kleijn, A.: Analyse der Folgezustände einseitiger Labyrinthexstirpation mit besonderer Berücksichtigung der Rolle der tonischen Halsreflexe. Pflügers Arch. ges. Physiol. **154**, 178–306 (1913).

Magnus, R., De Kleijn, A.: Körperstellung, Gleichgewicht und Bewegung bei Säugern. In: Hb. norm. pathol. Physiol. Vol. 15,1, p. 29–87. Berlin: Springer 1930.

Manni, E., Giretti, M.-L.: Vestibular units influenced by labyrinthine and cerebral nystagmogenic impulses. Exp. Neurol. **22**, 145–157 (1968).

McCabe, B.F., Ryu, J.H.: Experiments on vestibular compensation. Laryngoscope (St. Louis) **79**, 1728–1736 (1969).

McNally, W.J., Tait, J.: Ablation experiments on the labyrinth of the frog. Amer. J. Physiol. **75**, 155–179 (1925).

Menzio, P.: Rapporti fra la corteccia cerebrale ed i fenomeni di emislabirintazione. Arch. Fisiol. **49**, 97–104 (1949).

Meyer zum Gottesberg, A., Maurer, W.: Das Ewald'sche Gesetz. Z. Laryng. Rhinol. **29**, 532–540 (1950).

Mittelstaedt, H.: Physiologie des Gleichgewichtssinnes bei fliegenden Libellen. Z. vergl. Physiol. **32**, 422–463 (1950).

Mittermaier, R.: Über die Ausgleichsvorgänge im Vestibularapparat. Z. Laryng. Rhinol. **29**, 487–585 (1950).

Mowrer, O.H.: The electrical response of the vestibular nerve during adequate stimulation. Science **81**, 180–181 (1935).

Niven, J.I., Graybiel, A.: Directional sensitivity of semicircular canals following unilateral labyrinthectomy in man. J. appl. Physiol. **6**, 379–386 (1953–1954).

Northington, P.: Syndrome of bilateral vestibular paralysis and its occurence from streptomycine therapy. Arch. Otolaryng. **52**, 380–396 (1950).

Northington, P., Barrera, S.E.: Effects of unilateral and bilateral labyrinthectomy and intracranial section of eighth nerve. Arch. Neurol. Psychiat. (Chic.) **32**, 51–71 (1934).

Precht, W., Shimazu, H., Markham, C.H.: A mechanism of central compensation of vestibular function following hemilabyrinthectomy. J. Neurophysiol. **29**, 996–1010 (1966).

Russel, I.S.R.: An experimental investigation of eye-movements. J. Physiol. (Lond.) **17**, 1–26 (1894–1895).

Ruttin, E.: Funktionsprüfung des Vestibularapparates. In: A. Denker, O. Kahler, Eds. Handbuch der Hals-, Nasen- u. Ohrenheilk., p. 995. 1. Berlin: Springer, München: J. F. Bergmann 1926.

Schaefer, K.-P., Meyer, D.L.: Compensatory mechanisms following labyrinthine lesions in the guinea-pig. A simple model of learning. In: H. P. Zippel, Ed. Memory and transfer of information, p. 203–232. New York-London: Plenum Press 1973.

Schaefer, K.-P., Wehner, H.: Zur pharmakologischen Beeinflussung zentralnervöser Kompensationsvorgänge nach einseitiger Labyrinthausschaltung durch Krampfgifte und andere erregende Substanzen. Naunyn-Schmiedebergs Arch. Pharmak. exp. Path. **254**, 1–17 (1966).

SCHALTENBRAND, G., COBB, S.: Beobachtungen an halbseitigen Thalamuskatzen und Striatumkatzen sowie nach halbseitiger Extirpation des Frontal- und Occipitalpoles. Pflügers Arch. ges. Physiol. **222**, 589–612 (1929).

SCHÖN, L.: Quantitative Untersuchungen über die zentrale Kompensation nach einseitiger Utriculusausschaltung bei Fischen. Z. vergl. Physiol. **32**, 121–150 (1950).

SCHÖN, L.: Mikroableitungen einzelner zentraler Vestibularisneurone von Knochenfischen bei Statolithenreizen. Z. vergl. Physiol. **39**, 399–417 (1957).

SCHÖNE, H.: Die Regulation der Fehlbewegungen einseitig geblendeter Dysticuslarven. Z. Naturforsch. **5B**, 383–386 (1950).

SHIMAZU, H., PRECHT, W.: Tonic and kinetic responses of cat's vestibular neurons to horizontal angular acceleration. J. Neurophysiol. **28**, 991–1013 (1965).

SHIMAZU, H., PRECHT, W.: Inhibition of central vestibular neurons from the contralateral labyrinth and its mediating pathway. J. Neurophysiol. **29**, 467–492 (1966).

SPAMER, C.: Experimenteller und kritischer Beitrag zur Physiologie der halbkreisförmigen Kanäle. Pflügers Arch. ges. Physiol. **21**, 479–590 (1880).

SPIEGEL, E.A.: Labyrinth and cortex. The EEG of the cortex in stimulation of the labyrinth. Arch. Neurol. Psychiat. (Chic.) **31**, 469–482 (1934).

SPIEGEL, E.A.: Anatomy and physiology of the cortical projections of the labyrinth.In: Dizziness and vertigo. p. 25–38. New York: Grune and Stratton 1966.

SPIEGEL, E.A., ARONSON, L.: The interaction of cortical and labyrinthine impulses to ocular muscle movements. Amer. J. Physiol. **109**, 693–703 (1934).

SPIEGEL, E.A., DÉMÉTRIADES, T.D.: Die zentrale Kompensation des Labyrinthverlustes. Pflügers Arch. ges. Physiol. **210**, 215–222 (1925).

SPIEGEL, E.A., TESCHLER, L.: Experimentalstudien am Nervensystem. XII. Mitteilung. Über die Beziehung der Blickbahn zu den Vestibulariskernen. Pflügers Arch. ges. Physiol. **222**, 359–370 (1929).

SPRAGUE, J.M., CHAMBERS, W.W.: Regulation of posture in intact and decerebrate cat. I. Cerebellum, reticular formation, vestibular nuclei. J. Neurophysiol. **16**, 451–463 (1953).

SPRAGUE, J.M., CHAMBERS, W.W.: Control of posture by reticular formation and cerebellum in the intact, anesthetized and unanesthetized and in decerebrate cat. Amer. J. Physiol. **176**, 52–64 (1954).

SPRAGUE, J.M., CHAMBERS, W.W.: An analysis of cerebellar function in the cat, as revealed by its partial and complete destruction and its interaction with the cerebral cortex. Arch. ital. Biol. **97**, 68–88 (1959).

STENGER,H.H.: Erholungsnystagmus nach einseitigem Vestibularisausfall, ein dem Bechterew-Nystagmus verwandter Vorgang. Arch. Ohr.-, Nas.-, u. Kehlk.-Heilk. **175**, 545–549 (1959).

STENGER, H.H.: Schwindelanalyse, Untersuchung auf Spontan- und Provokationsnystagmus. In: Hals-, Nasen-, Ohrenheilk., Vol. III/1, p. 540–580. Stuttgart: Thieme 1965.

SZENTÁGOTHAI, J., RAJKOVITS, K.: Der Hirnnervenanteil der Pyramidenbahn und der prämotorische Apparat motorischer Hirnnervenkerne. Arch. Psychiat. Z. ges. Neurol. Psychiat. **197**, 335–354 (1958).

TEUBER, H.-L.: Perception. In: J. FIELD, H.W. MAGOUN, V.E. HALL, Eds. Handbook of Physiology, Sect. I. Neurophysiology III., 1965. Washington: Amer. Physiol. Soc. 1959.

THAUER, R., PETERS, G.: Der Einfluß operativer und pharmakologischer Eingriffe am Labyrinth auf Körperhaltung und Bewegung. Pflügers Arch. ges. Physiol. **235**, 316–329 (1935).

TRENDELENBURG, W.: Über die Bewegung der Vögel nach Durchschneidung hinterer Rückenmarkswurzeln. Arch. Physiol. **1906**, 1–126.

UEMURA, T., COHEN, B.: Vestibulo-ocular reflexes: Effects of vestibular nuclear lesions. Progr. Brain Res. **37**, 515–527 (1972).

Uffenorde, K.: Die chirurgischen Erkrankungen des inneren Ohres. In: Handb. der Chirurgie des Ohres, in: Katz-Blumenfeld II. pp. 178–365. Leipzig: Kabitsch 1924.

Ungar, G.: Inhibition of a brain protease by general anaesthetics. Nature (Lond.) **207**, 419–420 (1965).

Unterberger, S.: Vestibularisgrenzgebiet der Otiatrie und Neurologie. Fortschr. Neurol. Psychiat. **12**, 329–348 (1940).

Vogel, K.: Über den Nachweis des latenten Spontannystagmus. Z. Laryng. Rhinol. **22**, 202–207 (1932).

Vogel, K.: Über klinische Anhaltspunkte zur Unterscheidung von peripher und zentral bedingtem Nystagmus. Dtsch. med. J. **6**, 48–53 (1955).

Wilson, T.G., Pike, F.H.: The effects of stimulation and exstirpation of the labyrinth of the ear and their relation to the motor system. Phil. Trans. B. **203**, 127–160 (1913).

Winkler, C.: The central course of the nervus octavus and its influence on mobility. Verh. kon. Akad. v. Wetensch. Amsterdam, 2. Sectie, XIV/1 (1907).

Winston, J.: An experimental study of the toxic effects of streptomycin on the vestibular apparatus of the cat. Central nervous system. Ann. Otol. (St. Louis) **57**, 738–753 (1948).

G. General Interpretations

Chapter I.

A Systems Concept of the Vestibular Organs

By

R. Mayne, Tempe, Arizona (USA)

With 21 Figures

Contents

I. Introduction

This chapter examines the vestibular organs from a systems point of view in an attempt to describe their primary functions as well as the integrated operations of their essential elements. The examination is guided in large part by the analogy which is shown to exist between the vestibular system and the human-contrived inertial guidance system currently utilized in aerospace and submarine navigation. The operation of both systems can be shown to be based upon the same laws of physics, to embody analogous elements, to perform similar operations, and to provide analogous information.

A system has been defined as an assemblage of elements economically organized to perform of a given function or functions. A significant advance in the understanding of a biological system occurs when its elements can be shown to be so organized. The further investigation of the system can then proceed in a more purposive and effective manner. The Steinhausen model, for instance, was not only an important contribution in itself, but proved invaluable in subsequent investigations of the canals. Similarly it is hoped that whatever added precision the presently proposed model may bring to the integrated approach to the vestibular system will prove of value in future investigations.

It is an oversimplification to speak of the vestibular organs as organs of equilibrium. This description may apply to the primitive statocysts of lower organisms but it gives no indication of the greater range of functions of the vestibular organs or the extent of their vastly greater sophistication.

The simpler system provides data primarily related to the orientation of the organism relative to the vertical under static conditions, such as can be determined with a plumb bob, whereas various experiments reveal that the vestibular organs can provide information about the posture, orientation and displacement of the body during a complicated sequence of movements. It also provides the derivatives of these values for more effective body control. This information is updated at regular intervals by other sensory data, mainly those of vision, and is utilized to carry out preprogrammed acts of skill by the more advanced species of vertebrates. The flight of an airplane or of a spacecraft can be similarly programmed with the aid of inertial-guidance data analogous to those supplied by the vestibular organs. These data can also be corrected from time to time, for example by ground-based electronic navigation systems or radar.

Three distinct functions can be identified in both the inertial guidance and the vestibular organs. They are essential to the performance of the above functions, and include: angular movement-sensing elements, linear movement-sensing elements, and computational functions. In the case of the vestibular organs these elements correspond respectively with the semicircular canals, the otoliths and central processing. A description of the operation of the vestibular system must include the interplay of these three functions and cannot be restricted to the end organs in the inner ear.

One of the most important aspects of the operation of an inertial guidance system, as in the guidance of an airplane, is the independent measurement of the values of the components of gravity and acceleration acting on three orthogonal axes with respect to the plane. One set of measurements is required to determine the attitude of the airplane with respect to the vertical. The other set is needed to compute linear velocity and displacement. There must be no ambiguity between the two sets of measurements. Such requirements find a full parallel in the vestibular system but appear to have been generally overlooked in theories of vestibular function.

Mayne (1950) suggested that the vestibular organs operate basically as inertial systems. Barlow (1964–1966) proposed the same mode of operation for the long-range navigation of animals. Mayne (1966 A to D; 1969 A and B; 1970) developed various aspects of this theory.

The present chapter deals primarily with the uniform adaptation of the basic principles of inertial guidance to the vestibular organs of land animals. It is well known that variations of such an adaptation are found in lagfish, e.g. *Myxine* (LOWENSTEIN and THORNHILL, 1970).

An attempt is made to present the material from both a physical and a mathematical point of view. The non-mathematical reader may skip over the mathematical portion without losing the thread of the presentation. Those versed in mathematical techniques may wish to skip some of the verbal explanations.

It is hoped that the proposed systems concept, incomplete as it necessarily is, will provide a context within which much anatomical and experimental data can be integrated.

II. The Inertial Navigation System

A. General Description

Inertial navigation technology is a comparatively new development, its general practical application dating from since World War II. It has evolved into a highly specialized and sophisticated technology (e.g. DRAPER, 1960; MCLURE, 1960; BARLOW, 1964, 1966). The last two references are recommended as a lucid, more extensive treatment than the present one, suitable for the reader interested primarily in the application of inertial navigation principles to biology rather than in the technical details applicable to the physical system.

The basic principles of their operation, however, are simple. Complexity arises mainly because of the extreme accuracy which they must achieve, over long distances in the case of an airplane or a spacecraft, and over long periods of time in the case of a submerged submarine. In comparison, the biological system needs to be accurate only over short distances and time periods, at least insofar as normal body movements are concerned.

In a manner of speaking, an inertial navigation system consists of a system of speedometers and odometers such as is provided in an automobile, but geared to space instead of to the road. The instrumentation of the system is relatively simple.

B. Linear and Angular Accelerometer

All computations in an inertial guidance system must begin with a measurement of acceleration, both linear and angular. Velocity and position can then be computed from these measurements.

Newton's law to the effect that the force applied to a given mass is proportional to its acceleration is basic to the design of accelerometers. A linear accelerometer consists simply of a mass restricted to movement along a single axis against a spring. If the instrument is accelerated in any direction in space, a force proportional to the component of acceleration along the axis of freedom of the mass is exerted on the spring. The displacement of the mass may actuate an electrical transducer, the output of which would be a measure of this component.

In an angular accelerometer, the mass is symmetrical about a pivot and is constrained by the pivot to perform only rotary motions. Its rotation is again opposed by a spring. A small flywheel pivoted at the center and restrained by a torsional spring, with suitable "pick offs" to detect its displacement, constitutes an angular accelerometer.

It is convenient to describe the operation of an angular accelerometer in terms of the moment of inertia of the mass with respect to the pivot, and the resisting moment per unit angular displacement of the spring. The angular displacement of the mass can then be shown to be proportional to the component of angular acceleration about the pivot. A small amount of damping is usually included in linear and angular accelerometers.

C. Determination of Velocity and Position

Newton's laws of motion make it possible to determine the velocity and position of an object by simple operations based upon a knowledge of the history of its acceleration, initial velocity and position.

If the acceleration is constant it is enough to multiply the acceleration by the length of the period to obtain the change of velocity. An automobile traveling in a straight line with an acceleration of six miles per hour per second, will increase its speed by 60 miles per hour in 10 sec.

Similarly if the velocity is constant, it is enough to multiply the velocity by the length of the period to obtain the change of position. An automobile traveling at a constant speed of 60 miles per hour in a straight line will change its position by 300 miles in 5 hours. If the acceleration is not constant, an approximation of velocity can be obtained by a series of operations. Acceleration is measured at the beginning of small time intervals and multiplied by the length of the intervals, and the products are then added together. The further addition of the initial velocity at the beginning of the period would give the velocity at any time. Similarly, position with respect to a reference point can be obtained by the addition of three quantities: the initial distance to the reference point, the product of initial velocity by time, the sum of the products of velocity at the beginning of small time intervals and the length of the intervals. Exact measurements are theoretically possible with operations of this type if the time elements are short enough. These operations are known as integrations with respect to time, and can be expressed as follows in the notation of the integral calculus:

$$\ddot{x}_i(t) = c\,\varepsilon(t) \tag{1}$$

$$\dot{x}_i(t) = \dot{x}(0) + \int_0^t \ddot{x}(t)\,dt \tag{2}$$

$$x_i(t) = x(0) + \dot{x}(0)t + \int_0^t \int_0^t \ddot{x}(t)\,dt \tag{3}$$

where

$\ddot{x}_i(t)$ = acceleration input along X axis at time t
$\varepsilon\,(t)$ = elongation of accelerometer spring at time t
c = a constant of proportionality
$\dot{x}\,(0)$ = velocity along X axis at time $t = 0$
$\dot{x}_i(t)$ = velocity along X axis at time t
$x_i(t)$ = distance along X axis from a given reference point at time t
$x\,(0)$ = distance along X axis from the same reference point at time $t = 0$.

A similar set of equations could be written for angular acceleration, velocity and displacement. The operations represented in equations 1, 2 and 3 are easily instrumented in present-day technology.

D. Hypothetical Application of an Inertial System to an Automobile

For the purpose of illustrating the basic principles involved in inertial navigation, we may consider the hypothetical application of the system to an automobile. Instrumentation of equations 1, 2 and 3 would provide continous information about acceleration, velocity, and displacement of the automobile along the highway. Equation 1 would represent a simple linear accelerometer oriented along the long axis of the car and assumed to be horizontal, so as to be unaffected by gravity. It would provide information about linear acceleration along this axis. The instrumentation of equation 2 would include an integration of acceleration with respect to time and the addition of the initial velocity. It would then give continuous information about velocity along the highway. Equation 3 would represent, as indicated above, the computation and addition of the three quantities, as required for the determination of position.

The equipment would give information about the speed and the displacement with respect to the highway, assuming that the car always moves axially and does not skid in a curve. It would be unsuitable, however, for determination of the geographical bearings of the car in the general case of a nonrectilinear highway and, more particularly, for the programming of a specific path in a roadless territory along a circuitous course to avoid obstacles. These functions can only be performed if velocity and displacement are computed along earth rather than vehicle axes. This can be accomplished by mounting two linear accelerometers on a compass card, so that they will maintain north-south and east-west orientation. Displacements along these lines would provide the geographical bearings of the automobile at any time. Alternatively, a gyroscope could be used to maintain the proper orientation of the two accelerometers. Or again, the two accelerometers could be fixed to the automobile body. Their readings at any time could then be resolved into north-south and east-west components and integrated as before if the angle between the car axis and one of the geographical coordinates if known. This angle can be determined with a compass or gyroscope, or obtained by successive integrations of the readings of an angular accelerometer with its pivot oriented along the vertical.

One point needs to be emphasized, as it has a significant bearing on the later interpretation of otolith signals. The readings of the accelerometers must be resolved into their spatial components before they are integrated. If integrated first along vehicle axes they cannot subsequently be resolved into displacements along geographical axes.

A simple example will perhaps suffice to illustrate this point. Imagine that the automobile is traveling at constant angular speed ω along a circular course of radius R. The tangential accelerometer would read zero, the transverse accelerometer would measure a centripetal acceleration of ω^2R. The integration of the acceleration for n revolutions would cause the instrumentation to record a velocity of $2n\pi\omega$R toward the center. As a result of the second integration the instrumentation would register a transverse displacement of $2n^2\pi^2$R also toward the center. Actually the automobile would have returned to the same position after every full revolution, with zero transverse velocity. The correct measurement would have been effected if the centripetal acceleration had been resolved first into its geographical coordinates and then integrated around the circle. Its effect on velocity and displacement would have integrated to zero.

It will be seen that the angle of the vehicle with respect to a geographical axis is not only useful in the resolution of acceleration into orthogonal components, but also provides information about the orientation of the vehicle for directional steering and stabilization. This is of particular significance in an airplane or space vehicle or in the control of body movements.

E. The Three-Dimensional Case

The application of inertial navigation to an automobile is considerably simpler than its application to an airplane or spacecraft. The automobile moves only in two dimensions over the surface of the earth, so that only two accelerometers and processing schemes are needed to define its movements. Its attitude is determined by the four wheels, and the equipment does not have to be stabilized by a control system. The problem was arbitrarily simplified, also, by assuming that the accelerometers would remain horizontal so that their readings would be free of the effect of gravity. In the general case of the application of the system to an airplane or space craft, three linear and three angular accelerometers with associated computing elements are required to make necessary measurements in three dimensions.

But the greatest difficulty in the design and operation of inertial navigation arises because of the ambiguity between measurements of gravity and acceleration. Modern physics teaches us that the two phenomena are identical and must affect an accelerometer in precisely the same manner. The ambiguity, however, must be resolved if inertial navigation is to be at all feasible.

The values of the components of gravity acting on the vehicle must be determined without interference from acceleration in order to compute the direction of the vertical. The magnitude of the components of acceleration acting on the vehicle must be determined without interference from gravity in order to compute the velocity and displacement of the vehicle.

Most of the sophistication of inertial navigation is related to these problems. The biological system must resolve a similar dilemma.

Inertial navigation systems are divided into two classes, depending upon the manner in which the problem is resolved: the "stable-platform" and the "strapped-on" systems. In the stable-platform system, the accelerometers are mounted on a platform rigorously maintained in a horizontal position and orientation. Extremely accurate gyroscopes, capable of maintaining their orientation in inertial space with very little drift, are used to control the platform. As an airplane travels around the earth the platform must be precessed at the same angular rate to maintain its horizontal position. The rate is determined by dividing the linear velocity of the airplane, as computed in the system, by the radius of the earth. This "boot-strap" technique is called "Shuller tuning", and is the mathematical equivalent of tying the platform to a pendulum with a length equal to the radius of the earth. The system oscillates at the same frequency as such an hypothetical pendulum, with a period of 84 min. Other corrections of the system, e.g. for Coriolis acceleration, must be performed in a long-range navigation system but have little application to the short-term biological system. The oscillating halters of insects have some analogy with the stable-platform system (Barlow, 1966).

Because the sensors of the vestibule are rigidly attached to the head, it is more closely analogous to the strapped-on than to the stable-platform types of guidance systems. Computations are necessary in both the physical and the biological systems to separate the accelerometer signals into two sets of components related to acceleration and gravity and to resolve these components into space axes. It should be emphasized again that these operations must be performed first, before the acceleration measurements are integrated to obtain velocity and displacement with respect to space.

It would not be profitable to describe the operations performed in the physical system in any greater detail, as they are not fully analogous to those of the biological system. We should not approach biological functions with preconceived ideas based on the instrumentation of inertial guidance. We should, rather, become imbued with the relevant basic principles and relate them to available experimental and anatomical knowledge. There is a degree of flexibility in the instrumentation, but none in the basic principles.

F. The Basic Components of an Inertial System

Whatever the nature of the detailed instrumentation of the biological system may be, physical principles require that they include: a) angular sensors, b) linear sensors, c) data processing. A systems concept of vestibular functions should include a description of the integrated operation of these components.

III. The Contribution of the Vestibular System to Body Control

A vast literature is available on the responses of the body to various forms of disorientation and the effect of the destruction of parts or the whole of the vestibular apparatus. It is outside the scope of this chapter to attempt a review of the data. The gist of many studies is that labyrinthectomy performed on an animal causes severe postoperative disturbances, which become less severe as the animal apparently learns to substitute other sensors and possibly effects some central compensation for the destroyed vestibular organs. However the animal never seems to recover the full use of its former skills. These effects are well illustrated in a paper by Johnson et al. (1962) on the behavior of squirrel monkeys following labyrinthectomy.

It appears from these experiments that the vestibular organs provide an undetermined degree of refinement and precision in the control of body movements of a vertebrate but are not essential to its gross locomotion.

It may be well to cite here some evidence to the effect that the vestibular system also operates like an inertial system in the determination of the position of the body relative to the environment. The literature on this aspect is not extensive.

As we stand in a room, we can glance quickly at a given object some distance away, such as a doorknob, close our eyes, then walk across the room with eyes shut and come very close to touching the knob. We may well ask whether we perform this act by counting the number of our steps, or in response to vestibular signals.

In order to test these two possibilities, we placed subjects on a cart in a previous experiment (MAYNE, 1966a), and asked them to perform a similar task by giving verbal instructions to a person who pushed the cart as directed. The same approximate accuracy was achieved as in walking. These qualitative tests should be repeated with turns as well as straight-line movements, with both normal and labyrinthine-defective (L-D) subjects.

BERITOV (1957) performed a series of more extensive tests with animals, demonstrating the same capabilities of the vestibular organs. Blindfolded cats and dogs were placed in cages on a large table and moved from a starting point to feeding boxes along different paths, sometimes including right-angle turns. When brought back to the starting point and released from the cages, still blindfolded, the animals were able to retrace their steps, sometimes cutting corners to find the feeding boxes. Care was taken to eliminate odors as a means of guidance by applying petroleum to the table. Labyrinthectomized animals were unable to perform the task.

In order to perform as described, the animals must have constructed and retained a spatial representation of their passive movements, both linear and angular, without interference from the effect of gravity. Only this would make it possible to return to the feeding boxes when released from the cages. Since the animals could not perform this task following labyrinthectomy, only the vestibular organs could have supplied the necessary information by measurements and operations similar to those described earlier for the inertial system. Body movements in a somersault, a high dive, a game of basketball, or simply a walk from one room to another are probably monitored, in part, by the vestibular organs operating as an inertial system. Other evidence that the vestibular organs operate in this manner will be presented in the course of this chapter.

IV. The Semicircular Canals as Angular Sensors

A. General Description and History

The semicircular canals constitute the angular sensing elements of the vestibular system. There is a total of six canals, three on either side of the head. Each pair of canals is associated with one of the three mutually perpendicular axes of the head. The system of six canals is adapted, therefore, to respond to angular movement of the head about any of its axes.

A canal consists essentially of a small tube filled with a liquid, the endolymph, and wrapped around itself as in a doughnut except for its attachment to the utricle, as illustrated in Fig. 1. Its length covers approximately two-thirds of the circumference, and not half as its name would imply. An enlargement of the canal, the ampulla, accommodates an element functioning something like a water-tight spring door, the cupula, which is acted upon by the movement of the endolymph. The displacement of the cupula acts, in turn, upon the hair cells on the crista to generate the sensory signal. It will be shown later that the analogy between the

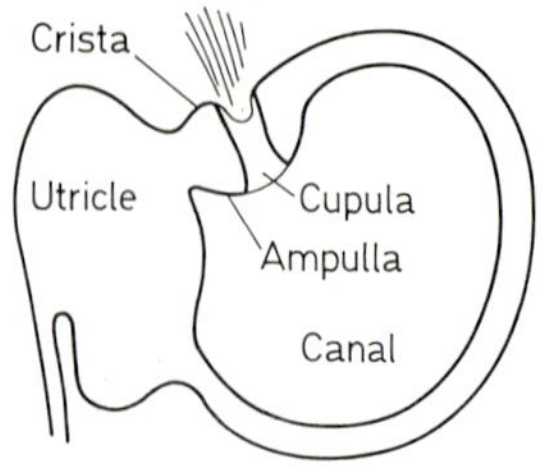

Fig. 1. Schematic representation of the semicircular canals (From Igaraski, 1960)

cupula and a "hinged" swinging door is only approximate, and its attachment to the crista is by no means a simple hinge.

Steinhausen (1931) was the first to propose an operational model of the canals. Schmaltz (1925) had proposed a similar model but the factor of elasticity of the cupula was not represented. Van Egmond et al. (1949) introduced mathematical techniques previously evolved for the torsional pendulum to the analysis of the canal response.

Both Steinhausen and Van Egmond showed that endolymph and cupula displacements are a measure of velocity rather than acceleration. Mayne (1950) computed the frequency response of the model, and showed that cupula displacement does indeed reflect velocity, but only within a given frequency range of input derived from head velocity. The computed frequency response predicted the error in phase and amplitude of the velocity measurements as a function of frequency.

An extensive literature demonstrates that the canal response is essentially related to the angular velocity of the head. Groen et al. (1952), recording from peripheral fibers in the ray, gave clear evidence that the responses were closely associated with the angular velocity of their preparations. Melvill Jones and Spells (1963) showed that the canals of various species are adapted to the frequency spectrum of their head movements through small but systematic alterations of their dimensions in the measurement of angular velocity of the head. Hixson and Niven (1961) and Young et al. (1966) computed the constants of the differential equation of the canal in experiments based on the Steinhausen model. Melvill Jones and Milsum (1965) showed that the canal signals are closely related to the velocity of the head in space within a given band of frequency, and are well adapted to monitor nystagmus of the eyes so as to cause a fixation of visual image on the retina during a head movement. Melvill Jones and Milsum (1971) and Melvill Jones (1971) reported on extensive recordings of canal-dependent units in the neural centers of the cat under sinusoidal rotational stimulation. They investigated primarily the range of frequencies below or slightly above ω_1, i.e. the lower normal range. They found that the response was generally in accord with that predicted by the Steinhausen model, and computed the values of ω_1 and ω_2 and of the elasticity of the cupula from their data. They showed that the signal available in neural centers is well adapted to monitor eye movements and body reflexes.

B. Operating Principle of the Steinhausen Model

The Steinhausen model is based on the following assumptions:

a) The canals encompass a full circle, b) cupular angular displacement is proportional to endolymph displacement with respect to the walls of the canal, c) the density of the cupula is equal to that of the endolymph, d) the friction of the cupula on the walls of the ampulla is negligible, e) the endolymph is considered as a solid mass moving as a whole against a viscous moment proportional to its velocity, f) the signal generated in the crista is proportional to the angular displacement of the endolymph. The analysis of the response of the model resolves itself into the derivation of the relation between input from angular motion of the head in space and endolymph displacement in the canals.

The qualitative operation of the canals can be visualized by simple physical considerations. If an angular acceleration is impressed on the head about an axis normal to the plane of a canal, say the horizontal canal, the endolymph within the canal will also be accelerated. The magnitude of its acceleration will be less than that of the head by an amount equal to the lagging acceleration with respect to the wall of the canals. This amount is negligible in normal head movements, and the acceleration of the endolymph with respect to space can be taken as equivalent to the acceleration of the head in space. Newton's laws interpreted for rotary motion state that the moment exerted on the endolymph is equal to the product of the moment of inertia and the angular acceleration. If the elasticity of the cupula is assumed to be negligible, as it is for normal head movements, the only appreciable moment acting on the endolymph to balance the inertial input moment must be due to viscosity. It follows from the above assumptions that the angular velocity of the endolymph with respect to the canal must be very nearly proportional to the angular acceleration of the head. SPEERS (1967) has shown, as indicated later, that these assumptions are not quite correct but that the basic operating principle of the canal is not impaired thereby.

The angular displacement must therefore be nearly proportional to an integration of acceleration with respect to time, or to velocity.

It will be seen that the semicircular canals differ from the angular accelerometer briefly described above in that the moment acting against the inertial moment is mainly viscous rather than elastic. The response to a given angular acceleration of the canal is a corresponding endolymph velocity, whereas it is a displacement in the case of a conventional accelerometer. The model assumes that the cells in the crista are responsive only to the displacement of the cupula and therefore of the endolymph. On the basis of these assumptions the measurement of acceleration is lost in the canals. It will be pointed out later, however, that this is not the case and that the canals are responsive to both acceleration and velocity. In terms of inertial guidance technology the Steinhausen model of the canals would be identified as an "integrating accelerometer" rather than an "overdamped pendulum." Overdamping is rather an anomaly in a pendulum, but a necessity in an integrating accelerometer.

Mathematical treatment is needed for a quantitative description of the performance of the canals and definition of the limits of their operating range.

C. Mathematical Treatment of the Steinhausen Model

1. Differential Equation of the Model

The response of the canals to different inputs of head movement can be determined by conventional mathematical techniques applicable to devices of this type that have inertia, viscosity, and elasticity. With reference to the preceding text and Fig. 1, the following equation can be written for any of the three canals:

$$I\,(\ddot{\theta}_i(t) - \ddot{\theta}_e(t)) = C\dot{\theta}_e(t) + K\theta_e(t) \tag{4}$$

and

$$\ddot{\theta}_i(t) = \ddot{\theta}_e(t) + \frac{C}{I}\,\dot{\theta}_e(t) + \frac{K}{I}\,\theta_e(t) \tag{5}$$

or

$$\ddot{\theta}_i(t) = \ddot{\theta}_e(t) + L\dot{\theta}_e(t) + P\theta_e(t) \tag{6}$$

where I = moment of inertia of endolymph

θ_i = component of angular displacement of the head with respect to a spatial axis normal to the plane of the canal.

C = moment of viscous force per unit angular velocity of endolymph with respect to the walls of the canals

K = moment of elastic restoring force per unit angular displacement of endolymph with respect to the walls of the canals

θ_e = angular displacement of the endolymph with respect to the walls of the canals

$$L = \frac{C}{I} \tag{7}$$

$$P = \frac{K}{I}\,. \tag{8}$$

We identify four important constants in terms of these parameters:

$$\omega_0 = \sqrt{P} \tag{9}$$

$$\tau_1 = \frac{L}{P} = \frac{C}{K} \quad \tau_2 = \frac{1}{L} \tag{10}$$

$$\varepsilon = \frac{L}{2\sqrt{P}} \tag{11}$$

where ω_0 = the natural undamped frequency of the system

τ_1 and τ_2 = the time constants of the system

ε = the damping factor of the system.

STEINHAUSEN (1931) was first to derive equation (6) and to understand its significance for the mode of operation of the canals as velocity transducers.

2. Laplace Transform Representation of the Model

Equation (6) can be written in terms of LaPlace transforms as follows:

$$s^2\theta_i(s) = s^2\theta_e(s) + Ls\theta_e(s) + P\theta_e(s) \tag{12}$$

The following transfer functions relating inputs of $\theta_i(s)$, $\dot{\theta}_i(s)$, and $\ddot{\theta}_i(s)$ to output $\theta_e(s)$ can be obtained from equation (12).

$$\frac{\theta_e(s)}{\theta_i(s)} = \frac{s^2}{s^2 + Ls + P} \tag{13}$$

$$\frac{\theta_e(s)}{\dot{\theta}_i(s)} = \frac{s}{s^2 + Ls + P} \tag{14}$$

$$\frac{\theta_e(s)}{\ddot{\theta}_i(s)} = \frac{1}{s^2 + Ls + P}\,. \tag{15}$$

3. Response to Sinusoidal Input of Velocity

The response of the canals as a function of $j\omega$ to an input of velocity can be expressed as follows:

$$\frac{\theta_e(j\omega)}{\dot{\theta}_i(j\omega)} = A_{\dot{\theta}_i}(\omega)e^{jB_{\dot{\theta}_i}(\omega)} \tag{16}$$

and

$$A_{\dot{\theta}_i}(\omega) = \frac{\omega}{[(P - \omega^2)^2 + L^2\omega^2]^{\frac{1}{2}}} \tag{17}$$

$$B_{\dot{\theta}_i}(\omega) = \frac{\pi}{2} - \tan^{-1}\frac{L\omega}{P - \omega^2} \tag{18}$$

where $A_{\dot{\theta}_i}(\omega)$ = amplitude ratio between θ_e and θ_i

$B_{\dot{\theta}_i}(\omega)$ = phase angle between θ_e and θ_i.

Equations (17) and (18) make it possible to compute the frequency response, or Bode plot, of the canals, as shown in Fig. 2 with assumed values for the constants.

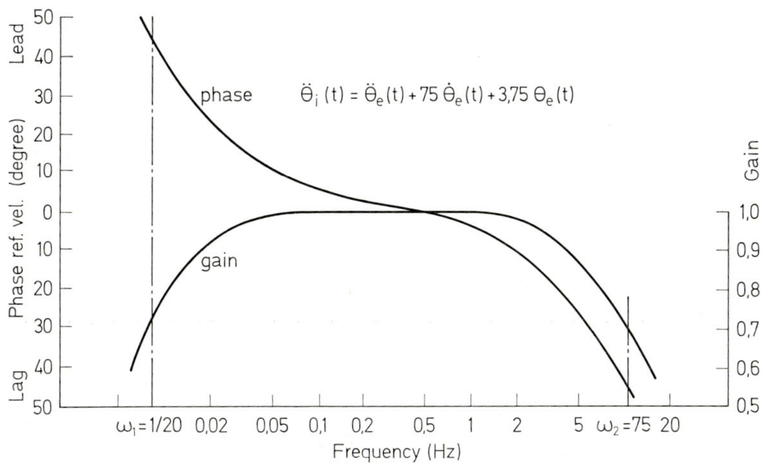

Fig. 2. Bode plot of canal response

The normal range of operation of the canals corresponds to the flat region of the curves. It is the region where ω^2 is approximately equal to P. From inspection of equations (17) and (18) it can be seen that for this region:

$$A_{\dot{\theta}_i}(\omega) \simeq \frac{1}{L} \tag{19}$$

$$\dot{\theta}_i(t) \simeq L\theta_e(t) \tag{20}$$

$$B_{\dot{\theta}_i}(\omega) \simeq 0. \tag{21}$$

Most head movements during normal body activity are in the range of frequencies where the canal response is flat, giving a nearly constant ratio between input and output and nearly zero phase shift.

4. Determination of the Long Time Constant τ_1 of the Model

The time constant $\frac{L}{P} \simeq \tau_1 = \frac{1}{\omega_1}$ has been evaluated by several methods with broad agreement between them. There is, however, no such agreement in the determination of the value of L and P as discussed later. If two step velocities, Ω_1 and Ω_2, are impressed on a subject and the time, T_1 and T_2, necessary for the effect (nystagmus or sensation) to die out is observed, we can write:

$$\Omega_t = \Omega_1 e^{-T_1/\tau_1}$$
$$\Omega_t = \Omega_2 e^{-T_2/\tau_1}$$

where Ω_t is assumed to be the threshold in the measurement of velocity by the canals. Equating of the right-hand sides of both equations and solving for τ_1 gives:

$$\tau_1 = \frac{T_1 - T_2}{\log \Omega_1 - \log \Omega_2}. \tag{22}$$

It will be shown later that the value of τ_1 derived in this manner does not represent that of the mechanical transducer alone, but also includes the effect of adaptation. The value of τ_1 determined from nystagmus is not the same as that determined from sensation (CAWTHORNE et al., 1956), indicating that the two phenomena cannot be explained by the same causal chain.

Variations of the above method, such as the determination of sensed displacement by subjects during postrotational experiments, are well-known. They have been described by GROEN and JONKEES (1948) and VAN EGMOND et al. (1949), and used by other experimenters, e.g. GUEDRY and CERAN (1959). They are, however, subject to the same error as the above method.

NIVEN et al. (1965), utilized the relation expressed in equation (18) to compute $\omega_1 = \frac{1}{\tau_1}$ by observation of the phase shifts of nystagmus with respect to two or more sinusoidal inputs of angular velocity at different frequencies. All these methods yield similar values for τ_1. They lie approximately between 8 and 15 for man, but, as indicated earlier, this value does not correspond to τ_1 for the mechanical end organ.

D. Modifications of the Steinhausen Model

Modifications proposed for the Steinhausen model will now be briefly reviewed.

1. Hydrodynamic Considerations

SCHMALTZ (1925, 1931) proposed a semicircular canal model similar to Steinhausen's but lacking the elasticity of the cupula. From application of the laws of laminar flow in small channels he derived the following expression for the value of $L = \omega_2$

$$L = \frac{A\mu}{r^2\varphi} \; 1/\text{sec} \tag{23}$$

where

μ = the coefficient of viscosity of the endolymph, 1×10^{-2} g/cm sec
φ = mass density of the endolymph, g/cm^3
r = internal radius of the canals, cm

STEER (1967) solved the Navier-Stokes equations for a step of acceleration input in a straight tube. Neglecting the effect of short time constants in the series, he obtained a value of $A = 5.8$. A similar value of $A = 6$ is obtained by assuming that the flow becomes instantaneously parabolic, with a resulting momentum 1.33 times that of uniform flow. The effect of the utricle may be approximated by assuming that it causes no viscous loss and no inertial moment output due to acceleration of the endolymph with respect to the walls of the canal but does create a pressure gradient during acceleration, leading to the following equation:

$$1.1\,\ddot{\theta}_i(t) = \ddot{\theta}_e(t) + L_1\dot{\theta}_e(t) + P_1\,\theta_e(t) \tag{24}$$

where $L_1 = \frac{L}{1.33} = \omega_2$ where L is as computed above in (23)

and $P_1 = 1.1P = \omega_0^2$.

STEER (1967) determined a value of 0.87 and RAUCH (1959) of 1.04 for the viscosity of human endolymph, the average of the two being 0.95. IGARASHI (1966) showed that the cross-section of the canal is elliptical with an average radius of 0.016 cm, yielding an approximate value of $\omega_2 = 220$. It appears from later considerations that equation (23) could overestimate ω_2 by a factor of two or three to 1. A different hydrodynamic system may have to be conceived in order to account for this large apparent discrepancy.

2. Experimental Determination of the Value of $L = \omega_2$

The above value of L is an order of magnitude greater than the values derived by a number of experimenters. VAN EGMOND et al. (1949) computed values of $L = 10$ and $P = 1$ for the horizontal canals of man. They based their calculations on a subjective estimate of the frequency of oscillation of the body when the phase shift between the sensation of maximum velocity is estimated by a subject to coincide with zero displacement of the swing. This would be the undamped natural frequency $\omega_0 = \sqrt{P}$ of the system. HIXSON and NIVEN (1961) obtained an average value of $L = 16$ for a number of subjects by objective measurements of the phase of nystagmus with respect to the oscillations of the body for two or more input frequencies. MAYNE (1965d) pointed out that these measurements were subject to serious errors as the phase shift is highly insensitive to the value of ω_2 in the frequency range in which these tests were performed. Nor can distal responses in the way of nystagmus or sensation be taken as representative of the response of the canal alone. It is rather the response of a system every component of which adds its own lag. The value of ω_2 computed from the responses of such a system could be only a fraction of that of any of its elements.

The value of ω_2 should preferably be determined from recordings taken at the periphery at a frequency significantly in excess of the natural frequency ω_0. FERNANDEZ and GOLDBERG (1971) did record from primary neurons of the semicircular canals of the squirrel monkey at a maximum frequency of 8 Hz, well above the probable value of ω_0. They concluded, however that this frequency was still not high enough to compute ω_2 from their data. It seems to this author that the difficulty in determining the value of ω_2 from the data arises mainly because the effect of a leading component in the response, cannot be distinguished from that of ω_2 at the higher frequencies.

The condition of a frequency of stimulation in excess of the natural frequency of the canals is more easily achieved in tests with fish than with mammal preparations because of the much lower frequency response of the canals of the fish (MELVILL JONES and SPELLS, 1963). GROEN et al. (1952) recorded from the primary neurons of the elasmobranch at a maximum frequency of 1.3 Hz and computed a value of $\omega_0 = 0.16$ Hz from their data. This value compares with the higher value of 1.2 Hz computed on the same basis for the squirrel monkey. These authors determined values of $\omega_1 = \frac{1}{35}$ rad/sec and $\omega_2 = 35$ rad/sec from the average observed phase shift of the responses. They measured the radius of the canal as 0.035 cm. If the value of $\mu = 1.20$ determined by KATE (1969) for the endolymph of the pike can be assumed to apply also to the elasmobranch, a value of $\omega_2 = 56$ can be computed from equation (23). This value is approximately the same as that determined experimentally. Unfortunately, it will be shown presently that even measurements performed under apparently ideal conditions may still be in error.

3. Adaptation

The word "adaptation" is generally used in vestibular theory to signify a reduction of sensory signals.

MALCOLM and MELVILL JONES (1969–1971) advanced an hypothesis intended to account for the adaptation of canal signals, as manifested by a reduction of the slow-phase velocity of nystagmus beyond that which can be accounted for in terms of the elasticity of the cupula. The hypothesis accounts for the secondary nystagmus which occurs after a step change of velocity (e.g. GRAYBIEL and BROWN, 1951), and is particularly pronounced after an extended period of constant acceleration (CRAMPTON, 1965). It was this phenomenon which led CAPPEL (1966) to suggest that the canals might be underdamped. The hypothesis proposed by MALCOLM and MELVILL JONES explains the overshooting of the canal signal in terms of a control function, rather than an underdamping of the canals. It assumes that the neural stimulus associated with a sensation of rotation or nystagmus is the difference between a signal proportional to cupula displacement and a shifting reference which tends exponentially toward the same value as the signal, so that the difference tends gradually toward zero. The effect, as pointed out by the authors, would not influence appreciably measurements of the velocity of the head in the normal range of frequencies of head movements, but would be noticeable during the long decay period of the response following a step change of velocity and during and following a period of constant acceleration. It would also affect the low-frequency response of the canals.

According to the hypothesis the signal would reduce to zero even with a constant cupula deflection such as may be caused by a constant acceleration. The interaction between the two effects of cupula elasticity and adaptation results in a very low-frequency, damped oscillation of the signal.

An analog computer simulation by the authors approximated very closely to the experimental data. An interesting result of the hypothesis is that the determination of the long time constant of the canals, as previously described, underestimates its value by 25 to 50%.

YOUNG and OMAN (1969) proposed a model of adaptation, corresponding essentially to the addition of a term of the form $\frac{M\theta_e(s)}{s}$ to the left member of equation (12). The technique of adding an integrative term in the control equation of a servo loop is frequently used in engineering to minimize the error. It is applicable, for instance, to the leveling of the floor of an elevator.

Both hypotheses are mathematically equivalent as pointed out by YOUNG and OMAN. If MALCOLM and MELVILL JONES' formulation is modified to include the effect of the short time constant which they neglect, they can both be expressed as follows:

$$\frac{\theta_e(s)}{\ddot{\theta}_i(s)} = \frac{k\,s}{(\tau_a s + 1)(\tau_1 s + 1)(\tau_2 s + 1)} \tag{25}$$

$K = \tau_a \cdot \tau_1 \cdot \tau_2$,
τ_a = the adaptation constant
τ_1 and τ_2 = the inverse of ω_1 and ω_2 as previously defined.

GOLDBERG and FERNANDEZ (I), FERNANDEZ and GOLDBERG (II), GOLDBERG and FERNANDEZ (III (1971)), recording from primary neurons in cats, demonstrated the presence of adaptation at the periphery. They showed that different cells vary greatly in their adaptive characteristics as defined by τ_a. GROEN et al. (1952) had previously reported a similar adaptation of primary neurons in the elasmobranch.

Another model of adaptation leading to the same mathematical expression is suggested later.

It must be noted that all experiments on adaptation appear to have been conducted in conditions where other sensory data would signify zero rotation of the body. It can be speculated that under other conditions which visual, otolithic, and somesthetic data would interpret as rotation of the body, the canal signal would tend to adapt to a value corresponding to a weighted average of all such data. Some evidence that such may be the case is presented later.

4. The Detection of Angular Acceleration by the Canals

The most significant challenge to the basic assumptions of the Steinhausen model came from the above series of papers by GOLDBERG and FERNANDEZ; FERNANDEZ and GOLDBERG II, and GOLDBERG and FERNANDEZ III (1971), which demonstrate that the response of the primary neurons of the canals of the squirrel monkey includes components related to the angular acceleration as well as to the velocity of the head. It follows that these neurons must be responsive to both the displacement and the velocity of the endolymph in the canals. This characteristic of the canals was also in evidence in early recordings from the primary neurons of the canals of the elasmobranch by GROEN et al. (1952), although the authors did not interpret it in this way.

4.1. Recordings from the Primary Neurons of the Squirrel Monkey

GOLDBERG and FERNANDEZ recorded from an extensive population of primary neurons from the canals of the squirrel monkey, with both constant acceleration and sinusoidal inputs. They showed that the two forms of stimulation are in accord, and demonstrate the presence of adaptation and of a leading component in the responses. They summarized their findings with the following transfer function:

$$H(S) = \frac{\tau_a S}{(1+\tau_a S)} \frac{1+\tau_L S}{(1+\tau_1 S)(1+\tau_2 S)} \tag{26}$$

where H(S) is referred to as an acceleration input,
τ_a = the adaptation constant,
τ_L = the leading component time constant,
τ_1 and τ_2 = the inverse of ω_1 and ω_2 as previously defined.

They found that the values of τ_a varied from cell to cell, from 30 sec to very large values when the cell is practically nonadapting. They found similarly that τ_L varied from cell to cell between 0.013 and 0.094 sec. τ_1 was determined from the low frequency response of non-adapting cells, τ_2 was determined from the hydrodynamic formula derived by STEER (1967) and dimensions of the canals by IGARASHI (1966). The average response of all cells was defined by the equation

$$H(S) = \frac{80s}{(1+80s)} \frac{1+.049s}{(1+5.7s)(1+.003s)}\,. \tag{27}$$

The average value of $\tau_a = 80$ corresponds approximately to that computed by MALCOLM and MELVILL JONES (1969) for man and the adaptation of nystagmus.

FERNANDEZ and GOLDBERG depicted the average canal response by means of a plot of equation (27) indicating the standard deviation for various points on the curve. This method of presentation gives a clear picture of the range of response variations as a function of frequency. It should not be interpreted, however, as signifying that the variations are artefacts caused by imperfection in the canal transducer, or that they result from experimental errors, as this method of presentation generally indicates. It may be helpful to visualize a canal transducer as an assemblage of distinct transducers sharing the same stimulating apparatus but coupled in different degrees to different modes of its motion. As indicated by the authors, the different responses can be visualized to serve distinct functions in the adaptation or optimization of the control of body movements.

4.2. Recordings from the Canals of Fish

The leading component of the response of the canals can only be demonstrated with relatively high-frequency stimulation such as was used by GOLDBERG and FERNANDEZ. It was not in evidence in the tests of MELVILL JONES and MILSUM (1971), who used a lower frequency. The recordings from the horizontal canals of the elasmobranch by GROEN et al. (1952) were also performed at a high frequency in relation to the probable value of ω_0. They also provide conclusive evidence of the presence of a leading component in the canal response.

The data are reproduced in Figs. 3 and 4, which indicates clearly that different cells exhibit different phase shifts with the same frequency of stimulation. The authors averaged the phase shift and computed values of $\omega_1 = \frac{1}{35}$ and $\omega_2 = 35$

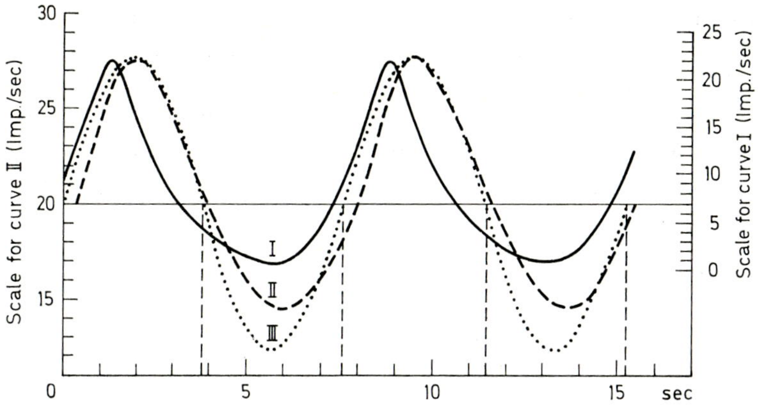

Fig. 3. Impulse frequency plotted against time, derived from two sensory units in the same preparation, recorded simultaneously during sinusoidal stimulation. I: distorted sine curve, leading phase $+24°$; II: less distorted sine curve, lagging phase $-13°$; III: pure sine curve for comparison, in phase $0°$. $T = 0.76$ sec, $\omega A = 18°/\text{sec}$. The turning points of the torsion swing are marked by broken vertical lines (From J.J. GROEN, O. LOWENSTEIN, A.J.H. YENDRIK: J. Physiol. (Lond.) **117**, 329–346 (1952))

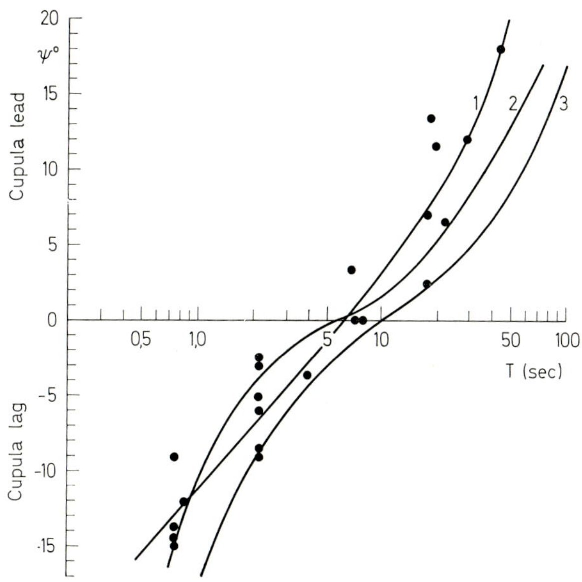

Fig. 4. Plot of phase shift of the response of a population of peripheral neurons in the horizontal canal of the elasmobranch v/s the period of a sinusoidal input of velocity (From GROEN, LOWENSTEIN and VENDRIK, 1952). Curve 1: average of responses by authors. Curve 2: Plot of response for $\omega_1 = 1/35$ and $\omega_2 = 35$. Curve 3: Plot of response for $\omega_1 = 1/50$ and $\omega_2 = 20$. See text for explanation

from the average. As indicated earlier, the latter value compares with 56 as computed from formula 23 with $\mu = 1.20$ and $r = 0.035$ cm.

The authors determined a value of $\tau_1 = \frac{1}{40}$ from the response of a single cell to a step change of angular velocity. This value, however, should be smaller because of adaptation. The value of $\frac{1}{50}$ was selected, although it would still be too high if the cell should exhibit average adaptation such as observed in man and monkey in the references quoted above.

A value of $\omega_2 = 20$ was selected to cause a plot of phase shift against frequency to pass through the points in the data with the greatest phase shift. This value would represent that of the canal proper if the cell responses corresponding to the points of greatest phase shift should contain no leading component. However, while GOLDBERG and FERNANDEZ found that some of the cells among the population they examined exhibited no adaptation, they apparently found none which did not contain a leading component. If the responses with the greatest lag in the fish data did contain a leading component, even one similar to the smallest one observed in the data on monkey, the value of $\omega_2 = 20$ obtained as indicated above would be grossly overestimated, by as much as one order of magnitude. This appears rather unlikely because of the wide discrepancy it would represent from the hydraulic determination of the constant and the difficulty of reconciling such a value with the data of Fernandez and Goldberg. In any case, the value of $\omega_2 = 20$ should not be overestimated and a lower value of perhaps 15 can be taken as more probable. It would appear on the basis of this data that equation (23) overestimates ω_2 by a factor of not less than 2 or 3 to 1.

GROEN et al. (1952) pinpointed the difference between the responses of different cells by recording simultaneously from two cells in the same preparation, one leading and the other lagging the velocity input. A cross-correlation was performed on the two cells with respect to a sinusoid in phase with velocity. The highly distorted leading response was found to correlate 96%, to have a high d.c. bias, a 10% second harmonic, and a small fourth harmonic component. It led the velocity by 28°, and therefore lagged acceleration by 62°. The other cell correlated nearly 100%, was quite free of harmonics, lagged velocity by 8° and acceleration by 98°. The stimulating frequency was 8.2 rad/sec and the value of τ_L was computed at 0.045 and 0.17 respectively for $\omega_2 = 15$, not too far out of line from the range of 0.013 to 0.094 found by FERNANDEZ and GOLDBERG for the squirrel monkey.

Returning to the value of ω_2 for man, estimated from hydraulic considerations at about 210, on the basis of the above discussion a more likely value would be about 75. At the same time, the value for ω_1 from MALCOLM and MELVILL JONES (1969) should be about 1/20. The Bode's plot of Fig. 2 was based on these values for ω_1 and ω_2.

5. Suggested Model of the Canals

There is a need for a model that is better able to reflect the complex response of the canals than the Steinhausen model. The model proposed in this paper was suggested primarily by a moving-picture film of cupula movement produced by

Dohlman in 1938 and kindly made available to the author. The film shows cupula movement in fish preparations. Professor Dohlman has pointed out that conclusions drawn from this film cannot be generalized to all species. We hope, however, that some of the principles evolved in a model based on this data can be adapted to other canal configurations. We shall first describe the modes of motion of the cupula revealed by this film.

5.1. The Modes of Motion of the Cupula

Figure 5a, traced from a frame in the film, shows an outline of the cupula following injection of ink into the canal. The pressure in the canal was successively raised and lowered, causing the cupula to move back and forth. The test showed that the cupula provides a watertight seal with the ampulla, as previously demonstrated by Steinhausen. A leak occurred, however, with extreme movements, presumably protecting the cupula from damage. Dohlman found that a pressure of 0.1 mm was sufficient to cause full deflection of the cupula. In Fig. 5b the center of the cupula was stained with india ink. It was again caused to move from side to side by raising and lowering the pressure in the canal. Figure 5b illustrates three positions of the cupula traced from the projections of different frames in the same sequence.

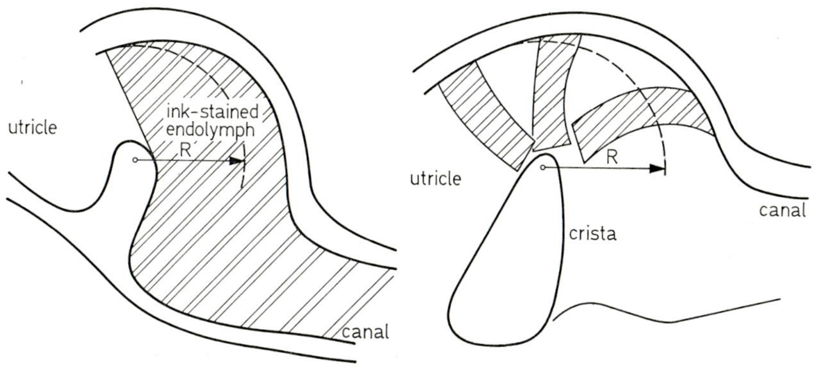

Fig. 5. Figures were traced from projections of single frames of film by Dohlman (1938). 5a: Injection of ink into the canal. 5b: Staining of the cupula. Note spiralling geometry of ampulla and unsymmetrical cupula movement. These features are associated in the proposed canal model with the Ewaldian nature of canal response

A number of observations can be made from the data.

a) Two modes of motion of the cupula are in evidence. The cupula bends as its tip slides with respect to the roof of the ampulla. At the same time its base slides with respect to the crista.

b) The roof of the ampulla is not concentric to the apex of the crista. This observation is corroborated by the lack of symmetry of the cupula movement.

c) When the cupula moves toward the enlarged channel, it tip moves through a greater angle than the base, indicating that there is little friction with the roof of the ampulla.

d) When the cupula moves toward the narrower channel the tip moves through a smaller angle than the base, indicating that the movement is opposed, in part, by friction with the roof.

e) Both the cupula and the subcupular region appear to be compressed for movement toward the narrower channel.

f) Vilstrup (1950) made a study of Dohlman's film and repeated some of his experiments. He noted that the resistance of the cupula to movement increases at high acceleration, and therefore high endolymph velocity. It is assumed, therefore, that the distortion of the cupula is resisted by viscous friction. Vilstrup showed that the cupula structure involves a mesh of fibrils encased in gelatinous material. The readjustment of the fibrils could thus be responsible for viscous friction, and might also provide some elastic restoring forces.

5.2. The Response of the Canals

Reconstruction of the operation of the canals of the fish can be attempted on the basis of the above observations although the model so evolved may not apply generally to the canals of different species.

According to the proposed model, the semicircular canal apparatus consists of a large number of distinct mechanical-to-electrical transducers sharing a common hydromechanical stimulating mechanism, but differently coupled to its motion. The cells of the apex of the crista would be primarily stimulated by the sliding mode of motion of the cupula and those at the base by the bending mode. The response of a specific cell would then be a function of both the angular acceleration input and the position of the cell on the crista.

(2) Measurement of Velocity

Within the normal frequency response of the canal the volume of displaced endolymph is assumed to be proportional to velocity. At a relatively low frequency, sliding with respect to both the crista and the ampulla is in phase with this displacement and therefore represents a measurement of velocity.

(3) Measurement of Acceleration

If, as assumed above, the bending of the cupula is resisted by viscous friction, it follows that this resistance is a function of the velocity of the endolymph flow. But this velocity is in turn proportional to the angular acceleration. With higher values of acceleration, the cupula would become stiffer, bend less and slide more, generating a leading component in the response. Such components would appear primarily in the cells at the apex.

5.3. Asymmetrical Response

It is well known that the canal responses of different cells are generally asymmetrical (Ewaldian law, see Fig. 4). Dohlman has reasoned (personal communication) that a cell which is responsive to an extremely small acceleration cannot also be responsive to the maximum acceleration to which the canals may be subjected. He has postulated a theory of recruitment, whereby different cells in the crista are stimulated successively during the movement of the cupula. A more complex operation must be visualized if the linearity of the total response is to be maintained over a wide range. This could be achieved by the successive, rather than simultaneous recruitment of the nonlinear individual cells as a function of ampulla displacement. Lack of symmetry of individual cell responses would then serve a function in the process. The unsymmetrical cell response may be associated with the lack of symmetry of the ampulla as revealed in Fig. 5. VILSTRUP (1950) commented on this same lack of symmetry. However, Dohlman pointed out (personal communication) that photomicrographs of various species do not support the generalization that Fig. 5 is typical of the geometry of all ampullae. The problem of the geometry of the ampulla and of its function in the canal response must therefore remain open, subject to further investigations.

5.4. Adaptation

The stimulation of the cells at the apex of the crista can be cancelled out without causing a flow of the endolymph in the canals. This can be achieved by a sliding of the cupula with respect to the crista, or by a change in the thickness of the subcupular region, with a slight compensatory bending of the cupula. Thus, adaptation could occur with constant endolymph displacement such as can be caused by a small constant acceleration. The cells on the sides of the crista would have a lesser degree of adaptability. If the process should take place as a result of elastic forces, and be resisted by viscous friction, the mathematical expressions derived by MALCOLM and MELVILL JONES (1969) and YOUNG and OMAN (1969) would apply.

The more sensitive, type I cells are said to constitute the major portion of the population of cells at the apex of the crista, while the less sensitive, type II cells are found primarily at the base (e.g. SPOENDLIN, 1965). It seems significant, therefore, that GOLDBERG and FERNANDEZ (1971) found a close correlation between the characteristics of sensitivity, leading component content, lack of symmetry, and adaptation among a population of cells. These cells, according to the present model, should be primarily those located at the apex. A mechanical model with a response to linear acceleration similar to the response of the canals to angular acceleration will be discussed later in the chapter. This response is generally described by transfer function 26, which was derived empirically by FERNANDEZ and GOLDBERG (1971).

E. Conclusions Drawn from Data on Semicircular Canals

The concept of the semicircular canals emerges from the above considerations as that of a multiplicity of distinct haircells operating as mechanical-to-electrical transducers, and coupled in different ways to a common stimulating hydromechanical apparatus.

Essentially, every cell combines the characteristics of a conventional and of an integrating angular accelerometer to different degrees, so that their responses combine components associated with angular velocity and acceleration.

In addition, the integrated response of the canals decays exponentially to zero for both constant velocity and constant acceleration. The adaptation for constant velocity is predicted by the simple Steinhausen model. Theories of the adaptation to constant acceleration and corresponding constant cupula displacement were proposed by MALCOLM and MELVILL JONES (1969–1970) and YOUNG and OMAN (1969).

It has been suggested that canal signals may adapt to a value corresponding to a weighted average of all sensory data relevant to body rotation, rather than to a zero value as assumed in the models described above.

The model we have proposed would account for the complex nature of the response, including its content of velocity- and acceleration-related components, its lack of symmetry and its adaptation. Further work is needed to determine whether or not the basic principles embodied in the model can be generalized to the canal configurations of different species.

A discrepancy between the values of ω_2 computed from hydromechanical considerations and determined experimentally is left unresolved.

The canal system is much more complex than is suggested by the Steinhausen model, which did however, prove invaluable in guiding the investigations which have led to a better understanding of the system. It still describes the prime function of the canals as angular velocity transducers.

V. The Otoliths as Linear Sensors

The otolith organs constitute the linear sensor components of the vestibular organs. Our understanding of these organs lags considerably behind our knowledge of the canals. It is well recognized that the otoliths must be responsive to both acceleration and gravity (e.g. JONGKEES and GROEN, 1946), as any inertial sensor must be. But the manner in which these two effects may be sorted out from the signal has received little consideration in vestibular theory. Still, as in the case os the analogous inertial navigation system, the independent values of these effecto must be known in order to determine the orientation of the head with respect to the vertical and the extent and direction of linear movements. Keeping this requirement in mind we shall examine anatomical and experimental data for cluef to how it can be met.

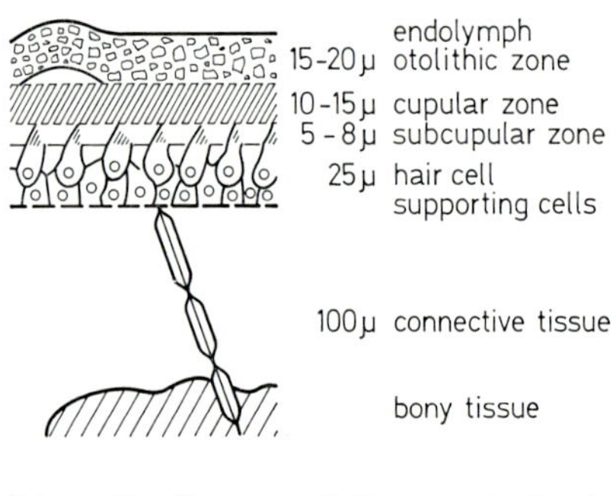

Fig. 6. Otolith Structure. Schematic diagram of the zonal structures of macula sacculi in the squirrel monkey. Reproduced from "Dimensional Study of the Vertibular and Apparatus" by IGARASHI and MAKOTO. Second Symposium on the Role of the Vestibular Organs in Space Exploration. NASA, SP-115, Washington, D.C.

A. Anatomical Structure

The reader is referred to other chapters in this handbook for a full description of the morphology of the otolith organs. However, a brief outline of their essential features may be appropriate here.

Two otolith organs are found on each side of the skull of vertebrates. They are situated in the membranes of the utricular and saccular sacs. With reference to Fig. 6, each organ comprises an otolithic zone loaded with calcareous crystals, the so-called otoconia, with a density greater than the endolymph. This zone is contiguous to the cupular and subcupular zones penetrated by the hairs of the haircells. The latter two zones are probably similar to the subcupular zone in the canals. This structure has suggested to many investigators that linear acceleration or gravity acting on the otoconia causes a shear movement of the otolithic zone with respect to the macula so that the hairs are bent, initiating the otolithic signals. It will be shown later that the effect of acceleration on the otolith organ must be more complex to account for the otolith response. It was also found earlier that the cupula movement must be more complex than a simple hinge action to account for the canal signals.

A large population of cells is distributed over the macula epithelium. A given cell has been found to respond only to a component of movement of the hairs along a specific axis, the direction of which is determined by the position of a so-called kinocilium hair with respect to a bundle of other hairs, the stereocilia. This finding made it possible to map the direction of maximum sensitivity of the population of cells in both the utricular and the saccular maculae, as shown in Fig. 7 (SPOENDLIN, 1965). The direction of maximum sensitivity of the cells changes systematically over the surfaces of the maculae. It can be assumed that for any pattern of acceleration and gravity in terms of magnitude and direction, there must be a corresponding pattern of stimulation. It would remain for neural centers to analyze this pattern and, presumably, resolve it into its components along three orthogonal axes with respect to the head. An inertial guidance designer would certainly have avoided the complexity of such analysis with the use of three independent transducers, each specialized with measurements along a single axis. But pattern analysis is easily performed by biological systems and the added complication may be well repaid in terms of some advantages, such as a more uniform sensitivity to the measurement of acceleration along any axis.

B. Characteristics of the Responses

We will now examine available data on the responses of otolithic cells to different forms of stimuli. As in the case of the semicircular canals it is highly desirable to examine responses from peripheral fibers to stimuli of appropriate frequency.

The present analysis is based primarily on recordings from fish preparations by LOWENSTEIN and ROBERTS (1950) which meet these requirements. However, other data (ADRIAN, 1943; CRAMER, 1962) from mammals lead to a similar interpretation (MAYNE and BELANGER, 1966). It will be shown also that the counterrolling response of the eyes in humans, long known to be monitored by the otoliths, reflects quite accurately the same patterns as those of fish preparations. We there-

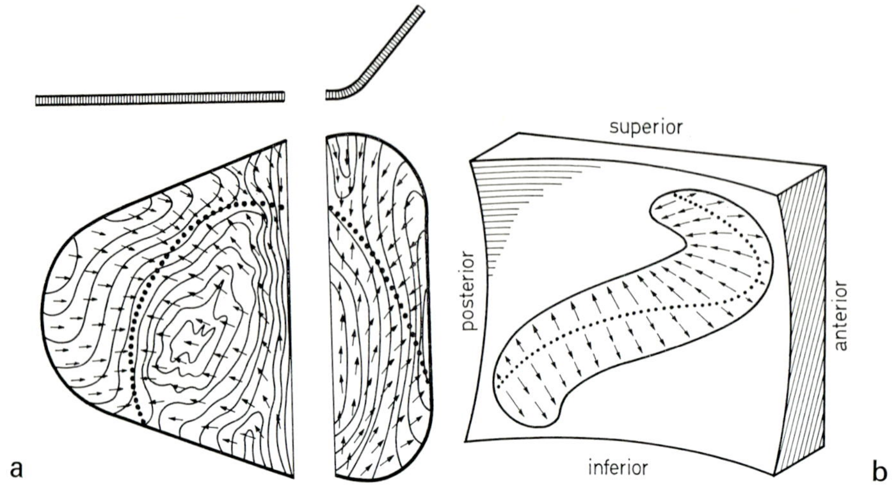

Fig. 7. Polarization of otolithic cells. 7a: Schematic drawing showing how reconstruction of surface of macula utriculi was done with serial sections of horizontal and inclined part of macula. Since surface of the macula utriculi is not entirely flat, each section of the serial sections hits actual surface of the sensory epithelium along a certain line which is indicated in this drawing by the fine curved lines. Arrows indicate direction of polarization of kinocilium as evaluated in each section with aid of phase contrast microscopy. 7b: Schematic representation of polarization pattern of sensory cells in macula sacculi of guinea pig. Here polarization is again reversed along a certain line going through entire macular surface (indicated as dotted line). In contrast to macula utriculi kinocilia on either side of this boundary line are not facing each other but facing away from each other. Reproduced from SPOENDLIN, H. H. "Ultrastructural Studies of the Labyrinth in Squirrel Monkeys". First Symposium on the Role of the Vestibular Organs in the Exploration of Space. NASA SP-77, 1965. National Aeronautics and Space Administration, Washington D.C.

fore hope to show that conclusions drawn primarily from the data of LOWENSTEIN and ROBERTS on fish otoliths are applicable to mammals. It has been shown above, similarly, that conclusions drawn from the responses of the canals of fish recorded by GROEN et al. (1952) apply to man and mammals.

The reader is referred to the chapter on physiology for a full description of the procedure in this series of tests. It is briefly summarized here, however, for the sake of continuity within this chapter.

The response of different fibers contiguous with the otolith organ and therefore representing the response of primary neurons were recorded under a number of conditions, including a) rotation of the preparations about the longitudinal axis of the fish, b) rotation about a transverse axis, c) static condition, with the preparations held motionless at different angular positions, d) rotation at constant speed, both counterclockwise and clockwise. In all cases the axis of rotation was horizontal. During rotation of the preparations, an otolithic cell was subjected to a sinusoidally varying component of gravity undistinguishable at the periphery from acceleration. The frequency of the stimulation in Hz was then equal to the angular velocity in revolutions per second. Some of the cells responded at twice this frequency, while the response of other cells had a pronounced second harmonic

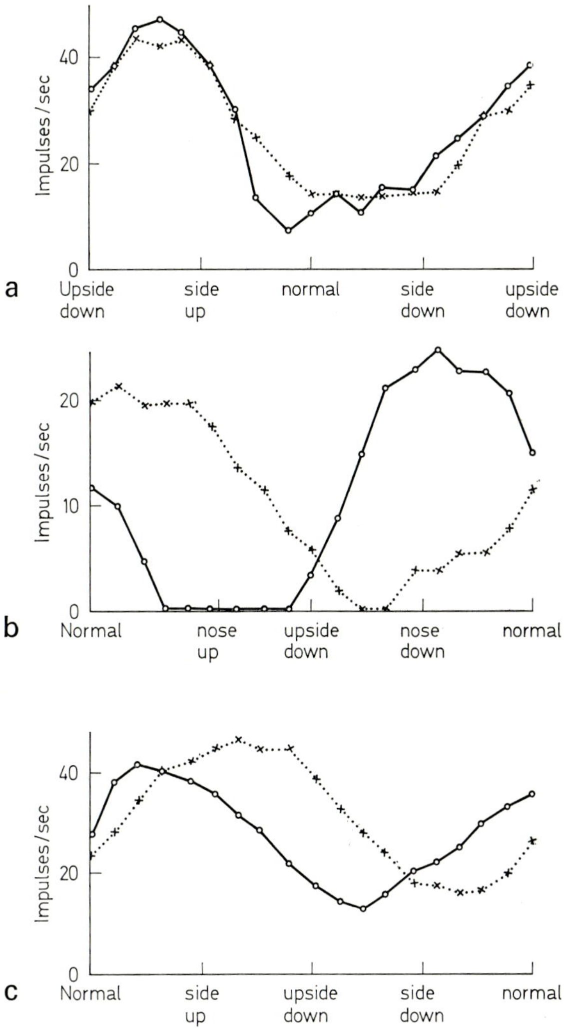

Fig. 8. Responses of three different types of otolithic cells in the thronback ray. 8a: Static response of type 1 cell. 8b: Dynamic response of type 2 cell. 8c: Mixed response of type 3 cell. Reproduced from: Lowenstein, O., Roberts, T. D. M.: J. Physiol. (Lond.) **110**, 399–415 (1950)

component. Flock and Wersäll (1962) have shown how this double frequency response can be caused by two cells in opposition. Higher harmonics may also result from variations in the sensitivity of the cells for different orientation of the gravity vector. We shall see later that such higher harmonics serve a useful purpose. The necessity of generating these harmonics may account, in part, for the cross-stimulation between cells. The present analysis, however, is only applicable to the first harmonic of the response.

The data shows that some cells respond to rotation about one axis other cells to rotation about the other axis, and still others, to rotation about either or both axis. This is in keeping with expectations based on the directional polarization of cells in the maculae. The responses of three cells that are most representative of characteristics observed in other cells are illustrated in Fig. 8. The following conclusions can be drawn from these responses.

1) The otolithic response can be one of three types: static, dynamic, or mixed.

2) A response is said to be static when its firing rate for any given angular position of the preparation is not affected by rotation. In other words, when the response is the same whether the preparation is stationary in one position or passing through the same position during continuous rotation. Also, the phase shift of the response for this type of cells must be the same for clockwise and counterclockwise rotation. Figure 8a illustrates such a static response.

3) A dynamic response is one that occurs only during a period of movement and dies down gradually when movement stops. It can be identified when the phase shift between clockwise and counterclockwise rotation is approximately 180° degrees, although this relation should occur only within a narrow band of frequencies. Figure 8b illustrates a cell which approximates such a response. The dynamic response leads the (g) stimulus. The output of this type cell returns nearly to zero for a constant value of the input, as shown in text Fig. 9 of the original paper.

4) The responses of other cells such as illustrated in Fig. 8c is mixed, including both a static and a dynamic component, the dynamic component, again, leading the static one.

LOWENSTEIN and ROBERTS recognized the presence in their data of the components of the responses defined here as "static" and "dynamic". They identified the first as position indicator and the second as a "positional change indicator". This is indeed a good intuitive description of the function of the two responses. More specifically, however, it can be said that:

a) The response of a type 1 cell and the static component of the response of a type 3 cell correspond to a measurement of the sum of the gravity and acceleration components acting along the responsive axis of the cells:

b) the response of a type 2 cell and the dynamic component of the response of a type 3 correspond to a measurement of the rate of change of the sum of the gravity and acceleration components acting on the responsive axis of the cells. These relations are approximately valid only within a certain band of frequencies.

There is an obvious analogy between the response of canal cells and those of the otolith. The canal cells combine a measurement of angular velocity with one of angular acceleration, while the otolith cells combine a measurement of the sum of gravity and acceleration with one of the rate of change of this sum. The former can be identified as a combination of conventional and integrating angular accelerometers, and the latter as a combination of conventional and differentiating linear accelerometers so that the response of both instruments must consist of two components, one leading the other by 90°. The relative emphasis on the measurement of these two modalities differs between the two instruments. As indicated earlier, data published by Fernandez and Goldberg show that the leading component in the canal response is only a significant factor at a high frequency of stimulation. The responses in Fig. 8a and Fig. 8b, on the other hand, represent respectively a nearly pure measurement of the component of gravity and of the rate of change of this component. There appear to be functional reasons for this response, as both components are required to determine both the extent and direction of linear movement and the direction of the vertical. At least they are required in the vestibular model currently proposed.

It was thought appropriate, therefore, to describe the responses of different cells in terms of these two components rather than in terms of a magnitude and a phase of their resultants, which is the usual practice in electrical engineering.

C. Mathematical Treatment

A physiological transducer can be described by a mathematical model relating input to output without regard to its possible anatomical structure. An attempt may then be made to conceive a structure which would fit both the mathematical model and the known anatomical features of the organ.

Two sets of axes are needed to describe the peripheral otolithic responses and the operation of the broader inertial system. Figure 9 illustrates the symbolism utilized in the representation of these two axes. For the sake of simplicity the linear movement of the head will be limited to the $x_\Sigma - z_\Sigma$ plane in space. At the same time the rotation will be limited to the y_π axis which will remain parallel to the y_Σ axis in space. The principles involved in this restricted degree of freedom can then be extended to the general case of three linear and three angular degrees of freedom, with respect both to space and to the head. The mathematics for this general case are complicated and beyond the scope of this paper. The basic principles involved, however, are the same as for the restricted case.

The following notation will be adopted to designate the otolithic inputs and outputs:

x_i, y_i, z_i = the components of acceleration acting respectively on the x_π, y_π and z_π head axes.
$g_{i_x}, g_{i_y}, g_{i_z}$ = the components of gravity acting respectively on the same axes as above.
$\ddot{u}_{i_x}, \ddot{u}_{i_y}, \ddot{u}_{i_z}$ = the sum of gravity and acceleration components acting respectively on the same axes as above.
x_o, y_o, z_o = the response of the otolith along corresponding axes.

The subscript π will be added to the above symbols only when confusion about which set of axes is used as reference is possible.

The subscript Σ will always be used whenever space axes are used as reference.

Velocity, displacement or rate of change of acceleration will be designated in the conventional way by the number of dots over a symbol, e.g.

$$\dddot{u}_{i_x} = \dddot{x}_i + \dot{g}_{i_x}.$$

Mayne and Belanger (1966) proposed the following transfer function to express the previously described relations between stimuli and responses of otolithic cells:

$$\frac{x_{o(s)}}{\ddot{u}_{i_x}(s)} = k_1 - \frac{k_2\,\omega_1\,\omega_2}{(s+\omega_1)\,(s+\omega_2)} \tag{28}$$

where k_1 and k_2 have the dimension of t^2 and ω_1 and ω_2 are the two break frequencies of the response. In the range of frequencies used in the tests in relation

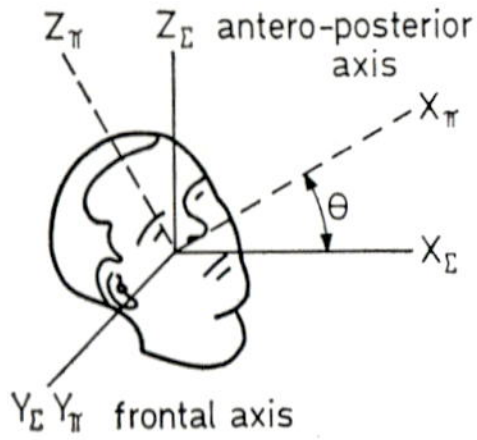

Fig. 9. Reference axes with respect to head (π) and space (Σ). (Y_Σ and Y_π remain parallel to each other in simplified head movements discussed in this chapter.) All measurements by vestibular organs must be made with respect to the head to which they are attached (π axes) and must be interpreted in terms of space (Σ axes) by processes described in text

to the value of ω_1, as computed later, the upper break frequency is of no significance and equation (28) can be written:

$$\frac{x_0(s)}{\ddot{u}_1(s)} = k_1 - k_2 \cdot \frac{\omega_1}{s + \omega_1}. \tag{29}$$

The expression can be visualized as describing the response of a transducer combining the characteristics of a conventional and of a differentiating accelerometer. When k_2 is zero the transducer is a conventional accelerometer corresponding to a type 1 cell. When $k_1 = k_2$ it approximates a differentiating accelerometer corresponding to a type 2 cell, for $k \leq \omega_1$. The response of the transducer can be expressed for the general case by the simple lead-lag expression:

$$\frac{x_0(s)}{\ddot{u}_{ix}(s)} = k_1 \frac{s + \frac{k_1 - k_2}{k_1}\omega_1}{s + \omega_1}. \tag{30}$$

The responses of different cells can be determined from this expression when the values of the different constants are known.

1. Computation of the Constants

Type 3 cell, Fig. 8c, $k_1 > k_2$.

Mayne and Belanger (1966) computed the constants for the above cells from data provided by Lowenstein and Roberts.

Introduction of these constants in 28 yielded:

$$\frac{x_0(s)}{\ddot{u}_{ix}(s)} = 24.25 - 15.6 \frac{0.232}{s + 0.232}. \tag{31}$$

Type 1 cell, Fig. 3a, $k_2 = 0$;
k_1 can be read directly from Fig. 3a, giving:

$$\frac{x_0(s)}{\ddot{u}_i(s)} = 20 \tag{32}$$

Type 2 cell, Fig. 8b. $k_1 \simeq k_2 \simeq k$.

The phase difference between clockwise and counterclockwise can be estimated at about 160°, and with the additional information that $\omega \cong 0.044$ rad/sec and $x_0 \cong 15$ impulses/sec the constants can be computed from equation 30 to give:

$$\frac{x_0(s)}{\ddot{u}_{i_x}(s)} = 86 \frac{s}{s + 0.25}. \tag{33}$$

The responses of the three cells are computed from equations (31), (32) and (33) for both sinusoidal and step input of acceleration, and are plotted on Fig. 10. These computed responses are similar to the first harmonic of the experimental responses of Fig. 8.

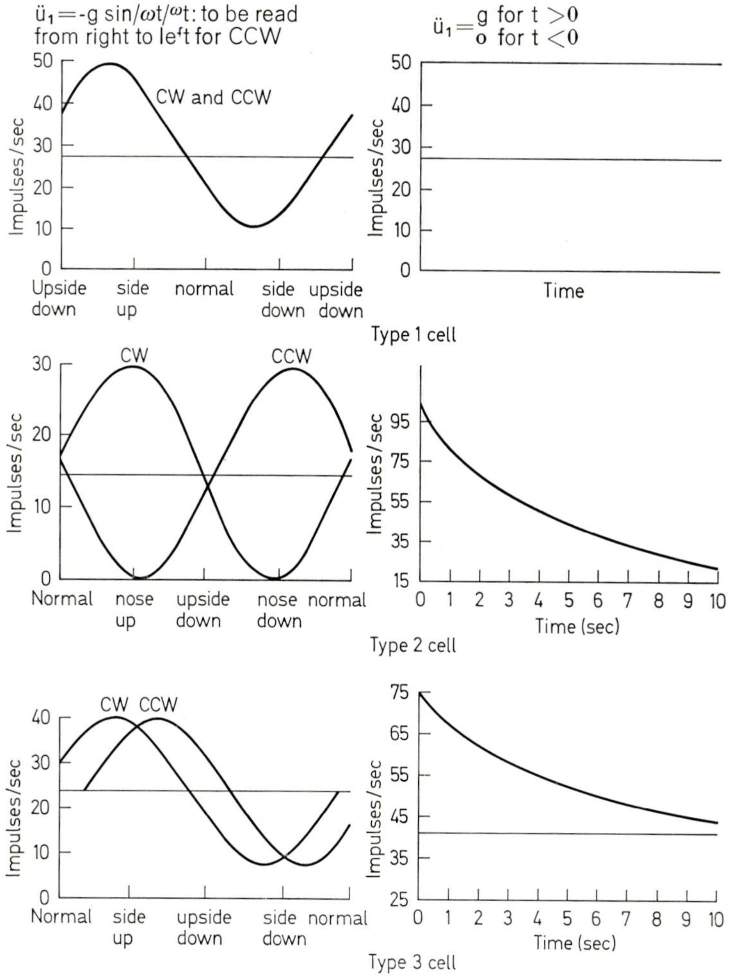

Fig. 10. Computed responses of fish otolithic cells depicted in Fig. 3 during continuous rotation both clockwise and counterclockwise and sudden 90° turn

D. Frequency Response of Type 2 Cells to a $\dddot{u}_i$ Input

If the type 2 cells are adapted to the measurement of the rate of change of the sum of acceleration and gravity input, they should exhibit a nearly flat response to this stimulus within the range of normal fish movements. This frequency response will now be computed for the cell.

For a $\ddot{u}_{ix}$ input the response of a type 2 cell can be written:

$$\frac{x_o(s)}{\ddot{u}_{ix}(s)} = \frac{k}{s + \omega_1}, \tag{34}$$

from which the amplitude ratio and phase can be computed as illustrated in Fig. 11. The band width of the transducer lies between $\omega = 0$ and $\omega = \omega_1$.

It will be noted that the value of ω_1 is approximately the same for both type 2 and type 3 cells, suggesting that cells differ only in terms of the constants k_1 and k_2. In a similar way, equation (27), by GOLDBERG and FERNANDEZ, assumes that the values of τ_1 and τ_2 are the same for all cells which differ only in τ_a and τ_L.

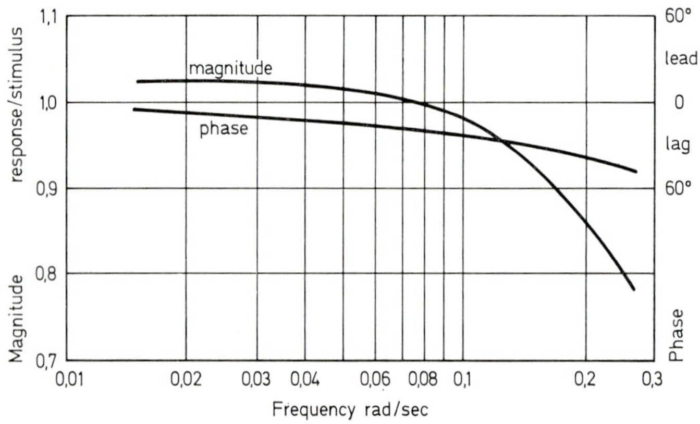

Fig. 11. Frequency response of type 2 otolithic cell for rate of change of acceleration input

$$\frac{x_o(s)}{\dddot{x}_i(s)} = \frac{1}{s + 0.25}$$

It will be noted from the data of LOWENSTEIN and ROBERTS that the speeds of rotation of the preparations were such as to cause a stimulation frequency of 0.044 rad/sec. It would be of interest to try to determine how these frequencies are related to the normal frequency range of fish movements. YOUNG et al. (1966) showed that in the case of man, the lower break frequency of the response of the organism to an input of linear velocity is the same as for the canals. If it can be assumed that this response reflects primarily that of the otoliths, and if the same relation between canal and otolith responses apply to fish as to man, then the previously estimated value of 0.02 rad/sec for the lower break frequency of the canals of the elasmobranch represents the lower range of the frequency content of the angular and linear movements of the fish. It appears, therefore, that the tests reported by LOWENSTEIN and ROBERTS were conducted well within both the frequency response of the otolith organs and the frequency range of normal fish movements.

E. Counterrolling of the Eyes

It has long been known that inclination of the head with respect to the vertical in the frontal plane causes the eyes to perform a slight rotary movement in the opposite direction. The effect is generally assumed to be the result of otolith stimulation (WOELNER and GRAYBIEL, 1959; MILLER and GRAYBIEL, 1965).

Early experimenters were concerned primarily with "static counterrolling", representing a measurement of the magnitude of roll v/s the value of the components of gravity acting in the x_π axis of the head. This relation was obtained by rotating subjects about a horizontal axis y_π to different angular positions between the vertical and x_π, and measuring counterroll with the subjects held stationary. The component of gravity acting on the x_π axis in the antero-posterior plane could then be computed from $g_{x\pi} = g \sin \theta$. The tests showed that counterroll is nearly proportional to this component, except in the case of higher harmonics. The electrical recording method used in the measurement of eyeball movements in the horizontal and vertical planes is inapplicable to roll. MILLER (1962) devised an ingenious and very precise technique for this purpose. It was utilized by KELLOGG (1965) to obtain a "dynamic counterrolling" response of the eyes during continuous rotation of the body. These data should provide information about the stimulus-response characteristics of the otoliths as nystagmus provides information about the characteristics of the semicircular canals.

The maximal speed of rotation used in Kellogg's tests was 15 rev/min, corresponding to a stimulus frequency of 1.57 rad/sec. This is quite accurately the upper break frequency determined by YOUNG et al. (1966) for the measurement of linear velocity, presumably by the otolith. It appears, therefore, that the tests were conducted approximately at the normal frequency response range of the otolith organs. We can assume that the dynamic counterrolling data of KELLOGG is a reasonably accurate image of the normal otolithic response, because a) it was obtained at frequencies corresponding to the normal frequency response range of the organ, and b) this range is very low as compared to that of the optomotor system and therefore should not suffer any significant additional phase shift in this system. The static counterrolling data should correspond to the static response of a type 1 cell, or to the static component obtained in the interrupted rotation of a type 3 cell, assuming, of course, that conclusions derived from fish data apply also to humans. The dynamic counterrolling, on the other hand, should represent the response of a type 3 cell to continuous rotation, including both a static and a dynamic component. Figure 12 shows a comparison of the two sets of data.

The static response of the type 1 cell depicted on Fig. 8a is plotted on the static counterrolling data of KELLOGG on the same scale. The agreement between the two sets of data is quite good. The plot also shows that both responses have nearly identical higher harmonic content. By reference to the data on fish and

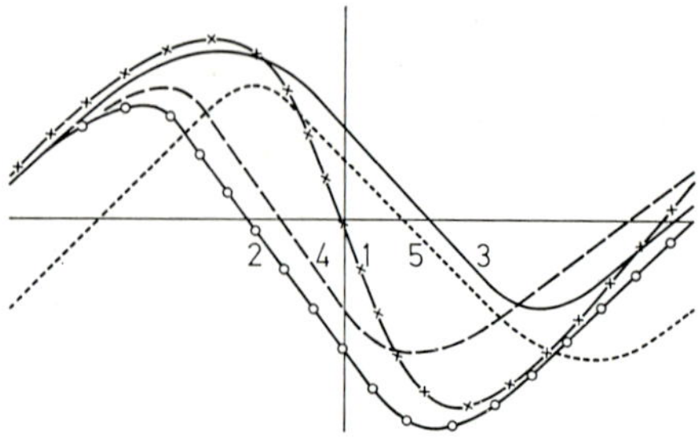

Fig. 12. Comparison of Counterrolling of the Eyes in Human and Fish Peripheral Otolithic Responses during rotation in the gravitational field. Counterrolling data from KELLOGG, R.S.: Dynamic Counterrolling of the Eye in Normal Subjects and in Persons with Bilateral Labyrinthine Defects. The Role of the Vestibular Organs in the Exploration of Space, NASA SP-77. Washington, D.C.: NASA 1965. Peripheral Otolith Data from: LOWENSTEIN, O., ROBERTS, T.D.M.: The Equilibrium Function of the Otolith Organs of the Thornback Ray. J. Physiol. (Lond.) **110**, 392–415 (1950). Curve 1: Static Counterrolling, Fig. 9, KELLOGG. +: Peripheral Otolithic Static response from type 1 cell, Fig. 3a of this report. Curve 2: Clockwise dynamic counterrolling Fig. 6, KELLOGG. Curve 3: Counterclockwise dynamic counterrolling Fig. 7, KELLOGG. Curve 4 and 5: Peripheral Otolithic mixed response from type 3 cell, for clockwise and counterclockwise rotation, Fig. 3c of this report. Human subjects are upright at 0° and upside down at 180°. Fish preparations are upright at 0° for type 1 cells and upside down for type 3 cells. In all cases curves are to be read from left to right for clockwise rotation and right to left for counterclockwise rotation. It follows that all dynamic responses for counterrolling and fish preparations *lead* the input. (See Fig. 3 for convention with fish preparations.) Convention with counterrolling from KELLOGG (personal communication)

man, it can be seen that the distortion of the response from a simple sinusoid has the effect of increasing the sensitivity of the response for the upright as compared to the inverted position. The dynamic responses for both fish and man are also quite similar. This is true, however, only if the counterrolling data is assumed to lead the gravity stimulus, as is the case for a type 3 cell. Actually, Kellogg's data is ambiguous in this regard for anyone not familiar with the conventions previously used by Miller in the reporting of counterrolling data, e.g. MILLER and GRAYBIEL (1965).

Without such conventions, it could not be ascertained whether rotation of the body and eyes of the subjects were specified with respect to observer or subjects. Personal communication with KELLOGG and MILLER cleared up these conventions and confirmed that the response was indeed leading the stimulus. This interpretation is corroborated by several other observations and makes it possible to apply the mathematical model evolved for fish to the data on counterrolling. Obviously, there would have been no fit between the two sets of data if one had led and the other lagged the stimulus.

The dynamic counterrolling data, however, is not exactly analogous to the fish response. The center of symmetry of dynamic counterrolling response shifts up or down depending on the direction of rotation. No such shift is observed in the fish data. A possible explanation is that the magnitude of counterrolling is affected by the "threat" experienced by the subjects, and that a cyclic variation of threat occurs during the rotation of the body. Such a modification of the gain would occur centrally.

Melvill Jones (1970) has commented on the difference of the extent of nystagmus exhibited by subjects during Coriolis stimulation in data published by Guedry and Montague (1961), when the head was inclined in one direction and returned to the initial position. Analysis of the effect of such head movements when the direction of body rotation is known shows that the more pronounced nystagmus corresponds to an illusion of falling forward. This is a more threatening situation than the illusion of rotating backward for the opposite head movement, because of the imagined protection of the back of the chair against a fall.

The dynamic counterrolling tests were in fact severely disturbing and several subjects became ill (personal communication from von Gierke, under whom the tests were conducted). It will be shown later that a severe conflict between vestibular and kinesthetic cues occurs in the upside-down position. It could be, then, that the portion of the cycle, from normal to inverted position is more threatening than the other half of the cycle. Possibly, however, the semicircular canals had an effect on the response, as discussed later. It is not clear from the data whether or not the canal signals were allowed to die down before counterrolling measurements were taken. It would be highly desirable to measure dynamic counterrolling as the result of side-to-side oscillations where the threat, if any, would be the same for acceleration in either direction and the canals response would not be involved.

Except for the shift of the center of symmetry, the response is closely analogous to that of a fish type 3 cell, assuming, as indicated earlier, that it leads the input. Kellogg performed a Fourier analysis of the data, determining the constant term and the sine and cosine components for first and second harmonics. Figure 13 illustrates the computations for first harmonic of the response for both the sine and the cosine versus speeds of rotations. The analysis was repeated by this author with similar results.

The sine, or static component, represents the approximate measurement of gravity acting upon the otolith.

The cosine, on the other hand, represents the rate of change of the static component. It will be noted that the static response is nearly constant within an error of 0.707 for all rates of rotation, and that the dynamic response increases linearly in nearly direct ratio with frequency, within the same approximate error. In the light of the previous discussion, the sine portion is a response to gravity, while the cosine is a response to the rate of change of gravity. An approximate fit of the response can be achieved with the simple lead-lag expression 30. A better fit can be obtained with equation (35) which includes two leading terms rather than one, as indicated in Fig. 13.

$$\frac{x_0(s)}{\ddot{u}_{ix}(s)} = 1.5 \frac{(s+2)(s+2)}{s+1.5}. \tag{35}$$

The equation fits the phase shift of the response quite accurately. The fact that another term must be added to fit the data may or may not be significant. The need for such a term cannot be established on the basis of available fish data, and a reliable formulation of the otolith response will only be possible when data comparable to these recorded by Fernandez and Goldberg for the semicircular canals are available for the otoliths. But it is perhaps enough to note from Fig. 13

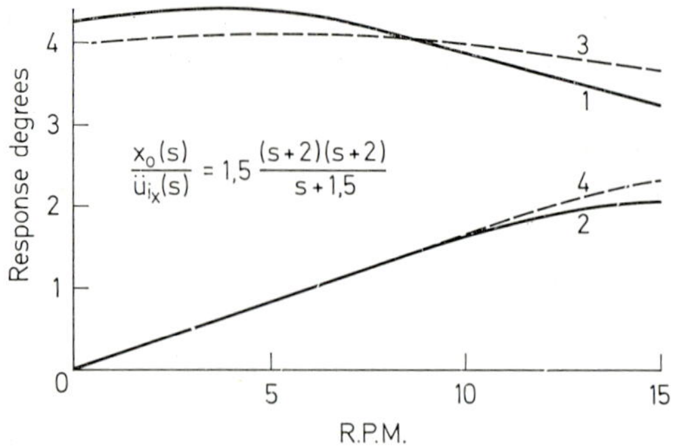

Fig. 13. Plot of computed values for the sine and cosine of dynamic counterrolling of the eyes v/s data by KELLOGG (1965). 1) Sine function (KELLOGG). 2) Cosine function (KELLOGG). 3) Sine function computed. 4) Cosine function computed

that the response of counterrolling approximates that of a type 3 cell and contains information about both gravity and the rate of change of gravity acting on thez π axis.

Obviously, if gravity is an adequate stimulus for counterrolling so is acceleration. It is difficult to conceive a functional requirement for the response to gravity. It might be thought that it would operate to maintain a constant orientation of the visual field on the retina when the head is inclined toward a shoulder. But the amount of counterrolling is too small for this purpose. MAYNE (1965d) suggested that it might generate an anticipatory visual signal for a sideways movement of the head and body to elicit a prompt muscular reaction to restore a threatened equilibrium. The vestibular signal, in this case, would not be used directly but would be added to the visual signal.

It would be interesting to fit subjects with an accelerometer and a control system designed to rotate the visual field by means of a prism in the same manner as counterrolling. It would then be possible to cancel out the effect of counterrolling in normal subjects, or produce normal counterrolling in the labyrinthine defective (L-D) subjects. The effect of the tests on the ability of the subjects to maintain their equilibrium would be a simple check of the above hypothesis.

The inferences drawn from considerations of the counterrolling of the eyes appear to be in full agreement with those previously drawn from experimental data on fish. They confirm the fact that the otoliths respond to both the sum of acceleration and gravity and to the rate of change of this sum. Counterrolling appears to be monitored by an otolithic response similar to that of a type 3 cell n the fish.

F. Physical Model of the Otolith

It may be of value to outline a physical model with a response similar to that described earlier mathematically. Figure 14 outlines such a model.

The device includes a number of simulated haircells coupled differently to the motion of the same stimulating apparatus. h_1, h_2, and h_3 correspond respectively to the cells described earlier as of the types 1, 2, and 3. The actuating mechanism consists of mass m, elasticity e, and damping c. The system is underdamped and its displacement is therefore proportional to acceleration within a given range of frequencies. The displacement of arm L_1, L_2 is resisted at one end by viscous friction c_2 and at the other end by elasticity e_3. If we assume that the effect of e_3 and c_2 is negligible on the displacement of the mass m, then the response of h_1, h_2, and h_3 can be shown to correspond to these derived earlier for the corresponding cells.

If the constants m, e_1 and c_1 are altered to cause the system to be overdamped, the displacement of the mass m will then be proportional to linear velocity, again within a certain range of frequencies, and the response of the system will be analogous to that of the canals for angular acceleration.

Both systems must have two modes of motion. In the case of the canals, as pointed out earlier they involve sliding of the cupula with respect to the ampulla, and sliding with respect to the crista. In the case of the otolith they may involve, as suggested by MAYNE (1966b), a shear of the otolith zone with respect to the

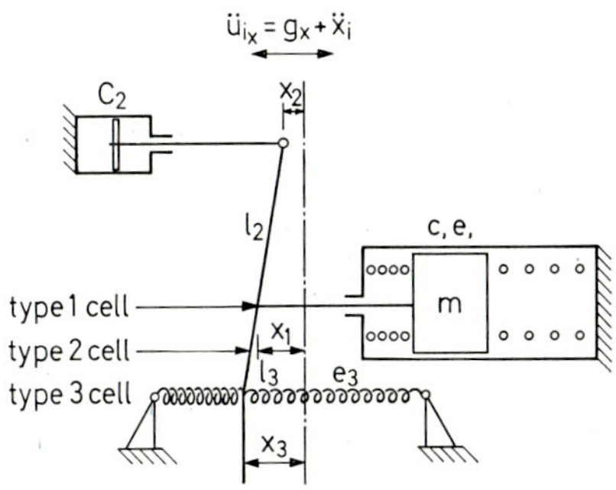

Fig. 14. Mechanical model of the otoliths and semicircular canals. x_1 is assumed to be determined solely by the constants m, c, and e for a given input of $\ddot{x}_{ix}$. In the case of the otolith the system would be underdamped so that within a normal range of frequencies $x_1 \simeq K_1 \ddot{u}_{ix}$. Transducers attached to arm L_3, as shown, would respond like type 1, type 2 and type 3 cells as described earlier. For the semicircular canals the system would be significantly overdamped so that within the normal range of frequencies: $X_1 \simeq K_2 \dot{u}_{ix}$. The system would respond to $\dot{u}_{ix}$ as the canals respond to angular velocity. Different transducers would have different leading component contents and different rates of adaptation. For closer analogy another lagging term should be added and c_2 should be made a variable, as by $c_2 = K_3 X_2$

macula, and a deformation of the entire organ with the membrane to which it is attached. It must be seen that because of the curvature of the organ, shear cannot occur without deformation. With proper constants of viscosity and elasticity of the different zones a response generally similar to that of the model may be possible. It may be expected that further data on the responses of a population of otolithic cells would reveal further similarities with the response of the canals. It may be found, for instance, that the lack of symmetry of the fish otolith response, as illustrated in Fig. 12, may be caused by a nonuniform stiffness of the macula, as the asymmetrical response of the canal was assumed earlier to be caused by a lack of symmetry in the geometry of the ampulla. The striola may play a part in determining the macula resistance to bending along different directions and speeds, as well as in the manner in which the two modes of motions, sheer and bending, may take place.

G. Other Proposed Mathematical Models

To the knowledge of the authors there have been few attempts to devise mathematical models of the otolith organs. YOUNG et al. (1966) proposed such a model, which they described by the following transfer function:

$$\frac{x_o(s)}{\dot{x}_1(s)} = \frac{ks}{(10s + 1)\,(.66s + 1)} \tag{36}$$

Expressed in terms of an acceleration stimulus and of the corner frequencies $\omega_1 = 0.1$ and $\omega_2 = 1.51$, our previous notation the equation becomes:

$$\frac{x_o(s)}{\ddot{x}_i(s)} = \frac{k_1}{(s + 0.1)\,(s + 1.51)}\,. \tag{37}$$

The function was obtained by oscillating subjects linearly and asking them to express their sensation of velocity by operating a control stick. The phase angle between the sinusoidal motion of the subjects and that of the stick determined the transfer function. The frequency band width represented by this function is surprisingly narrow: 0.1 to 1.51 rad/sec as compared to 0.1 and 10 to 200 for the canals depending on the accepted value for the constant ω_2. It will be noted that the lower portion of the band width is the same for both organs. Within the two corner frequencies, the model represents a linear integrating accelerometer, with a response similar to the canals for angular acceleration. Corroborating evidence will be presented later to the effect that the function does represent, indeed, a measurement of linear velocity involving the otoliths, although it is not believed to constitute a peripheral response of these organs.

The above equation was revised (YOUNG and MEIRY, 1967; YOUNG, 1969) to include a static component occurring in the counterrolling data of KELLOGG (1965) as follows:

$$\frac{x_o(s)}{\ddot{x}_i(s)} = \frac{1.5\,(s + 0.076)}{(s + 0.19)\,(s + 1.5)}\,. \tag{38}$$

The function differs from equation (30), proposed earlier by MAYNE and BELANGER (1966), in that the dynamic component of the response corresponds to an integration of the input between the two corner frequencies, instead of a differentiation.

The difference arises apparently from the interpretation by the authors of the phase shift in Kellogg's data as a lag, while it is taken here to represent a lead.

Actually this author (MAYNE and BELANGER, 1966; MAYNE, 1967) also assumed originally that the dynamic component of the response in the data of LOWENSTEIN and ROBERTS was an integration and represented a measurement of angular velocity by analogy with the canals. The data showed clearly that the dynamic portion of the response led the input; but in the absence of critical data on the response for different frequency inputs, it was thought possible that it could represent the negative of velocity. It became clear later that in the range of frequencies in which the tests were conducted, in relation to the computed value of the constant ω_1, the response represented a differentiation. The initial mathematical model remained valid, although its verbal description was in error. It was also found that the interpretation of phase shift as a lead was consistent with the established convention in the recording of counterrolling data (MILLER and KELLOGG, personal communication), the identification by KELLOGG of the dynamic component as a cosine as shown in Fig. 13, and the similarity of the fish data with the dynamic counterrolling response when both are taken to lead the input.

But there is an overriding functional requirement that rules out the possibility of an integration being performed at the periphery. As indicated earlier in the discussion of the inertial system, the response of the linear sensors must be separated into components related respectively to acceleration and gravity and resolved into space axes before they are integrated in the computation of velocity and displacement with respect to space. Expression 38 shows acceleration as the sole input to the otolith transducer and thus sidesteps this complication.

H. Conclusions of Otolith Considerations

Recordings by LOWENSTEIN and ROBERTS (1950) from the peripheral otolithic fibers of fish preparations during rotation were examined. They revealed that the cells can be divided into three types: those primarily responsive to the sum of acceleration and gravity, those responsive to the rate of change of this sum, and those responsive to both modalities.

A mathematical expression consisting of a simple lead-lag network was derived, describing the responses of the three types of cells by adjustment of the values of its constants. The responses computed from these expressions were found to be in close agreement with the first harmonic of the observed data. A physical model having the same transfer function as that proposed for the otolith was outlined.

When data on the response of a significant population of otolith cells become available it may be necessary to express them with a more complex function than proposed here. This possibility is suggested by the analysis of dynamic counterrolling.

It may be of interest to draw a comparison between the canal and otolith transducers in the light of the previously suggested modes of their operations.

Both organs comprise a population of distinct transducers differently coupled to the same stimulating apparatus.

In the case of the canals the endolymph is displaced as a function of head velocity. This displacement, in turn, reacts on the cupula to cause two modes of motion: one primarily related to the displacement itself, the other to the rate of chonge of displacement.

The cells stimulated by these two modes contain components related to head velocity and head acceleration. The ratio of the magnitude of these two components varies from unit to unit, depending on the prime mode of their stimulation.

In the case of the otolith, the otolithic zone is acted upon by the sum of acceleration and gravity components. This in turn causes two modes of hair stimulation related respectively to this sum and its rate of change.

There appears to be a greater variation in the relative magnitude of the two components of the response in the otolith than is the case for the canals.

It is assumed that the leading component in the canal response serves the primary function of broadening the band width of the apparatus by offsetting delays in various body control loops.

It was assumed that the primary function of the leading component in an otolithic cell is to provide a signal that is free of the effect of the constant value of the gravity component acting upon it.

The manner in which the data from all cells of both sets of organs is analyzed, integrated, and interpreted in the performance of body control is one of the more challenging problems of physiology.

A paper by FERNÁNDEZ et al. (1972) published subsequently to the submittal of the present chapter contributes significant further data on the otolith organs. Vector analysis is utilized in the paper to interpret the static response of otolithic units in the squirrel monkey. The authors infer from the analysis and morphological considerations that the polarization vectors of units associated with the utriculus lie near the horizontal plane, while those associated with the sacculus lie in the approximate sagittal plane. It is found further that the static response is nearly proportional to the component of gravity along the morphological polarization vectors as defined above. The static sensitivity of a cell is shown to be related in nearly direct ratio to its resting discharge. At the same time the response is found to be consistent with the theory that it is initiated by a shear of the otolith organ.

Although the investigation was limited to the observation of static responses it seems to corroborate various conclusions of the present chapter. The authors found it necessary, for instance, to hold a preparation in the same position for at least 30 sec after being rotated, to allow a transient effect to die down. The response of the otolithic cells of the squirrel monkey contain therefore both static and dynamic components as found to be the case in the fish and counter-rolling data. We have indicated that the static component of the otolith cell is proportional to gravity as found to be the case in the paper. It should be expected further that a cell with a high leading component content would have both a low resting frequency and a low sensitivity as found by the authors. Actually a cell of the pure type 2 would have zero resting frequency and zero static sensitivity. Examination of Fig. 16 of the original paper reveals that there are cells of very nearly this characteristic. In the light of the previous discussion a low resting discharge and sensitivity to a static input must be associated with a high dynamic component in the response.

Further, it is assumed in the next section of this chapter, that the dynamic component of the response is utilized primarily in the determination of the extent of linear movement, while the static component is utilized in the determination of the vertical. It is significant in this regard that the paper shows that saccular units, with a polarization vector in the sagittal plane, have a lower resting frequency and sensitivity than utricular units polarized horizontally. They must have, therefore, a greater dynamic, and a lower static component than the utricular cells. This is in accordance with functional requirements. Departure of the head from the vertical position would be best detected by the static response of utricular cells having their polarization vectors in the horizontal plane and having both a high resting rate and high sensitivity. At the same time movements of the body should occur mainly in the sagittal plane. Cells with a high dynamic content located in this plane would be best adapted for the detection of such movements.

The authors observed the same lack of symmetry noted above in data on static otolithic responses for both the fish and counter-rolling. This distortion of the response from a pure sine wave was assumed to be caused mainly by a second harmonic and to serve a function in providing a greater sensitivity for the upright, as compared to the inverted position of an animal.

It is hoped that the authors will continue their excellent series of investigations with measurements of the otolithic responses under dynamic conditions.

VI. Processing of the Otolith Signals

A. General Considerations

As indicated earlier, the response of the otoliths to an input of gravity and acceleration must be sorted out into components related to each modality. An initial processing takes place at the periphery through the rejection of the constant value of gravity in the dynamic portion of the signal by differentiation.

If the head is maintained in a constant position relative to the vertical, the dynamic signals related to three orthogonal axes with respect to the head can then be resolved along space axes. They can be then integrated once to give angular acceleration, twice for velocity, and three times for displacement, all with respect to space. The problem becomes more complicated, however, if the head is inclined relative to the vertical. The components of gravity acting on the otoliths are no longer constant and the dynamic portion of the responses then includes a measure of the rate of change of gravity. Integration of this portion of the responses as before would produce a false sense of movement of the head.

The static portion of the signal related to the sum of acceleration and gravity inputs cannot be utilized directly for the determination of the vertical. Any acceleration would modify the direction of the inertial vector and give a false sense of the vertical.

Further processings of the otolithic signals in the CNS is required for the vestibular system to provide information on both extent and direction of linear movements and the direction of the vertical.

The hypothesis regarding the nature of this processing, as initially proposed in the first draft of this chapter, has been summarized in subsequent publications (Mayne, 1969a, 1970). It will be presented below in two parts related to the determination of the vertical and the computation of linear velocity and displacement.

B. Determination of the Vertical

Several sensory organs are involved in the determination of the vertical. It may be said that our concept of the vertical corresponds to an invariant characteristic of the information supplied by these sensors. We will consider here, briefly, what operations must be performed on otolithic peripheral data to allow the vestibule to participate with other sensors in a joint determination of the vertical.

The system proposed is represented in Fig. 15, with numbered blocks to allow greater clarity in referring to them. The operations represented in these blocks are analogous to those performed in a physical system. Further experimentation and theoretical considerations are necessary to determine how these computations may be carried out by neural elements. The keys to the symbols used in the previous and following text are summarized in Table 1 for more convenient reference. As shown in the diagram, the input to the system includes otolithic signals related to the sum of the gravity and acceleration components acting on the x_π and z_π axis, and of semicircular canal signals corresponding to the angular velocity of the head about the Y_π axis.

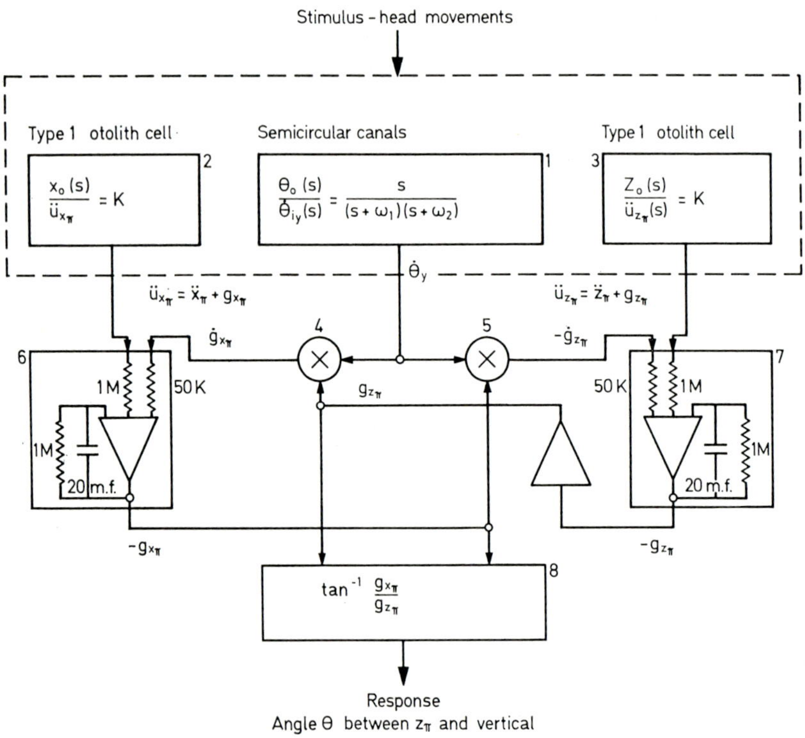

Fig. 15. Determination of the vertical constants of low pass-high pass filters are adjusted to give $\tau = 20$, found applicable to man

Table 1. *Summary of Keys to Symbols used in Block Diagrams*

θ:	angle of the vertical with longitudinal axes of the head
g:	gravity, 32 ft/sec^2
$g_{x\pi}$, $\dot{g}_{x\pi}$:	the component of gravity and rate of change of this component-along X_π head axis
$x_{i\pi}(s)$, $x_{o\pi}(s)$:	the input and output of a filter or transducer on the X_π head axis as a function of the operator (s)
x_π, $\dot{x}_\pi$, $\ddot{x}_\pi$, $\dddot{x}_\pi$:	displacement, velocity acceleration and rate of changes of acceleration the head along its X axis (X_π)
x_Σ, $\dot{x}_\Sigma$, $\ddot{x}_\Sigma$ $\dddot{x}_\Sigma$:	displacement velocity, acceleration rate of change of acceleration of the head along the X space axis (X_Σ)
$\ddot{u}_{x\pi}$:	the sum of acceleration and gravity component along the X_π axis
$\ddot{u}_{x\pi}$:	the sum of the rate of change of acceleration and gravity components acting on X_π axis
$K_1 =$	a constant
$\dot{\theta}_y =$	angular velocity of the about Y_π

Elementary
Low pass filter (a)

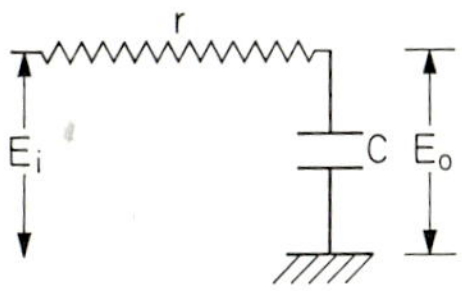

$$E_i(t) = \frac{1}{\omega_1}\dot{E}_o(t) + E_o(t)$$

$$\frac{E_o(s)}{E_1(s)} = \frac{\omega_1}{s + \omega_1}$$

Elementary
High pass filter (b)

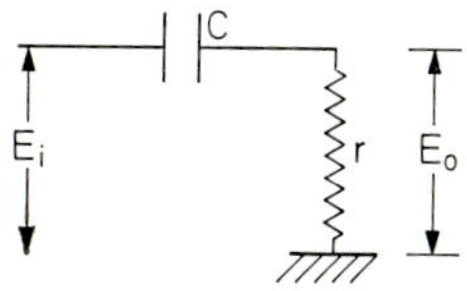

$$\dot{E}_i(t) = \omega_1 E_o(t) + \dot{E}_o(t)$$

$$\frac{E_o(s)}{E_i(s)} = \frac{s}{s + \omega_1}$$

where $\omega_1 = \dfrac{1}{rc}$

Responses to a step input as a function of s and t

$$E_o(s) = E_i(s)\left(\frac{1}{s} - \frac{1}{s + \omega_1}\right)$$

$$E_o(t) = E_i(t)\left[1 - e^{-\omega_1 t}\right)$$

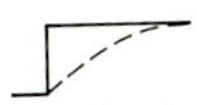

$$E_o(s) = E_i(s)\,\frac{1}{s + \omega_1}$$

$$E_o(t) = E_i(t)\, e^{-\omega_1 t}$$

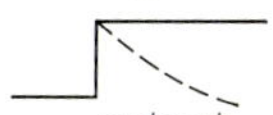

Responses *to a sinusoidal input* as a function of ω

$$\left|A_L(\omega)\right| = \frac{\omega_1}{\sqrt{\omega^2 + \omega_1^2}} \qquad \left|A_h(\omega)\right| = \frac{\omega}{\sqrt{\omega^2 + \omega_1^2}}$$

$$\beta_L(\omega) = -\tan^{-1}\frac{\omega}{\omega_1} \qquad \beta_h(\omega) = \tan^{-1}\frac{\omega_1}{\omega}$$

where $A_L(\omega)$ and $A_h(\omega)$ are the amplitude ratio of output over input for the low and high pass filters respectively and as a function of ω.
$\beta_L(\omega)$ and $\beta_h(\omega)$ are the corresponding phase shifts, lagging in the case of the low pass and leading in the case of the high pass filters.

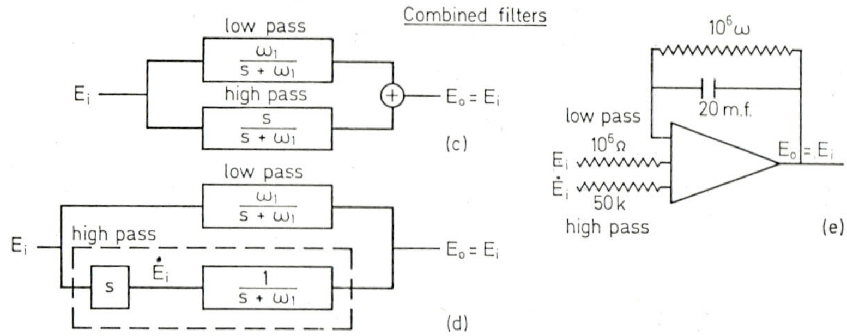

Fig. 16. Filtering techniques: Addition of the outputs of a low and high pass filter in (c) yields an output equal to the input. The high pass section may be broken up into two parts as indicated in Fig. (d). Equivalent circuit of (d) is shown in (e) using operational amplifier. The input of the circuit consists of E_i and $\dot{E}_1$ giving an output of E_i for either slow or fast change of the value of E_i

1. The Filtering Process

The operation of the proposed system depends primarily upon a filtering process. A few words about this process may be of value to the reader unfamiliar with basic electrical engineering circuitry and perhaps as a reminder to others. The proposed scheme involves a combination of low-pass and high-pass filtering.

Figure 16a illustrates an elementary low-pass filter. It is assumed that the input impedance is low and the output impedance high as compared to that of the filter, so that its characteristics will be determined mainly by the resistance r and the capacity c. It can be seen intuitively that if a step voltage is impressed on the filter the condenser will become charged gradually. The voltage output will also rise gradually from zero to a value equal to the input voltage as the condenser becomes fully charged. For a given amplitude of a sinusoidal input, the output will be greater for low than high frequencies. The filter imposes pronounced attenuation on high-frequency inputs and passes low frequencies with little loss of amplitude. For this reason it is called a low-pass filter. The relations between input and output for this circuit are shown in Fig. 16a.

Figure 16b shows a corresponding elementary high-pass filter. Reasoning intuitively again, it can be seen that if a step voltage input is impressed on the filter a current will immediately flow through the circuit causing an instantaneous rise of the voltage in the output. As the condenser becomes charged the current will drop and, with it, the output voltage. It will reach zero when the condenser is fully charged. At the same time it can be seen that for a given amplitude of a sinusoidal input the output will be greater for high than for low frequencies. The circuit imposes a marked attenuation on low-frequency inputs and passes those at high frequency with little loss of amplitude. For this reason it is called a high-pass filter. Relations between inputs and outputs are indicated in Fig. 16b.

Figure 16c shows how the two filters can be combined. The effect of one circuit cancels that of the other and the output is equal to the input of all times. Figure 16d shows an alternate way of achieving such a combination. The input E_i is first differentiated then put through a low pass filter which differs from the other only by the constant ω_1. The output is again equal to the input. Figure 16e shows another arrangement for a high-low pass filter using an operational amplifier. The values of resistance and capacity are adjusted to give a time constant of 20, found later to be applicable to the low-pass filter of man.

The reader may well question the purpose of such circuitry, with an output equal to the input. The point is that the processing rejects unwanted signals on the one hand, and provides for a rapid response when needed on the other. The application of this filtering technique to the otolith signals will be discussed below.

2. The Head Performs Linear Movements in the x_Σ z_Σ Plane with a Fixed Orientation to the Vertical

The otolith signals related to the x_π and y_π axes are fed to the low-pass section of filters 6 and 7. The portion of the signal associated with the constant value of gravity is passed unchanged by the filter. The portion due to the normally transient acceleration, to the left or right, forward or backward, is integrated over a period of time, and will normally add up to zero. The output of the filters is then a true representation of the magnitude of the components of gravity acting on the x_π and z_π axes. The direction of the vertical can be computed by simple trigonometric operations. It can be seen that if for any reason the output should drift away from a true measurement of the corresponding gravity component it will return gradually to the true value. Only the low-pass section is needed for the above operation. (The high-pass section is not operative because there is no semicircular signal.)

3. The Head is Turned about an Axis other than the Vertical

If the head is turned about an axis other than the vertical, there will be a corresponding rapid change in the magnitudes of the components of gravity acting on the z_π and x_π axes. The responses of the corresponding low-pass filters to such a rapid change will be slow, as indicated in Fig. 16b. Only after a substantial delay will the output of the two filters come to represent an accurate measure of the new values of the gravity components, so that disorientation would occur in the meantime. If the rates of changes of the components of gravity were known, the high-pass section of the filters could be utilized to effect a fast correction. It will be shown below that they can be computed if the angular velocity of the head is known at all times during the turn.

The following relation holds true at any time during a turn of the head for the restricted movements assumed here:

$$g_{x\pi} = g \sin \theta$$
$$g_{z\pi} = g \cos \theta$$

and since g is constant

$$\dot{g}_{x\pi} = \dot{\theta} g \cos \theta = g_{z\pi} \dot{\theta} \tag{39}$$
$$\dot{g}_{z\pi} = -\dot{\theta} g \sin \theta = -g_{x\pi} \dot{\theta}. \tag{40}$$

$\dot{g}_{x\pi}$ and $\dot{g}_{z\pi}$ can be obtained as shown in the diagram by multiplication of $g_{x\pi}$ and $g_{z\pi}$ by the output of the semicircular canal on the $y_{\pi\Sigma}$ axis as shown in Fig. 15. Signal processing by the combined high-pass and low-pass filters should keep the output at the proper value at all times within, of course, the frequency responses of the elements that are involved. The combination of the two filters would also operate to give an accurate measurement of $g_{x\pi}$ and $g_{z\pi}$ in the case of combined linear and angular movements.

The part played by other sensory organs in the determination of the vertical should also be included. The magnitudes $g_{x\pi}$ and $g_{z\pi}$ would then be obtained from the composite determination of the angle θ by all sensors and the value of the gravitational force on earth. Disturbances would then occur in space, as indicated later, with a different gravitational force. The scheme illustrated in Fig. 15 is used here for the sake of simplicity in illustrating a principle of operation. The part played by other sensory organs in the determination of the vertical belongs in the broader system of spatial representation and is thus beyond the scope of this chapter.

4. Determination of the Vertical in an Airplane Autopilot

The proposed processing model is somewhat analogous to the system used in an airplane autopilot for determination of the vertical. Both involve a slow and a fast response. The attitude of the airplane is determined by the angle between the axis of rotation of a gyroscope and the airframe. Light precessing torques are applied to the gyroscope as a function of the inclination of two pendulums along the longitudinal and transverse axes of the airplane. The pendulums are acted upon by gravity and acceleration during transient roll, pitch, side slips, increase or decrease of the speed of the plane. These transient inputs are integrated over a period of time, the duration of which depends on the strength of the precessing torques and the characteristics of the gyroscope. The process is similar to that of a low-pass filter in cancelling out the effect of random transient inputs. The constant value of the signal tends to maintain the gyroscope in a predetermined angle to the normal attitude of the airplane and therefore to the vertical. On the other hand, any deviation of the airplane attitude with respect to the normal is promptly detected by sensors for immediate correction by actuation of the appropriate control surfaces. It is such combinations of fast and slow responses that make it possible for the position of an airplane or of an animal to be properly monitored. As indicated later, both systems are subject to similar errors.

C. Determination of Linear Velocity and Displacement

In order to determine linear velocity and displacement, the otolithic data must be freed from the effect of gravity. Figure 17 illustrates an arrangement applicable to this function. The input otolithic signals to the system correspond to the rate of change of the sum of the acceleration and gravity components acting on the x_π and z_π axes. These, as indicated earlier, could be obtained from type 2 cells or extracted from the signals of all cells. The system also utilizes data from the previous block diagram, as indicated in the diagram.

The proposed processing will be considered briefly for the following conditions.

1. The Head Performs Linear Movement as Above

The $\dot{g}_{x\pi}$ and $\dot{g}_{z\pi}$ components in the output of the type (2) otolithic cells are zero. The $\dddot{x}_\pi$ and $\dddot{z}_\pi$ components can be multipled by the cosine of the angle θ obtained from block (8) in Fig. 15 and by the appropriate constant to give the

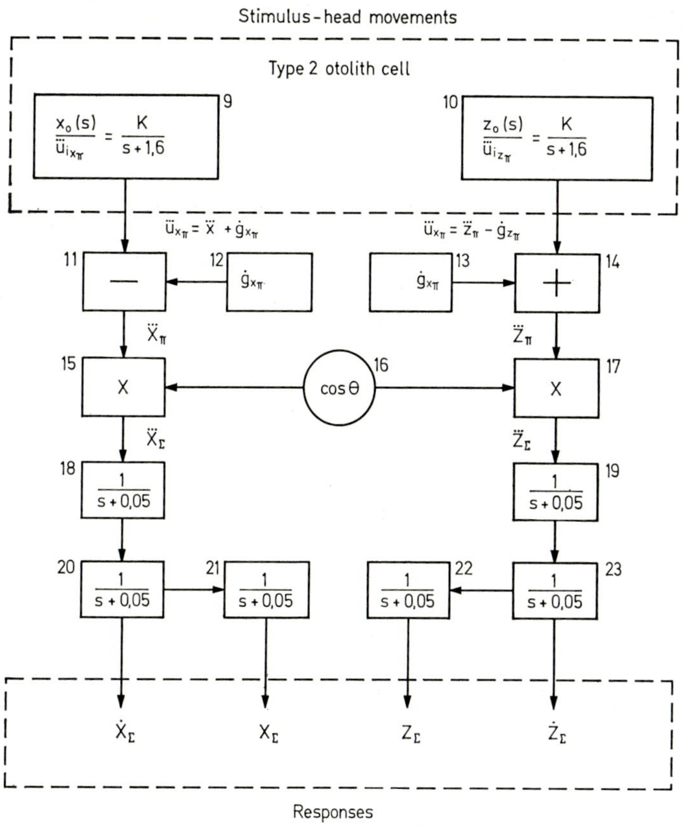

Fig. 17. Determination of velocity and displacement. Constants are selected to yield approximately the function. $\frac{x_0(s)}{\dot{x}_{i\Sigma}(s)} = \frac{s}{(s+1.60)\,(s+0.1)}$ Determined experimentally by Young et al. (1966)

rate of change of acceleration input with respect to space: $\ddot{x}_\Sigma$ and $\ddot{z}_\Sigma$. These values are processed by a lag network of the form $\frac{1}{s+a}$ to perform an approximate integration. For a value of $a = 0.05$, two such operations yield very closely expression 36 by Young et al. (1966) for velocity.

2. The Head is Turned, with or without Linear Movements

If the head is turned about an axis other than the vertical, with or without linear velocity, the output of the otolithic cells will acquire a $\dot{g}_{x\pi}$ and $\dot{g}_{z\pi}$ component which must be subtracted from the signal before integration takes place. These values were computed in blocks (5) and (4) of Fig. 15 by operation of the high-pass section of the filters and need only to be subtracted, as shown in diagram, to give $\ddot{x}_\pi$ and $\ddot{z}_\pi$. The operations can then proceed as in the previous case. Without the elimination $\dot{g}_{x\pi}$ and $\dot{g}_{z\pi}$ component from the otolithic signal, an erroneous velocity and displacement would be computed and an illusory motion would be sensed during inclination of the head.

The same basic operations depicted for a two-dimensional case are applicable to three dimensions, but their mathematical description is much more complicated.

D. Conclusions of the Considerations of Otolithic Signal Processing

The processing of the otolithic signals to separate the components due to gravity from those due to acceleration can only be based on one distinguishing characteristic, the constancy of one and the transient nature of the other. Gravity is identified by the system as the constant portion of the signal, acceleration as the transient portion.

Assuming, as before, that the peripheral otolithic signals can be separated into static and dynamic components, related respectively to the sum of gravity and acceleration and to the rate of change of this sum, the operations described above can be summarized as follows:

1) The differentiation of the sum of gravity and acceleration inputs at the periphery rejects the constant value of the signal representing the gravity input, as long as the head is maintained in the same attitude relative to the vertical.

2) The integration of the static signal in the low-pass section of the filter rejects transient acceleration, providing an accurate sense of the vertical, as long as the head maintains a fixed attitude relative to the vertical.

3) When the head is inclined with respect to the vertical, causing a rapid change of its orientation in the gravitational field, the above processing is no longer sufficient, because:

a) The low-pass filter cannot follow the rapid change, so that a false sense of the attitude of the head and body results, and;

b) The rate of change of the gravity components in the dynamic portion of the signal cannot be distinguished from those caused by acceleration, so that a false sense of movement results.

4) The slow response of the low-pass section of the filters can be corrected by means of the high-pass section. The rate of change of the gravity components acting on different axes of the head can be computed as shown in Fig. 15 and fed to the input of the high-pass section, so that the filter will provide a true measurement of the value of gravity for an accurate estimate of the direction of the vertical at all times. Without such a correction disorientation would occur during head movements.

5) Differentiation at the periphery eliminates only the constant component of gravity. It does not eliminate the varying effect caused by inclination of the head. Integration of the dynamic portion of the signal without correction for this effect would produce illusory sensations of movement. The rate of change of the gravity component is computed in 15. It can then be subtracted from the signal to give the rate of change of acceleration.

Correction for the effect of head movements can thus involve either the addition or the subtraction of a signal. Without such correction there may be illusions of body attitude or movement or both.

VII. Application of the Proposed Vestibular Model to Various Experimental Situations

An isolated empirical observation or an experimental finding acquires "meaning" when it can be correlated with other observations or findings in terms of a systems concept or a theory. The isolated discovery by Fabricius that veins are provided with one-way valves became meaningful in the light of Harvey's theory of the circulation of the blood. We shall examine briefly what degree of harmony and meaning the proposed model may bring to presently uncoordinated experimental data.

A. Parallel Swing Test

GUEDRY (1963) oscillated subjects lying supine on a parallel swing. The extent of the oscillation is pictured in Fig. 18. It can be computed from the length of the arms of the swing and the amplitude of the motion that the resultant inertial vector of gravity and acceleration oscillated by an amount of about $\pm 21°$ with respect to the head of the subjects. Guedry reported, however, that the subjects retained a clear sense of the direction of the vertical at all times. This observation is in

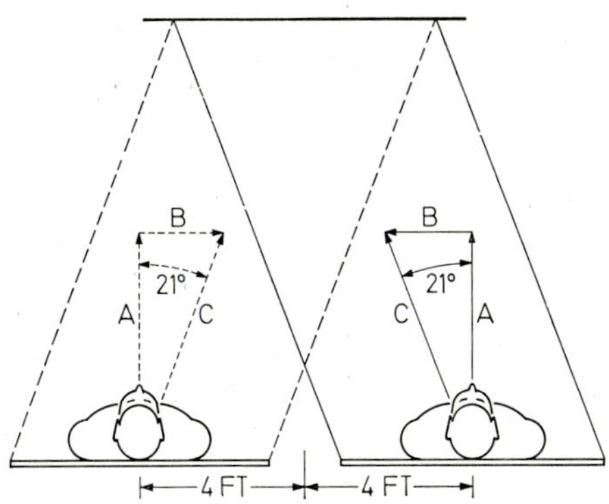

Fig. 18. Parallel swing experiments. Subject maintains a true perception of the vertical although the resultant of gravity and acceleration oscillates by an angle of 21°. Data source: GUEDRY, F. E., JR., and HARRIS, C. S.: "Labyrinthine Function Related to Experiments on the Parallel Swing," U.S. Naval Aviation Medical Center, Pensacola, Florida; 1963

agreement with the previous discussion of the effect of the low-pass filter when the attitude of the head is fixed with respect to the vertical. Similarly, we do not lose the sense of the vertical because of a sudden stop or start.

With a longer period of oscillation and a higher magnitude of acceleration the change in the direction of the inertial vector could have been detected by the subjects. The low-pass section of the filter is adapted to suppress only accelerations of a magnitude and frequency experienced in normal life activities.

B. Oculogravic Illusion

A subject seated on a platform rotating at constant velocity, with his frontal plane oriented axially, identifies the direction of the vertical with that of the constant resultant of centripetal and gravitational acceleration, in accordance with the principle stated previously. This phenomenon is known as the oculogravic illusion (GRAYBIEL and BROWN, 1951). If the platform is brought rapidly to a constant speed, effecting a near step change in the direction of the constant inertial vector, a corresponding step change in the sensed direction of the vertical does not occur. It is sensed, rather, to rotate slowly from the true to the illusory direction.

Figure 19 shows a plot of the sensed position of a subject with respect to the vertical v/s the time since the start of rotation, taken from data by CLARK and GRAYBIEL (1965). The plot shows that the sensed direction of the vertical approaches exponentially that of the inertial vector with a time constant of 20.

Under experimental conditions, the sudden change of direction of the inertial vector in the frontal plane of the subject is not accompanied by a canal signal in the same plane. The high-pass section of the filters is therefore inoperative, and the change can only be observed through the slow-reacting low-pass section. In accordance with the characteristics of such a filter the direction of the vertical must be sensed to approach exponentially that of the true direction of the inertial vector. The time constant 20 can therefore be taken to represent that of the biological low-pass filter in man.

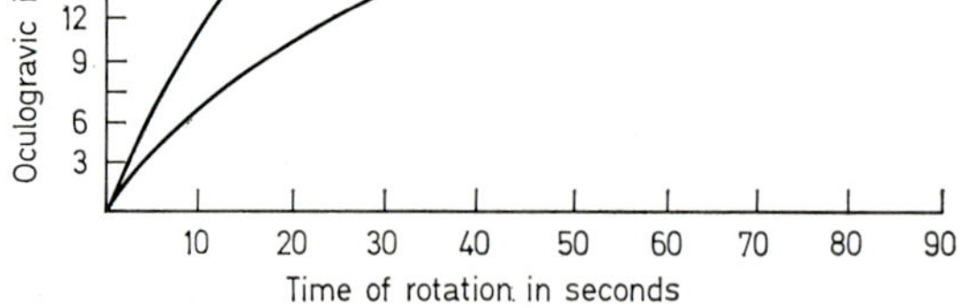

Fig. 19. Typical records of "oculogravic illusion delay". Illustration reproduced from: "Factors Contributing to Delay in Perception of Oculogravic Illusion," by B. CLARK and A. GRAYBIEL. NASA SP-77 National Aeronautics and Space Administration (1965). Curves represent the average estimates of the direction of the vertical by five subjects in a centrifuge following their rapid acceleration to a constant velocity. ∅ is the angle between the resultant of gravitational and centrifugal forces and vertical. Low-pass filters 6 and 7 in Fig. 15 with $\tau \simeq 20$ would account for the delay in the sensing of the true direction of the inertial vector by the subjects

Such a time constant seems well matched to that of the semicircular canals. In the case of the parallel-swing experiment discussed above, the oscillation of the inertial vector by $\pm 21°$ would be attenuated to $\pm 1°$ by a filter with this characteristic, and would be hardly noticeable.

The gyroscopic system described earlier for an autopilot also experiences an "oculogravic illusion" in a turn. The gyroscope tends to orient itself along the constant resultant of gravitational and centripetal accelerations, with a similar exponential change of the sensed vertical. Both systems interpret the direction of constant acceleration as vertical. It is standard practice to cut off the erection of the gyroscope in a turn to avoid building up an error in the determination of the vertical.

The oculogravic illusions of the physical and biological systems occur because it is impossible for any instrument to distinguish between constant acceleration and gravity. It is only possible to distinguish between constant gravity and a randomly transient acceleration. The delay of the illusion in man occurs because a change in the direction of a constant inertial vector is not accompanied by a corresponding canal signal, so that the change has to be detected by the slow reacting low-pass section of the filter. Incidentally, the experiment demonstrates that a sensation of rotation of the body, although lagging the input, can be generated by the otoliths.

C. Reactions of Animals with Inoperative Canals

The effect of changing the direction of the constant inertial vector on the head without corresponding semicircular canal signals can be demonstrated in animals by destruction of their canals or by rendering them in-operative.

Tait and McNally (1934) observed the reactions of frogs with extirpated canals but intact otoliths. They found that the frogs responded normally to a slow tilt, with appropriate compensatory reactions, but that they exhibited rather strong anticompensatory reactions in the case of the rapid tilt. They concluded:

"Thus we see that under conditions of quick tilt in the intact animal, the canals and the utricular maculae work in some complementary fashion."

It is this complementary working of the semicircular canals and otoliths that the present chapter is attempting to elucidate.

Money and Scott (1962) found a similar reaction with blindfolded cats having intact otolith organs but plugged canals. The reactions of blindfolded, normal and operated cats to quick tilt are illustrated in Fig. 20. The altered direction of the vertical cannot be perceived immediately by the animal on the basis of vestibular cues. Immediately following such rapid tilt the animal would sense itself still horizontal and would not initiate appropriate compensatory reactions. A moving picture of the test seems to show that it falls off or is thrown off the platform during a quick tilt. The anticompensatory reactions reported by Tait and McNally for the frog appear to be absent.

The model predicts that under the conditions of the test an illusory acceleration A_i of the indicated direction and magnitude in Fig. 20 should occur. The anti-compensatory reaction of the frog to the actual movement would be compensatory to this illusion. It may be that aquatic animals, such as frogs and fish, are adapted

a

b

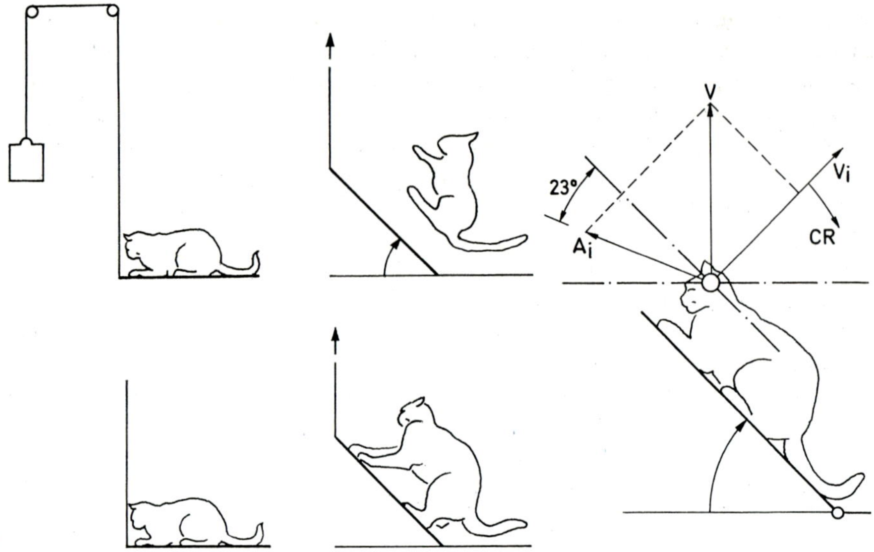

Fig. 20. Reflex reactions of normal and cat with plugged canals to quick tilt. 20a: Cat with plugged canals. 20b: Normal cat. 20c: Analysis of cat's illusion in (a), as predicted by model. V = Direction of true vertical with respect to cat; V_i = Direction of illusory vertical with respect to cat; A_i = Direction of illusory acceleration; C.R. = Compensatory reflex reaction (From MONEY and SCOTT, 1962)

to compensate for movements imposed upon them by waves, currents or eddies in their medium, while mammals have not acquired an adaptation of this kind. This would explain the presence of anticompensatory reactions with frogs and their absence in cats. The problem of fish behavior will be discussed later.

In the case of a slow tilt, the low-pass portion of the filter can follow the gradual changes of the values of the components of gravity acting on different head axes, and both frogs and cats compensate adequately for the tilt without cues of rotation from the canals and are able to maintain their equilibrium on the platform.

D. Rotation of Immersed Subjects

It would be hardly possible to design a more appropriate and dramatic experiment to demonstrate the operation of the model than one performed by STONE and LETKO (1964), in which they rotated subjects immersed in water.

Figure 21 illustrates one of the experimental conditions of the test where the axis of rotation passes approximately through the two ears of the subjects. The true motion and the illusion experienced by the subjects are depicted in this figure. The illusions of both attitude and motion are fully explained by the model currently proposed.

Under the test conditions the subjects are completely dependent upon otolith sensory data to determine either their position or movements in space. Flotation in water practically eliminates somesthetic cues. The tank in which they are enclosed blocks the view to the outside, and there are no canal signals because of the constant angular velocity. The otoliths are acted upon by gravity in the same manner as in the previously discussed tests of LOWENSTEIN and ROBERTS (1950) with fish preparations. The components of gravity acting along the z_π and y_π axes are oscillatory and 90° out of phase with each other. The static otolith signals corresponding to these components of gravity are not passed by the low-pass filter, and since the high-pass section is incapacitated because of lack of semicircular canal signals, the subjects do not perceive the rotation of their body.

At the same time the rates of changes of the gravity components acting on x_π and z_π axes must be interpreted as rate of change of acceleration, without semicircular canal signals to cancel out the effect of gravity. Integrated three times they produce an illusion of movement of the head around a circle. This illusion combines with that of no rotation of the body to produce the ferris wheel illusion. The sensed radius of the circle should be g/ω^2, where ω is the angular

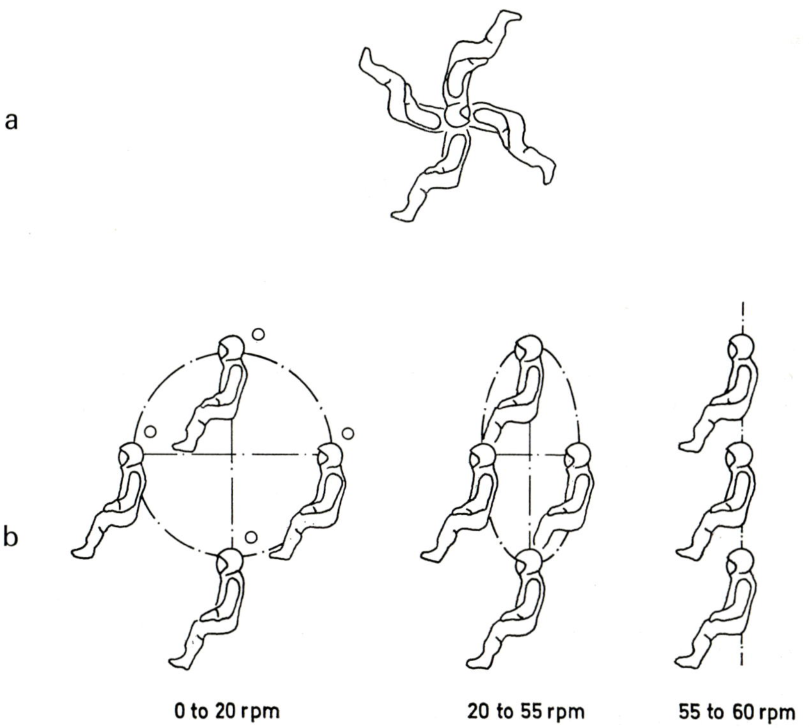

Fig. 21. Rotation of subjects immersed in water. From: "Some observations during weightlessness simulation with subjects immersed in a Rotating Water Tank" NASA-TN-2195, by STONE, R.W., and LETKO, W., 16 pp. Sept. 1964. Fig. a shows the successive positions assumed by the subject during rotation of the tank. Fig. b shows the illusory movement sensed by the subject. See text for explanation of illusion

velocity in radians per second. It may be interesting to note that the illusion is unaffected by the subject's cognitive knowledge of the "true" experimental situation.

Figure 21 shows that as the frequency of rotation is increased the sensed path of the body becomes elliptical and ultimately, a straight, vertical line. This was interpreted by STONE and LETKO to signify that the frequency response of the otolith organs along the longitudinal axis z_π is higher than along y_π axis. Another test, not illustrated here, shows that the response along the x_π axis is similar to that on the y_π axis. The difference in the responses of the otoliths along the normally vertical and horizontal axes of the head seems functionally consistent, as leg muscles can be applied more effectively along the former than the latter.

It may be estimated from the drawings that the illusory displacement on the y_π axes reaches 0.707 of the maximum amplitude at about 20 rev/min. The upper corner of frequency response of the corresponding transducer according to linear theory would then be $\omega_2 = 2.1$ radians, in approximate agreement with that of 1.5 in equations (37) by YOUNG et al. (1966) for the determination of linear velocity. According to the present model this function represents the responses of blocks 9 through 20 in Fig. 17. It is also in approximate agreement with the value estimated above from dynamic counterrolling data.

The experiment provides strong evidence for the validity of the present model. It indicates also that equation (37) by YOUNG et al. (1966) is a reasonably accurate representation of the measurement of linear velocity, although it cannot represent the peripheral response of the otoliths in the light of the above discussion.

E. Stimulation of the Canals by Linear Acceleration

A number of experiments on the response of the canals are not accountable in terms of conventional canal theory. Various explanations have been proposed, but the more interesting possibility is that the canals may be responsive to linear acceleration. We shall review briefly some of the pertinent experiments and attempt to interpret their results.

1. Stimulation by a Rotating Linear Vector of Acceleration

Such stimulation is most conveniently achieved with the rotation of a subject or preparation about a horizontal axis, barbecue-spit fashion (e.g., CORREIA and GUEDRY, 1964; GUEDRY, 1965a, b; GUEDRY, 1966; BENSON and BODIN, 1966). The findings of these experiments may be summarized briefly as follows:

Upon the start of rotation a normal subject experiences a normal nystagmus. As a constant velocity of 60°/sec is reached and maintained, the slow phase velocity of nystagmus decays but is not totally suppressed as is the case for rotation about a vertical axis. It then persists for the duration of the test, undergoing cyclic changes at a frequency of once per revolution. Upon cessation of the rotation the nystagmus decays faster than in the case of rotation about a vertical axis. L-D subjects do not experience continuous nystagmus, only a reversing cyclic fluctuation of the slow phase. At speeds of over 30 rev/min the nystagmus of normal subjects resembles that of L-D subjects.

Normal subjects experience a sensation of continuous rotation, generally combined with an illusory movement of the head and body about a circle in an approximately vertical plane. At speeds of over 30 rev/min the subjects experience only the motion of the body as a whole. The sensed orientation of the long axis of the body is generally realistic as horizontal. L-D subjects do not experience continuous rotation, only the movement of the body as a whole about a circle. The sensed orientation of the long axis of the body may be highly unrealistic, sometimes reaching the vertical.

The above observations are obviously not proof of canal stimulation. Nystagmus can be stimulated optokinetically when a stationary subject observes a rotating environment (e.g. MELVILL JONES, 1966; COLLINS et al., 1970). At the same time, it was pointed out earlier that otolith stimulation can cause a sensation of rotation in the oculogravic illusion when the canals are silent. A central perceptual scheme must be assumed to be responsible for the interpretation of all sensory data in terms of either a rotation of the body in space, and/or a rotation of the environment with respect to the body. The first creates a sensation of rotation useful in monitoring body reflexes, the second monitors eye movements for clearer vision.

Canal signals are only one of a number of possible inputs to this central scheme. They generally can be interpreted as a rotation of the body in space as well as with respect to the environment, and they generally cause both a sensation of rotation and nystagmus, but not always. In the postrotational situation, for instance, the evidence of the canals is rejected when it conflicts with visual sensory data in a lighted room. It may be surmised that if one or more sources of sounds were disposed around a rotating subject, or if he was allowed to touch a close-fitting concentric wall, he would experience an indefinite sensation of rotation and nystagmus in the absence of canal signals.

There seems to be no reason why the otoliths and somesthetic sensors should not be adequate inputs to perceptual functions in the determination of rotation of the body in the barbecue situation. This author was given a ride on the equipment used in the tests, (courtesy Guedry) and can vouch that the sensation of rotation in his case was unmistakable and appeared to originate mainly from somesthetic sensory data, as the body successively rested on a metal frame and hung from the straps. It must be clear that the filtered otolith signals would give no information on rotation, and if the otoliths have a part in the sensation, it must be through their unfiltered signals.

In the light of the above remarks, the experimental results of the barbecue-spit rotation can be interpreted as follows:

At the beginning of rotation the canals give true information regarding the rotation of the body. As the canal response decays the somesthetic sensors, and perhaps the unfiltered signals from the otoliths may indicate rotation. There would be, however, a loss of "credibility" of this interpretation with a reduction of nystagmus, because of the loss of canal signals.

At the same time, without canal signals, the rate of change of the gravity components acting on the type 2 cells must be interpreted as rate of change of acceleration. Integrated once, they are sensed as two oscillatory linear acceleration vectors at right angles with each other in space, and 90° out of phase in time. Integrated twice more they produce an illusion of body rotation in a vertical plane, as in the case of the immersed subjects. Perceptual processes interpret these cues as best they can, in terms of a combined movement of the body as a whole in a modified ferris wheel illusion, and continuous rotation, with different emphasis on one type of illusion or the other with different individuals. At the same time a reversing nystagmus corresponding to the illusory acceleration is superimposed on the continuous one.

During the deceleration, a canal signal is generated signifying rotation in a direction opposite to that indicated by somesthetic or otolithic cues. Nystagmus is extinguished rapidly because of the conflict.

It may be surmised that somesthetic signals are adapted to signify rotation for a normal subject by correlation with canal signals. Such adaptation cannot take place in the case of an L-D subject and he interprets the forces of gravity on his body only as acceleration. Integration, as before, causes a sensation of body movement about a circle without continuous rotation. Incidentally, the fact that L-D subjects experience reversing nystagmus indicates that somesthetic cues might be a factor in linear acceleration nystagmus. They are perhaps also a factor in normal subjects.

The otoliths of the normal subjects can also be effective in determining the angle of the long axis of the body with respect to the horizontal. The signals from cells polarized along the long axis of the body should not be affected by the rotation and should reverse sign for a head-up, as compared to a feet-up position. The normal subject, as indicated earlier, maintains a realistic estimate of the orientation of the long axis of his body, while the L-D subjects do not.

Nystagmus of indefinite duration could only be caused by a constant deflection of the cupula. Steer (1967) has proposed a model which would account for such a deflection when the canals are stimulated by a rotating linear vector of acceleration. However, the theory of adaptation discussed earlier predicts that a canal signal due to a constant deflection of the cupula, should adapt to a zero value. According to this theory it could not be the cause of a nystagmus of indefinite duration.

It seems, therefore, that the barbecue-spit rotation experiments do not provide evidence of canal stimulation by a rotating linear vector of acceleration. In the view of this author they are better explained in terms of central functions.

2. Recordings from the CNS of a Cat during Stimulation by a Rotating Linear Vector of Acceleration

Benson et al. (1970) examined the responses from units in the neural centers of the cat during stimulation by a rotating linear vector of acceleration. The stimulus was provided by a platform suspended by four parallel wires, which was made to move bodily in a circle without angular rotation. The cells selected for examination had to meet the criteria of being unresponsive to linear acceleration along two orthogonal axes, and being responsive to angular acceleration. Responses elicited from these cells under the conditions of the test could be taken as evidence of their stimulation by a rotating linear vector of acceleration.

However, the cells that were so selected could have been "rotation-dependent" rather than "canal-dependent", reflecting the output of the central perceptual scheme discussed earlier. This scheme would have interpreted a canal signal during the diagnostic tests as signifying rotation, but would have interpreted other appropriate sensory signals similarly. Possibly also the response may have represented the actual canal response, adapted, as suggested earlier, to a central estimate of body rotation, based on the weighted responses of other sensors. The effect, however, would have been one of adaptation, not of direct stimulation by linear acceleration.

Some observations by BENSON et al. tend to support the view that the canals are not directly stimulated by the linear acceleration vector. They showed that units which responded with an increase of the resting frequency for, say, clockwise angular acceleration, would respond with a higher frequency for parallel counterclockwise rotation. The opposite response is observed for cells responding with increased frequency for counterclockwise angular acceleration.

In the case of the rotation of the body as if on a spit it can be seen that the gravity vector is fixed in space and therefore rotates with respect to the body in the opposite direction to the body in space. In the case of the parallel swing, however, the linear vector rotates with respect to the cat preparation in the same direction as that of the swing. It follows that a cat adapted in normal activity to interpret somesthetic and otolith signals as rotation would sense this rotation in a direction opposite that of the swing.

A rotation-dependent cell which increases its frequency for counterclockwise rotation in the barbecue situation would be expected to reduce it for the same direction of parallel swing rotation. Actually the record shows that this occurs for some units but that in general the frequency of the cell only increases more for one direction than the other. We must learn more about central processes before we can hope to make accurate predictions of the behavior of central units. The direction of the change, however, is in accord with the above interpretation. This view is further borne out by tests with a normal cat, which show that the slow-phase nystagmus beats in the same direction as that of the swing rotation.

It is well known that slow phase nystagmus normally beats in a direction opposite to the sensed rotation which must therefore be opposite to that of the swing. BENSON et al. noted a cyclic component in the response, which will be discussed later.

The recordings from the CNS of cat during parallel-swing rotation, like those from humans during "barbecue-spit" rotation, provide no clear evidence of the stimulation of the canals by linear acceleration.

3. Stimulation in a Counterrotating Centrifuge

Stimulation by a rotating linear vector of acceleration can also be achieved in a counterrotating centrifuge. In this experiment, a subject is seated on a rotating chair located on the arm of a centrifuge. The chair and the arm are rotated at the same speed but in opposite directions so that the subject always faces in the same direction. He experiences, therefore, no angular stimulation, only a rotating centripetal vector. In contrast with barbecue stimulation, the subject experiences no angular rotation at the beginning of the test.

MONEY (1966) used experiments of this kind to investigate the possible effect of the initial angular stimulation at the beginning of the barbecue tests. He reported that nystagmus was observed in six out of eight subjects. An illustration of the response of one subject shows reversing nystagmus, while another illustration shows continuous nystagmus with a superimposed one per revolution cyclic variation.

MONEY reported (personal communication) that his subjects experienced no sensation of continuous rotation, and only exhibited nystagmus. Similarly GRAYBIEL and JOHNSON (1963) reported sensations of modified ferris wheel illusions among their subjects, but did not report that they experienced sensations of continuous rotation. As indicated earlier, sensations of continuous rotation and nystagmus are the normal response for barbecue-spit rotation.

Counterrotating and barbecue-spit rotation produce precisely the same vestibular and nearly the same somesthetic stimulations. Yet, the former situation is not interpreted as body rotation in space, while the latter is. There must, be, therefore, other inputs to the central evaluation scheme besides sensory data. Rotation of the body about a horizontal axis is apparently given a higher probability of occurrence than rotation about a vertical axis, probably because of previous life experiences such as rolling in bed. The presence of nystagmus is a reflection of the fact that perceptual functions interpret sensory data to signify rotation, assumed rather illogically to occur in the environment about a fixed body. Central processes are rather heuristic in nature and not always rational.

Examination of data on counterrolling in experiments by STEER (1967) on humans indicates that humans, like cats, judge the direction of the rotation of their body (assuming the usual correspondence between nystagmus and sensation of rotation) to be in a direction opposite to that of the centrifuge.

Counterrotation stimulation does not throw new light on the possible stimulation of the canals by a rotating linear vector of acceleration. It emphasizes the fact that the response to a given stimulation involves complex central processes and inputs other than sensory.

4. Stimulation by Constant Linear Acceleration

Such stimulation is best achieved in a centrifuge. The literature on the subject is quite extensive (e.g. BENSON and WHITESIDE, 1961; BENSON, 1962; CRAMPTON, 1962; LANDSBERG et al., 1965; BENSON and BODIN, 1966; CRAMPTON, 1966). The last two references present a clear summary of previous findings.

One of the more puzzling aspect of these experiments is the dependence of nystagmus upon the orientation of the subject on the centrifuge. BENSON (1962) showed that for a clockwise rotation of the centrifuge, and a terminal centripetal acceleration of 3.07 g, a subject facing to the right of the radius would experience a greater nystagmus than one facing toward the center. Nystagmus would then continue indefinitely in the same direction. If the subject should face to the left of center, the initial nystagmus would be reduced, would reverse direction and would also last indefinitely. The nystagmus is not accompanied by a sensation of rotation.

CRAMPTON (1966) pointed out that the discrepancy between the two responses is more marked when the subjects are facing tangentially. A subject will sense accurately the direction and magnitude of his movement during the initial period of the centrifuge acceleration. As the oculogravic illusion asserts itself, the subject feels that he is being tilted sideways. For a clockwise rotation of the centrifuge a subject facing in the direction of rotation will feel that his body is inclined towards his right. His sensed direction of rotation due to canal stimulation would still be about the long axis of his body. This axis, however, is now tilted with respect to his sensed vertical so that oscillatory otolith and somesthetic signals would be expected to occur. Because of the lack of such signals, central processes "conclude" that the body has stopped rotating. But the subject may experience the illusion that the centrifuge has tilted with the chair and has continued its rotation about the body now fixed in space. The nystagmus caused by such an illusion would be in the same direction as that caused originally by the rotation of the centrifuge. The initial nystagmus is then increased in strength and persists indefinitely in the initial direction. There are, however, no sensations of body rotation. If the subject faces in the opposite direction, the nystagmus due to the above illusion is opposite to that due to the centrifuge rotation. The initial nystagmus is reduced in strength and is reversed after the canals have become silent.

The above perceptual interpretation of sensory data is not without conflicts, but it is probably the best that can be achieved under the conditions of the test. Not much credibility is placed on its validity in perception as the nystagmus is very slight. The theory of the adaptation of the canal signals to a constant deflection of the cupula would also argue against a constant response of the canals. Plausible explanations of the results of tests in the centrifuge can be formulated without invoking the stimulation of the canals by a linear vector of acceleration.

F. Models for the Direct Stimulation of the Canal by Acceleration

The above discussion has emphasized central processes in accounting for observed responses. It does not, however, rule out a possible contributory effect of direct stimulation of the canals.

Correia and Money (1970) found that cats with plugged canals still exhibited nystagmus, but of reduced magnitude, when rotated barbecue fashion. Janeke (1968) reported that severing the utricular nerve bilaterally in the rabbit abolished nystagmus. On the other hand, continuous nystagmus was abolished in cats with plugged canals in a counterrotating centrifuge (Money, 1966).

The discrepancy between the responses of cats with inoperative canals in the barbecue and counterrotating situation was explained by Money (personal communication) in terms of the greater acceleration force in the former over the latter type of stimulation. He also pointed out that cats in which continuous nystagmus was suppressed by plugging the canals when tested in the counterrotating centrifuge exhibited nystagmus, although of lesser amplitude, in barbecue stimulation. On the basis of the above limited experimental data it can be argued that direct stimulation is a contributory factor in the observed response but that the otoliths are the principal one. It could be, however, that the difference of response before and after blocking the canals is the result of damage to the overall organ by the surgery.

LOWENSTEIN (1970) pointed out that the problem can only be settled by recording directly from primary neurons under stimulation of the canals by linear acceleration, and undertook such an experimental program. He reported that preliminary tests with elasmobranch canal preparations had demonstrated a definite response of some units to a tilting of the preparation about an axis passing through the plane of the canals. Although preliminary, these tests seem to constitute the most convincing evidence to date regarding the response of the canals to linear acceleration.

The author reported some success in observing a response to a rotating linear vector of acceleration. However, he found that fewer cells were responsive to this form of stimulation than they were to tilting, and to a lesser degree. It is hoped that continuing investigations will throw new light on this type of response.

A central problem is that of determining the mechanism of the stimulation of the canal to linear acceleration and the function it may serve if any.

It has been suggested that the effect may be caused by a difference between the density of the cupula and that of the endolymph. CRAMPTON (1966) investigated this hypothesis. He observed the response of canal units in the brainstem of rats differently oriented on a centrifuge. The theory would call for either an increase or decrease of the initial response during the acceleration period, then a constant excitatory or inhibitory response with constant angular velocity, depending on the orientation of the animal with respect to the radius. CRAMPTON found a cell which responded approximately as predicted by the theory and one which did not, the latter response adapting to a nearly zero output. Because of the conflicting responses, he concluded that the canals did not respond to linear acceleration and that the effects observed were of central origin.

It could be, however, that the cell which responded in accordance with the theory was nonadaptive, while the other was highly adaptive. Experiments such as those conducted by MALCOLM and MELVILL JONES (1969) seems to show that the integrated effect of all cells, as measured by nystagmus, adapts to a zero response for a condition of constant deflection of the cupula, in the case of constant angular acceleration. FERNANDEZ and GOLDBERG (1971) have shown, however, that some cells are nonadaptive.

STEER (1967) proposed an ingenious model which would account for the fact that linear acceleration in the diagnostic tests of BENSON et al. (1970) did not affect the cells while a rotating vector of acceleration supposedly did. He postulated that a difference between the gravity of endolymph and perilymph may cause a "pumping action," pushing the endolymph toward the ampulla and causing a permanent deflection of the cupula. The mechanism would not predict any effect in the Lowenstein or Crampton experiments.

Another explanation may be suggested, based on the canal model presented earlier. As postulated in this model the roof of the ampulla has a spiral shape with respect to the crista. It follows that the cupula has a larger area toward the wider side than it has toward the narrower one. An equal increase of pressure on both sides, caused by a step input of linear acceleration or gravity, would then cause a resultant force in the direction of the narrower channel. This force would act directly on the apex of the cupula without appreciable endolymph displacement, and would be proportional to acceleration or gravity acting in the plane of the canals.

The signal would then be expected to decay as a function of the constant of adaptation of the particular cell.

Melvill Jones (1967) reported that during diagnostic tests intended to single out cells responsive only to the canals, some cells were observed to respond to both linear and angular acceleration and were rejected. However, in view of the findings of Lowenstein (1970), the responses could have been purely canal-dependent. According to the present model of the canal, they would have been associated, then, with primary units near the apex of the crista. They would be expected to have a high degree of adaptability, with a high leading component content. On the other hand the cells responding purely to angular acceleration should be associated with cells near the base of the crista with relatively low adaptability.

A canal system in accordance with the presently proposed model, or one involving a different density between cupula and endolymph, would respond sinusoidally to stimulation by a rotating linear vector of acceleration. It should give no information about continuous rotation which would have to be derived from central interpretation of other sensory data. Steer's model could not account for an oscillatory response, nor as indicated earlier for the response to the tilt of a preparation about an axis in the plane of the canals.

Melvill Jones (1967) and Benson et al. (1970) recorded such an oscillatory response. It is not clear, however, why the cells responding in this manner should not have responded similarly during the diagnostic tests with sinusoidal linear acceleration. It may be that adaptation of the canals to other sensory data by a process suggested earlier could have caused the cupula to move to a position of greater sensitivity in the ampulla. But the possibility that angular movement may have been excited in the swing in spite of all precautions to avoid it cannot be ruled out.

It is difficult to imagine a specific function which may be served by the response of the canals to linear acceleration. Possibly it may be of value in canceling out Coriolis effects during combined rotation and inclination of the head in the course of normal body movements. But it could also be a useless response, inherent in a scheme adapted primarily to the generation of a leading component in the canal signal and detectable only with single units. According to the model the effect on one canal should be opposed by that on the opposite side of the head, so that linear acceleration would have no effect on the integrated canal response. It is hoped that further investigations will throw further light on the problem, particularly insofar as it may affect a model concept of the canals.

The operation of the vestibular system can only be described in terms of the integrated response of canals, otoliths and central functions. An attempt was made earlier to model the functions responsible for the separation of sensory signals related to acceleration from those related to gravity. A model of the perceptual functions that interpret various modalities of sensory data in terms of rotation of the body with respect to space and/or with respect to a background of interest, with sensation and/or nystagmus as outputs must be formulated.

G. Coriolis Illusion

The vestibular reactions discussed above have illustrated some of the disturbances that occur when the high-pass section of the filter is inoperative because of the absence of semicircular signals. It is appropriate to examine cases where the low-pass section is inoperative. The so-called Coriolis illusion illustrates this condition.

This well-known illusion is caused by cross-coupling between canals during combined turns of the head about two orthogonal axes, outside the frequency response of one or both canals (e.g. GUEDRY and MONTAGUE, 1961; MAYNE, 1965c). Experiments have shown that the effect is to cause a strong illusory sensation of rotation of the body about an axis other than the other two.

A subject seated in a chair which is rotating counterclockwise, for instance, will experience an illusion of forward rotation if he inclines his head toward his left shoulder, and of rotation backward if he inclines it toward the right. These illusions are predicted by present theory. However a linear, as well as a rotary illusory movement, has been observed (POWELL, 1964).

The proposed model accounts for both the linear and the rotary illusions. In accordance with previous discussion any stimulation of the canals must cause an input to the high-pass section of filters 6 and 7 in Fig. 15. The inclination of the head to the right or to the left causes a normal corresponding input to both the low-pass and high-pass sections. The extent of head movement in this direction is then properly interpreted. The cross-coupling stimulation of the canals, having angular acceleration components in the sagittal plane, will similarly cause an input to the high-pass section of the appropriate filters. There will be no corresponding input from the otoliths, however, since the head has not rotated in this plane. It can be shown that the overall effect will be a sensation of rotation about a transverse axis (assuming an inclination of the head by 45°) and of a sinusoidal linear acceleration in the sagittal plane.

This latter effect is clearly demonstrated in a series of tests by LETKO and STONE (1967). They rotated subjects lying on a platform with the long axis of their body oriented either axially or tangentially. In the case of a tangential orientation, the authors show by conventional cross-coupling theory that a nod of the head should cause a sensation of rotation about the long axis of the subject's body. A motion-picture record, a copy of which was kindly supplied to the author by Langley Research Center, shows that the eyes of the subjects perform a horizontal nystagmus as expected from this prediction, but that they also perform an oscillatory counterrolling movement. The situation is quite analogous to horizontal rotation discussed earlier, except that in the case currently under discussion the semicircular canals are stimulated but the otoliths are not, while the reverse is true for horizontal rotation. Both types of stimulation should cause counterrolling. No attempt was made to observe it in the barbecue tests, but its occurrence was demonstrated in the tests by KELLOGG (1965) during the rotation of subjects, also about the horizontal. Real or illusory sensation of acceleration, in other words the "perception" of acceleration, on the transverse axis of the head is the adequate stimulus for counterrolling. The tests bear out the prediction of the model to the effect that such a perception should occur during Coriolis stimulation.

H. Space Sickness

It is a well documented fact that space can cause disturbances similar to motion on earth (BILLINGHAM, 1966; YUGANOV et al., 1966). The present model accounts for these disturbances in that it shows that space can cause conflicts in spatial perception (Mayne, 1966d, 1969a–b, 1970).

Two such modes will be considered:

1. The Inverted Illusion

The feeling of standing in an inverted position has been experienced by astronauts in a space environment and by subjects during sub-g maneuvers in an airplane (Graybiel and Kellogg, 1966). Sjoberg (1970) proposed an hypothesis for this illusion in terms of the effect of zero g on the otolith organs. Dzendolet (1971) reported on the experiences of subjects during parabolic sub-g flights in support of this hypothesis. His point of view is not far from that proposed by Mayne (1966d) in terms of the present model.

With the head held erect and motionless in a 1 g environment the dynamic portion of the otolith signal on the z_π axis is zero, while the static signal corresponds to the 1 g input. The otoliths are silent on the other two axes. In the case of a jump from a platform to the ground, a short downward acceleration is experienced, then a deceleration as the body is brought to rest as gently as possible by flexion of the legs. There is an immediate response from the dynamic portion of the otolith transducer. This response is interpreted properly through central processing as downward movement, then a return to a motionless state. The rapid change of the input does not affect the static response because of the low-pass filter, and there is no alteration to the sense of the vertical.

In the case of zero g there is a constant reduction of the static signal on the z_π axis over that occurring on earth, while the static signals on the other two axes are zero. The reduction of the static signal on the z_π axis can be interpreted as a constant acceleration and therefore as gravity directed toward the feet. There are two situations that are analogous to this pattern of stimulation on earth: a prolonged constantly accelerated free fall, and standing in an inverted position. An approximation of the first occurs during the first part of a delayed parachute jump or in a ski jump. Standing on the head is analogous to the zero g situation in that the static component of the response on the z_π axis is reduced and that the signal is zero on the other two axes. It differs, however, in the magnitude of the reduction: two g for the inverted position on earth, one g for the weightlessness situation. Qualitatively, however, the two otolithic responses are similar, and are interpreted in the same manner. It is significant that zero g is not necessary to produce the illusion, only a reduction of the constant value of acceleration (Graybiel and Kellogg, 1966), although the magnitude of the reduction necessary to produce the illusion has not been established.

It is significant that blind goldfish will swim in an inverted position during a period of zero g in a parabolic airplane flight (von Baumgarten, 1970).

The "credibility" of the illusion at the perceptual level may not be very high, at least among astronauts, as it is unstable and is not experienced by all subjects. It would be interesting to test two sets of subjects in parabolic airplane flights; one set selected among parachute or ski jumpers, and another set selected from yoga practitioners, and see whether one set would experience primarily an illusion of falling and the other an inverted position.

DZENDOLET (1971) made an interesting observation. Upon entering the reduced g portion of the parabola, during the pull up of the airplane, subjects facing forward sensed that they were being rotated backward, subjects facing to the rear felt that they were rotated forward until they reached the inverted position. The direction of the sensed rotation was, therefore, the same with respect to the airplane and independent of the way the subjects were facing. In the transition between the dive and the climb of the airplane, during the pull up, there is a sharp change of the direction of the inertial vector with respect to the airplane and to the subject. The change is made up of the pitch up of the airplane and of its deceleration in the climb. The author points out that the rate of turn of the airplane is too slow to be detected by the semicircular canals. The change due to deceleration occurs, of course, without rotation of the airplane. The total effect is one of rotating the apparent vertical, as determined by the nearly constant inertial vector, in a forward direction with respect of the plane. The change is not detected immediately by the otolith and, as in the case of the oculogravic illusion, there is a slow sensed rotation toward the back of the airplane to bring the body in proper angular relation with the illusory direction of the vertical. The rotation caused by this process cannot exceed 90° and probably would not exceed 45° or 60°. The effect of reduced g, as explained above, comes into play bringing the subject to the illusory, fully inverted position. It must be clear, as pointed out by DZENDOLET, that since astronauts are subject to the inverted illusion, it is not essential to approach zero g in a parabolic flight in order to create it.

2. Disorientation due to Head Movements

In order to account for disorientations in space due to head movements we must assume, as indicated earlier, a somewhat different processing from that illustrated in Fig. 15. The angle θ between the vertical and the z_π axis must be taken from the joint determination of this value by different sensors. The values of $g_x = g \sin \theta$ and $g_z = g \cos \theta$ can then be computed by appropriate trigonometric operations and a multiplication by the g value to which the organism is adapted. Inclining the head in a different g environment should then cause errors in the processing for the attitude of the head and for its linear movement. The processing indicated in Fig. 15 would interpret a head movement in any g environment properly.

That the disturbance may occur in space as the result of head movements is well documented. BILLINGHAM (1966), for instance, quotes as follows from a Russian report about the reactions of the Russian cosmonauts FEOKTISTOV and YUGATOV in the voskhod flight (see also YUGANOV et al., 1966). "Alongside illusions, especially in the middle of the flight, an unpleasant sensation of slight, short-term giddiness was observed when the head was turned sharply." We shall examine the illusions predicted by the model for an astronaut without previous adaptation to space immediately following an inclination of his head to his left by 20° while standing on the moon.

The canal signals are the same as they would be on earth. The high-pass section of the filter responding to the canal input operates to reduce the output of the filter associated with the z_π axis and increase that on the x_π axis by amounts corresponding to those required in a 1 g environment for a 20° turn. But the initial values of the filter output before the turn correspond only to 1/6 g. The correction effected by the high-pass section of the filter will, therefore, be in error. The illusion in the attitude and linear movement can be computed under these conditions for the proposed model. We can write:

$$
\begin{aligned}
\Delta z_\pi &= -(1-\cos 20°)\mathrm{g} = -0.06\, g \\
\Delta x_\pi &= \mathrm{g} \sin 20° = 0.342\, g \\
z_{\pi o} &= 0.16\ \mathrm{g} \\
x_{\pi o} &= 0 \\
z_{\pi o} + \Delta z_\pi &= (0.16 - 0.06)\mathrm{g} = 0.10\ \mathrm{g} \\
x_{\pi o} + \Delta x_\pi &= 0.34\ \mathrm{g} \\
\theta_i &= \tan^{-1}\frac{0.342}{0.1} = 74°,
\end{aligned}
$$

where

Δz_π and Δx_π = change in filter outputs effected through high-pass sections on z_π and x_π axes.

$z_{\pi o}$ and $x_{\pi o}$ = initial output signal of filters on z_π and x_π axes.

θ_i = illusory rotation of the head.

The astronaut would experience an illusory rotation 54° greater than the actual rotation.

There would be also an error in canceling out the effect of the rate of change of the gravity component, resulting in an illusory acceleration. The effect would be the difference between the actual change of the component of 1/6 g acting on each axis, and the correction that would have been effected on earth on the basis of 1 g. We would have:

$$
\begin{aligned}
\ddot{z}_{\pi i} &= -(1-\cos 20°)\ 0.16\ \mathrm{g} + \Delta z_\pi = 0.09\, g \\
\ddot{x}_{\pi i} &= 0.16\ \mathrm{g} \sin 20° - \Delta x_\pi = -0.284\, g
\end{aligned}
$$

where $\ddot{z}_{\pi i}$ and $\ddot{x}_{\pi i}$ = the illusory acceleration experienced on each axis.

These two illusions would combine to produce an illusion of a magnitude:

$$A_i = \sqrt{0.09^2 + 0.284^2} = 0.30\, g$$

The prediction of the model for the operation of the vestibular organs in space, should be no more surprising than the illusions demonstrated experimentally during the rotation of immersed subjects, also predicted by the model, and also involving illusions of both attitude and movement. The space illusion, as described, could only be perceived in the absence of other sensory data. Under normal visual stimulus, the inclination of the head would cause a brief unpleasant sensation, as described in the above quotation. But brief unpleasantness can easily add up, in time, to severe nausea. Extensive experience in the piloting of jet aircrafts during aerobatic maneuvers appear to reduce space disturbances. The Russians, Feoktistov and Yugarov, mentioned earlier as having suffered disorders in space, were nonpilots. Other members of the same crew, who were jet pilots, were undisturbed. On the other hand Titov and Schwickhart, both jet pilots, were disturbed. While the training of astronauts in jet airplaned aerobatics has provided some adaptation to the space situation it does not appear to have fully resolved the problem.

I. The Effect of Head Movements on Motion Sickness

JOHNSON et al. (1951) found that the incidence of motion sickness can be increased by head movements. It follows from the previous discussion that when the head is subjected to linear acceleration outside the normal response of the otoliths, a head movement will be improperly corrected, causing a perceptual conflict.

K. Fish Behavior

There are obvious similarities between the vestibular organs of fish and mammals. The Steinhausen model of the canals applicable to man was evolved from experiments on the organs of fish and subsequently tested by various investigators in fish preparations. The canal response of monkeys resembles that of fish in so far as adaptation and leading component content are concerned. Counterrolling data and references in the literature about recordings from the otolith organs of mammals indicate, as discussed earlier, that the otolith responses of earth- and water-bound species are similar. The conclusions drawn here from the responses of the otoliths of fish, seem to lead to a consistent systems concept of the vestibular functions of land animals as an inertial system.

It would be tempting, therefore, to extend this systems concept to the fish, and look for a similar central processing of peripheral sensory data by a low pass-high pass filtering technique. Some recent experiments by VON BAUMGARTEN et al. (1971) demonstrate that this concept is not simply and directly applicable to the fish. The authors observed the movements of blinded goldfish in a tank of water during acceleration in an automobile. They recorded the movements of the fish and the readings of an accelerometer, by means of a motion picture camera. From their data, they plotted the magnitude of the resultant acceleration and gravity, the direction of an apparent horizontal (taken as normal to the resultant of gravity and acceleration) and the fish attitude v/s time. It is apparent from these data that the fish responds quickly to a change in the direction of the inertial vector. The authors also presented a photograph of two fish, one facing toward the front of the car and the other toward the rear. Both turned in the direction of the apparent horizontal, with only a small delay, one fish pitching up while the other dived. This is in contrast to the reaction of man to a sudden change of the direction of the inertial vector in the oculogravic illusion experiments where, as noted earlier, the change is only perceived gradually with considerable delay. Actually, the control system of fish for attitude and movement would be expected to have undergone a different adaptation from those of land animals. The head of the fish is attached to its body so that independent head movements need not be taken into account. The true direction of the vertical should have far less significance for the fish than for a land animal. It is not threatened with a fall, and the gravitational vector of force on its body need not be taken into account in the programming of body movements, as it is *cancelled* out by its buoyancy.

The apparent horizontal, on the other hand, is a very significant parameter in the behavior of the fish, corresponding, as it does, to a locus of constant water pressure. It is easy to imagine (particularly when it has been already demonstrated) that the fish would monitor its body position to remain parallel to the continually varying apparent horizontal as the result of waves, currents or eddies. There is no need for filtering the otolith signal in the determination of its direction, as it follows quite accurately any of its disturbances.

The fish possesses an otolith organ, the lagena, that land animals do not have. LOWENSTEIN and ROBERTS (1952) found that the response of this organ is highly sensitive to small inclinations of their preparations with respect to the vertical. It can be speculated that it fulfills a significant function in the more complex problem of the fish stabilization in cooperation with other organs. MCNAUGHTON and MCNALLY (1946) pointed out that the lagena has "an equilibrium function in the frog." There is a need for the fuller development of the interrelated functions of the more complex vestibular organs of the fish. In any case, the problems of differentiating between the effects of gravity and those of acceleration appear to be as real under water as on land. HARDEN JONES (1956), for instance, found that if the tank in which a fish is swimming is accelerated linearly, the fish will turn in the direction of the acceleration vector. If accelerated along its body axis toward its head, it will not turn; but it will make a 180° turn if accelerated toward its tail. VON BAUMGARTEN et al. confirmed this observation and found that the stimulus for the reaction was the rate of change of acceleration. As indicated earlier, the otoliths of the fish provide a measurement of this modality. But the fish must react to rate of change of acceleration, not rate of change of the gravity vector. The above authors determined that the threshold for the reaction was of the order of 4.5 g/sec. A fish pitching down at a rate of 250°/sec, will experience a gravitational acceleration directed toward its tail, of the same order of magnitude. Yet it must not be caused to make an immediate 180° turn. A cancellation of this effect can be performed as proposed here for land animals, in terms of canal signals.

It can be speculated further that the fish must rely on its vestibular apparatus to a greater degree than land animals in carrying out programmed movements, as in the pursuit of a smaller fish or the escape from a larger one, the reaching of a bit of food, or simply maneuvering about in the water for no apparent reason. There, again, a distinction must be made between gravity and acceleration. It can be speculated that the normal stabilization control may be cut off during such movements, and that the fish maintains a perception of space and of the vertical. When the fish dashes forward, for instance, the control must not cause it to dive as it does in the accelerated tank.

VON BAUMGARTEN et al. showed a plot of the response of the fish in a tank of water to oscillations on a parallel swing. The fish altered its attitude with very little lag, and by an amount corresponding quite closely to the alteration of the direction of the apparent horizontal. When accelerated in the automobile, however, there was a large overshoot of the fish response. A change in the angle of the inertial vector by 25° was accompanied by a change of the attitude of the fish by 85°. Biological controls are normally more accurate in the performance of an intended function. It must be that some factor, other than an intent to maintain the fish in an apparently horizontal position, enters into the control equation. We can speculate that the fish turns, first, under the normal stabilizing control in response to the inclination of the apparent horizontal. Acceleration and velocity, measured by the rest of the system and interpreted on the basis of previous adaptation, can only signify to the fish that it has been caught in a swift current. A reflex reaction to escape it by continuing its rotation beyond horizontal may then be generated. Whatever the explanation, the phenomenon seems to require the postulation of another mechanism besides that of a faulty control loop, normally intended to maintain horizontality.

Von Baumgarten et al. argued that a fish was very unlikely to be exposed to a rate of change of acceleration in the order of 4.5 g/sec and that the reaction of turning toward the direction of the acceleration would therefore be useless. It does not seem impossible, however, that a fish would experience a rate of change of acceleration of this magnitude when caught in a swift current in a stream or in breakers in the sea. It may be good strategy for the fish to turn in the direction of the current, rather than "buck it", in order to see where it is going so that it may perform an avoidance maneuver if necessary before crashing into a rock. That the fish tends to swim with the current is indicated by another observation of Harden Jones (1957). He noted that if any part of the body of the fish should happen to touch the bottom or sides of the tank while being carried by the water, the fish would instantly turn in the direction of the water movement. Whether the direction of the movement is sensed by actual contact with a fixed object, or by the vestibular organs, the reaction is the same, serving apparently the same function. But again the magnitude and direction of the fish velocity can only be sensed properly by the vestibular organs if gravity is excluded from the computations.

No account of the fish vestibular system can exclude the complicated interaction between eye movements and vestibular stimulation demonstrated by Lee (1894–1895). Blinding the fish must not only eliminate visual sensory data, but must also eliminate vestibular signals which are normally added to vision. Mayne (1965b) suggested that vision and the vestibular apparatus may collaborate in the pursuit of a fish to set up a collision course through a constant bearing navigation, similar to that applicable to a missile air-to-air guidance system.

The vestibular apparatus of the fish appears to be more highly evolved than that of land animals. Neither can escape the physical requirement of distinguishing between signals related to gravity and those related to acceleration, although, as demonstrated by von Baumgarten et al. (1971), such a distinction is not needed or made in monitoring the attitude of the fish. Further experimentation is needed, as well as observations of fish in their natural habitat in relation to movement of the water, to elucidate the vestibular organs of fish.

L. Pathologic Disorders

Hopefully, the present model may be of value in the investigation of pathologic disorders of the vestibular system, and in the development of improved diagnostic techniques. A few guarded comments based primarily on theoretical considerations of the present model, and only on a most cursory review of clinical literature may be permitted.

1. Positional Nystagmus

The facts that linear acceleration is an adequate stimulus for nystagmus (Niven et al., 1966), and that illusions of accelerations are equally adequate, as indicated earlier, are of significance to the problem. It is also significant that such illusions can be produced by improperly coordinated responses between otoliths and semicircular canals.

If, for instance, the canals should be inoperative and the otolith normal, the syndrome would be similar to that observed by Money et al. (1962) in cats with plugged canals. It can be further speculated that for an inclination of the head toward the right shoulders, the vestibular signals would tend to cause illusions of both attitude and acceleration as indicated earlier for the space situation. The lack of canal signal about the turn and the presence of proprioceptive data to the effect that the body has rotated with respect to the head could be interpreted as signifying that the body stands at an angle with respect to the head fixed in space. On the other hand, without canal signals the rate of change of the components of gravity on the otoliths would be interpreted as rate of changes of acceleration. Integrated once, these signals should produce a sensation of acceleration to the left and a horizontal nystagmus, with the slow phase beating toward the right. If the peripheral otolith signals are missing, and the canal response is normal, inclination of the head to the right, as before, should again produce both illusions but the slow phase of nystagmus should beat toward the left. Counterrolling of the eyes should occur in the first case as a result of the sum of the effect of gravitational and illusory acceleration. Counterrolling may also occur in the latter case by a reduced amount and in the opposite direction, as a result of a difference between the effect of gravity and of the illusory acceleration.

The integrity of the canal or otolith peripheral signals can be checked, of course, by standard means such as a rotary stimulus about either a vertical or a horizontal axis. But a useful diagnosis may be possible on the basis of the above observations. The model predicts that nystagmus caused by inoperative canals or otoliths should be suppressed shortly after a head movement. This nystagmus would be identified as "direction-changing", Bergstedt (1961). A direction-fixed positional nystagmus, independent of head movement, would probably point to a central pathology.

It would be helpful in the diagnosis of the location of the disturbance to create a situation in which the patient could sense and describe his illusions of attitude and acceleration under various stimuli. A situation of this kind would involve deprivation of other sensory data.

2. Hydrops

It has long been recognized that a vestibular disorder can be caused by hydrops in the endolymphatic cavity. Knapp (1871) identified the pathology as a form of labyrinthine glaucoma. G. Portman (1927) punctured the endolymphatic sac to relieve excess pressure of the endolymph. M. Portman (1969) reported a high incidence of relief of dizziness following this type of surgery, but continued instability in many cases.

Dohlman (1964) showed evidence that the endolymph flows from the endolymphatic cavity into the endolymphaticus sac where it appears to be absorbed.

He argued that there must be a delicate regulatory process to maintain a balance of pressure between the endolymphatic and perilymphatic fluids. It may be surmised that the regulatory factor could be the distension of the endolymphatic sac.

The hydraulic model suggested earlier for the utricular otolithic transducer requires a close regulation of the relative volume of the two cavities since its response is a function of the distortion of the sac membrane. An organ sensitive only to shear between the otolithic zone and the maculae, as it is conventionally assumed to be, would be much less sensitive, if at all, to slight deformation of the membrane. It also seems that the organ would adapt to a small and constant distortion, but that severe symptoms would be caused if the endolymph pressure built up slowly and was suddenly released. The puncturing of the endolymphaticus sac would insure a more constant condition with regard to the distortion of the otolith organ.

That the surgical intervention does not fully restore the proper functioning of the organs may have a number of causes. It has been found, for instance, that together with hydrops, pathologic conditions are generally associated with a large increase in the protein content of endolymph (VOLDRICH, 1970). Computations by this author based on data by HERSHEY (1967) shows that in the ranges of the rate of shear of the canal, an increase of protein content in the endolymph to that of blood plasma, could increase the coefficient of viscosity by a factor of more than 40 to 1. Such an increase would correspond to a practical blockage of the canals.

It would be of particular interest to attempt to determine the responses of the utricular otolith with fish or mammals following the plugging of the endolymphaticus canal or the puncturing of the endolymphaticus or utricular bag, as was suggested earlier. These tests may provide a better understanding of the otolithic transducer, the effect of hydrops, and of surgical interventions.

It would not be profitable to speculate further on the theoretical application of the present model to pathologic disorders. It is only by close interaction between modeling and experimentation that progress can be made, both in the modeling and in the understanding of a particular syndrome.

M. Conclusions of Applications of Model

Hopefully a case has been made for the general validity of the proposed model, although further investigations will certainly bring out the need for modifications.

The oculogravic illusion is evidence that man perceives a sudden change in the inertial vector as a gradual one with considerable delay.

Parallel-swing experiments show that man does not lose the sense of the direction of vertical when subjected to transient acceleration. Both observations are explained by the presence of a low-pass filter.

The immersed rotation of subjects demonstrates the illusion of both movement and attitude, which are predictable from the model when the high-pass section of the filter is inoperative because there are no semicircular canal signals.

The reaction of cats with plugged canals to slow and fast tilt is in agreement with the model prediction when the high-pass section is inoperative because of lack of semicircular canal signals.

The counterrolling of the eyes, and the observation of an illusory linear sensation of motion during Coriolis stimulation can be predicted from the model when canals are stimulated without a corresponding stimulation of the otolith.

The illusions of body movements as a whole during stimulation by a rotating linear vector can be predicted from the model because of the absence of semicircular canals. Other observed sensations and nystagmus can be explained in terms of central phenomena of perception.

The model predicts illusions of both attitude and movement when the head is inclined in space, accounting for observed disturbances in space as the result of such head movements.

The fish reacts without delay to a change in the direction of the inertial vector, in contrast to the slow reaction of man in the oculogravic illusion. But the need to distinguish between acceleration and gravity during a dive remains. Further investigations are needed to determine how the fish performs this function.

The model was shown to be of possible value in accounting for pathologic disturbances of the vestibular apparatus.

There is a need for a direct method of evaluating the qualitative effect of gravity and acceleration on the otoliths without complicated mathematical computations. It is suggested that the stimulus be considered to act on two axes with respect to the head, say the x_π and z_π axes. Two transducers should be assumed to be associated with each axis, including a conventional and a differentiating accelerometer. The outputs of the conventional accelerometers would provide a direct measurement of the inputs of the sum of acceleration and gravity along the two axes, and would be used for the determination of the vertical. If the inputs are due to transient acceleration, they would be canceled out by the low-pass filter. If they are caused by a turn of the head, the high-pass section would come into play by interaction with the semicircular canals, causing a prompt response. The output of the differentiating accelerometers on the other hand would be utilized in determining sensations of linear movements. The effect of constant gravity would be eliminated by differentiation when the head is not rotated. During a rotation the effect of the rate of change of the gravity component must be eliminated as a function of canal signals. Abnormal responses such as those discussed above can easily be interpreted in this manner.

VIII. Summary and Discussion

A. The Separation of Gravity and Acceleration – Dependent Otolith Signals

Experimental data reported in the literature show that the vestibular system, operating alone or jointly with other sensors, can supply the following information:

a) the angular acceleration, velocity, and position of the head with respect to the vertical and two other mutually perpendicular axes with respect to a fixed environment;

b) the linear acceleration, velocity, and position of the head along three axes with respect to a fixed environment.

This information is utilized in the control of body movements, in relation to gravitational forces and the environment.

The proposition that the vestibular system provides information about the direction of the vertical under dynamic conditions of body movements and also about the extent and direction of linear movements leaves no choice regarding the physical principles applicable to their operation. They are Newton's laws of motion and the equivalence of gravity and acceleration; the same principles applicable to an inertial-navigation system which supplies analogous information. There are choices, however, regarding the precise manner in which these principles can be instrumented. Anatomical considerations must determine this choice, insofar as the biological system is concerned. The present model is an attempt to satisfy both physics and anatomy.

The most central and challenging problem in the design of inertial-guidance systems arises because of the necessity of making independent determinations of the values of gravity and acceleration which are acting on the system. The difficulty arises primarily because of the equivalence of these two modalities.

Inertial-guidance designers resolved the problem by two basic approaches embodied in the "stable-platform" and the "strapped-on" systems. The latter system is more closely analogous to the vestibular apparatus than is the former. This is because the sensors are fixed with respect to the vehicle, as the vestibular end organs are fixed with respect to the head. The linear sensors in both systems must respond to varying gravitational forces whenever the attitude of their supporting structure is altered. At the same time, they may be acted upon by varying acceleration forces. Similar operations must be performed in both to sort out signals into two sets of components related respectively to gravity and acceleration inputs. Only then is it possible to determine the attitude of the supporting structure with respect to the vertical, and the extent and direction of its linear movements.

These sorting out, or filtering, operations are based on the only distinguishing characteristic between gravity and acceleration: gravity is constant in direction and magnitude with respect to the earth's surface, while acceleration can act in any direction and is generally of transient nature. It follows that any angular movement of the supporting structure of the sensors about an axis other than the vertical must be followed by a predictable change of the components of gravity acting along its various axes. Acceleration, on the other hand, occurs independently of such movements. Beyond these basic principles, applicable to both the man-contrived and the biological systems, the detail of their instrumentation must differ, each adapted to its specific requirements: High accuracy over long distances and extended periods of time, in one case, high mobility with accuracy limited to short distances and time periods in the other. It is the difference between guiding a missile over a distance of 5,000 miles and monitoring a body movement in the return of a tennis serve.

B. The Systems Approach to Vestibular Functions

Integration of essential functions takes precedence over thoroughness, unity over rigor, in a systems approach to a given problem. And, if essential functions are first accounted for, the chances are that the details will fall into place. The blood must circulate or else where would it come from, and where would it go. And if the blood circulates, there must be a connection between arteries and veins. The attempt to comply with these logical necessities led Harvey to the system of blood circulation, and Malpighi to the discovery of the capillaries. The present model is an attempt to meet a similar imperative in the performance of vestibular functions.

The reader is invited to consider whether he can discover any escape from the necessity of making independent measurements of gravity and acceleration in an inertial scheme of guidance, physical or biological. Inertial guidance designers have not found any. He may then decide whether this particular function, if required, deserves a similar hierarchical rank to that of the canals and the otoliths in a systems concept of the vestibular apparatus.

The reader can further determine whether the model presently proposed fulfills this required function, and whether it has been tested satisfactorily in a sufficient number of independent situations to warrant the expectation that it would also account for the behavior of the system in situations not considered here. If so, fitness of the model may be taken as a tentative criterion of the validity of an hypothesis, before an attempt is made to test it experimentally. Considerable labor in the performance of unprofitable experiments may be saved by this means. At the same time the model may provide significant leads for fruitful experimental and theoretical explorations.

The model leaves many unexplained problems and, indeed, may raise more questions than it resolves. However it may "bracket" areas in which the solution of these problems may be found. The full accounting of the response of the canal may be achieved by refinement of the model proposed here. A model of the otolith organs may be evolved within the constraints that they must respond generally as described mathematically, and in a manner analogous to a proposed mechanical model. Systems considerations would also require that this explanation account for available morphological data, including the organization of cells in the maculae, their spatial polarization, the function of the striola, the preponderence of type 1 cells along its ridge, the modes of attachment of the membraneous sacs to the osseous cavity, the structures and the interconnections of the membraneous labyrinth, etc.

The model may provide leads in the interpretation of recordings from neural centers (e.g. Melvill Jones, 1967, 1969; Crampton, 1965, 1971) and of the tracings of nerve fibers between end organs and neural centers (e.g. Brodal et al., 1969) in terms of functions.

Melvill Jones (1969), for instance, recorded the responses from units to otolith stimulation by linear sinusoidal acceleration. These responses can be interpreted as delays of the stimulus by different amounts for different cells. Such delays are not in evidence in the peripheral recordings discussed earlier. They do not fit, either, the present conceptualization of the end organs. On the other hand, they could be taken as evidence of the hypothesized low-pass filter which may be conceived to consist of a delay line made up of lag networks in series. If the signal should decay exponentially along the line, a summation of a number of taps along its length would constitute a low pass filter. This possibility deserves further consideration and investigation.

The model raises also a number of questions about neural operations and organization. How is an integration performed centrally? Does it correspond to an analog or a digital processing? A neuron model, such as that proposed by Hiltz (1965), could provide a lag network of the character illustrated in Fig. 17 to effect the integration of the otolith signal. It would be interesting in this connection to search in neural centers for evidence of the successive steps in the processing of the signal, also illustrated in the diagram.

The vestibular system itself is a component of spatial representation which interprets and organizes sensory information into two sets of data regarding the position of the head with respect to objects in the environment, and the position of various parts of the body with respect to the head. Ultimately a systems concept of the control of body movement must be evolved. This should include the system of spatial representation, experimental data and theory of the role of different neural centers (e.g. Kornhuber, 1971), and the "black box" response (e.g. Mayne, 1951; Mayne and Mead, 1953). The neuron-glial cell interactions might also be included (Hyden, 1967), which may account for programming. Hopefully, the present model may be of value in this attempt.

Beyond the systems with which the vestibular organs are most directly associated, they can be also shown to be enmeshed with practically every aspect of life.

C. Perception and the Vestibular System

It is not possible, as indicated earlier, to understand the response of the organism to vestibular stimulation without consideration of perceptual processes associated with the classic works of Boring (1942) and Ames (1960). What we see, or perceive, is not determined solely by a physical image on the retina, and neither is there a one-to-one relation between vestibular stimulation and the response of the organism. Similar perceptual processes are interposed in both cases between the sensory organs and the response. The same image of the moon on the retina corresponds to a different perceived size depending on its position in the sky; and a man appears to be the same size regardless of his distance and, therefore, of the size of his image on the retina of an observer. Similarly, an angular stimulation of the canals may or may not cause nystagmus, depending on factors such as the illumination of a room, "interest," "threat," etc. The same somesthetic stimulation may carry the meaning of rotation for man with greater certainty in a barbecue pit rotation than in a counterrotating room. The cat's otolithic signals may be passed through a low-pass filter before they are utilized or they may be used directly, as illustrated by the reactions of animals with blocked canals to slow and fast tilt in one experiment, and to barbecue rotation in another.

If confirmed, the identification by Benson et al. (1970) of cells associated with the perception of rotation rather than direct stimulation by the canals should be a significant contribution to the neurological aspect of perceptual theory.

It would be interesting to try to determine at what level a canal-dependent signal becomes rotation-dependent and by what process. The problem is, of course, one of the most central and least understood in neurology, involving as it does memory, conditioning or, in general, the permanent modification of neural networks. Benson et al. (1970) found a number of rotation-dependent cells in the neural centers of the cat. Does this mean that for every primary neuron, or at least for a large number of them, there is a corresponding rotation-dependent unit? This appears to argue for a chemical, rather than a network theory of conditioning and memory at the level of single neurons. The experiments of Hyden (1967) on the interplay between glial cells and neurons, and other experiments on the conditioning of a single neuron (e.g. von Baumgarten, 1968) suggest this possibility. But, the reader may ask, where does the next step take place, and by what mysterious process does a pattern of neural events become a sensation of rotation?

The normal processes or perception are perhaps best brought to light by their malfunctions in the creation of illusions which are in conflict with reality, as interpreted by conscious processes. Vestibular physiology has a rich catalog of such illusions, well suited for the investigation of the logical mechanics of these processes, their monitoring agencies, their interaction with conscious processes, etc. The ferris wheel illusion for instance, may be said to constitute the "unconscious" formulation of a conceptual scheme, within which sensory data can be interpreted consistently. What then is the relation between this process and that of a consciously directed creative function? And what is the relation between the perceptual functions and the "unconscious" in psychology? Vestibular physiology, like psychology, needs the assumption of two levels of the mind, two ways of knowing, to account for the ferris wheel illusion.

D. Adaptation

Vestibular physiology offers some of the best illustrations of biological adaptation. It is indeed remarkable that man, the end product of an evolutionary process which has taken place strictly in an environment of 1 g linear acceleration and negligible rotation, should adapt as readily as he does to an environment of zero g, of constant rotation or of a maneuvering airplane. The last adaptation is perhaps the most remarkable, requiring that a pilot should maintain a perception of the orientation, velocity and approximate position of his body as part of the airplane structure, with respect to three sets of axes, associated respectively with the earth, the inertial vector in a turn and the air mass, when only one set is required on the earth. More remarkable yet is the fact that he must perform this feat by substitution of artificial sensors for his vestibular organs which are quite useless in the airplane situation. Hardly less remarkable is the adaptation to a rotating environment, because of the severe errors caused in the perception of position and the movement by cross-coupling of the canals during an inclination of the head, and by the Coriolis effect during body movements. The many experiments conducted on adaptation to this environment (e.g. Graybiel et al., 1960; Guedry and Graybiel, 1962; Graybiel et al., 1965) give a clue to some of the mechanics of adaptation to a specific environment. They appear to involve the resolution of sensory conflicts either by suppression of the less probable data, or by correction of these data by the generation of an internal signal, a so-called compensatory reaction.

Vestibular physiology offers a rich field for the investigation of sensory organization, the manner in which unity is achieved between different sensors, and how, in the words of Sherrington, the nervous system performs its "integrative action".

E. Motion Sickness – a Syndrome of Rejection

We generally explain a particular phenomenon by showing that it fits logically into an existing context. If the context does not exist, the explanation must supply it. The explanation of motion sickness is believed faced with this necessity.

There are two prevalent theories of motion sickness: the overstimulation of the vestibular organs and the conflict theory. MONEY (1968) pointed out that neither theory is consistent with the facts, and that neither gives any hint regarding the possible function of this reaction. (See chapter on motion sickness by W. H. JOHNSON in this handbook.)

MAYNE (1970) proposed a theory of motion sickness which may be briefly summarized herein. He showed that many situations associated with a high incidence of the disturbance, and said to be non-conflicting, actually are conflicting. The present chapter illustrates how conflicts can arise in situations where gravity is interpreted as acceleration. Without such explanation it could be easily assumed that these situations are non-conflicting although they are known to be disturbing. It is believed possible to demonstrate on the basis of these studies, or at least reasonably infer, the presence of a conflict in all situations conducive to motion sickness. All conflicts, however, do not cause the disturbance. Some of them may be even "amusing". The organism does not respond uniformly to conflict or disharmony.

We can perhaps define a conflict as a divergence between the interpretation in perception of various sensory data available to us at any given time, or as a divergence between an expected and a predicted response. Motion sickness related conflicts are mainly associated with the vestibular organs. According to the present view, this is only because such conflicts are difficult to resolve and involve the threat of a fall. There are examples in the literature of motion sickness without motion and therefore without vestibular stimulation. At the same time, distorting glasses are also known to produce nausea reactions. Much work remains to be done in order to discover what are the characteristics of conflicts which may cause the organism to respond in one way or in another. It is known that subjective factors such as threat, a mood of interest or depression, the facility with which a conflict may be resolved, previous adaptation, as well as personal traits are factors in the incidence of motion sickness.

With the above reservations, the conflict theory of motion sickness is taken here as valid. However, the assertion that a conflict is a necessary condition for the occurrence of motion sickness is not a satisfactory explanation of the disturbance, even if proved in all possible cases. Our reason demands that a full explanation of the phenomenon must also include a description of what useful function it performs.

Money (1968) wrote in this regard: "The powerful central mechanism for this response" (vomiting) "can perhaps be considered as one would consider a prominent anatomical structure without a known function." In other words, according to Money, it is equally difficult to assume that the motion sickness reaction is without function as to imagine that breathing or a lung structure would be, had not their functions already been demonstrated. Money added that the elucidation of the vomiting reaction could lead to a significant advance in biology.

The history of physiology is replete with examples of structures which were thought at one time to be vestigial and useless, and which were discovered later to be indispensable to the normal functioning of the organism. Significant advances were indeed made when such functions were discovered.

In a search for the possible function of the motion sickness reaction, we note that this type of reaction is not uniquely associated with motion. It occurs frequently in many life situations. It is a good scientific methodology to try to discover inductively a unique explanation for similar events.

A medical student may become ill upon his first introduction to the dissecting room. The idea of homosexual practices may disturb a person with a heterosexual outlook of acceptable behavior. We may become nauseated when readiing about the treatment of the inmates of a concentration camp. A witness to a severe accident may be caused to vomit. An acquaintance of this author became physically ill upon learning of the fall of Singapore during World War II. Another asked "Can you explain why I am perfectly comfortable in a Washington trolley car, but I am nauseated in a Pittsburgh trolley car?" It was not difficult to suggest that he must associate the city of Pittsburgh with an unpleasant experience which he was trying to forget. Whereupon he admitted that he was indeed trying to drive out of his mind the memory of a very unhappy marriage consummated in Pittsburgh. The introductory sentence to a recent magazine review of an article read: "The material has a distinct emetic quality." We may also be nauseated and caused to vomit by indigestion or food poisoning. Nausea, therefore, is a rather ubiquitous response of the organism.

We ask then, what common cause can we discover between such instances as moving the head in a rotating room, seeing a cadaver, being told about abnormal sexual practices, reading about the brutal treatment of human beings, witnessing an accident, hearing about the fall of Singapore, recalling an unhappy occurrence, and having indigestion?

The idea that comes through this enumeration is one of conflict and rejection. It is easy enough to visualize the usefulness of the rejection of the indigestible content of the stomach. But how about the other forms of rejection? It can be shown that they contribute to the stability of various previously established responses of the organism.

Man is born with few fixed patterns of behavior but with a high capacity to acquire them. Such pseudo-instincts have validity in regulating behavior. They have been acquired after repeated occurrences in which they have proved of value during so-called "conditioning" or "learning". In the interest of the organism, they should not be altered too easily. The negative reinforecment of nausea can cause the rejection of material in conflict with such modes of response. The rejection of the sight of a cadaver by a medical student may allow him to preserve his "belief" in the permanence of his own life. The rejection of the news of the fall of Singapore, by the man who became ill upon hearing it, may permit him to preverse his idea of white supremacy. The rejection by an astronaut of the conflicting sensory data he experiences upon the inclination of his head may make it possible for him to preserve his previously organized response to vestibular sensory data. It may be said further that the nausea reaction, or repugnance, plays a role in what Sherrington has called "The Integrative Action of the Nervous System" by rejecting the nonintegrable. Integration and unity have intrinsic values of their own. The concept of rejection and repression originated with FREUD. However, he saw repression and the disturbances it may create as an essentially sexual manifestation. In contrast the present theory is set in a multidimensional context.

Under normal life situations only light sensations of nausea are needed to protect the organism against the intrusion of incompatible material. Feelings associated with expressions such as revolting, repulsive, nauseating, loathsome, disgusting, repugnant, sickening are conscious evidence of the operation of a mechanism of rejection. The same feelings may be generated by the intake of an emetic drug or the stimulation of a vomiting center. We infer that the same stimulation of the same mechanism takes place in both instances since the output in the way of a feeling of nausea is identical. In a similar way adrenalin is released concomitantly with the feelings of fear, while saliva and gastric juices are released in association with the consciousness of food. Both reactions could also be caused by proper chemical or physical stimulation. Behaviorists may not agree with the propriety or usefulness of such inferences. But more about this later.

The protection afforded the organisms against the intrusion of conflicting "psychic" material is not unlike that afforded by immunological reactions against the intrusion of an incompatible chemical substance. It may happen in both the repugnant and the immunological reactions that the invading "material" resists rejection, and that the organism persists in trying to reject it. A positive feedback process may then be initiated whereby an increased tendency toward rejection causes an intensification of the unpleasant nausea and a further magnification of the tendency toward rejection. Both the immunological and the repugnant reactions may then cause severe stresses in the organism because of the overfunctioning of mechanisms normally intended to protect it. We may identify the disturbances as a "rejection syndrome." It may be significant in this connection that both the repugnant and the immunological reactions respond to antihistamine medication.

It is suggested that the rejection syndrome plays a role in shock. Shock is an ill-defined reaction. It is identified primarily with disturbances which occur following an injury and loss of body fluids. But shock, or shock-like disturbance can also occur without apparent physiological injury or loss of blood. They can be triggered by psychic factors (e.g., WIGGERS, 1950). The symptomatology of shock is similar to motion sickness involving depression, sweating, circulatory disturbances, palor of the cheeks and sometimes vomiting. The possibility that the rejection syndrome plays a part in shock should not be overlooked. Such rejection could involve a "psychic" attempt of the organism to repress the consciousness of a trauma, physiological or mental, as well as other purely physiological reactions.

Selye (1956) postulated that reactions which he called "stresses" are present in all diseases. Such stresses may be accounted for, in part, by rejection. It is interesting in this connection that a car-sick passenger can be relieved if he takes over the wheel. We may theorize that the "interest" attendant to the task is a reaction opposite that of rejection, which is then inhibited. It could be, therefore, that many therapies without a medical theoretical basis, such as physical therapy, Indian yoga, Japanese moxa, Chinese acupuncture, faith therapy have a similar rationale. They could operate to create "interest," "hope" and thereby inhibit rejection.

We have gone far afield in our search for a context in which the motion sickness reaction could be fitted. In the process we have tied together, more or less loosely, a good many previously unrelated reactions. The simplification effected thereby appears to justify the provisional acceptance of the theory for further development.

F. Toward a System Concept of Life

There is a need for a system concept of life which would integrate various approaches to life science. The scientific approach to life, however, involves epistemological and methodological problems which have not been fully resolved.

The scientific process begins in all fields with the recordings of individual observations. In time an attempt is made to integrate these observations into a theoretical construction that is both simple and logically consistent. Physical scientists have not found that these two requirements are incompatible. The simplification of a theory often results in a more logical formulation, and a search for greater rigor often leads to greater simplicity. The mind of man is well adapted to function in a world the elements of which are organized simply and consistently. Only in such a world could man come to trust in the "truth-value" of the simplicity and logical consistency of his conceptualizations.

Man possesses only one mind which must serve in all his attempts to understand the world about him. Whatever may be "a priori" and whatever "adaptation" in physical science methodology, it would appear reasonable to expect that it must serve in life science as well. It is true that life science must deal with the "subjective" while physical science deals only with the "objective." We can infer, however, as indicated earlier that any distinct subjective feeling, such as nausea, corresponds to the operation of distinct "objective" physiological mechanisms. Clynes (1968) has given evidence that such is the case. Such mechanisms may then be inferred, simulated in a computer program, and finally identified in neural centers. Actually, it can be said also that our concept of the objective is only an assumed common cause between a specific consciousness of our own and a similar consciousness inferred to occur in the minds of others. In this sense Berkeley's idealism applies to science. The elements of all scientific constructions in the physical or the living world: energy, mass, time, space, a feeling of nausea, a totthache, a pleasurable reaction must be found in consciousness. There is then no basic distinction between the scientific process in the physical and living world.

The use of the physical science methodology in the investigation of a biological structure or of a set of biological reactions implies that they are simply organized. This in turn implies the existence of a unifying principle in their organization, a function or a goal. It follows that the most important initial step in the investigation of a structure is the formulation of the proper hypothesis regarding function or functions it must perform.

The present chapter started with the inference that the functions of the vestibular organs could be identified with the well established ones of an inertial guidance system. What followed was in part an attempt to recreate or reinvent a system which would perform these functions as simply as possible and would fit available experimental and morphological data.

Similarly the theory of motion sickness was evolved to fit an assumed function. If this function was chosen properly the ambiguities and inconsistencies it may contain will be ultimately resolved.

Perhaps the most significant contribution of the theory, if confirmed, will be its implications. It must be seen, for instance, that repugnance is only one regulatory mechanism among a system of others. Modalities such as aesthetic, humor, drive, love, aggression, hunger, sex, etc. besides repugnance are visualized as part of the system. It may be inferred from the classical experiments of MILLER (1968) that the system is effective in regulating all functions in man and animals and perhaps all life. The theory of repugnance suggests that it operates also through the creation and the relieving of somatic stresses. There have been individual theories of the above modalities. Without a clearly perceived central function, however, they cannot be integrated into neurological and behavioral sciences in which they appear to belong. It must be seen first that have a part in the organization of sensory data, adaptation and perception as discussed earlier in connection with the vestibular organs. They may serve also as the basis for theories of stresses and psychosomatic disorders, and the formulation of systems of reason or ethics.

It is only with the adoption of the full physical science methodology that a system concept of life can be evolved. The assumption that the living world like the physical one is constructed simply must be part of the scientific approach to life regardless of its teleological implications. Of course, simplicity is not the only criterion in science and it is sometimes over-emphasized. There is a substantial body of opinion, for instance, to the effect that theories which attempt to account for physical phenomena in terms of mathematical transformations based on the constancy of the velocity of light, for all behavior in terms of sex, or for all creation in terms of natural selections, are unsatisfactory because, although simple, they do not account for the functions they are intended to perform.

We should not forget, also, that while a necessary condition for the evolution of life as we know it must have included the presence of water, of an atmosphere, and a proper range of temperatures, it must also have included the existence of principles and laws such as those of gravitation, thermodynamics, electromagnetism, quantum mechanics as well as those which make it possible for a neural structure to transduce an electrical or chemical input into a toothache or an aesthetic experience. All these principles are necessary at least in the higher forms of life.

Acknowledgments

The initial study leading to the preparation of this chapter was conducted under contract No. Nas9-4460 from the Manned Spacecraft Center NASA, Houston, Texas, 1965–1966 to the Goodyear Aerospace Corporation, with the author as principal investigator.

The author is indebted to Professor G. MELVILL JONES for assistance in the preparation of the initial draft of this chapter in 1968 and to Professor OTTO LOWENSTEIN for helpful comments on the original draft and subsequent revisions. The work was greatly influenced by the opportunity of witnessing tests in progress in various laboratories, including those of the U.S. Naval Aerospace Institute at Pensacola, Florida, under Dr. ASHTON GRAYBIEL, the Aviation Medical Research Unit at McGill University, Canada, under Dr. G. MELVILL JONES, the Vestibular Research Unit of the Defence and Civil Institute of Environmental Medicine, Canada, under Dr. K.E. MONEY, the Department of Zoology and Comparative Psychology of the University of Birmingham, England, under Dr. OTTO LOWENSTEIN. The author is grateful to Professor G.F. DOHLMAN for making available to him his moving picture film on the movement of the cupula and for his many pertinent comments. Professor L.G. WRENN, visiting Professor of Psychology at Arizona State University, and Professor PAUL W. PRUYSER, HENRY MARCH PFEIFFER Professor at the Menninger Foundation, made valuable criticisms of the section on motion sickness. Dr. JOHN BILLINGHAM's helpful cooperation with the initial research program, the reading of the chapter by Professor TRUET B. THOMPSON of the Electrical Engineering Department and by Professor ERNEST LINDHOLM and ROBERT C. HAYGOOD of the Psychology Department, the valuable criticisms of the section on fish behavior by Dr. HOWARD C. HOWLAND of Cornell University, are acknowledged. The author is also indebted to investigators who have kindly cleared up miscellaneous questions raised in personal communications, as acknowledged in the body of the chapter. Discussions with members of the faculty of the Electrical Engineering Department of this University, including Professors PAUL E. RUSSELL, JOHN D. PATTERSON, WILBUR C. CLARK and MURRAY D. SIRKIS, proved stimulating and helpful in clearing up technical problems. The work was made possible through the support and understanding of Professor T.E. TICE, chairman of the Department of Electrical Engineering. Professor H.H. KORNHUBER, editor of this handbook, has been very helpful throughout the several revisions of the work. The author must remain solely responsible for any errors or erroneous views in this chapter.

References

ADRIAN, E.D.: Discharges from vestibular receptors in the cat. J. Physiol. (Lond.) **101**, 389–407 (1943).

AMES, A.: The Morning Notes of Adelbert Ames. New Brunswick, N.J.: Rutgers University Press 1960.

ANSOM, B.J.: Endolymph hydrops. Arch. Otolaryng. **89**, 70–83 (1969).

BARLOW, J.S.: Inertial navigation in relation to animal navigation. J. Inst. Navig. **19**, 3 (1966).

BARLOW, J.S.: Inertial navigation as a basis for animal navigation. J. theor. Biol. **6**, 76–117 (1964).

BELANGER, F., MAYNE, R.: Report No. GERA-1085, Contract No. NASA-4460, 46 pp., Manned Spacecraft Center, NASA, Houston, Texas 1965.

BENSON, A.J., WHITESIDE, T.C.: The effect of linear acceleration on the response to angular acceleration in man. J. Physiol. (Lond.) **156**, 6 (1961).

BENSON, A.J.: Effect of Linear Acceleration on Labyrinthine Nystagmus in Man. Communication 1016, Proc. 22nd Int. Congress. Physiol. Sci. 1962.

BENSON, A.J., BODIN, M.A.: Interaction of linear and angular acceleration on vestibular receptors in man. Aerospace Med. **37**, 144–154 (1966).

Benson, A.J., Guedry, F.E., Melville Jones, G.: Response of semicircular canal-dependent units in vestibular nuclei to rotation of a linear acceleration vector without angular acceleration. J. Physiol. (Lond.) **210**, 475–494 (1970).

Bergstedt, M.: Studies of positional nystagmus in the human centrifuge. Acta oto-laryng. (Stockh.) Suppl. No. 166, 144 pp. (1961).

Beritov, I.S.: Spatial projection of perceived environmental objects by means of labyrinthine receptors. Fiziol. Zh. (Mosk.) **43/7**, 600–610 (1957).

Billingham, H.T.: Russian experience in vestibular physiology related to space environment. Second Symposium on the Role of the Vestibular Organs in Space Exploration, NASA SP-115, 5–9, National Aeronautics and Space Administration, Washington, D.C., 1966.

Boring, E.G.: Sensation and Perception in the History of Experimental Psychology. New York, London: Appleton-Century 1942.

Brodal, A.: Anatomical points of view on the alleged morphological basis of consciousness. Acta Neurochirurgica. Sonderdruck aus Vol. XII, FASC. 2. Berlin-Heidelberg-New York: Springer 1964.

Brodal, A., Pompeiano, O., Walberg, F.: The vestibular nuclei and their connection, anatomy and functional correlations (Ramsey Henderson Trust Lectures). Edinburgh, London: 1962. Oliver and Boyd.

Brown, J.H.: Modification of vestibular nystagmus by change of task during stimulation. U.S. Army Med. Res. Lab. Report No. 667, (1966), Fort Knox, Ky.

Cannon, W.B.: Bodily changes in pain, hunger, fear and rage. Boston: Charles T. Branford 1953.

Cappel, K.L.: Determination of physical constants of semi-circular canals from measurements of single neural unit activity under constant angular acceleration. NASA SP-115, 229–236, Washington, D.C.: NASA 1966.

Cawthorne, T., Dix, M.R., Hallpike, G.S., Hood, J.D.: The investigation of vestibular functions. Brit. med. Bull. **12**, 131 (1956).

Clark, B., Graybiel, A.: Some factors contributing to the delay in the perception of the oculogravic Illusion. NASA SP-77, 151–162. Washington, D.C.: NASA 1965.

Clynes, M.: Toward a theory of man: precision of essentic form in living communication. Information processing in the nervous system. K.N. Leibonic, Ed. New York-Berlin: Springer 1968.

Collins, W.E.: Effects of mental activity on vestibular nystagmus and the electroencephalogram. Nature (Lond.) **190**, 47771, 194–195 (1961).

Collins, W.E., Schröder, D.J, Rice, N., Mertens, R.A., Kranz, G.: Some characteristics of optokinetic eye movements. Aero space Med. **41**, 1251–1262 (1970).

Correia, M.J., Guedry, F.E., Jr.: Modification of vestibular responses as a function of the rate of rotation about an earth horizontal axis. Acta oto-laryng. (Stockh.) **62**, 297 (1966).

Correia, M.J.: Nystagmus and eye deviation in the environments of flight and spale travel proc. NINTH IHT. Congress, Mexico, D.F. 1969, Excerpta Medica, Amsterdam 449–455 (1970).

Correia, M.J., Money, K.E.: The effect of blockage of all six semicircular canal ducts on nystagmus produced by dynamic linear acceleration of the cat. Acta oto-laryng. (Stockh.). **69**, 7–16 (1970).

Correia, M.J., Guedry, F.E.: Influence of gravity on responses elicited by stimulation of the horizontal semicircular canals. Report NSAM-905, Order R-93, Naval Aerospace Medical Institute Pensacola Fla. 1964.

Cramer, R.L.: Response of mammalian gravity receptors. Aerospace Med. **33**, 663–666 (1962).

Crampton, G.H.: Centripetal acceleration and vestibular nystagmus in man. Paper read before the Psychonomic Society, St. Louis (1962).

Crampton, G.H.: Response of single cells in cat brain stem to angular acceleration in the horizontal plane. NASA SP-77, Washington, D.C.: NASA 1965.

CRAMPTON, G.H.: Does linear acceleration modify cupula deflection? Second Symp. on the role of the vestibular organs in space exploration. NASA SP-115, 169–181, Washington, D.C.: NASA 1966.

CRAMPTON, G.H., GALL, K.J.: Responses of single cells within the cat medulla during prolonged acceleration. EHTR-4505, (1971), Dept. of the Army, Edgewood Arsenal, Md.

DOHLMAN, G.: Investigations in the functions of the semi circular canals. Acta oto-laryng. (Stockh.). Suppl. **51**, 211–218 (1944).

DOHLMAN, G.F.: Secretion and absorbtion of the endolymph. Ann. Otol. (St. Louis) **73**, 708–723 (1964).

DRAPER, C.S., WRIGLEY, W., HOVORKA, J.: Inertial Guidance. New York: Pergamon Press 1960.

DZENDOLET, E.: Comments on Sjoberg's hypothesis for the mechanism of the inversion illusion under zero-gravity conditions. Aerospace Med. **42**, 11: 1211–1213 (Nov. 1971).

FERNÁNDEZ, C., GOLDBERG, J.M.: Physiology of peripheral neurons innervating semicircular canals of the squirrel monkey, Part II. Response to sinusoidal stimulation and dynamics of peripheral vestibular system. J. Neurophysiol. **34**, 4: 661–675 (1971).

FERNÁNDEZ, C., GOLDBERG, J.M., ABEND, W.K.: Response to static tilt of peripheral neurons innervating otolith organs of the squirrel monkey. J. Neurobiol. **35**, 978–997 (1972).

FLOCK, A., WERSÄLL, J.: A study of the orientation of the sensory hairs of the receptor cells in the lateral-line organs of fish, with special reference to the function of the receptors. J. Cell Biol. **15**, 1–19 (1962).

GILBRETH, D.A.: Fluid mechanics. Belmont, Calif.: Wadsworth 1965.

GOLDBERG, J.M., FERNANDEZ, C.: Physiology of peripheral neurons innervating semicircular canals of the squirrel monkey. Part I: Resting Discharge and Response to Constant Angular Acceleration. 635–661. Part II: Variations Among Units In Their Discharge Properties. 676–684. J. Neurophysiol. **34**, 4 (1971).

GRAYBIEL, A., WHITESIDE, W.H.: Comparison of the symptomatology experienced by healthy persons and subjects with loss of labyrinthine function when exposed to unusual patterns of centrifugal force in a counter-rotating room. Ann. Otol. (St. Louis) **72**, 357 (1963).

GRAYBIEL, A., BROWN, R.H.: The delay in visual reorientation following exposure to a change in direction of resultant force on a centrifuge. J. gen. Physiol. **45**, 143–150 (1951).

GRAYBIEL, A., MEEK, J.C., BEISCHER, D.E., RIOPELLE, A.J.: Observations of canal sickness and adaptation in chimpanzees in a "slow rotation room." Report No. 55, U.S. Naval School of Aviation Medicine, MR005.13-6001, Subtask 1, 10/31/1960.

GRAYBIEL, A., CLARK, B., ZARRIELLO, J.J.: Observations on human subjects living in a "slow rotation room" for periods of two days. Arch. Neurol. **3**, 55 (1960).

GRAYBIEL, A., KENNEDY, R.S., KNOBLOCK, E.C., GUEDRY, F.E., MERTZ, W., MCLEOD, M.E., COLEHOUR, J.K., MILLER, E.F., FREGLY, A.R.: Effects of exposure to a rotating environment (10 rev/min) on four aviators for a period of twelve days. Aerospace Med. **36**, 8: 733–754 (1965).

GRAYBIEL, A., KELLOGG, R.S.: The inversion illusion in parabolic flight: its probable dependence on otolith function. In: Second symposium on the role of the vestibular organs in space exploration. NASA SP-115. Washington, D.C.: U.S. Government Printing Office 1966.

GROEN, J.J., JONGKEES, L.B.J.: The turning test with small regulable stimuli. IX. The cupulogram obtained by subjective angle estimation. J. Laryng. **62**, 236–240 (1948).

GROEN, J.J., LOWENSTEIN, D., VENDRIK, A.J.H.: The mechanical analysis of the response of the horizontal semicircular canal in the isolated elasmobranch labyrinth. J. Physiol. (Lond.) **117**, 329–346 (1952).

GUEDRY, F.E., CERAN, S.J.: Derivation of subjective velocity from angular displacement estimates made during prolonged angular acceleration: adaptation effects. Army Med. Res. Lab. Report No. 376 (1959).

Guedry, F.E., Montague, E.K.: Quantitative evaluation of the vestibular coriolis reaction. Aerospace Med. **32**, 487–500 (1961).

Guedry, F.E., Graybiel, A.: Compensatory nystagmus conditioned during adaptation to living in a rotating room. J. appl. Physiol. **17**, 398 (1962).

Guedry, F.E.: Comparison of vestibular effects in several rotating environments. The Role of the Vestibular Organs In Space Exploration. NASA SP-77, p. 243–255. Washington, D.C.: NASA 1965a.

Guedry, F.E.: Orientation of the rotation axis relative to gravity: its influence on nystagmus and the sensation of rotation. Acta oto-laryng. (Stockh.) **60**, 30 (1965b).

Guedry, F.E., Harris, C.S.: Labyrinthine function related to experiments on the parallel swing. Report No. 86, U.S. Naval School of Aviation Medecine, MR005, 13–6001. Subtask 1, P. 12 (1963).

Guedry, F.E.: Some vestibular problems related to orientation in space. Acta oto-laryng. **69**, 174–185 (1968).

Guedry, F.E.: Influence of Linear and Angular Acceleration on Nystagmus, NASA SP-115 185–198. Washington D.C.: U.S. Gov. Print. Office 1966.

Hallpike, C.S., Cairns, H.: Observations in pathology of Meniere disease. J. Laryng. **53**, 625–655 (1938).

Harden Jones, F.R.: An apparent reaction of fish to linear acceleration. Nature (Lond.) **178**, 642–643 (1956).

Hershey, Daniel, Ed.: Chemical engineering in medicine and biology, p. 69. London: Plenum Press 1967.

Hiltz, F.F.: Simulated membrane functions and additional feedback characteristics for an artificial neuron. I.E.E.E. Trans. on Bio-Med. Electronics, **BME-42**, No. 2, 94–104 (April 1965).

Hixson, W.C., Niven, J.I.: Steady-state nystagmus response to semicircular canal stimulation by angular acceleration. U.S. Naval School of Medicine Rep. No. 57 (1961).

Hyden, Holger, Ed.: The neuron. Amsterdam-London-New York: Elsevier 1967.

Igarashi, M.: Dimensional studies of the vestibular end-organs apparatus. NASA SP-115, Second Symposium on the Role of the Vestibular Organs in Space Exploration, p. 47–54. Washington, D.C.: NASA 1966.

Janeke, M.: On nystagmus and otoliths. Thesis Amsterdam: Cloeck En Moedigh 1968.

Johnson, W.H., Stubbs, R.H., Keck, G.F., Franks, W.R.: Stimulus required to produce motion sickness. I. Preliminary Report dealing with importance of head movements. Aviation Med. **22**, 365–374 (1951).

Johnson, W.H., Meek, J.C., Graybiel, A.: Effect of labyrinthectomy on canal sickness in squirrel monkeys. Ann. oto-rhino-laryng. **71**, 2: 389–402 (1962).

Jongkees, L.B.W., Groen, J.J.: The nature of the vestibular stimulus. J. Laryng. **61**, 529–541 (1946).

Kate, J.H.: The oculo-vestibular reflex of the growing pike. A biophysical study (thesis). Groningen: Rijksuniversiteit T E 1969.

Kellogg, R.S.: Dynamic Counterrolling of the Eye in Normal Subjects and in Persons with Bilateral Labyrinthine Defect. NASA SP-77, 195–202, Washington, D.C.: NASA 1965.

Knapp, H.: Clinical analysis of inflammatory affections of inner ear. Circh. Ophthal. Otolaryng. **2**, 204–283 (1871).

Kornhuber, H.H.: Motor functions of cerebellum and basal ganglia. Kybernetics **8**, 157–162 (1971).

LANDSBERG, M.P., GUEDRY, F.E., GRAYBIEL, A.: Effect of changing resultant linear acceleration relative to the subject on nystagmus generated by angular acceleration. Aerospace Med. **36**, 456–460 (1965).

LEE, F.S.: Study of the senses of equilibrium. J. Physiol. (Lond.) **15**, 311–348 (1894).
IBID, **17**, 192–210 (1895).

LETKO, W., STONE, R.W.: The effect of the plane of vestibular stimulation on task performance and involuntary eye motion. NASA SP-152. Washington, D.C.: NASA 1967.

LOWENSTEIN, O., ROBERTS, T.D.M.: The equilibrium function of the otolith organs of the thornback ray (Raja Clanatee). J. Physiol. (Lond.) **110**, 392–415 (1950).

LOWENSTEIN, O.E.: The electrophysiological study of the responses of the isolated labyrinth of the lamprey (Lampretra Fluviatilis) to angular acceleration, tilting and mechanical vibration. Proc. roy. Soc. B **174**, 410–434 (1970a).

LOWENSTEIN, O.E.: Electrophysiological experiments on the isolated surviving labyrinth of elasmobranch fish to analyze the response to linear acceleration. Vestibular function on earth and in space. J. STAHLE, Ed.; Wenner Gran Symposium No. 15, p. 35–41. Oxford and New York: Pergamon 1970b.

LOWENSTEIN, O., THORNHILL, R.A.: The labyrinth of Myxine, anatomy, ultrastructure, and electrophysiology. Proc. roy. Soc. B **176**, 21–42 (1970).

MALCOLM, R., MELVILL JONES, G.: A quantitative study of vestibular adaptation in humans. Canadian Forces Institute of Environmental Medicine, 69-RD-1, pp. 37, (May 1969). *Also* Acta oto-laryng. (Stockh.) **70**, 126–135 (1970).

MATHOG, R.H., CRAMER, R.L.: Testing of the Vestibular System. Aerospace Med. **42**, 7: 741–745 (1971).

MAYNE, R.: The operating principle of the vestibular mechanism. Symp. Psychophysiological Factors in Spatial Orientation, Pensacola, Fla, 1950, Navexos P-965 (1950).

MAYNE, R.: The dynamic characteristics of the semicircular canals. J. comp. Physiol. **43**, 309–319 (1950).

MAYNE, R.: Engineering aspects of the mechanism of body control. AEII J. 6 pp., March, 1951.

MAYNE, R., MEAD, R.: Analog Computer Simulation of the Airplane Pilot. Second Piloted Aircraft Flight Control System Symp. Buaer Report AE-61-5 Part 1. AD 208765 (1952).

MAYNE, R.: Research Contract No. 4460, Manned Spacecraft Center, NASA, Houston, Texas. Functional Aspects of the System of Spatial Representation. GERA-1040, p. 47, 1965a.

IBID. The functional parameters of the semicircular canals, GERA-1056, 32 pp. (1965b). The constants of the semicircular canals, GERA-1083, 18 pp. (1965c).

IBID. Nystagmus and body control for inputs of repeated pattern. GERA-1080, 28 pp. (1965d).

IBID. Three-dimensional aspects of the operation of the semicircular canals. GERA-1057, 26 pp. (1965e).

IBID. The functions of the otolith organs. GERA-1100, 30 pp. (1966a).

IBID. The mechanics of the otolith organs. GERA-1112, 30 p. (1966b).

IBID. Summary Report. GERA-1158, 50 pp. (1966c).

IBID. MAYNE, R., BELANGER, F.: The interpretation of single or few fiber recordings, 18 pp., GERA-1113 (1966).

MAYNE, R.: Discussion of Paper by Young and Meiry. NASA, SP-152, Washington, D.C.: NASA 1967.

MAYNE, R.: The biological inertial system. Proc. I.E.E.E. Resources Round-up, Region 6, P.O. Box 869, Phoenix, Arizona, 209–222 (1969a).

MAYNE, R.: The Analogy of the Vestibular Organs to an Inertial Guidance System. Proc. Ninth Int. Congress, Oto-Rhino-Laryngology, Mexico City, 1969. Excerpta Med. Amsterdam 407–415 (1970).

MAYNE, R.: Space sickness — its causes and possible prevention. First Western Space Congress, Santa Maria, Calif., 1970.

McClure, C.L.: Theory of inertial guidance. Englewood Cliffs, N.J.: Prentice-Hall (1960).

McMitchael, A.E., Graybiel, A.: A Rorschach indication of emotional instability and susceptibility to motion sickness. Aerospace Med. **34**, 997–1000 (1963).

McNaughton, I.P.S., McNally, W.S.: Some experiments which indicate that frog's tagend has equilibrium function. J. Laryng. **61**, 204–214 (1946).

Melvill Jones, G., Spells, K.E.: A theoretical and comparative study of the functional dependence of the semicircular canal upon its physical dimensions. Proc. roy. Soc. B **157**, 403–419 (1963).

Melvill Jones, G.: Predominance of anti-compensatory oculomotor response during rapid head rotation. Aerospace Med. **35**, 965–968 (1964).

Melvill Jones, G., Milsum, J.H.: Spatial and dynamic aspects of visual fixation. I.E.E.E. Transactions on Biomedical Eng. **BME-12**, 2: 54–62 (1965).

Melvill Jones, G.: Interactions between optokinetic and vestibulo-ocular responses during rotation in various planes. Aerospace Med. **37**, 2: 172–177 (1966).

Melvill Jones, G.: Neutral Reflection of Vestibular Mechanics, 169–179, NASA SP-152, Washington, D.C.: U.S. Gov. Print. Office 1967.

Melvill Jones, G., Milsum, J.H.: Neural response of the vestibular system to translational acceleration. Conference on System Analysis Approach to Neurophysiological Problems, Brainerd, Minnesota (June 1969).

Melvill Jones, G.: On the Organization of Neural Control in the Vestibulo-ocular Reflex Arc. Symp. on the Control of Eye Movements. P. Bach-y-Rita and C.C. Collins, Eds., p. 25. San Francisco: Academy Press 1969.

Melvill Jones, G.: Origin significance and amelioration of Coriolis illusions from the semicircular canals. A Nonmathematical Approach. Aerospace Med. **41**, 5: 483–490 (1970).

Melvill Jones, G., Milsum, J.H.: Frequency response analysis of central-vestibular unit activity resulting from rotational stimulation of the semicircular canals. J. Physiol. (Lond.) **218**, 1–25 (1971).

Melvill Jones, G.: Transfer Function of Labyrinthine Volleys through Vestibular Nuclei. Basic Aspects of Central Vestibular Mechanisms. O. Pompeiano and A. Brodal, Eds. Symposium, Pisa, Italy (1971) In press.

Miller, E.F. II, Graybiel, A.: Otolith function as measured by ocular counterrolling. NASA, SP-77, 121–130, Washington, D.C.: NASA 1965.

Miller, E.F. II: Counterrolling of the human eyes produced by head tilt with respect to gravity. Acta oto-laryng. (Stockh.) **54**, 480–501 (1962).

Miller, N.E.: Learning of visceral and glandular responses. Science **163**, 434–445. (1968).

Minsky, M. Ed.: Semantic Information Processing, Cambridge-London: MIT 1968.

Money, K.E., Scott, J.W.: Functions of separate sensory receptors of nonauditory labyrinth of the cat. Amer. J. Physiol. **202**, 6: 1211–1220 (1962).

Money, K.E.: Discussion of F.E. Guedry's paper. "Influence of Linear and angular acceleration on Nystagmus", p. 196. NASA, SP-115, Government Printing Office. Washington, D.C. (1966b).

Money, K.E.: Motion sickness. Physiol. Rev. **50**, 1: 1–39 (1970).

Newell, A.: Computer programs that simulate human congnitive behavior. Conference on Cerebral Systems and Computer Logic. Pasadena, Cal, Cal. Inst. of Tech. and The Rockefeller Found. **64**, 7 (1960).

Niven, J.I., Hixson, W.C., Correia, M.J.: An experimental approach to the dynamics of the vestibular mechanism. NASA, SP-77, 43–67. Washington, D.C.: NASA 1965.

NIVEN, J.I., HIXSON, W.C., CORREIA, M.J.: Elicitation of horizontal nystagmus by periodic linear acceleration. Acta oto-laryng. (Stockh.) **62**, 429 1966.

PORTMAN, G.: Recherche sur le sac endolymphatique: résultat et applications chirurgicales. Gronningen: Collegium Oto-Rhino-Laryngologicum 1927.

PORTMAN, M.: Endolymphatic sac surgery. Arch. Otolaryng. **89**, 101–103 (1969).

POWELL, T.J.: Acute motion sickness induced by angular acceleration. Royal Air Force Institute of Aviation Medicine. FPRC. p. 865 (Feb. 1964).

RAUCH, S.: La biochemie de l'endolymphe et de la périlymphe. C.R. Soc. franç. Oto-Rhyno-Laryng. **56**, 238 (1959).

SCHMALTZ, C.: Über die Reizvorgänge an den Endorganen des Nervus octavus. Arch. ges. Physiol. **208**, 424–444 (1925).

SCHMALTZ, C.: The physical phenomena occurring in the semicircular canals during rotary and thermic stimulation. Trans. roy. Soc. Med. **25**, 359–381 (1931).

SELYE, H.: The stresses of life. New York, Toronto, London: McGraw-Hill 1956.

SHERRINGTON, C.S.: The integrative action of the nervous system. New Haven: Yale Univ. Press 1947.

SJOBERG, A.: Experimental studies of the eliciting mechanism of motion sickness. In: Fourth Symposium on the Role of the Vestibular Organs in Space Exploration. NASA SP-187. Washington, D.C.: U.S. Government Printing Office 1970.

SPOENDLIN, H.H.: Ultra-structural studies of the labyrinth in squirrel monkeys. NASA SP-77, 7–22. Washington, D.C.: NASA 1965.

STEER, R.W.: The influence of angular and linear acceleration and thermal stimulation on the human semicircular canals. Sc.D. Thesis, M.I.T., (1967).

STEINHAUSEN, W.: Über den Nachweis der Bewegung der Cupula in der intaken Bogengangs-ampulle des Labyrinthes bei der naturtichen rotatorischen und calorschen Reizung. Pflügers Arch. ges. Physiol. **228**, 322 (1931).

STONE, R., JR., LETKO, W.: Some observations during weightlessness stimulation with Subject Immersed in a rotating water tank. NASA TND-2195, 16 pp. Langley Field, Va.: NASA 1964.

SUGIE, N., MELVILL JONES, G.: A model of eye movements induced by head rotation, I.E.E.E. Transactions Systems, Man, Cybernetics, S.M.C.I., No. 3 (1971).

TAIT, J., MCNALLY, W.J.: Some features of the action of the utricular maculae (and of the associated action of the semicircular canals) of the Frog. Phil. Trans. roy. Soc. **224**, 241–286 (1934).

VAN BUSKIRK, W.C.: Experimental and theoretical model studies of some dynamic response characteristics of the semicircular canals. Sc.D. Dissertation, Stanford University (1960).

VAN DISHOECK, H.A.E., SPOOR, A., NIJHOFF, P.: The opto-gyral illusion and its relation to the nystagmus of the eyes. Acta oto-laryng. (Stockh.) **44**, 597–607 (1954).

VAN EGMOND, A.J., GROEN, J.J., JONGKEES, L.B.W.: The turning test with small regulable stimuli: I. Method of Examination. J. Laryng. **62**, 63–68 (1948).

VAN EGMOND, A.J., GROEN, J.J., JONGKEES, L.B.J.: The mechanics of the semicircular canals. J. Physiol. (Lond.) **110**, 1–17 (1949).

VILSTRUP, T.: Studies of the complete structure and mechanism of the cupula. Ann. Otol. (St. Louis) **59**, 46–71 (1950).

VOLDRICH, L.: Present-day view on endolymph production. Proceedings of the Ninth International Congress on Oto-Rhino-Laryngology, Mexico City 1969. Excerpta Medica, Amsterdam, 641–642 (1970).

VON BAUMGARTEN, R.J.: Mechanism of biological memory. Agard Bionics Symposium, Brussels, 1968. In press.

Von Baumgarten, R.J., Atema, J., Hukuhara, J., Rocker, M.: Behavioral responses of blind goldfish to short periods of weightlessness. Space Life Sci. **1**, 554–564 (1969).

Von Baumgarten, R.J.: Vestibular research in space. Progress Report No. 2, Contract No. NAS 2-6057, NASA, Ames Research Center (1970).

Von Baumgarten, R.J., Baldrighi, G., Atema, J., Shillinger, G.L.: Behavioral responses to linear accelerations in blind goldfish. Space Life Sci. **3**, 25–33 (1971).

Wiggers, C.J.: "Physiology of shock". New York: Commonwealth Fund 1950.

Woelner, R.C., Graybiel, A.: Counterrolling of the eyes and its dependence on the magnitude of gravitational or inertial force acting laterally on the body. J. appl. Physiol. **14**, 4: 632–634 (1959).

Vallenstein, E.S.: The anatomical locus of reinforcement. Progress in physiological psychology. E. Stellar and J.M. Sprague, Eds. New York: Academy Press 1968.

Young, L.R., Meiry, J.L., Yao, T.Li: Control engineering approaches to human dynamic space orientation. NASA SP-115, 217–227. Washington, D.C.: NASA 1966.

Young, L.R., Meiry, J.L.: A revised dynamic otolithic model. NASA SP-152, 363–366. Washington, D.C.: NASA 1967.

Young, L.R.: The current status of vestibular system models. Automatica **5**, 369–383 (1969a).

Young, L.R., Oman, C.R.: Model of vestibular adaptation to horizontal rotations. Aerospace Med. **40**, 1076–1080 (1969).

Yuganov, E.M., Gorshikov, A.L., Kasyian, I.I., Bryanov, I.I., Kolosov, I.A., Kopanev, V.I., Lebeden, V.I., Popov, N.I., Solodovnik, F.A.: Vestibular reactions of cosmonauts during the flight in the voskhod spale ship. Aerospace Med. **37**, 691 (1966).

Chapter II.

The Vestibular System and the General Motor System*

By

H.H. KORNHUBER, Ulm

With 20 Figures

Contents

I. Introduction

A chapter on the general motor system might seem out of place in a handbook of sensory physiology. However, while in other systems sensory and motor mechanisms are integrated to some extent, in the vestibular system motor mechanisms predominate, so that it has been questioned whether it is a sensory system at all (GRIFFITH, 1922).

---

* In memory of ERICH VON HOLST.

The vestibular system is the head system of proprioception, determining the posture of the whole animal. Animals such as fish, frog, and rabbit are extremely disturbed after bilateral labyrinthine loss, and even in man there is severe disturbance of equilibrium in the acute stage following unilateral loss of a labyrinth. Furthermore, in phylogenesis the cerebellum has developed out of the vestibular nuclei (JOHNSTON, 1902; for review, see NIEUWENHUYS, 1967). It is difficult to understand how the vestibular nuclei relate to the spinal cord and the cerebellum, or the function of the neck reflexes and the motor cortex, without some general understanding of the motor system.

About 50 years ago the student of motor mechanisms was confronted with a profusion of segmental and higher static and dynamic reflexes — a situation to which ERICH VON HOLST reacted with sarcasm. However, the contemporary situation is not so different in principle. On the one hand we are offered cybernetic models far from biologic reality and on the other hand many papers are published describing functionally unrelated details of excitatory or inhibitory neuronal effects, often without any consideration of what is functionally necessary in a given system. Some synthesis of the methods of neurophysiology and systems theory might not be inappropriate here. Concepts like reflex, regulation, learning, conditioned reflex, or control are not sufficient to explain the motor behavior of a spider or a man. As will be shown, concepts like integrator, program, nad function generator are also necessary.

To supplement DOTY's excellent description of the pitfalls in interpreting the consequences of lesions in the visual system (this handbook, vol. VII/3, pp. 483–486), a few remarks regarding the motor system might be in order. Without some prior knowledge of the function of a given system, it can be misleading to record from neurons with a limited set of sensory stimuli. First, one might miss the adequate stimuli, and second, even if they are found, a functionally correct interpretation might be impossible without some knowledge of the connections and the specific function of the given class of neurons. For instance, all parts of the motor system receive sensory messages directly or indirectly, so that their neurons respond to vestibular, somatosensory, visual, or auditory stimuli similar to neurons in sensory areas.

A powerful method for the analysis of motor systems is to record the activity of single neurons during active motor behavior. However, in order to avoid misinterpretations, it is necessary to make a complete record of the movements and how the neuronal behavior relates to them in time. For instance, a movement of the hand often begins with a contraction of the shoulder muscles and may be accompanied by eye movements. Furthermore, movements of a given part of the body (e.g. the eyes) are often organized in quite different ways according to the velocity, amplitude, and type of stimulus received.

The effects of electrical stimulation within the central nervous system may differ with the structure of the tissue stimulated. In motor areas of the cerebral cortex the elements that respond to near-threshold stimuli are the efferent fibers, while in the cerebellum efferent, afferent, and intra-cerebellocortical fibers may be stimulated, depending on electrode position and type of current used.

The effects of lesions seem to be simpler, the closer the lesion is to the final common path; with more distant lesions the effects become difficult to interpret without additional information about the system.

Species differences have to be taken into account. Because of the difference in eye position and the presence or absence of a fovea, the oculomotor-vestibular systems of rabbit and monkey show characteristic differences. The visual and oculomotor systems of man differ from those of the rhesus monkey, at least with respect to predictive ability. Man is distinguished from other living species more than anything by the sophistication of his central nervous system. Therefore, in studying the biology of the central nervous system, we must make more use of clinical experience to learn about physiology than we do in any other field. Furthermore, the lesions induced in the human brain by genetic errors of metabolism or by viruses are sometimes more complete and more limited than those that can be produced surgically in animal experiments. For instance, it is virtually impossible to remove the cerebellar cortex completely without damaging the intracerebellar nuclei; yet in the initial stages of certain acute or subacute types of cerebellocortical atrophy in man (e.g. the Louis-Bar syndrome of children or the subacute cerebellar cortical atrophy of middle-aged or elderly patients) the lesion is limited to the cerebellar cortex and may be rather complete. The use of clinical findings to support a physiological argument should, however, be restricted to typical cases which correlate with known pathologic anatomy. Unusual findings are often due to additional atrophy. The attribution of a severe disorder of eye movements to basal ganglia disease was probably a misinterpretation of this sort (for discussion, see KORNHUBER, 1973a).

There are several ways of gathering initial information about the function of a motor system: for instance, noting of the results of lesions, with limited attempts at functional interpretation; systematic recording and consideration of the activities, responses and connections of a given subsystem and of the available knowledge about functionally related parts; and relation of the overall function of the motor system in a given animal to its typical behavior and environment. All of these approaches have contributed to the functional interpretation presented here.

II. The Holding Function of the Vestibular System

The basic function of the vestibular system is to stabilize body and eye positions in order to ensure precise, goal-directed movements and clear vision. This resembles the stabilization of a gun platform on a battleship; platform and gun, however, are identical in the case of the eye, and partly identical in the case of the body and the limbs. Furthermore, the degree of motor freedom is greater in a freely moving animal than in a battleship. For these reasons, it is necessary to set limits to the vestibular stabilization of eye and body postures by means other than vestibular afferents.

1. Vestibular Stabilization of Body Posture

In higher vertebrates that have a freely moving head, the labyrinths indicate body position only in conjunction with the afferents from the neck receptors. Therefore the vestibular afferents cannot be used as a stabilizing feedback signal for body position unless the position of the head relative to the body is taken into account. von Holst and Mittelstaedt, 1950 concluded that neck afferents must be subtracted from labyrinthine messages to yield the right signal for maintaining equilibrium both in tilting situations and when only the head is moved. The neck reflexes are the exact opposite of the labyrinthine tilting reflexes (Fig. 1), which depend on the vertical channels and otoliths. Unfortunatley,

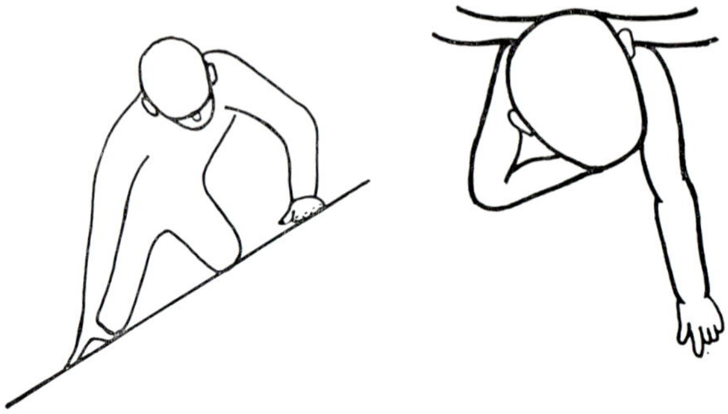

Fig. 1. The asymmetric tonic neck reflexes (to the right, in a child) are the antagonistic partners of the labyrinthine tilting reflexes (to the left). When the head is turned with the nose toward the left, the neck reflex induces extension of the left arm and flexion of the right arm. Rapid lateral tilt with the nose to the left, however, causes extension of the right and flexion of the left arm. Labyrinthine tilting reflexes prevent falling during rapid tilt; neck reflexes prevent falling due to labyrinthine reflexes when only the head is moved. From Kornhuber, Arch. Ohrenheilk. **194** (1969)

Magnus, who discovered the neck reflexes, failed to appreciate this fact and his erroneous functional interpretations of the neck reflexes persist in physiological textbooks up to the present. The vestibular tilting reflexes (McNally and Tait, 1925; Rademaker, 1931; Rademaker and Garcin, 1933) and the tonic neck reflexes are independent of the cerebellum. The vestibular and neck afferents converge in the vestibular nuclei (Fredrickson, Schwarz and Kornhuber, 1965).

Tonic neck reflexes occur as independent phenomena in a normal child only in the first year of life, yet their prominent role in maintaining body equilibrium in adults (as opposed to regulating eye position, see Kornhuber, 1966, 1970, and this volume, Chap. F.I.) is clear from experimental section of the upper three dorsal cervical roots in cat (Magnus and Storm van Leeuwen, 1914) and monkey (L. A. Cohen, 1961). The resulting body disequilibrium is as severe as that found after bilateral labyrinthectomy. A man can hardly do a handstand without dorsiflection of the head (Fukuda, 1961).

In addition to receptor afferents of the upper neck joints, there are also many afferents from joints in the limbs to the vestibular nuclei, predominantly from proximal limb joints (Fredrickson, Schwarz and Kornhuber, 1965). As these responses are not abolished by cerebellectomy nor by deep barbiturate anesthesia, they are not mediated by the cerebellum and probably not by the reticular forma-

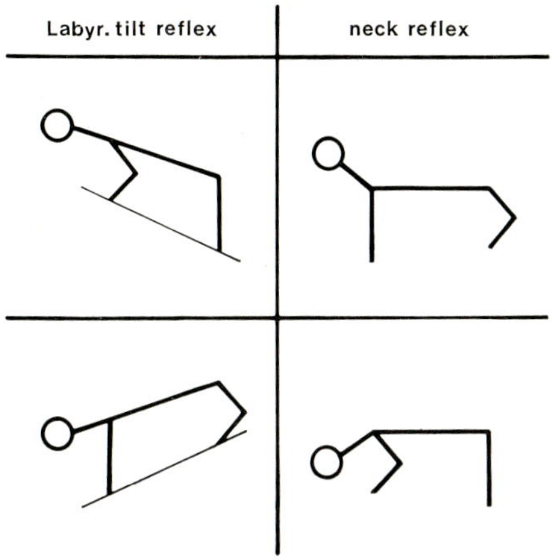

Fig. 2. The symmetrical neck reflexes as antagonistic partners of labyrinthine tilting reflexes with tilt in a rostrocaudal direction (around a transverse axis)

tion. These deep somatic afferents from the limbs need not surprise us in view of similar feedbacks to other motor centers, such as the motor cortex. The absence of group-Ia muscle afferents in the vestibular nuclei (in contrast to the presence of joint afferents) has been confirmed by Barness and Pompeiano (1971) and Pompeiano and Barness (1971).

The vestibular regulation of body posture is, of course, superimposed on spinal regulations. In the long term, the most prominent reflex found in man after spinal transection is the nociceptive flexion reflex (with flexion paraplegia as the consequence). Following supramesencephalic lesions, however, reticular facilitation of the antigravity stretch reflex (resulting in extensor spasticity) is dominant in the human leg, while flexion (belonging to grasp and cling reflexes) dominates spasticity in the hand and arm, resulting in the Wernicke posture. It is important that we understand these mechanisms, which differ in man and in quadrupeds, because they are basic not only for motor physiology, but also for everyday clinical practice. For instance, following spinal injury or cerebral stroke, the development of severe spasticity and contracture can be prevented by appropriate counterpositioning of the patient's limbs.

2. Vestibular Stabilization of Eye Position

As pointed out in the introduction to this volume (Kornhuber, part. 1), the main advantage of vestibular as opposed to visual stabilization of eye position is the better frequency response of vestibular stabilization in the higher frequency range. The frequency-response characteristics of the semicircular canal apparatus have been adjusted by natural selection so as to operate in the normal range of the motor system (Mayne, 1950; Jones and Spells, 1963).

Between the labyrinths and the extraocular muscles is an elementary three-neurons reflex arc (Cohen, Suzuki and Bender, 1964; Ito, Nisimaru and Yamamoto, 1973). The effects of electrical stimulation of single ampullar nerves agree well with the analysis of the afferents from these nerves following rotational stimuli (Lowenstein and Sand, 1940). However, there are several reasons why natural vestibular eye movements cannot be fully accounted for by this elementary reflex arc. First, an integration of the velocity signal provided by the vestibular nerve is necessary. Second, in order to stabilize the position of the eye in the orbit, several muscles must contract together and the amount of co-contraction will vary with the position of the eye. Third, the function of the individual eye muscles varies with the position of the eye. Fourth, reflex movements of the eyes cannot be continued indefinitely. The vestibular system itself is unable to measure or determine the position of the eyes over a long period of time, therefore some independent signal of eye position must exist to produce meaningful vestibular eye movements. Unfortunately, little is known about this important point.

Some nystagmus rhythm can still be recorded from the proximal end of the abducens nerve after all oculomotor nerves have been cut and the eyes extirpated (McIntyre, 1939). Local anesthesia of the extraocular muscles does not abolish vestibular nystagmus (De Kleyn, 1922). There is no stretch reflex in the extraocular muscles of the monkey (Keller and Robinson, 1971). These observations favor the hypothesis that the onset of rapid phases of nystagmus may be determined by signals from motor outflow rather than from spindle feedback. A signal of this kind could perhaps come from the reticular formation and cerebellar nuclei, since they perform the necessary integration (see below). So far, tonic neurons that indicate eye positions and are not engaged in saccadic-burst activity have been found only in the frontal eye field of the monkey (Bizzi, 1968) (these neurons presumably receive this information from the cerebellar nuclei via the dorsomedial thalamus), and in the paramedian pontine reticular formation (Fuchs and Luschei, 1972) where the quick phases of horizontal nystagmus originate. Furthermore, some incomplete integration of vestibular velocity signals in the horizontal plane is probably performed by neurons of the paramedian pontine reticular formation since the second integration is not completely abolished by cerebellectomy (D. Robinson, person. comm.). Probably there is feedback from the reticular neurons to the vestibular nuclei which modulates their activity corresponding to the nystagmus rhythm (Duensing and Schaefer, 1958; Horcholle-Bossavit and Tyč-Dumont, 1972). None of these observations exclude the possible influence of extraocular muscle afferents upon eye movement, and especially upon the time of onset of rapid phases of nystagmus. Except for a few neurons driven by vestibular stimuli but also influenced by eye muscle stretch in the vestibular nuclei (Weber and Steiner, 1965), extraocular muscle afferents have so far been found only in structures related to rapid phases of nystagmus or saccadic eye movements. Gernandt (1968) found that eye muscle stretch inhibited reticular neurons driven by vestibular stimuli; no such inhibition was observed in fibers of the medial longitudinal fasciculus. Fuchs and Kornhuber (1969) found afferents from passive stretch of extraocular muscles in the cerebellar cortex of the cat. They also observed a large short-latency field potential to passive eye muscle stretch in the brainstem below the nodulus.

III. Visual Stabilization of Eye Position and Smooth-Pursuit Eye Movement

Vestibular regulation of eye position is better than visual regulation at higher frequencies, but worse in the low-frequency range (see chapter A.I.). Since the vestibular apparatus is unable to hold the eyes constant for long periods, continuous visual regulation is also necessary for stabilization of eye position. This visual regulation is to some extent identical with optokinetic regulation or the smooth-pursuit eye movement.

In man, continuous visual regulation of eye position is largely mediated via the cerebral cortex. Consequently, unilateral lesions of the corticofugal fibers from the visual and association areas of the occipital, temporal and parietal lobes to the brainstem result in impairment of optokinetic nystagmus towards the contralateral side and of smooth-pursuit eye movement to the ipsilateral side, leading to unilateral weakness of visual eye stabilization against vestibularly induced eye shifts. This weakness appears as a directional preponderance of caloric nystagmus when tested under conditions of visual fixation (BADER and KORNHUBER, 1965; see Chap. F.I. this volume). Contesting the sampled data model of YOUNG and STARK (1963), ROBINSON (1965) showed that human smooth-pursuit eye movement is continuously regulated by visual feedback. It was shown by COLLEWJIN and VAN DER MARK in the rabbit that without continuous visual regulation eye position is unstable. It is similarly unstable in blind humans. Stabilization of eye position with respect to environment is a function which is already present in animals like the rabbit that have panoramic vision but do not possess a fovea. Foveate species, like monkey and man, have in addition foveal smooth tracking of small stimuli moving across a steady visual background.

The neural mechanisms of both peripheral and foveal smooth pursuit and fixation include the cerebellar nuclei, since slow atrophy of the whole cerebellum including the nuclei causes gaze nystagmus and optokinetic disturbance (JUNG and KORNHUBER, 1964). Moreover, certain lesions of the cerbellar nuclei or their fiber connections with the brainstem cause pendular fixation nystagmus (ASCHOFF, CONRAD and KORNHUBER, 1974), while cerebellar cortical lesions do not cause gaze nystagmus, fixation nystagmus, or disturbance of smooth pursuit (KORNHUBER, 1968). The disturbance of smooth pursuit and the presence of gaze nystagmus was confirmed by total cerebellectomy in the monkey (WESTHEIMER and BLAIR, 1973), whereas such disturbances were not found after cerebellar cortical lesions (ASCHOFF and COHEN, 1971). These findings lend support to the theory (KORNHUBER, 1970, 1971, 1974) that the nuclear and cortical functions in the cerebellum are different. The nuclei add continuous hold regulation to cerebello-cortical function.

It is this stabilization of positions by means of continuous feedback regulation which distinguishes the function of the cerebellar nuclei from that of the cerebellar cortex (as will be pointed out later), whereas it is analogous to that of the vestibular nuclei (KORNHUBER, 1970, 1971, 1974). The cerebellar nuclei and the vestibular nuclei are similarly related to the cerebellar cortex: both are monosynaptically inhibited by the Purkinje cells (ITO and YOSHIDA, 1964; ITO et al., 1964). Phylogenetically, the vestibular nuclei provide the model for the cerebellar nuclei, because the oldest part of the cerebellar cortex was derived from the vestibular nuclei. The function of the vestibular nuclei directed by the labyrinths was to stabilize the position of the whole body; the cerebellar nuclei, however, stabilize the positions of parts of the body (eyes or limbs) as directed by the visual system, the cerebral cortex, or the optic tectum.

It was presumably because this visual holding function requires integration (COLLEWIJN, 1972) that the vestibular system transferred part of its function, namely the second integration, to the cerebellar nuclei. Since the adequate stimulus for the cupula is angular acceleration of the head, a double integration has to be performed in order to stabilize eye position. The first integration is done

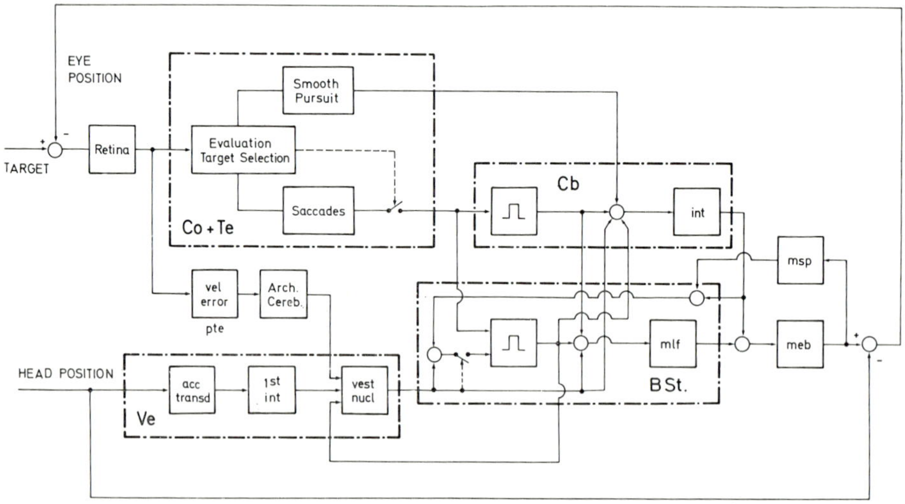

Fig. 3. Block diagram of the neural mechanisms of eye position control (vestibular eye stabilization, smooth-pursuit eye movement, rapid phases of nystagmus, and saccades). *Ve* vestibular apparatus and vestibular nuclei, *BSt.* brainstem, *mlf* medial longitudinal fasciculus, *Co* cerebral cortex, *Te* tectum opticum, *Cb* cerebellum, *int* integrator, *EM* eye muscles, *meb* muscles and eye-ball, *msp* muscle spindles, *pte* pretectal area. In the vestibular apparatus, the first integration of head acceleration is performed mechanically. There is visual motion feedback (via the accessory optic tract and the archicerebellum) for adaptation of gain and elimination of drifts prior to the second integration which is performed in the reticular formation and cerebellum. The vestibular system has two pathways to the oculomotor nuclei: direct feedforward via the medial longitudinal fasciculus and a multisynaptic pathway through the brainstem reticular nuclei. There are two step generators for rapid phases of nystagmus and saccades, one in brainstem reticular nuclei, which perhaps provides preemphasis of force, the other in the cerebellum (probably for fine control of saccadic duration and size). There is feedback from the eye muscle spindles to the cerebellum and to the step generator in the brainstem reticular nuclei, but probably the cerebellar integrator also feeds back to the brainstem step generator (since nystagmus rhythm persists after section of the eye muscles). The reticular and cerebellar integrators are leaky and therefore need continuous visual input in order to hold eccentric eye positions. The smooth-pursuit and saccadic branches of visuomotor information processing in the forebrain make use of a common mechanism for evaluation and target selection. The tectum opticum closely cooperates with the cortical visual system in designing saccades (W. BECKER and H.H. KORNHUBER, unpubl.)

mechanically in the semicircular canals. The discharge rate of the first-order vestibular fibers is proportional to the velocity of the head. Since the eye muscles (and other mechanical factors of the orbit) are incapable of performing the second integration, there must be a neural integrator between the vestibular and oculomotor nuclei (ROBINSON, 1968; CARPENTER, 1971; SKAVENSKI and ROBINSON, 1973). This integrator has been shown to be located at least in part in the cerebellum (CARPENTER, 1971); it is obviously not in the cerebellar cortex, for cerebello-cortical lesions do not affect the holding function (KORNHUBER, 1968). The migration of the second integration into the cerebellar nuclei might account for the projection of primary and secondary vestibular fibers to the nuclei (for review, see BRODAL, Chap. D.I., this volume). The removal of the integrator causes a marked reduction of low-frequency gain in the vestibular frequency response (CARPENTER, 1971). Simple bedside clinical tests in patients reveal disturbance of smooth-pursuit eye movement and gaze nystagmus (JUNG and KORNHUBER, 1964). Some incomplete integration of vestibular velocity signals is, however, done outside the cerebellar nuclei (probably in the reticular formation) since after cerebellectomy the time constant of eccentric gaze positions is still in the order of 1 sec (D. ROBINSON, pers. comm.). Integrated signals are obviously fed back to the vestibular nuclei. The activity of many neurons of the vestibular nuclei in the non-decerebrate animal corresponds to eye position rather than head velocity, while in the decerebrate preparation all cells of the vestibular nuclei indicate head velocity.

IV. Predictive Tracking

When a regular (predictable) square-wave motion is used as the visual stimulus, the human brain (which initially responds with a delay of 0.2 to 0.3 sec) rapidly detects the periodicity and predicts the motion, so that the eyes may be in phase with stimuli of moderate frequencies (around 0.4–1.0 Hz). Similarly, gain and phase relations of smooth-pursuit tracking work much better for predictable sine waves than for unpredictable stimuli (STARK, VOSSIUS and YOUNG, 1962). It is very interesting that predictive square-wave tracking, which seems to require nothing but a phase shift of a simple internal rhythm, is not present in the rhesus monkey (FUCHS, 1967). One might speculate that the evolution of predictive eye tracking could have had something to do with the hunting behavior of man; the rhesus monkey is not a hunter. Several authors have tried to fit mathematical models to the predictive capacities of human eye movements, but the situation turned out to be more complex than anticipated (DALLOS and JONES, 1963; MICHAEL and JONES, 1966; ST.-CYR and FENDER, 1969). The prediction behaves nonlinearly in the sense that it is not possible to estimate the response to one class of stimulus motions by a linear combination of responses to other classes of stimuli. However, one point seems to be clear: unlike head, trunk, arm, or hand movements, which are capable of reproducing complicated patterns by long-term prediction, eye movements have only short-term predictive ability. This important difference is, of course, not due to the visual system, which analyzes stimulus motions for both hand and eye movements, but rather corresponds to the inability of the oculomotor system to perform voluntary ramp movements (see below).

V. Visual Control of the Vestibulo-Ocular Reflex Arc via the Archicerebellum

Unlike stabilization of body posture, which is effected by vestibular feedback, vestibular stabilization of eye position occurs by negative feedforward, since the labyrinths are not influenced by eye position. Systems of this sort tend to drift and are sensitive to quite small internal changes; therefore some visual adjustment is useful. It is advantageous to eliminate drift and adjust gain prior to the second integration; this is done in the vestibular nuclei by means of a visual pathway that runs via the accessory optic tract, the pretectal nuclei, and the central tegmental tract to the flocculus and nodulus (MAEKAWA and SIMPSON, 1973); these in turn inhibit neurons in the vestibular nuclei. This pathway has been found in the rabbit, and it may also be important in man since lesions of the flocculonodular lobe cause positional nystagmus (see KORNHUBER, Chap. F.I., this volume).,

VI. Rapid Phases of Nystagmus and Saccadic Eye Movements

Slow phases of vestibular nystagmus and smooth-pursuit eye movements on the one hand, and rapid nystagmic phases and saccadic eye movements on the other hand, differ not only in their relative velocities, but also in their neural organization, the stimuli that evoke them, and their sensory consequences. An early observation (BÁRÁNY, 1907) of a patient who as a consequence of a pontine tuberculoma lost the rapid phase of ipsilateral nystagmus while the slow phase was preserved, indicated that different neural structures might underlie the rapid and slow phases of vestibular nystagmus. LORENTE DE NÓ (1928, 1931, 1933) in his classic experiments showed that the quick phase of horizontal nystagmus originates in the paramedian pontine reticular formation and not in the vestibular nuclei; his conclusion was confirmed by later observations (DUENSING and SCHAEFER, 1957, 1958; BENDER and SHANZER, 1964; COHEN and HENN, 1972; FUCHS and LUSCHEI, 1972). Similarly, the origin of the quick phases of vertical vestibular nystagmus seems to lie in the mesencephalic nuclei, whose destruction leads to vertical gaze paralysis. The slow phases of optokinetic nystagmus, on the other hand, are selectively impaired by barbiturate intoxication whereas the rapid phases are far less affected. RASHBASS (1961) has shown that the reaction times of smooth-pursuit and saccadic eye movements vary independently. Smooth-pursuit eye movements begin after a reaction time of about 125 to 150 msec, while saccades need about 200 msec. Repeated saccades will occur instead of smooth-pursuit eye movements if the mechanisms controlling the latter are upset. Smooth-pursuit eye movements are determined by target velocity, saccadic movements by displacement. ROBINSON (1965) has shown that smooth-pursuit eye movements are continuously regulated by vision, while rapid nystagmic phases and saccades are too fast for this. The visual determination of the angle to be moved occurs before the onset of the saccade; once a saccade has started, it follows a predetermined course which cannot be changed at will (ballistic type of movement) (WEST-

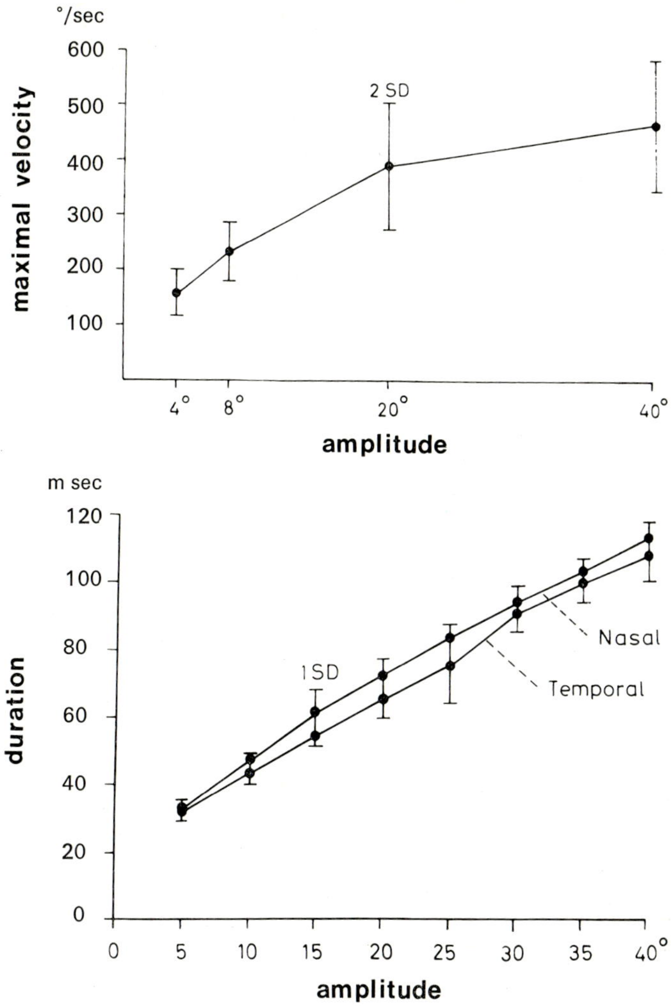

Fig. 4. The relationship between maximal angular velocity and amplitude of human saccadic eye movements is nonlinear with saturation at about 40° (from KORNHUBER, KREJCOVA and SCHMIDT, unpubl.). The relationship between the duration and amplitude of saccades, however, is linear up to 40° (from ROBINSON, J. Physiol. (Lond.) **174** (1964))

HEIMER, 1954). The duration of both saccades and rapid nystagmic phases up to about 40° is a linear function of their amplitude. Saccades of 5° have a duration of about 30 msec; 35° saccades last about 100 msec. The relation is similar for quick nystagmic phases and saccades (RON, ROBINSON and SKAVENSKI, 1972), but rapid phases of vestibular nystagmus are slightly faster than saccades of similar length under the same visual conditions. Furthermore, the velocity of both saccades and quick phases is similarly reduced (and the duration consequently prolonged) by darkness or lack of structure in the visual field (BECKER and FUCHS, 1969; RON, ROBINSON and SKAVENSKI, 1972).

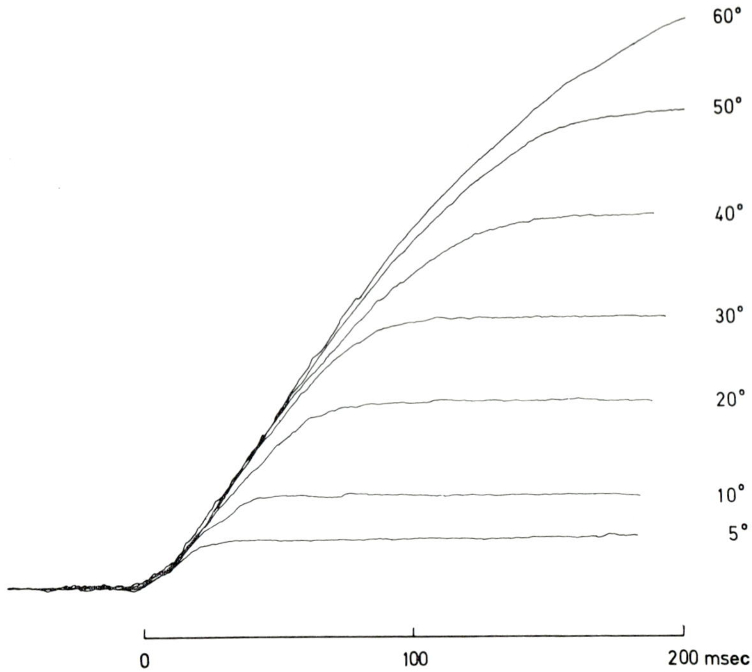

Fig. 5. Average course of human saccadic eye movements of different amplitudes. Bitemporal electrooculogram from a normal subject, looking forth and back between two points on a horizontal line. The first 16 saccades to the right were averaged. Some reduction of saccadic velocity due to slight drowsiness is unavoidable under these experimental conditions without alerting drugs like amphetamines. By courtesy of W. BECKER (unpubl.)

Both rapid nystagmic phases and saccades have a refractory period of about 80 msec in man (from start to start) when they run in the same direction (GAEFKE, 1968; ROBINSON, 1968). In the monkey, a somewhat shorter refractory period has been observed after electrical stimulation of the frontal eye field (ROBINSON and FUCHS, 1969). When the frontal eye fields are stimulated in both hemispheres, the refractory period exists only for saccades of the same direction, and not for vertical saccades that follow horizontal ones, or for saccades in the other horizontal direction. Similar results were obtained with electrical stimulation of the optic tectum in the monkey (ROBINSON, 1972). Thus, the refractory period is introduced between the optic tectum and the extraocular motoneurons. Such a long refractory period may have evolved for internal reasons concerning the pulse generator (e.g. in order to ensure that programming of the next step was not biased by foregoing events), but it is also useful to allow undisturbed visual information processing between jumps since, if saccades occurred more often, this would result in a "masking" effect.

Rapid nystagmic phases and saccades similarly affect visual perception of motion. Motion is fully perceived during stimulus-bound, passive smooth eye movements, such as slow phases of vestibular or optokinetic nystagmus and

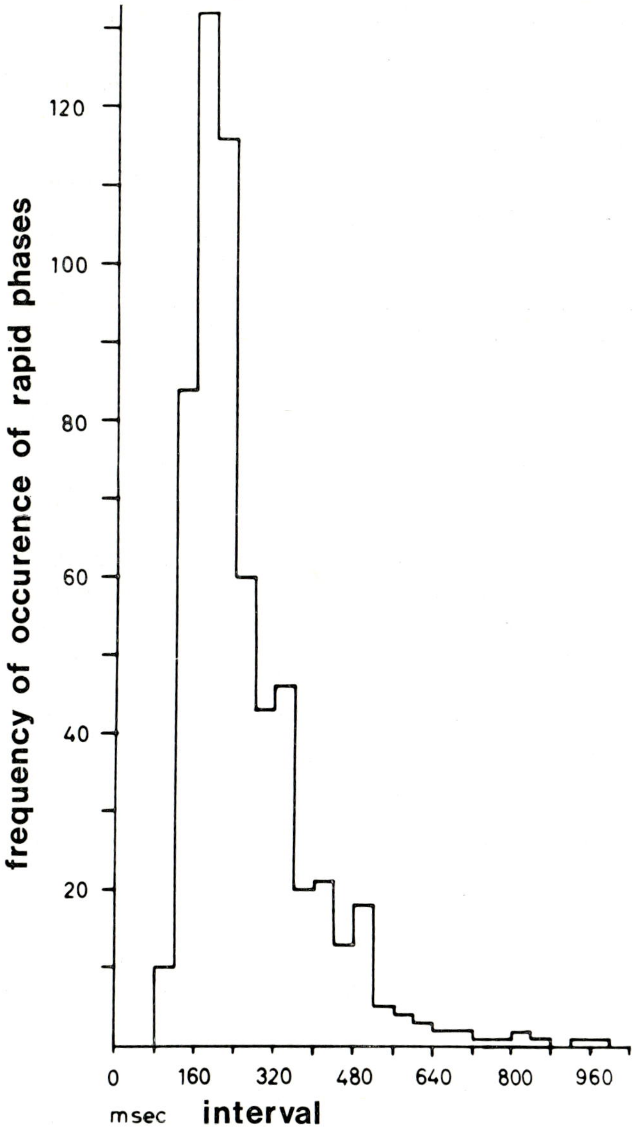

Fig. 6. The distribution of intervals between the rapid phases of human horizontal vestibular nystagmus under conditions of strong rotatory acceleration shows a refractory period of 80 msec when measured from onset to onset of the rapid phases. A similar refractory period exists after rapid phases of optokinetic nystagmus and saccades (from GAEFKE, Thesis, Freiburg i.Br. 1968)

smooth-pursuit eye movements, as well as during eye movements induced by external pressure upon the eyeball. However, during saccades and fast nystagmic phases, visual motion perception is inhibited in the direction contrary to these eye movements. Therefore, vestibular nystagmus induces apparent motion of the visual surroundings in the direction contrary to the slow nystagmic phases but not in the same direction. This is not due to differences in the velocity of the eye movements, since slow phases of vestibular or optokinetic nystagmus may be as fast as 100°/sec yet visual motion perception is preserved, whereas small saccades may be as slow as 4°/sec but there is no apparent movement.

Despite all these similarities between the rapid phases of vestibular nystagmus and saccades, there is one important difference: rapid phases of vestibular nystagmus in nonfoveate animals like the rabbit are not exactly programmed by visual targets whereas saccades in foveate animals are. Several findings suggest that the evolution of this new function not only required an interface between the visual system and the old saccadic pulse generator, but also induced the development of another, more precise pulse generator in the cerebellum. Indeed, it seems as if saccades are not only basically different from non-visually guided rapid phases of nystagmus, but are also of two different kinds, coarse and fine, depending on the optic tectum and the visual cortex, respectively.

Let us begin with the last finding. YOUNG's sampled data model (1963) suggested that the visual information used for programming saccadic eye movements is gathered discontinuously at intervals of about 200 msec. However, YOUNG's model did not agree with experimental findings. Saccades may occur at intervals of 80 msec, and visual information usually seems to be gathered continuously, although there are special situations in which saccades are inhibited for about 200 msec in order to avoid "masking" of visual information processing in situations where no further information could be obtained by additional saccades (BECHINGER et al., 1974). Further research along these lines has revealed another interest-

---

Fig. 7. Features of human correction saccades following coarse saccades upon targets stepped randomly in the horizontal plane. A: Magnitude of correction saccade (ordinate) as a function of target distance (abscissa) in one subject. Each point represents the average of 24 movements; correction saccades for undershooting of coarse saccade were entered as positive samples into the average, corrections for overshoot as negative ones, and if no correction saccade occurred the sample was considered as a zero. SY denotes saccades travelling between positions that are symmetrical with respect to the primary position, AXO saccades that return from an eccentric position to the primary position, and AOX saccades that start from the primary position to reach an eccentric one. Note the absence of further increase of the amplitude of correction saccades beyond target angles of 50°, so that the average magnitude of the correction saccade does not exceed 6°. B: Latency of correction saccades, measured from the end of the main saccade (ordinate) as a function of magnitude of the correction. Same subject as in A. Each point represents one movement. Solid line gives the average, broken line shows average optomotor reaction time (latency between target step and onset of main saccade) in the same experiment. The latency of corrections exceeding 3° of amplitude is almost independent of the size of the correction and is 80 msec shorter than the optomotor reaction time. Smaller corrections need more time on average; note, however, that the lower limit of latency (about 130 msec) is fairly independent of the correction amplitude (From BECKER, Bibl. ophthal. 82, (Basel) Karger, 1972). C: The amplitude information in the saccadic system is continuously updated. If a first step of the target is followed by a second one prior to the onset of the saccadic reaction that is being prepared as a response to the first step, the second step can modify the amplitude of the saccade under preparation. In the present example, a double step sequence consisting of horizontal 30°-step forth followed after 50, 100, 150 or 200 msec by a 15°-step back was presented at random together with other plain and double step patterns. About 50 responses were recorded at each of the 4 step separations. Each response saccade is represented by one point; the ordinate gives its amplitude and the abscissa its time of occurence

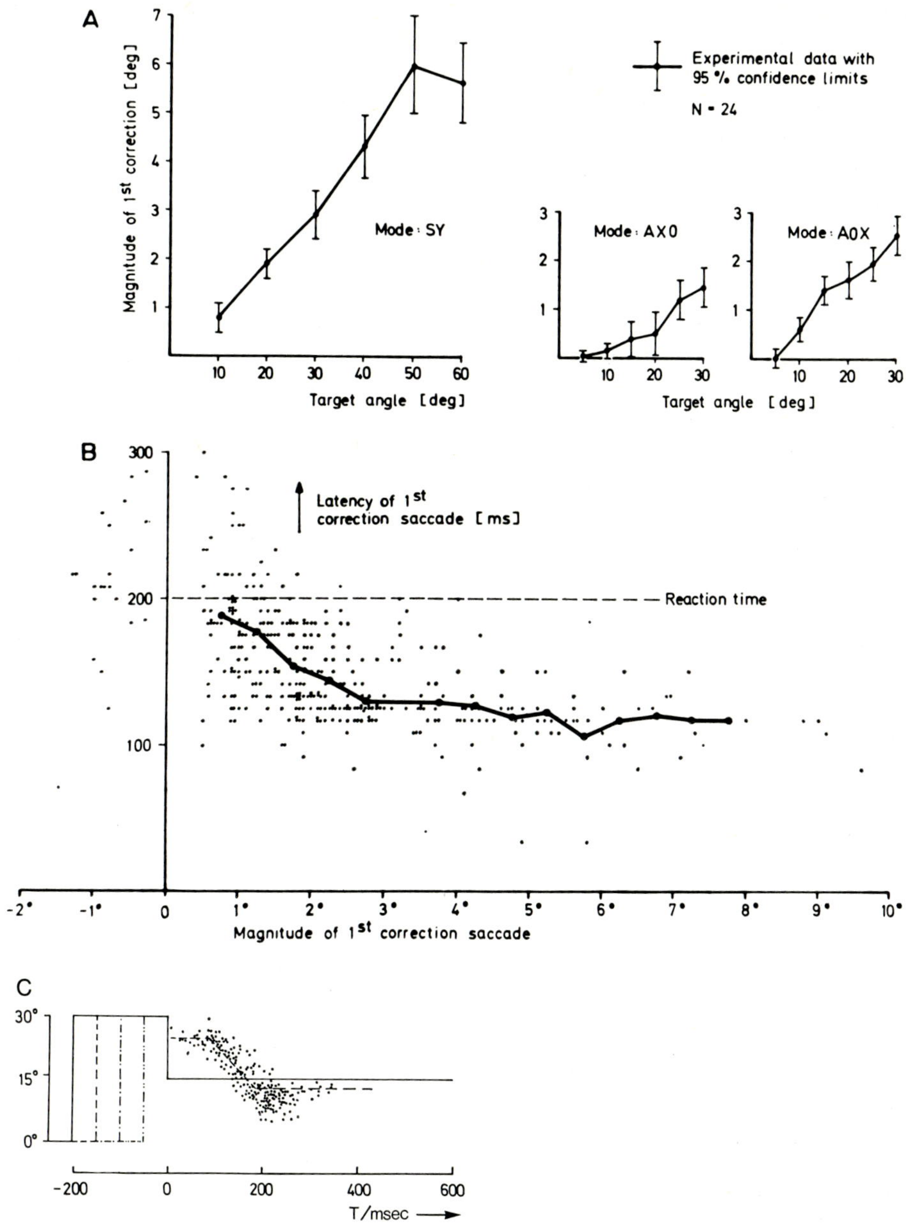

with respect to the second target step. Three straight line segments have been fitted to the data (broken line): the left horizontal segment represents the average amplitude of saccadic reactions to plain steps of 30°, the right horizontal segment corresponds to saccades aiming 15°-targets. The oblique segment has been fitted by eye and represents the time course in which the programming of the saccadic amplitude is changed by the second step. Modification of the amplitude starts already 85 msec after the second step and is completed within about 200 msec. In the present example, the second target step required a shortening of the saccadic amplitude; if the second step calls for a prolongation of the saccade, it needs about 200 msec in order to initiate the amplitude modification. From BECKER and JÜRGENS, 1974

ing finding. BECKER and FUCHS (1969) and BECKER (1972) showed that with large target displacements the saccadic system seems to know that it cannot with high precision match a large angle by a single step. Therefore it uses a double-step approach: first a coarse saccade, which covers about 90% of the distance to the target, then a fine correction saccade of 1–6°, which has a latency of only 130 msec; this is much shorter than the main saccadic reaction time (200 msec or more). Visual information is gathered during this 130 msec interval and is used to program the fine correction saccade. When the target displacement is further increased, the fine correction saccade usually does not exceed 5–6°. This saccadic behavior might be related to the fact, that in the monkey the peripheral visual field projects in a retino-topic manner to the superior colliculus while the central 5° to 7° have no direct retino-tectal connections. There is, however, a dense projection to the superior colliculus from the part of the striate cortex that serves the central 5° of the visual field (WILSON and TOYNE, 1970).

Although the data seem somewhat controversial at present, the cerebellum is probably more important for saccadic eye movements than was thought a few years ago. KORNHUBER (1968) reported that dysmetria of saccadic eye movement is a consequence of cerebellar cortical atrophy. In such cases there is no paralysis of gaze and no gaze nystagmus; the smooth-pursuit eye movement seems to be normal and the vestibular nystagmus is intact. The saccadic eye movements, however, are grossly dysmetric, usually hypometric. Instead of one main move-

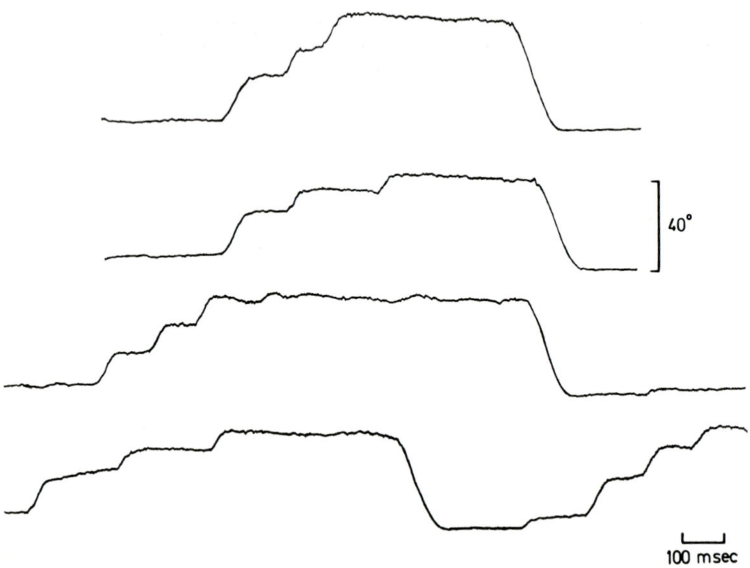

Fig. 8. Cerebellar dysmetria of saccadic eye movements. Hypometria of saccades towards the right in a case of a cerebellar tumor. Normal (large) saccades to the left. The patient was asked to look forth and back between two targets symmetrical to midposition. There is no gaze paresis and no nystagmus. The speed of the hypometric eye movements is normal (From KORNHUBER, in: Vorträge der Erlanger Physiologentagung 1970 (KEIDEL and PLATTIG, Eds.) Berlin-Heidelberg-New York: Springer)

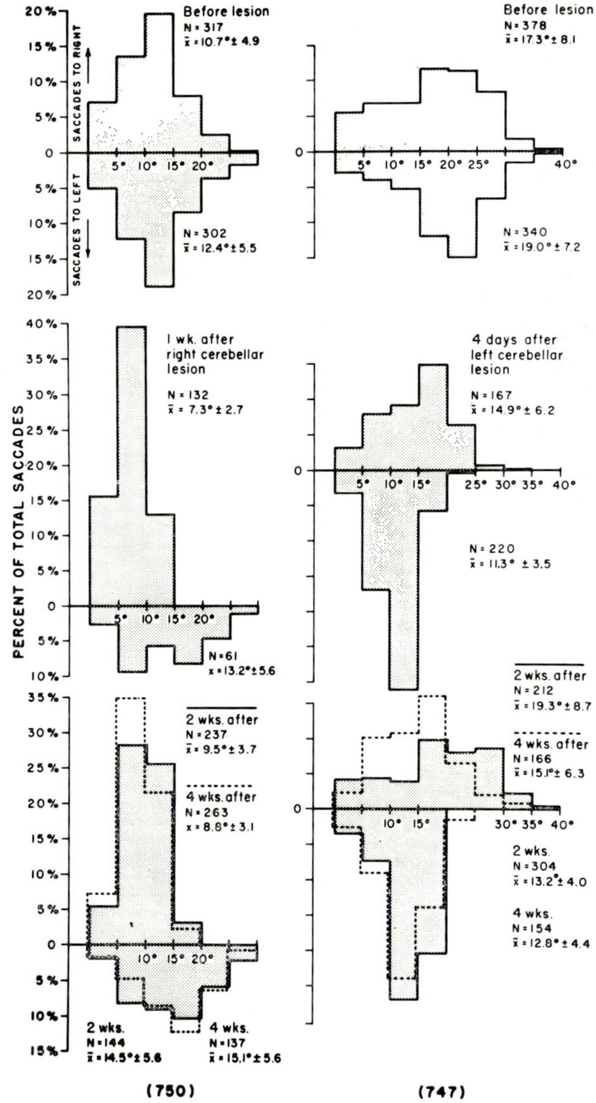

Fig. 9. Distribution of amplitudes of spontaneous horizontal saccadic eye movements before and after cerebellar cortical lesions in the paravermis and vermis (lobuli V, VI and VII) of two monkeys (monkey 750 = graphs on left, monkey 747 = graphs on right). N indicates total number of saccades to either side during the same period of time. x is mean amplitude, ± standard deviation. The bottom graphs show the distribution in each animal after 2 weeks (solid lines) and 4 weeks (dotted lines). Differences in mean amplitude and number of saccades to either side were significant after operation ($p < 0.05$). While the saccades are symmetrically distributed to the right and left before operation, after operation the mean amplitude of saccades is significantly smaller towards the side of the lesion (From Aschoff and Cohen, Exp. Neurol. **32** (1971))

ment to the goal there are several small or medium-sized saccades. In unilateral lesions the dysmetria is ipsilateral. The velocity of the hypometric saccades may be normal. This pure cerebellar dysmetria of saccadic eye movements is best seen in cases of subacute atrophy of the cerebellar cortex e.g. the Louis-Bar syndrome of children or the subacute cerebellar cortical atrophy of middle-aged or elderly patients. At more advanced stages of the disease or in patients with slowly progressing atrophy, e.g. Friedreich's atrophy, there is usually gaze nystagmus and a disturbance of smooth pursuit and optokinetic nystagmus in addition to dysmetria, indicating involvement of the cerebellar nuclei. Eventually, the saccade may be slowed down, which would correspond to transneuronal atrophy of the oculomotor neurons in the brainstem. The saccadic dysmetria accompanying cerebellocortical atrophy has been atrributed to the lobuli Vb and c, VI, and VIIA (Kornhuber, 1970), since afferent projection from the eye muscles was found here (Fuchs and Kornhuber, 1969) and this region yielded eye movements upon electrical stimulation (Hampson, Harrison and Woolsey, 1952) (Fig. 10). The dysmetria

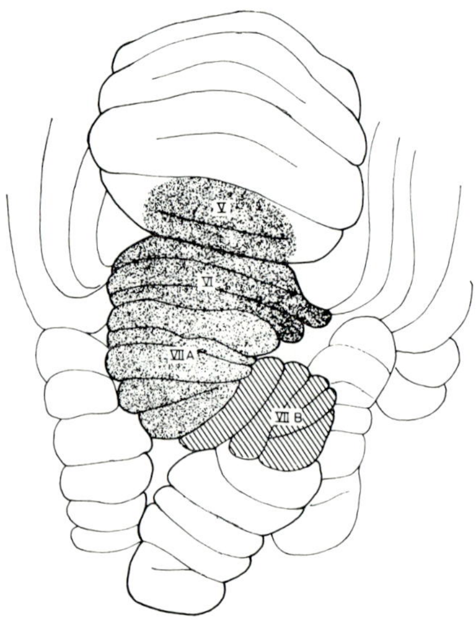

Fig. 10. The projection of eye muscle afferents to the cerebellar cortex of the cat is located in lobuli Vb and c, VI, and VIIA. There is a weaker projection to VII B. Based on potentials evoked by small step stretch of extraocular muscles in barbiturate anesthesia. The projection of visual afferents is located in the same region, which also yields saccadic eye movements upon electrical stimulation (From Fuchs and Kornhuber, J. Physiol. (Lond.) **200** (1969))

of saccadic eye movements has been reproduced experimentally in the monkey by lesions of the vermis and adjacent paravermis including lobules VI and VII (Aschoff and Cohen, 1971); the defect was not so severe as in clinical cases of cerebellocortical atrophy because the experimental lesions were incomplete. A severe defect of the initiation of fast phases of optokinetic nystagmus was also observed in rabbits after total cerebellectomy (COLLEWIJN, 1970), but in the monkey cerebellectomy failed to abolish the fast phases of nystagmus (WESTHEIMER and BLAIR, 1973), perhaps due to better visual facilitation of fast phases in this animal. The authors claimed that cerebellectomized monkeys could execute saccades with good precision, although the severe gaze nystagmus present in these animals precluded an exact study. The theory of cerebello-cortical involvement in programming fast (step) movements (KORNHUBER, 1970, 1971, 1974) acquired further support from the finding that in the rhesus monkey Purkinje cells discharge prior to saccades and fast phases of optokinetic nystagmus but not during slow phases (LLINÁS and WOLFE, 1972). RON and ROBINSON (1973) found that saccades evoked by electrical stimulation of lobuli V to VII of the monkey's vermis had direction and amplitude independent of pulse train frequency, pulse width, and pulse train length; above threshold, however, saccadic amplitude increased with increasing stimulus current. This result might be interpreted by the assumption that threshold stimuli excite large-diameter parallel fibers and stronger stimuli excite thinner parallel fibers. From a region in the cerebellar hemisphere, RON and ROBINSON evoked saccades together with smooth eye movements. The smooth components could be due to inhibition of cerebellar nuclear neurons via Purkinje axons, or to excitation of nuclear neurons via antidromic firing of collaterals of climbing or mossy fibers.

The cerebellar cortex seems to have evolved as a more precise step generator, providing the higher motor resolution demanded by the visual acuity of the central part of the fovea. Fixation must be maintained within about 10 min of arc, a task for which the older step generator in the reticular nuclei of the brainstem was presumably not precise enough, although it can compensate in part for the oculomotor defect resulting from cerebellar lesions. The nature of the normal coordination of these two systems has still to be clarified. Theoretically, the termination of large saccades might be regulated by proprioceptive feedback from the eye muscles (FUCHS and KORNHUBER, 1969).

VII. The Forebrain and the Vestibulo-Reticulo-Cerebellar System

What is the origin of the motor commands that make use of the automated functions of the vestibulo-reticulo-cerebellar system? Is the motor cortex able to control all kinds of voluntary movement, as usually stated in textbooks? In order to answer these questions, let us consider the overall function of the motor system in an animal within its environment.

1. Strategy and Tactics of Action. Sensory Association Areas and Apraxia

Movements are usually part of actions, and actions serve the needs of the organism and the survival of the species. They are therefore guided by messages both from the internal milieu and from the environment. Let us classify these messages as strategic or tactical. If we are thirsty, our strategy is to search for water. This strategy is determined by the osmoreceptive neurons of the hypothalamus and by the volume receptors of the left atrium. The tactics of our search, however, depend on the environment and are laid down in the sensory (primary and association) areas of the occipital, temporal and parietal lobes of the forebrain and their thalamic nuclei. Lesions of these sensory and association areas induce errors of spatial orientation, failure to recognize objects, and apraxia (inability to perform skilled aimed movements in the absence of paralysis of limb or eye).

2. Cerebral Potentials Preceding Voluntary Movements

Evidence obtained in man from cerebral potentials preceding movements by the method of reverse analysis (KORNHUBER and DEECKE, 1965) is in good agreement with the results recorded from lesions in sensory association areas of the forebrain. In such experiments the first event preceding voluntary movement is not a localized potential over the motor cortex but the bilateral Bereitschafts-potential (readiness potential), which is greatest over the parietal cortex and at the vertex when it precedes voluntary saccadic eye movements (BECKER et al., 1972). The second potential, the pre-motion positivity, is also bilateral and wide-spread. Even movements most dependent on the motor cortex (human finger movements) are preceded by a bilateral Bereitschaftspotential and a bilateral pre-motion positivity, and both of these are larger over the parietal than over the precentral area of the ipsilateral hemisphere. It is only after these events have taken place that a unilateral potential appears; it is greatest over the hand area of the contralateral motor cortex. The unilateral potential starts about 50 msec before the movement, the pre-motion positivity starts about 80 to 90 msec, and the Bereitschaftspotential about 800 msec prior to onset of fast finger movements (DEECKE, SCHEID and KORNHUBER, 1969).

3. Is a Cortical Reflex Arc to the Motor Cortex the Basis of Voluntary Movements?

When apraxia was discovered, it was assumed by analogy with the spinal reflex arcs that the disorder was caused by disruption of a cortico-cortical reflex arc that sends information from the sensory association areas of the occipital, temporal and parietal lobe to the motor cortex. This hypothesis became so popular that it is treated as a self-evident fact in textbooks and even in recent papers, although the available anatomical and physiological evidence argues against it. The work of PANDYA and KUYPERS (1969) and JONES and POWELL (1970) shows that the primary and association areas of the visual and auditory system do not project to the motor cortex. There might be a very indirect route from the posterior association areas to the motor cortex via the frontal lobe; however, apraxia (the origin of the belief that cortico-cortical reflex arcs are the basis of voluntary movement) does not occur with frontal lesions. In accordance with these anatomical findings, neurons of the cat's motor cortex do not respond to visual stimuli (KORNHUBER and ASCHOFF, 1964); the contradictory results of BUSER and IMBERT (1961) were probably due to chloralose anesthesia. When neurologists jumped to the conclusion that a cortico-cortical reflex arc is the basis of voluntary movements, they forgot that voluntary movements are technically quite different from spinal reflexes, because voluntary movements require the active creation of a spatio-temporal pattern. For instance, the movement of a light spot on the screen of an oscilloscope requires a function generator; its biological equivalent is the step (or pulse, or burst) generator that underlies saccadic eye movements or rapid

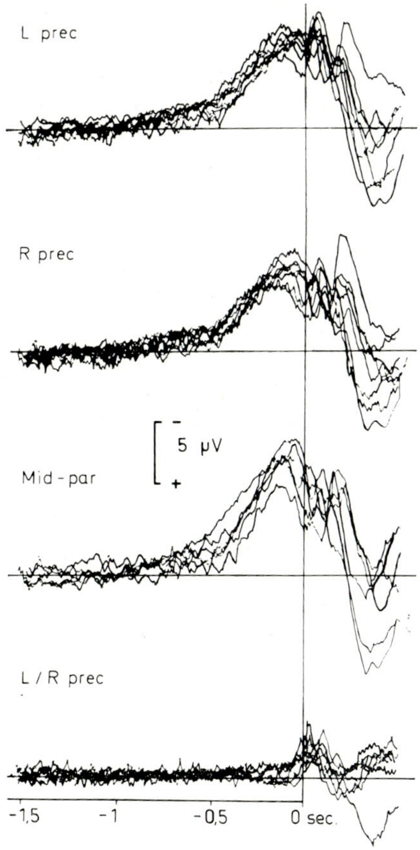

Fig. 11. Cerebral potentials, recorded from the human scalp prior to voluntary rapid flexion movements of the right index finger. The potentials were obtained by the method of reversed analysis (Kornhuber and Deecke, 1965). Eight experiments with the same subject on different days; about 1000 movements per experiment. Upper 3 rows: monopolar recording, with both ears as reference; the bottom trace is a bipolar record, left versus right precentral hand area. The Bereitschaftspotential (readiness potential) starts about 0.8 sec prior to onset of movement; it is bilateral and widespread over precentral and parietal areas. The pre-motion positivity, bilateral and widespread too, starts about 90 msec before onset of movement. The motor potential appears only in the bipolar record; it is unilateral over the left precentral hand area, starting 50 msec prior to onset of movement in the electromyogram. Experiment of W. Becker, L. Deecke, B. Grözinger, and H.H. Kornhuber, first presented at the German Physiological Society meeting 1969; Pflügers Arch. **312**, R 108

phases of nystagmus. The cerebral cortex is an analyzer for the detection of features, similarities, patterns, etc.; it is also a synthesizer and categorizer and a large memory core, but it is clearly not a function generator for spatio-temporal patterns of movement. Judging from the severe akinesia seen in the final stages of diseases of the basal ganglia or cerebellum, it is probably safe to conclude that voluntary movement is impossible without basal ganglia, cerebellum and brain-stem reticular nuclei, although this dependence has never been demonstrated directly.

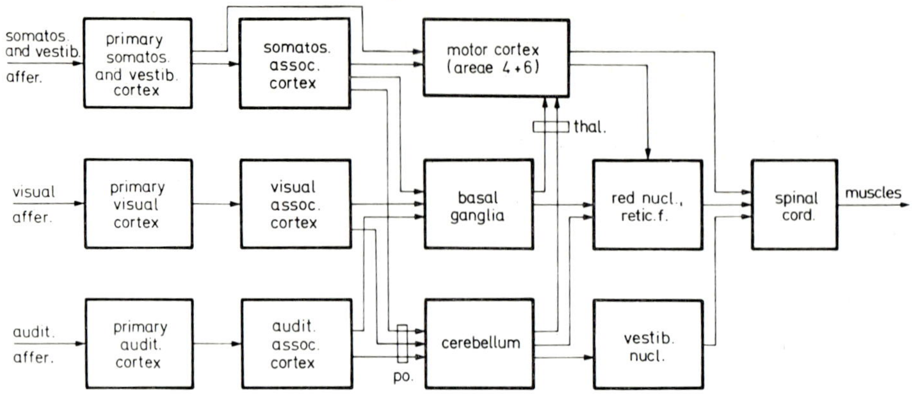

Fig. 12. Information flow diagram showing tactics of voluntary movements. The sensory messages processed in the primary and association areas of the cerebral cortex give rise to motor commands that are transformed into spatio-temporal patterns by the function generators in the cerebellum and basal ganglia. For simpler movements, their output goes directly via the old supranuclear motor centers of the brainstem (the vestibular nuclei, the red nucleus, and the reticular formation) to the spinal cord. For movements that need sophisticated tactile analysis of objects, their output goes via the motor cortex (From KORNHUBER, in: F.O. SCHMITT and F.G. WORDEN, Eds. The Neurosciences, Third Study Program, Cambridge, Mass., and London: MIT Press 1974)

4. Fiber Connections between Cerebral Cortex, Cerebellum and Basal Ganglia

Anatomically, the cerebellum (NYBY and JANSEN, 1951) and the basal ganglia (the strio-nigro-pallidum) (KEMP and POWELL, 1970) — considered here as a functional unit for the sake of simplicity — are connected in parallel between nearly the whole cerebral cortex (input source) and the motor cortex (output target), with a synapse in the ventro-lateral thalamus, of course. In other words, although there is input from the motor cortex to both the cerebellum and the basal ganglia, most afferents to these structures come from sensory and association areas of the cortex. Thus, for the most part, the motor cortex follows the basal ganglia and cerebellum in the direction of information flow. It is not surprising that the motor cortex also projects to the cerebellum and basal ganglia, since the motor cortex is a sensory (somatosensory and vestibular) association area (KORNHUBER and ASCHOFF, 1964).

This consideration brings us back to the cerebellum, which will now be considered in a wider framework, starting again with saccadic eye movements.

VIII. Discontinuous (Saccadic) Function of the Cerebellar Cortex

Cerebellar function is usually supposed to come into play after a movement has been triggered by the motor cortex and to function to make the movement smooth and free from oscillations. Despite this common belief, I consider that the cerebellum does not merely regulate movements programmed and initiated by the motor cortex, but that it participates in the design of rapid movements prior to their initiation. I base this idea on the observation of dysmetria of saccadic eye movements due to atrophy of the cerebellar cortex (KORNHUBER, 1968). In the case of saccades, the whole course of the movement is programmed prior to onset, and it is similar with rapid arm movements, as shown by their dysmetria after cerebello-cortical lesions. The angle to be covered by a saccade is measured by the visual system prior to onset. For the movement, however, the spatial data must be converted into temporal data, i.e. the duration of the saccade, since its angle depends largely upon its duration. Inability to determine the duration of a

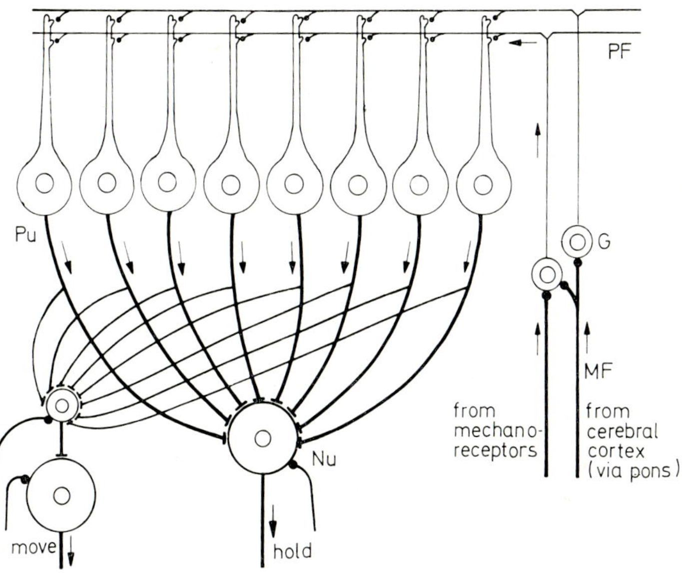

Fig. 13. The parallel fiber (PF) delay line in the cerebellar cortex with the row of Purkinje cells (Pu) converging on a neuron of the cerebellar nuclei (Nu). This arrangement acts as a step function generator, timing the duration of fast preprogrammed (open-loop) movements that are too quick to be regulated continuously (saccadic-type movements). The intervals between different fast movements can be timed by this clock. At the granular cells (G) that give rise to the parallel fibers, the afferents converge from the cerebral cortex (via the pons) and from the spinal cord and mechanoreceptors. The inhibitory action of the Purkinje cell output stops the holding function of a hold neuron and disinhibits (by means of an inhibitory interneuron) a move neuron (From KORNHUBER, in: KEIDEL and PLATTIG, Eds. Vorträge der Erlanger Physiologentagung 1970. Berlin-Heidelberg-New York: Springer)

saccadic burst must therefore result in a disturbance of saccadic amplitude. It has been suggested that the translation of spatial into temporal data (angle into burst duration) is effected by selective excitation of appropriate granular cells in the cerebellar cortex. The granular cells run into parallel fibers which excite a row of Purkinje cells. If the axons of such a row of Purkinje cells converge onto a common neuron in the cerebellar nuclei (which has been hypothesized, see Fig. 13), this nuclear neuron will be inhibited (or disinhibited by an inhibitory neuron) for as long as the action potentials are traveling down the parallel fibers (KORNHUBER, 1970, 1971, 1974). With fibers up to 5 mm long (in one direction) and conduction velocities down to 0.05 m/sec, eye movements lasting up to 100 msec are possible. BRAITENBERG and ATWOOD (1958) concluded on anatomical grounds that the parallel fibers of the cerebellar cortex constitute a delay line having the ability to transform spatial into temporal patterns. Unfortunately, BRAITENBERG's papers on the cerebellum have not received the attention they deserve, because he failed to consider that a row of Purkinje cells might converge at the next neuronal stage and consequently attributed an inappropriate function to the climbing fibers (BRAITENBERG, 1961; BRAITENBERG and ONESTO, 1960).

If the parallel fibers act as a delay line, this would explain why it is usually hypometria rather than hypermetria that accompanies atrophy of the cerebellar cortex. Any metabolic deficiency probably first affects the thinnest and longest parallel fibers — those responsible for the large-amplitude saccades, according to our theory. The discontinuous, saccadic nature of cerebello-cortical activity sheds some light on the function of the elaborate inhibitory network found by ECCLES et al. (1967) in the cerebellar cortex. Discontinuous action calls for a clearing command after each operation to erase the traces of the previous action and to ensure exact limitation of movement.

In the visual pathway to the cerebellum there is a synapse in the optic tectum. The cells here only become active before saccadic eye movements of a specific direction and size; they are not involved in smooth-pursuit movements (SCHILLER and KÖRNER, 1971; WURTZ and GOLDBERG, 1972). However, the duration of the saccades is not coded in the discharge of these neurons, because many of them fire for a period two to three times longer than the duration of the corresponding saccade.

1. Parametric Gain Adjustment via Climbing Fiber Action

As has been pointed out (p. 590), the vestibulo-ocular feedforward needs adjustment of gain by visual feedback. GONSHOR (1971) has shown in man that in experiments with reversing prisms the vestibulo-ocular reflex shows slow, but considerable plasticity resulting in reduction and even reversal of gain. ROBINSON (1974) found in the cat that this plasticity is abolished by removal of lower parts of the cerebellar cortex (including the nodulus, uvula, paraflocculus, lower half of the pyramis and of the paramedian lobes). The reason why visual feedback to the vestibular system causes parametric adjustment and why it is not simple direct feedback is probably that there is not enough time for meaningful conventional feedback. Head movements are usually fast (up to 200° per sec and more), and retinal action is slow.

Obviously the adjustment of gain in the cerebellar cortex is done by climbing fiber action since visual input to the archicerebellum comes via climbing fibers (MAEKAWA and SIMPSON, 1973). Extrapolating the results from the vestibulo-cerebellum and combining the ideas of KORNHUBER (1970–1974) about cerebellar step and holding functions, on the one hand, with those of BRINDLEY (1964), MARR (1969), ITO (1974) and ROBINSON (1974) about motor learning, on the other hand, one might draw the tentative conclusion that the cerebellum is an apparatus for designing and adjusting fast movements and for holding the positions in between.

2. Role of Peripheral Mossy Afferents to the Cerebellar Cortex. Adiadochokinesis and Sequential Programs

In addition to dysmetria of fast step movements, adiadochokinesia, or the inability to perform rapid repetitions of fast movements, is a symptom of cerebello-cortical lesions. This brings us to the function of the peripheral afferents to the cerebellum from receptors in the skin, joints, and muscles and from spinal motor centers. The function of these afferents cannot be to provide negative feedback in a continuous servo-regulation because the cerebellar cortex acts like a clock, programming the duration of fast movements. One function of the afferents from mechanoreceptors might be to participate in the selection of the appropriate granular cells. Movements from different starting positions need different durations. For instance, saccadic eye movements from the midposition to a lateral position have a longer duration than saccades from the lateral to midposition. The selection of granular cells is, of course, mainly the task of afferents signalling messages from the cerebral cortex (via the pontine nuclei). However, afferents from mechanoreceptors could also influence the selection of granular cells so as to take into account the starting position of the limb or eye to be moved. Another function of the peripheral afferents to the cerebellar cortex might be to time the start of the next parallel-fiber volley. Temporal coordination of successive rapid movements is important in writing or speaking or (for birds) flying. The activity of many small birds consists mainly of rapid movements that are too fast to be regulated continuously by sensory feedback. When a bird flies through the branches of trees, its survival depends on the temporal coordination of rapid movements; it is perhaps because of this that birds have such a large cerebellum (most of all the humming bird). Adiadochokinesis, slowing down of handwriting, and a hesitatant type of speech are signs of cerebello-cortical lesions in man. To use internal feedback from preceding motor actions or reafferent sensory signals is a more reliable way of timing successive movements than to have a temporal superprogram that times the start of each single movement component, independently of the actual end of the preceding movement. The cerebral cortex presumably provides a sequential program of movements with rather general commands about speed; the exact timing must depend on the reafferent messages, which converge with the signals from the forebrain at the granular cells of the cerebellar cortex (see Fig. 14).

IX. Function of the Cerebellar Nuclei

Unlike the cerebellar cortex with its discontinuous, saccadic function, the cerebellar nuclei have a continuous holding function (Kornhuber, 1970, 1971, 1974), as can be inferred from holding tremor, pendular fixation nystagmus, and gaze nystagmus resulting from cerebello-nuclear lesions, and from the functional analogy with the vestibular nuclei. These facts help us to understand why the cerebellar Purkinje cells are inhibitory in action, as found by Ito et al. (1964).

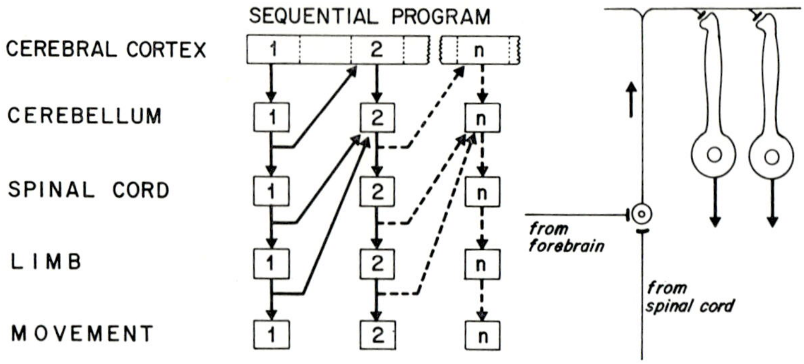

Fig. 14. Timing of a series of rapid movements by reafferent volleys. Instead of constructing a temporal superprogram to start each single component of movement irrespective of the occurrence and timing of the preceding movement, the cerebral cortex presumably provides only a sequential program with specification of direction, amplitude, overall speed, etc., while the cerebellum effects the exact timing of the components of movements, using reafferent signals from lower motor centers or mechanoreceptors (From KORNHUBER, in: F. O. SCHMITT and F. G. WORDEN, Eds. The Neurosciences, Third Study Program, Cambridge, Mass., and London: MIT Press 1974)

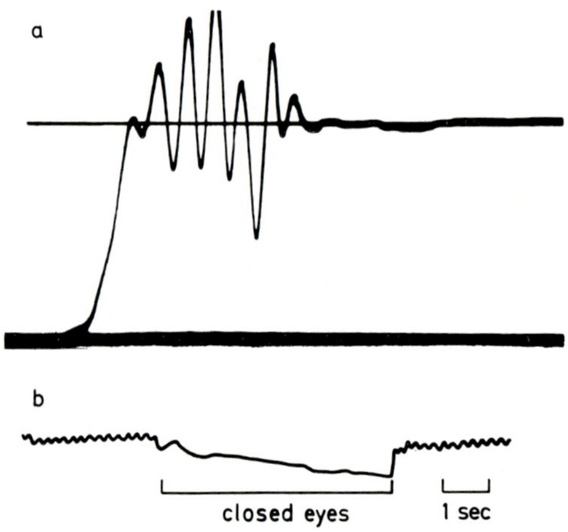

Fig. 15. Holding tremor of the arm (a) or eye (b) in a patient with lesions of the cerebellar nuclei or their efferent fiber connections with the thalamus (a) or brainstem (b). In a, the arm was rested on a lever to allow movements in the horizontal plane only. The oscillation appears when holding a position after rapid step movement. In b, the pendular eye nystagmus (which is an acquired symptom in multiple sclerosis) is present during fixation and disappears when the eyes are closed. a is a record made by Dr. B. CONRAD; b from the study by ASCHOFF, CONRAD and KORNHUBER, 1974. (From KORNHUBER, in: KEIDEL and PLATTIG, Eds. Vorträge der Erlanger Physiologentagung 1970. Berlin-Heidelberg-New York: Springer

The holding function has to be inhibited to make movement possible, although inhibition of holding still falls short of movement. In the vestibular and cerebellar nuclei, however, there are in addition to large neurons small interneurons which may be inhibitory. Inhibition of these inhibitory interneurons would release the main neurons for action.

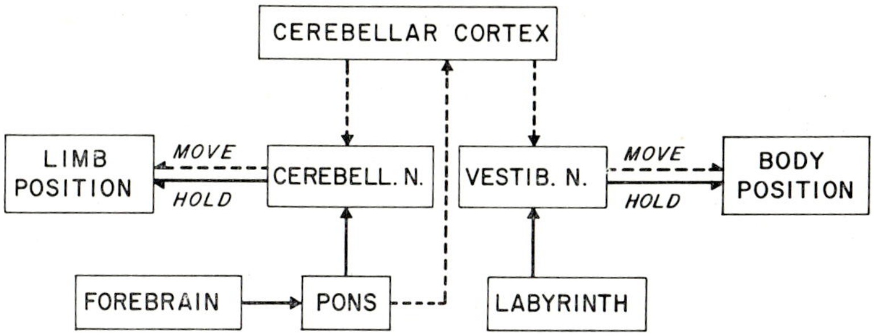

Fig. 16. Analogy (in function and in connections with the cerebellar cortex) of the vestibular nuclei and the cerebellar nuclei. Phylogenetically, the vestibular nuclei must have been the model for the cerebellar nuclei (From KORNHUBER, in: F.O. SCHMITT and F.G. WORDEN, Eds. The Neurosciences, Third Study Program, Cambridge, Mass., and London: MIT Press 1974)

X. Archicerebellum and Motion Sickness

Although complex psychological and even Freudian psychoanalytical explanations of motion sickness are current, motion sickness is strictly due to physiological mechanisms. Bilateral labyrinthectomy abolishes motion sickness (SJÖBERG, 1931) whereas blindness does not. Extirpation of the lower vermis including the nodulus relieves the susceptibility to motion sickness (BARD et al., 1947) whereas, contrary to the predictions of psychoanalysis, lesions of the fronto-basal neocortex, which remove higher drives and release primitive drives like hunger, do not bring relief. Motion sickness is mainly caused by head movements during rotation (JOHNSON and MAYNE, 1953); this is a situation in which the Coriolis effect causes labyrinthine stimulation in a plane different from that of head movement. The effect of vermal lesions may be explained as follows: like the visual or the somatosensory system, the vestibular system has the problem of distinguishing between messages from the environment and stimuli due to active movements. Apparently, it solves this problem like other sensory systems by inhibiting certain sensory effects of active movements. In the frog the labyrinthine receptors are under the direct efferent inhibitory control of the cerebellum (LLINÁS and PRECHT, 1969) but in the cat the vestibular nuclei are inhibited by the cerebellum. There is a figure in the literature (R. S. SCHMIDT, 1965) displaying a similar hair cell mechanoreceptor in amphibians, the lateral-line stream receptor, that shows a short burst of efferent inhibitory impulses to the receptor preceding each active gill movement. Similar results have been obtained with the goldfish vestibular nerve (C.L. SCHMIDT et al., 1972). Inhibitory signals of this kind sent by the archicerebellum during fast head movements must be inappropriate in the Coriolis situation and perhaps even more confusing when attempting adjustment of gain in the wrong plane. This could be the cause of motion sickness and might explain why it is relieved by removal of the archicerebellum (KORNHUBER, 1970, 1971, 1974).

XI. The Basal Ganglia as Ramp Generator

If the cerebellum is a generator for fast (open-loop step) movement, then where are the continuous smooth movements at various voluntary speeds produced? Movements of this kind can be made at will and at any speed (within limits) with hand, arm, leg, head, trunk, etc., but not with the eyes. Voluntary eye movements are saccadic; a smooth-pursuit movement of the eyes is possible only when the target is moving, or for short-term prediction in connection with a moving stimulus in the external world. Voluntary slow eye movements independent of the moving stimulus are not only unnecessary but would interfere with visual perception: Therefore, in the intervals between the microsaccades used to overcome retinal adaptation, the eyes are kept relatively steady.

Ramp movements, i.e. smooth movements at voluntary speeds, are apparently generated in the basal ganglia (KORNHUBER, 1970, 1971, 1974). The evidence is as follows. First, the basal ganglia are important for movements of parts of the body other than the eyes. Second, eye movements are not represented in the motor cortex to which the basal ganglia project via the ventrolateral thalamus. The frontal eye field receives thalamic afferents from mediodorsal but not from the ventrolateral nucleus. Third, while most of the symptoms of lesions in the basal ganglia are signs of release (rigidity, resting tremor, chorea, athetosis, torsion dystonia, and ballism), the only deficiency symptom is akinesia. In the monkey severe akinesia results from bilateral lesions of the internal pallidum, which is the output stage of the basal ganglia (METTLER, 1945). Akinesia is the only symptom of basal ganglia disease that cannot be relieved by stereotactic surgery in the pallidum or thalamus. On the contrary akinesia is usually more severe after bilateral lesions in the ventrolateral thalamus or pallidum. Whereas athetosis and torsion dystonia clearly involve released ramp movements, akinesia in parkinsonism consists of a defect in ramp generation. Akinesia predominantly affects actions which require initiation or change of ramp movements, such as rising from a sitting or a lying position, turning over, starting to walk, stopping walking, or turning during walking. Because of the defective ramp initiation in Parkinson patients, some ramp movements are performed very slowly; the ramp components of the leg movements during walking, however, are replaced by small rapid movements of the cerebellar type, because very slow leg movements would endanger equilibrium. Finally, direct testing of the theory presented here revealed that neurons of the putamen are active only prior to and during slow movements and are not engaged in fast arm movements (DELONG, 1974), while cerebellar Purkinje cells are active only preceding saccadic eye movements and rapid nystagmic phases and not during smooth eye movements (LLINÁS and WOLFE, 1972). The different contributions made to a movement by the step (saccadic), ramp (smooth) and hold functions can be demonstrated by a simple experiment, the finger-to-nose test. If the movement is performed as fast as possible, three components can be distinguished: (1) a rapid (preprogrammed) movement which brings the finger near the nose; (2) a short hold with a little oscillation; (3) a slow ramp movement to the nose. The first component depends on the cerebellar cortex, the second on the cerebellar nuclei, and the third on the basal ganglia. The first component may be disturbed by dysmetria, the second by large oscillations ("intention" tremor, postural tremor or holding tremor), and the third by akinesia and rigidity.

XII. The Motor Cortex: Tactile Adjustment

The motor cortex is often said to be the system for producing voluntary movements. This widespread assumption is certainly erroneous since, after bilateral removal of the motor cortex, cats show almost normal motor behavior, including many actions which would doubtless be classified as "voluntary" in man. Similarly, electrical stimulation of the cerebral cortex (often adduced to demonstrate that the motor cortex alone is motor in nature) clearly shows that the whole

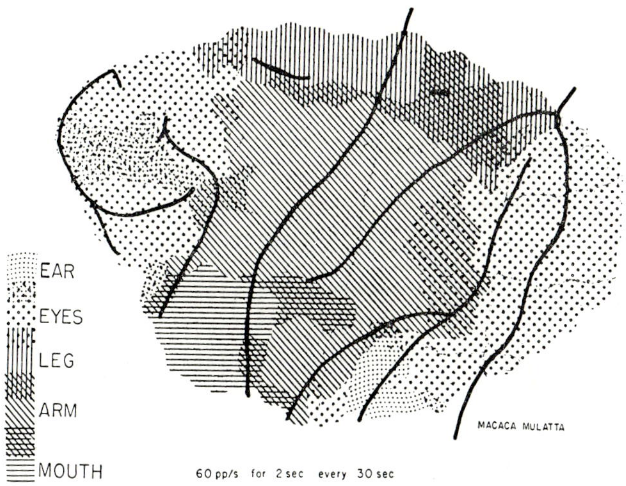

Fig. 17. Map of the movements elicited at threshold by electrical stimulation from the cortex of an unanesthetized monkey. All of the 610 stimulation electrodes used yielded responses at about the same threshold. This map is very similar to that published by WAGMAN, 1964 (see article by FREDRICKSON, KORNHUBER and SCHWARZ in this handbook, D.VI.). According to these motor maps of the monkey cortex and similar results from the VOGTS (1919), the whole of the cerebral cortex is "motor" in nature. Finger, arm, leg, face, mouth or tongue movements are elicited from the Rolandic sensory motor region only, while eye, head, ear or adversive trunc movements are elicited from widespread areas in the occipital, posterior parietal, temporal and frontal lobes (From LILLY, in: HARLOW and WOOLSEY, Eds. Biological and Biochemical Bases of Behavior, Madison: University of Wisconsin Press 1958)

cortex yields movements. This is not the result of current spread (as argued by the Montreal School in contesting these results), since the pattern of the movements evoked by stimuli outside the sensorimotor cortex is specific and differs from that of the Rolandic area (VOGT and VOGT, 1919; FOERSTER, 1936; LILLY, 1958; WAGMAN, 1964; ALBE-FESSARD and DONALDSON, 1970). Obviously, these motor effects are mediated by the cerebellum and basal ganglia to which the whole cerebral cortex projects (to the cerebellum via the tectum, pontine nuclei, or reticular nuclei).

While electrical stimulation outside the sensorimotor Rolandic area yields eye, hand, ear and adversive trunk movements, the motor and somatosensory fields on both sides of the Rolandic fissure produce limb, face, and especially finger, toe, lip, and tongue movements. This is in full agreement with what is known of the effects of lesions in the motor cortex. The movements most affected are those of the hand, especially the fingers, while eye, head, and trunk movements remain intact. There is a quantitative correspondence between the representations of the different parts of the body in the somatic and motor cortical areas. From the anatomical point of view the motor cortex is a somatic association area, for it receives strong afferents from the somatic fields but not from visual or auditory primary or association areas (PANDYA and KUYPERS, 1969; JONES and POWELL, 1970). Recordings from single units in the cat's motor cortex fully support this view: somatic afferents are the most common sensory afferents at neurons of the motor cortex; the next most common are the vestibular afferents, but visual affer-

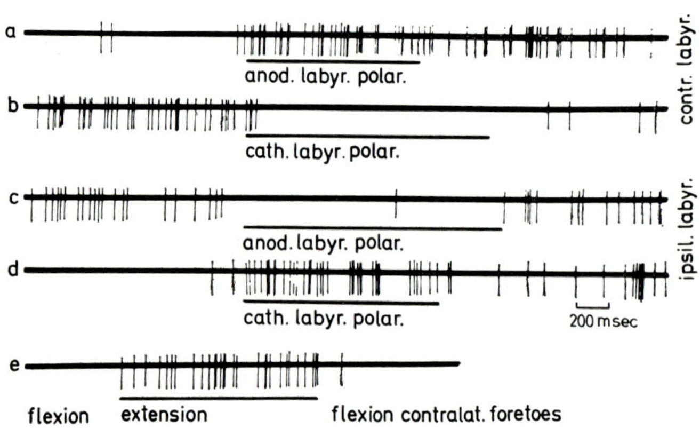

Fig. 18. Typical neuron of the cat's motor cortex showing convergence of deep somatic (e) and vestibular afferents (a to d). In the awake cat two thirds of the neurons of the motor cortex responded to somatic, half of the neurons to vestibular stimuli, but none to visual stimuli (From KORNHUBER and ASCHOFF, Naturwissenschaften **51** (1964))

ents have never been found (KORNHUBER and ASCHOFF, 1964). With respect to the vestibular afferents, it should be noted that the vestibular cortical projections are special subdivisions of the first somatosensory cortical area (see Chap. D.VI., this volume). The reactions induced by sensory stimuli that are lost after extirpation of the motor cortex are the somatic and vestibular ones: tactile placing and hopping (BARD, 1938), tactile grasping (DENNY-BROWN, 1960), and vestibular placing of the forelegs (BARD and ORIAS, 1933) while e.g. the visual placing reaction is preserved. These facts imply that the special task of the motor cortex is not voluntary movement. The motor cortex is a specialized device for making tactile and proprioceptive adjustments of the motor patterns generated by the cerebellum and basal ganglia for movements that need a higher tactile control

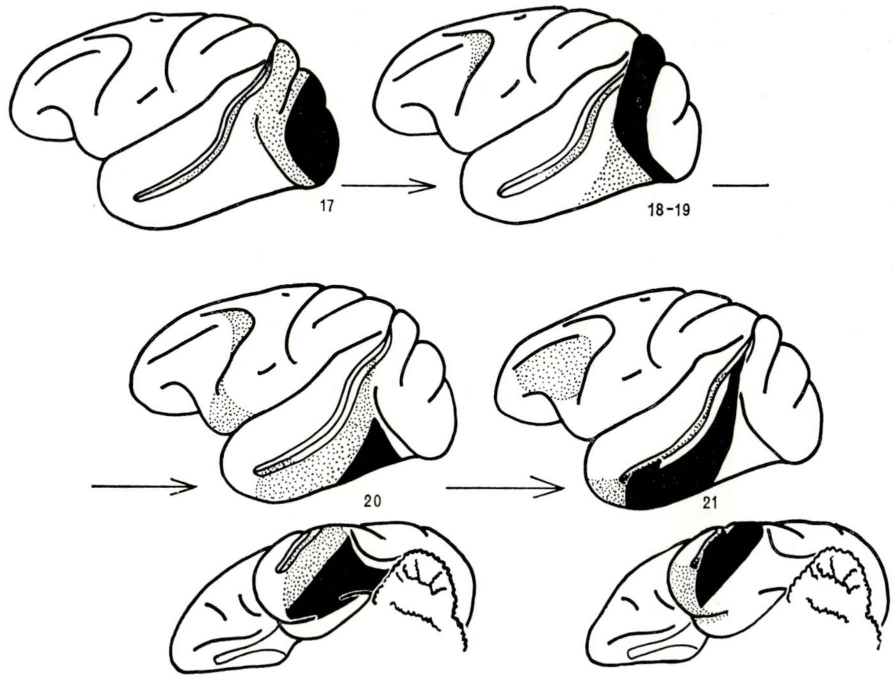

Fig. 19. Schematic summary of the outward progression of cortico-cortical connections emanating from the striate cortex. The progression reaches the infero-temporal, temporo-basal and frontal cortex, but not the motor cortex. Similarly, there is no projection from the auditory sensory and association cortex to the motor cortex (From E.G. JONES, in: F.O. SCHMITT and F.G. WORDEN, Eds. The Neurosciences, Third Study Program, Cambridge, Mass., and London: MIT Press 1974)

(KORNHUBER, 1970, 1971, 1974). From the phylogenetic point of view, one could say that only movements able to take advantage of the enormously elaborate analysis of tactile messages provided by the development of the somatosensory cortex ascended during evolution to the motor cortex, while movements that work just as well without sophisticated tactile regulation (such as eye movements) maintained their centers at the older, lower levels of the central nervous system: i.e. the vestibular nuclei, reticular formation, and red nucleus; all three receive afferents from the cerebellum and the last two also from the basal ganglia (see Fig. 12).

XIII. The Function of the Frontal Eye Field

The function of the frontal eye field (area 8) is not yet clear, but some suggestions can be made on the basis of the available data. Its function is certainly not to produce all saccadic (as opposed to smooth-pursuit) eye movements, nor does the frontal eye field create all the voluntary (as opposed to visually guided) eye movements. Bilateral lesions of the frontal eye field (area 8) do not seem to impair eye movements, or at the most result in a slight inattentiveness (KENNARD and ECTORS, 1938; METTLER, 1945; DENNY-BROWN, 1951; PRIBRAM, 1955; BRUCHER,

1966). Optokinetic nystagmus is normal after bilateral lesions of the frontal eye fields (Henderson and Crosby, 1952; Pasik and Pasik, 1964). Unilateral lesions of the frontal eye field, however, result in (1) neglect of contralateral visual stimuli, (2) transient eye and head deviation to the ipsilateral side and ipsilateral circling gate, and (3) neglect of the contralateral and preference for the ipsilateral hand (Kennard and Ectors, 1938; Kennard, 1939; Clark and Lashley, 1947; Welch and Stuteville, 1958; Denny-Brown, 1966; Brucher, 1964; Latto and Cowey, 1972). The neurons of the frontal eye field do not fire prior to saccadic or other eye movements; most of the neurons related to eye movements represent eye position without adaptation, a few fire during saccades, but not before saccades (Bizzi, 1968). The frontal eye field projects to the superior colliculus (Kuypers and Lawrence, 1967). The cortico-cortical association fibers from the region of area 8 seem to project to the arm-hand region of the motor cortex (Pandya and Kuypers, 1969). The thalamic afferents to area 8 (unlike those of the motor cortex) run from the mediodorsal nucleus, specifically from its paralamellar part (Scollo-Lavizzari and Akert, 1963). The afferents to the paralamellar part of the dorsomedial nucleus are not known; however, the dorsomedial nucleus is known to receive afferents from the hypothalamus and limbic system. Nauta (pers. comm.) believes that the paralamellar part receives some of its afferents from the cerebellum.

From these data we may infer that the frontal eye field receives information from the motivational centers of the hypothalamus and limbic system. Unilateral inattention to visual stimuli, similar to that observed after lesions of area 8, has also been observed after unilateral hypothalamic lesions. The influence of area 8 on visual attention or search may be mediated via a facilitatory influence on the optic tectum. Another function of the frontal eye field may be to represent at cortical level the position of the eyes that is important for the coordination with goal-directed hand movements. The projection to area 6 and the neglect of the contralateral hand favor this hypothesis.

Electrical stimulation of the frontal eye field yields saccadic eye movements the size of which is spatially coded in this area (Robinson and Fuchs, 1969). However, despite the strong projection of area 8 to the optic tectum, the pathway for saccades from the frontal eye field bypasses the tectum, because with frontal eye field stimulation saccadic latency is shorter than with tectal stimulation (Robinson, 1972). After ablation of the tectum, frontal eye field stimulation still yields saccadic eye movements whereas visual cortex stimulation no longer elicits any saccades (Schiller, 1972). Thus, a saccadic pathway from the frontal eye field independent of the tectum does exist, but it is obviously little used under most viewing conditions as demonstrated by the single-unit results of Bizzi (1969).

XIV. Neural Organization of the Strategy of Action

It has been known since the experiments of W.R. Hess and Ph. Bard that some of the nervous substrates underlying the various drives to act are located in the diencephalon (for reviews, see Bard, 1939; Hess, 1954; von Holst, 1958; Ploog, 1964; Vanderwolf, 1971). Hess was able to elicit exploratory behavior, feeding, flight, aggression, vomiting, relaxation, sleep, urination and other activities by means of hypothalamic stimulation. Unilateral hypothalamic lesions produce inattention to visual, tactile and proprioceptive stimuli occurring on the opposite side, in which they resemble large subcortical lesions of the hemisphere. Orientation, feeding or attack behavior to contralateral stimuli is lost for several weeks after lateral hypothalamic lesions. In the clinical literature this loss of drives is called akinetic mutism. Mutism and immobility are part of this syndrome, except that the eyes are often kept open and moved. The lesions leading to akinetic mutism are bilateral and are located in the central gray matter, the hypothalamus, the medial thalamus or the cingulate gyrus, and nearby structures. Lesions of the frontal lobes, to which the hypothalamus projects via the medio-dorsal thalamus, do not cause akinetic mutism, but bilateral lesions of the orbital cortex often result in disinhibition of primitive drives (hunger, or the drive to collect e.g. money or other strange things). In contrast, lesions of the frontal convexity may

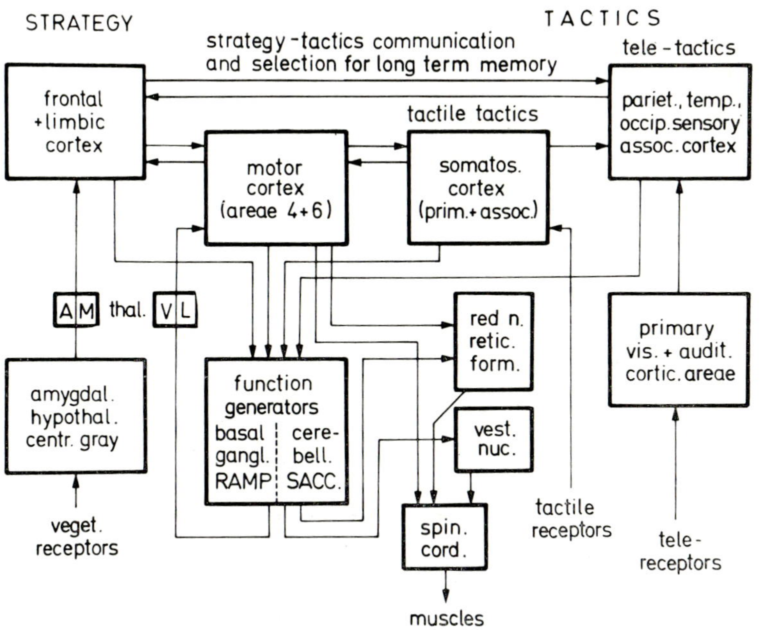

Fig. 20. Information flow diagram showing strategic and tactical mechanisms in voluntary actions. The mechanisms of strategy (represented at cortical level in the frontal lobe and cingulate gyrus) and the mechanisms of tactics (in the posterior association cortex) both have access to the motor function generators in the cerebellum and basal ganglia. *A* anterior, *M* mediodorsal, *VL* ventrolateral thalamus. The communication lines between frontal and sensory association cortex are also important for selecting data for tranfer from short- to long-term memory. The neural mechanisms underlying the strategy of actions (e.g. hypothalamus, amygdala and orbitofrontral cortex) of course receive both exteroceptive and vegetative information; the former arrives in preprocessed format from the sensory association areas, while the hypothalamus gets this information indirectly via the cingulate gyrus-hippocampus loop (From Kornhuber, in: F.O. Schmitt and F.G. Worden, Eds. The Neurosciences, Third Study Program, Cambridge, Mass., and London: MIT Press 1974)

induce apathy and reduction of all activities. It seems that the need for homeostasis of the internal milieu and the drives underlying the survival of the species are represented in the mesencephalon, the hypothalamus, and the limbic system, and that the activity of these structures is mediated into action, at least in part, via the frontal and cingulate cortex.

The frontal cortex has direct access to the basal ganglia and (via the pontine nuclei) to the cerebellum, but a great deal of the influence the frontal and cingulate cortex has on actions is probably effected via the fronto-parietal, fronto-occipital and fronto-temporal connections, and via fibers from the cingulate gyrus to the latero-posterior thalamic nucleus, which in turn projects to the parietal lobe. In other words, the mechanisms of the strategy of action, represented at the cortical level in the frontal and limbic areas, and the mechanisms of tactics, represented in the temporal, parietal and occipital lobes, are in communication with each other. This communication of motivational and intellectual functions of the brain is, of course, necessary not only for actions but also for orientation, thinking, and the selection of information for storage in the long-term memory (KORNHUBER, 1973b). The best-known frontal lobe syndrome in monkeys, failure in delayed-response or delayed-alternation tests, is a sign of partial disconnection of these systems.

XV. The Lesson of Speech

The frontal aphasia due to lesions of BROCA's field consists largely of a defect in the strategy of speaking; in BROCA's aphasia the language is ungrammatical and monotonic. WERNICKE's type of aphasia, due to lesions of the temporal lobe, is characterized by disordered lexical details, the nouns, which are part of the tactics of speaking. In BROCA's aphasia, the nouns are usually preserved but cannot be activated and organized into sentences; this shows that in the integrated brain BROCA's field acts on WERNICKE's. In WERNICKE's aphasia the strategy of speaking is preserved and often released, resulting in much meaningless speech; this suggests that normally WERNICKE's field also acts on BROCA's. The old assumption that the basis of speech is a cortico-cortical reflex arc from WERNICKE's to BROCA's field and then via the motor cortex to the motoneurons is contradicted by the speech disorders characteristic of lesions in the cerebellum, basal ganglia, and thalamus. Obviously, both BROCA's and WERNICKE's fields have direct access to the motor function generators (cerebellum and basal ganglia), and the cortico-cortical interaction between them is bidirectional.

XVI. Shifting Focus of Actions and Unity of Personality

There is no single superhomunculus in the brain, nor a single superdrive like FREUD's libido. Man and animals have many drives, and the unity of the human personality or the conscious self cannot be localized in a small anatomical structure of the dominant hemisphere; it is a process that depends on many fiber connections. During everyday life, the leading focus of action shifts frequently between the four lobes of the forebrain, between right, left and bilateral, and between the cortex and several subcortical structures.

We are still far from understanding this complex interplay. Fortunately we do not need to understand it in order to diagnose a case of stroke. But those of us who are physicians should keep an open mind relative to the whole phenomenon of man — his motivations, his high degree of freedom, and his creative abilities — in order to avoid pointless therapeutic activity. To cite an example: in the affluent Western countries, overeating is a major cause of disease and death.

References

ALBE-FESSARD, D., DONALDSON, J.M.L.: Relation of movements induced by intracortical stimulation to receptive fields of points in the perirolandic and parietal cortex of the monkey. J. Physiol. (Lond.) **210**, 57P (1970).

ASCHOFF, J.C., COHEN, B.: Changes in saccadic eye movements produced by cerebellar cortical lesions. Exp. Neurol. **32**, 123–133 (1971).

ASCHOFF, J.C., CONRAD, B., KORNHUBER, H.H.: Acquired pendular nystagmus with oscillopsia in multiple sclerosis: a sign of cerebellar nuclei disease. J. Neurol. Neurosurg. Psychiat. **37**, 570–577 (1974).

BADER, W., KORNHUBER, H.H.: Großhirnläsionen und vestibulärer Nystagmus. Vergleichende elektronystagmographische Untersuchungen bei geschlossenen Augen und mit visueller Fixation. Acta oto-laryng. (Stockh.) **60**, 197–206 (1965).

BARD, P.: Studies in the cortical representation of somatic sensibility. Harvey Lect. **33**, 143–169 (1938).

BARD, P.: Central nervous mechanisms for emotional behavior patterns in animals. Res. Publ. Ass. nerv. ment. Dis. **19**, 190–218 (1939).

BARD, P., ORIAS, O.: Localized cortical management of visual and labyrinthine placing reactions. Amer. J. Physiol. **105**, 2–3 (1933).

BARD, P., WOOLSEY, C.N., SNIDER, R.S., MOUNTCASTLE, V.B., BROMILEY, R.B.: Delimitation of central nervous mechanisms involved in motion sickness. Fed. Proc. **6**, 72 (1947).

BÁRÁNY, R.: Physiologie und Pathologie des Bogengangsapparates. Leipzig: Deuticke 1907.

BÁRÁNY, R.: Die Untersuchung der reflektorischen vestibulären und optischen Augenbewegungen und ihre Bedeutung für die topische Diagnostik der Augenmuskellähmungen. Münch. med. Wschr. **54**, 1072–1075, 1132–1135 (1907).

BARNESS, C.D., POMPEIANO, O.: Effects of muscle afferents on brainstem reticular and vestibular units. Brain Res. **25**, 179–183 (1971).

BECHINGER, D., KONGEHL, G., KORNHUBER, H.H., WALTHER, C.: What do the eye movements contribute to the visual perception of length? Pflügers Arch. ges. Physiol. **347**, R 63 (1974).

BECKER, W.: The control of eye movements in the saccadic system. Bibl. ophthal. (Basel) **82**, 233–243 (1972).

BECKER, W., FUCHS, A.F.: Further properties of the human saccadic system: eye movements and correction saccades with and without visual fixation points. Vision Res. **9**, 1247–1258 (1969).

BECKER, W., HOEHNE, O., IWASE, K., KORNHUBER, H.H.: Bereitschaftspotential, prämotorische Positivierung and andere Hirnpotentiale bei sakkadischen Augenbewegungen. Vision Res. **12**, 421–436 (1972).

BECKER, W., JÜRGENS, R.: Reactions to double step stimuli: evidence for model feedback and continuous information uptake. Wenner Gren Center Symposium, 1974.

BENDER, M.B., SHANZER, S.: Oculomotor pathways defined by electrical stimulation and lesions in the brainstem of monkey. In: The Oculomotor System, BENDER, Ed., pp. 81–140. New York: Hoeber 1964.

BIZZI, E.: Discharge of frontal eye field neurons during saccadic and following eye movements in unanesthetized monkeys. Exp. Brain Res. **10**, 69–80 (1968).

BRAITENBERG, V.: Funktionelle Deutung von Strukturen in der grauen Substanz des Nervensystems. Naturwissenschaften **48**, 489–496 (1961).

BRAITENBERG, V., ATWOOD, R.P.: Morphological observations on the cerebellar cortex. J. comp. Neurol. **109**, 1–34 (1958).

BRAITENBERG, V., ONESTO, N.: The cerebellar cortex as a timing organ. Discussion of a hypothesis. Atti I. Congr. intern. med. cibern., pp. 239–255. Napoli: Soc. intern. med. cibern. 1960.

BRINDLEY, B.G.S.: The use made by the cerebellum of the information that it receives from sense organs. Int. Brain Res. Org. Bull. **3**, 80 (1964).

BRUCHER, J.M.: L'aire oculogyre frontale du singe. Ses fonctions et ses voies efférents. Editions Arscia, Librairie maloine Bruxelles-Paris 1964.

BUSER, P., IMBERT, M.: Sensory projections to the motor cortex in cats: a microelectrode study. In: Sensory Communication, W. ROSENBLITH, Ed. Cambridge, Mass.: MIT Press, New York: Wiley 1961.

CARPENTER, M.B.: Ascending vestibular projections and conjugate horizontal eye movements. pp. 150–189. In: Neurological aspects of auditory and vestibular disorders, FIELDS, ALFORD, Eds. Springfield/Ill.: C.C. Thomas 1964.

CARPENTER, R.H.S.: Cerebellectomy and the transfer function of the vestibulo-ocular reflex in the decerebrate cat. Proc. roy. Soc. B **181**, 353–374 (1972).

CLARK, G., LASHLEY, K.S.: Visual disturbances following frontal ablations in the monkey. Anat. Rec. **97**, 326 (1947).

COHEN, L.A.: Role of eye and neck proprioceptive mechanisms in body orientation and motor coordination. J. Neurophysiol. **24**, 1–11 (1961).

COHEN, B., HENN, V.: The origin of quick phases of nystagmus in the horizontal plane. Bibl. ophthal. (Basel) **82**, 36–55 (1972).

COHEN, B., SUZUKI, J., BENDER, M.B.: Eye movement from semicircular canal nerve stimulation in the cat. Ann. Otol. (St. Louis) **73**, 153–170 (1964).

COLLEWIJN, H.: Dysmetria of fast phase of optokinetic nystagmus in cerebellectomized rabbits. Exp. Neurol. **28**, 144–154 (1970).

COLLEWIJN, H.: An analog model of the rabbit's optokinetic system. Brain Res. **36**, 71–88 (1972).

COLLEWIJN, H., VAN DER MARK, F.: Ocular stability in variable feedback conditions in the rabbit. Brain Res. **36**, 47–57 (1972).

DALLOS, P.J., JONES, R.W.: Learning behavior of the eye fixation control system. IEEE Trans. Automatic Control AC – **8**, 218–227 (1963).

DEECKE, L., SCHEID, P., KORNHUBER, H.H.: Distribution of readiness potential, pre-motion positivity, and motor potential of the human cerebral cortex preceding voluntary finger movements. Exp. Brain Res. **7**, 158–168 (1969).

DENNY-BROWN, D.: The frontal lobes and their functions. In: Modern Trends in Neurology, Feiling (Ed.) pp. 13–81. London: Butterworth 1951.

DENNY-BROWN, D.: The general principles of motor integration. In: Handbook of Physiology, Section I: Neurophysiology. J. FIELD, H.W. MAGOUN, V.E. HALL, Eds. Washington: Amer. Physiol. Soc. 1960.

DENNY-BROWN, D.: The cerebral control of movement. Liverpool: Liverpool University Press 1966.

DUENSING, R., SCHAEFER, K.P.: Die Neuronenaktivität in der Formatio reticularis des Rhombencephalons beim vestibulären Nystagmus. Arch. Psychiat. Nervenkr. **196**, 265–290 (1957).

DUENSING, R., SCHAEFER, K.P.: Die Aktivität einzelner Neurone im Bereich der Vestibulariskerne bei Horizontalbeschleunigungen unter besonderer Berücksichtigung des vestibulären Nystagmus. Arch. Psychiat. Nervenkr. **198**, 225–252 (1958).

ECCLES, J.C., ITO, M., SZENTÁGOTHAI, J.: The cerebellum as a neuronal machine. Berlin-Heidelberg-New York: Springer 1967.

FOERSTER, O.: Motorische Felder und Bahnen. In: Handbuch der Neurologie VI, BUMKE, O., O. FOERSTER, Eds. Berlin: Springer 1936.

FREDRICKSON, J.M., SCHWARZ, D., KORNHUBER, H.H.: Convergence and interaction of vestibular and deep somatic afferents upon neurons in the vestibular nuclei of the cat. Acta oto-laryng. (Stockh.) **61**, 168 (1965).

FUCHS, A.F.: Periodic eye tracking in the monkey. J. Physiol. (Lond.) **193**, 161–171 (1967).

FUCHS, A.F., KORNHUBER, H.H.: Extraocular muscle afferents to the cerebellum of the cat. J. Physiol. (Lond.) **200**, 713–722 (1969).

FUCHS, A.F., LUSCHEI, E.S.: Unit activity in the brainstem related to eye movement. Bibl. ophthal. (Basel) **82**, 17–27 (1972).

FUKUDA, T.: Studies on human dynamic postures from the viewpoint of postural reflexes. Acta oto-laryng. (Stockh.) Suppl. **161** (1961).

GAEFKE, H.: Die Intervallverteilung der raschen Augenbewegungen des Menschen beim optokinetischen und vestibulären Nystagmus und bei Bildbetrachtung. Freiburg i. Br.: Thesis, Med. Fak. 1968.

GERNANDT, B.E.: Interactions between extraocular myotatic and ascending vestibular influences. Exp. Neurol. **20**, 120–134 (1968).

GONSHOR, A.: Habituation of natural head movement in man. Proc. Internat. Union Physiol. Sci. **9**, 211 No. 619 (1971). German Physiol. Soc. 1971.

GRIFFITH, C.R.: A historical survey of vestibular equilibration. Urbana, Ill.: Univ. Illinois Press 1922.

HAMPSON, J., HARRISON, C., WOOLSEY, C.: Cerebro-cerebellar projections and the somatotopic localization of motor function in the cerebellum. Res. Publ. Ass. nerv. ment. Dis. **30**, 299–316 (1952).

HENDERSON, J.W., CROSBY, E.C.: An experimental study of optokinetic responses. Arch. Ophthal. **47**, 43–54 (1952).

HESS, W-R.: Induzierte Störungen der optischen Wahrnehmung. Nervenarzt **16**, 57–66 (1943).

HESS, W.R.: Das Zwischenhirn, Syndrome, Lokalisationen, Funktionen. 2nd Edition. Basel: Schwabe 1954.

HOLST, E. VON: Die Arbeitsweise des Statolithenapparates bei Fischen. Z. vergl. Physiol. **32**, 60–120 (1950).

HOLST, E. VON: Die Funktionsstruktur des Zwischenhirns. Fortschr. Zool. **11**, 245–275 (1958).

HOLST, E. VON, MITTELSTAEDT, H.: Das Reafferenzprinzip (Wechselwirkungen zwischen Zentralnervensystem und Peripherie). Naturwissenschaften **37**, 464–475 (1950).

ITO, M.: The control mechanisms of cerebellar motor systems. In: The Neurosciences, Third Study Program. F.O. SCHMITT and F.G. WORDEN (Eds.), p. 293–303. Cambridge and London: MIT Press 1974.

ITO, M., YOSHIDA, M.: The cerebellar-evoked monosynaptic inhibition of Deiters' neurons. Experientia (Basel) **20**, 515–516 (1964).

ITO, M., YOSHIDA, M., OBATA, K.: Monosynaptic inhibition of the intracerebellar nuclei induced from the cerebellar cortex. Experientia (Basel) **20**, 575–576 (1964).

ITO, M., NISIMARU, N., YAMAMOTO, M.: The neural pathways mediating reflex contraction of extraocular muscles during semicircular canal stimulation in rabbits. Brain Res. **55**, 183–188 (1973).

JOHNSON, W.H., MAYNE, J.W.: Stimulus required to produce motion sickness. Restriction of head movement as a preventive of air sickness. J. Aviat. Med. **24**, 400 (1970).

JOHNSTON, J.B.: The brain of Petromyzon. J. comp. Neurol. **7**, 2–82 (1902).

JOHNSTON, J.B.: An attempt to define the primitive functional divisions of the central nervous system. J. comp. Neurol. **7**, 87–106 (1902).

JONES, G.M., SPELLS, K.E.: A theoretical and comparative study of the functional dependence of the semicircular canal upon its physical dimensions. Proc. roy. Soc. B **157**, 403–419 (1963).

JONES, E.G., POWELL, T.P.S.: An anatomical study of converging sensory pathways within the cerebral cortex of the monkey. Brain **93**, 793–820 (1970).

JUNG, R., KORNHUBER, H.H.: Results of electronystagmography in man: the value of optokinetic, vestibular and spontaneous nystagmus for neurologic diagnosis and research. pp. 428–482. In: The Oculomotor System, M.B. BENDER, Ed. New York: Hoeber 1964.

KELLER, E.L., ROBINSON, D.A.: Absence of a stretch reflex in extraocular muscles of the monkey. J. Neurophysiol. **34**, 908–919 (1971).

KEMP, J.M., POWELL, T.P.S.: The cortico-striate projection in the monkey. Brain **93**, 525–546 (1970).

KENNARD, M.A.: Alterations in response to visual stimuli following lesions of frontal lobes in monkeys. Arch. Neurol. Psychiat. (Chic.) **41**, 1153–1165 (1939).

KENNARD, M.A., ECTORS, L.: Forced circling in monkeys following lesions of the frontal lobes. J. Neurophysiol. **1**, 45–54 (1938).

KLEYN, A. DE: Experimentelle Untersuchungen über die schnelle Phase des vestibulären Nystagmus beim Kaninchen. Graefes Arch. Ophthal. **107**, 480 (1922).

KORNHUBER, H.H.: Physiologie und Klinik des zentralvestibulären Systems (Blick- und Stützmotorik). In: Hals-Nasen-Ohren-Heilkunde, ein kurzgefaßtes Handbuch, Bd. III, Teil 3, pp. 2150–2351. J. BERENDES, R. LINK, F. ZÖLLNER, Eds. Stuttgart: Thieme 1966.

KORNHUBER, H.H.: Neurologie des Kleinhirns. Zbl. Neurochir. **191**, 13 (1968).

KORNHUBER, H.H.: Physiologie und Klinik des vestibulären Systems. Arch. Ohr.-, Nas.-, u. Kehlk.-Heilk. **194**, 111–148 (1969).

KORNHUBER, H.H.: Das vestibuläre System, mit Exkursen über die motorischen Funktionen der Formatio reticularis, des Kleinhirns, der Stammganglien und des motorischen Cortex sowie über die Raumkonstanz der Sehdinge. In: Vorträge der Erlanger Physiologentagung 1970, W.D. KEIDEL, K.H. PLATTIG, Eds. Berlin-Heidelberg-New York: Springer 1971.

KORNHUBER, H.H.: Motor functions of cerebellum and basal ganglia: the cerebello-cortical saccadic (ballistic) clock, the cerebello-nuclear hold regulator, and the basal ganglia ramp (voluntary speed smooth movement) generator. Kybernetik **8**, 157–162 (1971).

KORNHUBER, H.H.: Cerebellar control of eye movements. Advanc. Oto-rhino-laryng. **19**, 241–253 (1973a).

KORNHUBER, H.H.: Neural control of input into long term memory: limbic system and amnestic syndrome in man. In: Memory and Transfer of Information, pp. 1–22. H.P. ZIPPEL, Ed. New York: Plenum Press 1973b.

KORNHUBER, H.H.: Cerebral cortex, cerebellum, and basal ganglia: an introduction to their motor functions. In: The Neurosciences, III. Study Program, pp. 267–280. F.O. SCHMITT, F.G. WORDEN, Eds. Cambridge and London: MIT Press 1974.

KORNHUBER, H.H., ASCHOFF, J.C.: Somatisch-vestibuläre Konvergenz und Interaktion an Neuronen des motorischen und des somatosensiblen Cortex der Katze. Pflügers Arch. ges. Physiol. **278**, R 72 (1964).

KORNHUBER, H.H., DEECKE, L.: Hirnpotentialänderungen bei Willkürbewegungen und passiven Bewegungen des Menschen: Bereitschaftspotential und reafferente Potentiale. Pflügers Arch. ges. Physiol. **284**, 1 (1965).

KUYPERS, H.G.J.M., LAWRENCE, D.G.: Cortical projections to the red nucleus and the brainstem in the Rhesus monkey. Brain Res. **4**, 151–188 (1967).

LATTO, R., COWEY, A.: Frontal eye-field lesions in monkeys. Bibl. ophthal. (Basel) **82**, 159–168 (1972).

LILLY, J.C.: Correlations between neurophysiological activity in the cortex and short term behavior in the monkey. In: Biological and biochemical bases of behavior, HARLOW, WOOLSEY, Eds. Madison/Wisc.: Univ. Wisconsin Press 1958.

LLINÁS, R., PRECHT, W.: The inhibitory vestibular efferent system and its relation to the cerebellum in the frog. Exp. Brain Res. **9**, 16–29 (1969).

LLINÁS, R., WOLFE, J.W.: Single cell responses from the cerebellum of Rhesus proceeding voluntary, vestibular and optokinetic saccadic eye movements. Soc. Neurosci, **2**, (1972).

LOWENSTEIN, O., SAND, A.: The individual and integrated activity of the semicircular canals of the elasmobranch labyrinth. J. Physiol. (Lond.) **99**, 89–101 (1940).

DELONG, M.R.: Motor functions of the basal ganglia: single-unit activity during movement. In: The neurosciences, III. Study Programm, pp. 319–325. F.O. SCHMITT, F.G. WORDEN, Eds. Cambridge and London: MIT Press 1974.

LORENTE DE NÓ, R.: Die Labyrinthreflexe auf die Augenmuskeln nach einseitiger Labyrinth-Exstirpation, nebst einer kurzen Angabe über den Nervenmechanismus der vestibulären Augenbewegungen. Wien: Urban and Schwarzenberg 1928.

LORENTE DE NÓ, R.: Vestibulo-ocular reflex arc. Arch. Neurol. (Chic.) **30**, 246–291 (1933).

LORENTE DE NÓ, R.: Ausgewählte Kapitel aus der vergleichenden Physiologie des Labyrinthes. Die Augenmuskelreflexe beim Kaninchen und ihre Grundlagen. Ergebn. Physiol. **32**, 73–242 (1931).

MAEKAWA, K., SIMPSON, J.E.: Climbing fiber responses evoked in vestibulocerebellum of rabbit from visual system. J. Neurophysiol. **36**, 649–666 (1973).

MAGNUS, R.: Körperstellung. Berlin: Springer 1924.

MAGNUS, R., STORM VAN LEEUWEN, W.: Die akuten und die dauernden Folgen des Ausfalles der tonischen Hals- und Labyrinthreflexe. Pflügers Arch. ges. Physiol. **159**, 157 (1914).

MARR, D.: Theory of cerebellar cortex. J. Physiol. (Lond.) **202**, 437–470 (1969).

MAYNE, R.: The dynamic characteristics of the semicircular canals. J. comp. physiol. Psychol. **43**, 309–319 (1950).

McINTYRE, A.K.: The quick component of nystagmus. J. Physiol. (Lond.) **97**, 8–16 (1939).

McNALLY, W.J., TAIT, J.: Ablation experiments on the labyrinth of the frog. Amer. J. Physiol. **75**, 155–179 (1925).

METTLER, F.A.: Effects of bilateral simultaneous subcortical lesions in the primate. J. Neuropath. exp. Neurol. **4**, 99–122 (1945).

MICHAEL, J., JONES, G.M.: Dependence of visual tracking capability upon stimulus predictability. Vision Res. **6**, 707–716 (1966).

NIEUWENHYS, R.: Comparative anatomy of the cerebellum. In: The Cerebellum. C.A. FOX, R.S. SNIDER, Eds. Progr. Brain Res. 25. Amsterdam: Elsevier 1967.

NYBY, O., JANSEN, J.: An experimental investigation of the cortico-pontine projection in Macaca mulatta. Norske Vid. Akad. SKR I. Math. Naturw. Kl. **3**, 475 (1951).

PANDYA, D.N., KUYPERS, H.G.J.M.: Cortico-cortical connections in the Rhesus monkey. Brain Res. **13**, 13–36 (1969).

PASIK, P., PASIK, T.: Oculomotor functions in monkeys with lesions of the cerebrum and the superior culliculi. In: The Oculomotor System. M.B. BENDER, Ed. New York: Hoeber 1964.

PLOOG, D.: Verhaltensforschung und Psychiatrie. In: Psychiatrie der Gegenwart, pp. 291–443. Vol. I/1, B. GRUHLE, JUNG, MAYER-GROSS, MÜLLER, Eds. Berlin-Göttingen-Heidelberg-New York: Springer 1964.

POMPEIANO, O., BARNESS, C.D.: Effect of sinusoidal muscle stretch on neurons in medial and descending vestibular nuclei. J. Neurophysiol. **34**, 725–734 (1971).

PRIBRAM, K.H.: Lesions of 'frontal eye field' and delayed response of baboons. J. Neurophysiol. **18**, 105–112 (1955).

RADEMAKER, G.G.J.: Das Stehen. Statistische Reaktionen, Gleichgewichtsreaktionen und Muskeltonus unter besonderer Berücksichtigung ihres Verhaltens bei kleinhirnlosen Tieren. Berlin: Springer 1931.

RADEMAKER, G.G.J., GARCIN, R.: L'épreuve d'adaption statique. Suite à l'étude de quelques réactions des extremités d'origine labyrinthique. Rev. neurol. **60**, 566 (1933).

RASHBASS, C.: The relationship between saccadic and smooth tracking eye movements. J. Physiol. (Lond.) **159**, 326–338 (1961).

ROBINSON, D.A.: The mechanics of human saccadic eye movement. J. Physiol. (Lond.) **174** 245 (1964).

ROBINSON, D.A.: The mechanics of human smooth pursuit eye movement. J. Physiol. (LOND.) **180**, 569–591 (1965).

ROBINSON, D.A.: The oculomotor control system: a review. Proc. IEEE **56**, 1032–1049 (1968).

ROBINSON, D.A.: Eye movements evoked by collicular stimulation in the alert monkey. Vision Res. **12**, 1795–1808 (1972).

ROBINSON, D.A.: Physiology and control aspects of supranuclear oculomotor systems. Wenner-Gren Center Symposium, 1974.

ROBINSON, D.A., FUCHS, A.F.: Eye movements evoked by stimulation of frontal eye fields. J. Neurophysiol. **32**, 637–648 (1969).

RON, S., ROBINSON, D.A.: Eye movements evoked by cerebellar stimulation in the alert monkey. J. Neurophysiol. **36**, 1004–1022 (1973).

RON, S., ROBINSON, D.A., SKAVENSKI, A.A.: Saccades and the quick phase of nystagmus. Vision Res. **12**, 2015–2022 (1972).

SCHILLER, P.H.: Some functional characteristics of the superior colliculus of the Rhesus monkey. Bibl. ophthal. (Basel) **82**, 122–129 (1972).

SCHILLER, P.H., KÖRNER, F.: Discharge characteristics of single units in superior colliculus of the alert rhesus monkey. J. Neurophysiol. **34**, 920–936 (1971).

SCHMIDT, R.S.: Amphibian acoustico-lateralis efferents. J. cell. comp. Physiol. **65**, 155–162 (1965).

SCHMIDT, C.L., WIST, E.R., DICHGANS, J.: Efferent frequency modulation in the vestibular nerve of goldfish correlated with saccadic eye movements. Exp. Brain Res. **15**, 1–14 (1972).

SCOLLO-LAVIZZARI, G., AKERT, K.: Cortical area 8 and its thalamic projection in Macaca mulatta. J. comp. Neurol. **121**, 259 (1963).

SJÖBERG, A.A.: Experimentelle Studien über den Auslösungsmechanismus der Seekrankheit. Acta oto-laryng. (Stockh.) Suppl. **14** (1931).

SKAVENSKI, A.A., ROBINSON, D.A.: Role of abucens neurons in vestibulo-ocular reflex. J. Neurophysiol. **36**, 724–737 (1973).

STARK, L., VOSSIUS, G., YOUNG, L.R.: Predictive control of eye tracking movements. IRE Trans. Human Fact. in Electronics. HFE **3**, 52–56 (1962).

ST.-CYR, G.J., FENDER, D.H.: Non-linearities of the human oculomotor system: gain. Vision Res. **9**, 1235–1246 (1969).

ST.-CYR, G.J., FENDER, D.H.: Non-linearities of the human oculomotor system: time delays. Vision Res. **9**, 1491–1503 (1969).

VANDERWOLF, C.H.: Limbic-diencephalic mechanisms of voluntary movement. Psychol. Rev. **78**, 83–113 (1971).

VOGT, C., VOGT, O.: Allgemeinere Ergebnisse unserer Hirnforschung. IV. Die physiologische Bedeutung der architektonischen Rindenfelderung auf Grund neuer Rindenreizungen. J. Psychol. Neurol. (Lpz.) **25**, 399 (1919).

WAGMAN, J.H.: Eye movements induced by electric stimulation of cerebrum in monkeys and their relationship to bodily movements. In: The Oculomotor System. M.B. BENDER, Ed. New York: Hoeber 1964.

WEBER, G., STEINER, F.A.: Labyrinthär erregbare Neurone im Hirnstamm und Kleinhirn der Katze. Helv. physiol. Acta **23**, 61–81 (1965).

WELCH, K., STUTEVILLE, P.: Experimental production of unilateral neglect in monkeys. Brain **81**, 341–347 (1958).

WESTHEIMER, G.: Eye movement responses to a horizontally moving visual stimulus. A.M.A. Arch. Ophthal. **52**, 932–941 (1954).

WESTHEIMER, G., BLAIR, S.M.: Oculomotor defects in cerebellectomized monkeys. Invest. Ophthal. **12**, 618–621 (1973).

WILSON, M.E., TOYNE, M.J.: Retino-tectal and cortico-tectal projections in Macaca mulatta. Brain Res. **24**, 395–406 (1970).

WURTZ, R.H., GOLDBERG, M.E.: Superior colliculus cell responses related to eye movements in awake monkeys. Science **171**, 82 (1971).

WURTZ, R.H., GOLDBERG, M.E.: Activity of superior colliculus in behaving monkey. III. Cells discharging before eye movements. J. Neurophysiol. **35**, 575–586 (1972).

YOUNG, L.R., STARK, L.: Variable feedback experiments testing a sampled data model for eye tracking movements. IEEE Trans. of the Prof. Tech. Grp. on Human Factors in Electronics HFE-**4**, 38–51 (1963).

Author Index

Page numbers in *italics* refer to the bibliography

Subject Index

Volume VI:
Vestibular System
Part 1: **Basic Mechanisms**
Editor: H. H. Kornhuber
251 figures. VIII, 676 pages. 1974
Cloth DM 239,–; US $97.60
Subscription price
Cloth DM 191,20; US $78.00
ISBN 3-540-06889-9

Part 2:
Psychophysics, Applied Aspects and General Interpretations
Editor: H. H. Kornhuber
198 figures. VIII, 680 pages. 1974
Cloth DM 249,–; US $101.60
Subscription price
Cloth DM 199,20; US $81.30
ISBN 3-540-06864-3

Volume VII:
Part 1: **Photochemistry of Vision**
Editor: H. J. A. Dartnall
296 figures. XII, 810 pages. 1972
Cloth DM 238,–; US $97.10
Subscription price
Cloth DM 190,40; US $77.70
ISBN 3-540-05145-7

Part 2:
Physiology of Photoreceptor Organs
Editor: M. G. F. Fuortes
342 figures. X, 765 pages. 1972
Cloth DM 244,–; US $99.60
Subscription price
Cloth DM 195,20; US $79.70
ISBN 3-540-05743-9

Part 3:
Central Processing of Visual Information
Editor: R. Jung
A: **Integrative Functions and Comperative Data**
208 figures. XI, 775 pages. 1973
Cloth DM 248,–; US $101.20
Subscription price
Cloth DM 198,40; US $81.00
ISBN 3-540-05769-2

B: **Visual Centers in the Brain**
216 figures. VIII, 738 pages. 1973
Cloth DM 248,–; US $101.20
Subscription price
Cloth DM 198,40; US $81.00
ISBN 3-540-06056-1

Part 4:
Visual Psychophysics
Editors: D. Jameson, L. M. Hurvich
297 figures. X, 812 pages. 1972
Cloth DM 248,–; US $101.20
Subscription price
Cloth DM 198,40; US $81.00
ISBN 3-540-05146-5

Part 5:
A: **The Visual System in Evolution: Vertebrates**
Editor: F. Crescitelli
In preparation

B: **The Visual System in Evolution: Invertebrates**
Editor: H. Autrum

Volume VIII:
Perception
Editors: R. Held, H. W. Leibowitz, H. L. Teuber. In preparation

Volume IX:
Development of Sensory Systems
Editor: M. Jacobson. In preparation

Prices are subject to change without notice

Springer-Verlag
Berlin Heidelberg New York